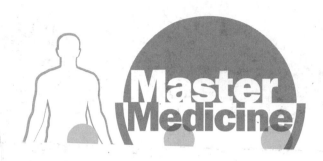

Master Medicine

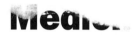

Medi...

...wn below.

ditor: Laurence Hunter
: Barbara Simmons
mma Riley
Larking
Gardner

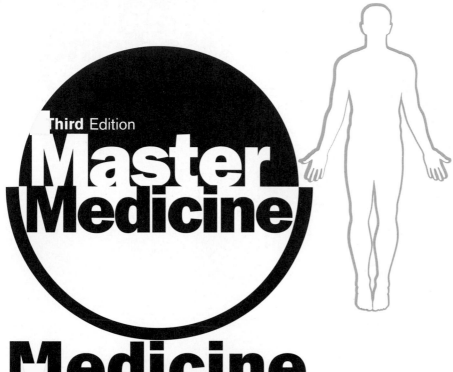

Third Edition

Master Medicine

Medicine

A clinical core text
with self-assessment

Paul O'Neill

BSc (Hons) MB ChB
FRCP MD

Professor of Medical Education
and Head of Medical School,
University of Manchester;
Consultant Physician, South
Manchester University Hospitals
NHS Foundation Trust,
Manchester, UK

Tim Dornan

DM FRCP MHPE PhD

Professor of Medicine,
University of Manchester and
Director of Medical Education,
Salford Royal NHS Foundation
Trust, Manchester, UK

David Denning

MB BS FRCP FRCPath
DCH

Professor of Medicine and
Medical Mycology,
Education and Research Centre,
University of Manchester,
South Manchester University
Hospitals NHS Foundation
Trust, Manchester, UK

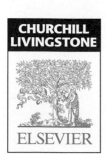

CHURCHILL
LIVINGSTONE

ELSEVIER

Edinburgh London New York Oxford Philadelphia St Louis Sydney Toronto 2008

CHURCHILL
LIVINGSTONE
ELSEVIER

© Pearson Professional Limited 1997
© Harcourt Publishers Limited 2002
© 2008, Elsevier Limited. All rights reserved.

First edition 1997
Second edition 2002
Third edition 2008

ISBN: 978-0-443-10320-9

British Library Cataloguing in Publication Data
A catalogue record for this book is available from the British Library

Library of Congress Cataloging in Publication Data
A catalog record for this book is available from the Library of Congress

Note
Knowledge and best practice in this field are constantly changing. As new research and experience broaden our knowledge, changes in practice, treatment and drug therapy may become necessary or appropriate. Readers are advised to check the most current information provided (i) on procedures featured or (ii) by the manufacturer of each product to be administered, to verify the recommended dose or formula, the method and duration of administration, and contraindications. It is the responsibility of the practitioner, relying on their own experience and knowledge of the patient, to make diagnoses, to determine dosages and the best treatment for each individual patient, and to take all appropriate safety precautions. To the fullest extent of the law, neither the Publisher nor the Authors assume any liability for any injury and/or damage to persons or property arising out of or related to any use of the material contained in this book.

The Publisher

 ELSEVIER your source for books, journals and multimedia in the health sciences

www.elsevierhealth.com

The publisher's policy is to use **paper manufactured from sustainable forests**

Working together to grow libraries in developing countries

www.elsevier.com | www.bookaid.org | www.sabre.org

ELSEVIER   BOOK AID International   Sabre Foundation

Printed in China

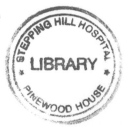

Contents

Acknowledgements

We are grateful to the following for reviewing and commenting on the chapters for the new edition: Alan Fitchet (Cardiovascular disease), Jeremy Dick (Neurological disease), John Houghton (Haematology), Phil Kalra (Renal disease), Tara Kearney (Endocrinology and metabolism), Paul Miller (Gastrointestinal disease), Jon Miles (Respiratory disease), Penny Chandiole (Genitourinary disease section of Infectious diseases chapter), Ariane Herrick (Musculoskeletal disease) and Matthew Helbert (Immunology chapter and for a useful allergy case history).

We would also like to thank our wives, Jo, Ceri and Merian, for their patience and support, without which nothing would have been written at all.

Using this book

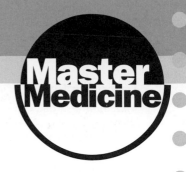

Philosophy of the book

This third edition has been extensively revised in the light of changes in medical practice and in consultation with subject experts. A key development has been the widespread availability of guidelines based on best available evidence and consensus. We strongly recommend that you develop the habit of consulting these in your studies and also as you start your clinical career. Excellent examples can be found at:

- the British Thoracic Society — http://www.britthoracic.org.uk
- the British Society of Gastroenterology — http://www.bsg.org.uk.

This chapter aims to help you:

- understand how the emphasis on self-assessment in this book can make learning easier and more enjoyable
- use this book to increase your understanding as well as knowledge
- plan your learning.

How much do you know about diabetes? Are they the right things? Can you answer exam problems on diabetes? This book aims to help you with these questions. You probably have some knowledge of medicine, perhaps a bit patchy, and some clinical experience. We want to help you to be better at integrating knowledge and solving either real problems or simulated ones in examinations. We have tried to present essential information, for doctors practising in the UK, in a concise and ordered fashion. Principles are illustrated and mechanisms explained rather than simply giving you lots of facts to memorise.

Do not think, though, that this book offers a 'syllabus'. It is impossible to draw boundaries around medical knowledge, and learning is a continuous process carried out throughout your career. As we see it in 2007, this book includes all that you *must* know, most of what you *should* know about, and some facts of which you *might* be aware.

We assume that you are working towards one or more examinations, probably in order to qualify. Our purpose is to show you how to overcome these barriers. As we feel strongly that learning is not simply for the purpose of passing exams, the book aims both to help you to pass and to develop *useful* knowledge and understanding.

Layout and content

The first part of each chapter sets out the key learning objectives: those things which anyone starting a medical career needs to know and an examiner expects them to know. More detailed learning objectives are to be found at the start of each major section. One starting point might be to look at these objectives and then test yourself in the self-assessment section at the end of each chapter. This will help to steer you towards areas that you need to work on. Alternatively, you can go straight into the main body of the chapter and check that you have achieved the objectives at the end; if not, then you will need to do further work and perhaps read about the topics elsewhere.

In all the chapters, we have included a clinical case study at the start of each major section. These vignettes are designed to stimulate thought and curiosity about what you know and understand and what you need to focus on in your learning. They are drawn from the authors' clinical experience and illustrate common problems and challenges. We have not provided 'answers' to these and the approach is for you to draw these out from the text and also the self-assessment that concludes each chapter.

The main part of the text describes important topics in major subject areas. Within these sections, we have put down the essential information in a logical order with explanations and links. In order to help you, we have used lists to set out frameworks and to make it easier for you to put facts in a rational sequence. Tables are used to link quite complex information.

There are some situations in medicine that require you to act immediately and senior help may not be available. For some of these emergencies, we have put the steps that you must take into an 'emergency' summary box. These are based on current guidelines at the time of writing, but guidelines do change.

You have to be sure that you are reaching the required standards, so the final section of each chapter is there to help you to check out your knowledge and understanding. The self-assessment is in the form of multiple choice questions (including single best answers), case histories, extended matching questions (EMQs), short notes, data interpretation, key features questions, picture questions and sample stations that might be included in objective structured clinical examinations (OSCEs). Questions are designed to integrate knowledge across different chapters and to focus on the decisions you will have to take in a given clinical situation. Detailed answers are given with reference to relevant sections of the text; the answers also contain information and explanations that you will not find elsewhere, so you have to do the assessments to get the most out of this book.

Using the book

Your first task before using the book is to map out on a sheet of paper a series of three lists dividing the major subjects (corresponding to our chapter headings) into an assessment of your strong, reasonable and weak areas. This gives you a rough outline of your learning schedule, which you must then fit in with the time available. Clearly, if your examinations are looming large, you will have to be ruthless in reducing the time allocated to your strong areas. The major subjects should be further classified into individual topics. Encouragement to store information and to test your ongoing improvement is by the use of the self-assessment sections. You must keep checking your current level of knowledge.

Overall the aim is to help you to learn through the use of interlinked steps:

- What do you already know about the subject?
- Why do you want to learn more about the subject? You will acquire knowledge much more easily if you can put it in a framework.
- What things needs explaining? What do you not understand?
- Can you expand on these things? You should explain as much as you can from different aspects.
- Set yourself goals for where your knowledge is lacking.
- Check that you have achieved these.

If you can, discuss problems with colleagues/friends. The areas which you understand least well will become apparent when you try to explain them to someone else. You will also benefit from hearing a different perspective on a problem.

Approach to examinations

The discipline of learning is closely linked to preparation for examinations. Many of us simply opt for remembering facts because full understanding is often not required, such as in multiple choice questions. We would prefer it if you acquired a deeper knowledge and understanding but, recognising constraints on your time, advocate a pragmatic approach that combines the necessity of passing examinations with longer-term needs.

The hardest step is to determine what will be in the exam; medicine does not draw boundaries around knowledge either in breadth or depth. The best approach is to combine your lecture notes, textbooks (not reference) and past examination papers. From the last, for example, you may find out that not only are the pulmonary manifestations of HIV infection a possible examination topic but you will also get an indication of the depth of knowledge required.

You then have to choose what sources you are going to use for your learning and revision. Textbooks come

in different forms. At one extreme, there is the large reference book, which includes extensive literature citation. At the other end of the spectrum is the condensed 'lecture note' format, which often relies heavily on lists. In the middle of the range are the medium-sized textbooks. You should choose the book(s) that suits your needs (and that of the examination!) and that you find readable.

You should now have a rough syllabus, your own lecture notes and some books that you feel comfortable in using. The next stage is to map out the time available for preparation. You must be realistic in this, allowing time for breaks and working steadily, not cramming. If you do attempt to cram, you have to realise that only a certain amount of information can be retained in short-term memory, so as the classification of the lipid disorders moves in, then the terminology of the renal tubular acidoses moves out! Cramming is simply retention of facts. If the examination requires understanding, you will be in trouble.

You might be tempted to do general reading of a large textbook. Even if this was feasible in the time available (the number of pages to be read tends to increase as the examination gets closer), it is not very effective in that often you cannot remember anything of the topic you have just covered. An analogy would be driving a car along a familiar route, arriving, but being unable to recall anything of the journey.

We advise an approach, as outlined above, based on the use of key steps, learning objectives and self-assessment. For a subject such as endocrinology, we would recommend setting out the topics to be covered and then attempting to summarise your knowledge about each in note form. By this means, gaps in your knowledge/understanding become apparent. Use of 'mind-maps' may be appropriate in helping to make connections: for example, between the physiological control of thyroxine, secretion and thyrotoxicosis. It is much more efficient to go to textbooks having thought about what you know, as you are then 'looking' for information and explanation.

Self-assessment will help in determining the time to be allocated to each system. If you are consistently scoring excellent marks in a particular subject, it is not cost-effective to spend a lot of time trying to achieve the 'perfect' mark. In an essay, it is many times easier to obtain the first mark (try writing your name) than the last. You should also try to decide on the amount of weight to be assigned to each subject; this should be heavily biased to the likelihood of it appearing in the examination! It is not sensible to devote large amounts of time to the ocular manifestations of systemic disease if ophthalmology is not included in the 'syllabus' you have devised.

As the examination draws near you should attempt practice questions and complete papers. It is not sufficient to have the necessary knowledge and understanding; you need to demonstrate these to the examiners. Many people pay insufficient attention to the type of question they are going to encounter: Moving the focus away from books and lecture notes to actual questions helps in identifying where knowledge is still lacking and what work is still to be done.

Methods of examination

Multiple choice questions

Unless sophisticated, multiple choice questions test recall of information. The aim is to gain the maximum marks from the knowledge that you can remember. You should read the stem with great care, highlighting the 'little' words such as *only, rarely, usually, never* and *always*. You will often lose marks because of 'negatives', such as *not, unusual* and *unsuccessful*. If the stem is phrased *may occur*, this has entirely different connotations to *characteristic*. The latter may mean a feature which should be there and the absence of which (for example, central chest pain in myocardial ischaemia) would make you question the correctness of the diagnosis. Alternatively, it can also be used to describe rare features that would suggest the diagnosis: for example, yellow vision (xanthopsia) in digoxin toxicity. If the stem is long with several lines of text or data, then you should try to summarise it by extracting the essential elements.

You must check the marking method before starting as it may employ a negative system in which marks are lost for incorrect answers. The temptation is to adopt a cautious approach, answering a relatively small number of questions. However, this can lead to problems as we all make simple mistakes or even disagree vehemently with the answer in the computer! Caution may lead you to answer too few questions to pass after the marks have been deducted for incorrect answers.

Distracters are the technical term for parts of questions which sound as though they are correct but are definitely incorrect. A good example would be symptoms and signs of *hyper*natraemia being included in a question on *hypo*natraemia. This is the most common cause of losing marks even though you know the answer.

Extended matched questions

In this third edition, we have included examples of extended matching questions (EMQs), as these are becoming increasingly common in undergraduate and postgraduate examinations. They consist of a theme (e.g. weight loss), a series of options and then a question (e.g. for each patient, select the most likely diagnosis from the list of options). You then have to read each patient vignette and decide the most likely cause. EMQs test your ability to recall knowledge and **apply** it to a clinical problem. They are not negatively marked. EMQs seem to separate out those students who can use their knowledge from those who have simply learned facts by rote.

Short notes

Short notes are not negatively marked. The system is for a 'marking template' to be devised which gives a mark(s) for each important fact. You will gain nothing for style or superfluous information. Your aim is to set out your knowledge in an ordered *concise* manner. The common faults are, first, devoting too much time to a single question thereby neglecting the rest and, second, not limiting the answer to the question asked. For example, in a question about the management of diabetes mellitus, you should not list all facts about diabetes, only those relevant to management.

Key features questions

A new format for assessment is the 'Key features' question, which is designed to assess how you filter and connect information, as opposed to simply coming up with the right answer. These questions are based on the concept of critical steps in decision-making and ask you to identify, from a clinical vignette, the important things that have lead you to a particular decision, which could be a diagnosis or concerned with investigation or management. Mostly, we have left the questions open (e.g. 'what features support this diagnosis?'), but you will encounter questions that ask for a certain number of responses (e.g. 'what are the three most important features supporting this diagnosis?'). These questions add to the variety in the book and should stimulate further thinking and learning.

Essays

Similar comments apply to essays, but you may get marks for logical development of an argument or theme. Conversely, you will not obtain good marks for an essay that is a set of unconnected statements. Length matters little if there is no cohesion. Most people are aware of the need to 'plan' their answer yet few do this. It is important in an examination based on essays that you manage your time and all questions are given equal weight, unless stated otherwise in the instructions. A brilliant answer in one essay will not compensate you for not attempting another because of time. Nobody can get more than 100% (usually 75%) on a single answer!

Data interpretation

Data interpretation involves the application of knowledge to solve a problem. In your revision, you should aim for an understanding of principles; it is impossible to memorise all the different data combinations. In the exam, a helpful approach is to translate numbers into a description: for example, a serum potassium of 2.8 mmol/l is *low* and the ECG tracing of a heart rate of 120/min shows a *tachy*cardia. Pattern recognition can then be attempted.

Data questions are not usually negatively marked so put down an answer even if you are far from sure that it is right. Conversely, there is no point in listing four possibilities if the question asks for one response. The examiner will not choose from your answers; the first response will be taken!

Image/picture questions

Pattern recognition is the first step in a picture question. You should couple this with a systematic approach looking for abnormalities. For example, you should check the breast shadows, bony skeleton, soft tissues, retrocardiac space, etc. in a chest radiograph. Describe in your mind what you see and try to match it with common problems. Again, even if doubtful, put an answer down. Images often come with an accompanying statement or data. You should use this alongside the visual image as it may give a clue as to the answer required; it may be essential in distinguishing between two conditions which give a similar slide appearance.

Case history questions

A more sophisticated form of examination question is an evolving case history with information being presented sequentially; you are asked to give a response at each stage. They should be constructed so that a wrong response in the first part of the question still means that you can obtain marks from the subsequent parts. Patient management problems are designed to test the recall and application of knowledge through an understanding of the principles involved. As with the data interpretation, you should always give answers unless the exam instructions indicate the presence of negative marking.

Viva

The viva examination can be a nerve-wracking experience. You are normally faced with two examiners who may react with irritation, boredom or indifference to what you say. You may feel that the viva has gone well and yet you failed, or, more commonly, you think that it has gone badly simply because of the apparent attitude of the examiners.

Your main aim during the viva should be to steer the questioning of the examiners so that they are constantly asking you about things you know about. Despite what is often said, you can prepare for a viva. Questions are liable to take the form of one of a small number of types centred around subjects that cannot be examined in the traditional clinical exam:

- emergency medicine (e.g. diabetic coma)
- management of common conditions (e.g. hypertension)
- clinical sciences (e.g. control of blood pressure).

For each heading, you can prepare a list of the *common* problems.

Another approach used by examiners is to invite you to start the viva by asking what you have read recently or what you think is an important recent medical advance. Prepare something along these lines beforehand.

During the viva there are certain techniques that will help you to make a favourable impression. When discussing the management of something, it is better to say 'I would do this' rather than 'the book says this'. You should try to strike a balance between saying too little and too much. It is hard on examiners when you will not expand on any of your answers and it is equally difficult if you refuse to shut up! Remember, the longer you talk without stopping, the more likely it is that you have either gone off the topic or are showing the examiners the inadequacy of your knowledge.

In a viva, the examiners are likely to want to explore the *limits* of your knowledge; do not be upset if they push you hard. It is alright to say you do not know something; most examiners will want to change tack to see what you do know about.

Objective structured clinical examinations

Clinical examinations are not the main focus of this book. However, we have included some examples of objective structured clinical examination (OSCE) stations in the self-assessment to help *you* to develop the right balance between academic work and gaining clinical experience. For more help, you should look at Dornan and O'Neill *Core Clinical Skills for OSCEs in Medicine* (Churchill Livingstone, 2006), which we consider to be a companion book to this edition.

Normal values

In both examinations and clinical practice, most test results are given together with the normal reference range for that laboratory. However, you are expected to know certain normal ranges as they are essential for making decisions in an emergency. Furthermore, familiarity with the ranges for common indices will help you a obtain a 'feel' for data interpretation and abnormal patterns. Thus, a serum potassium of 1.9 mmol/l has a greater significance than one of 3.1 mmol/l even though both are low.

In the list of normal values in Tables 1 and 2, we have indicated with an asterisk the indices for which you would be expected to be able to give an approximate normal range. Remember that laboratories do vary and a normal range is simply that which 95% of the normal population served by that laboratory would fit into.

Conclusions

We have set out a framework for using this book, but you should amend this according to your own needs and the examinations you are facing. Whatever approach you adopt, the aim should be for an understanding of the principles involved rather than rote learning.

Table 1 Normal values for haematology

Index	Range	Unit
White blood cell*	4.0–11.0	$\times 10^9$/l
Neutrophils	2.0–7.5	$\times 10^9$/l
Lymphocytes	1.5–4.0	$\times 10^9$/l
Eosinophils	0.04–0.4	$\times 10^9$/l
Monocytes	0.2–0.8	$\times 10^9$/l
Basophils	<0.1	$\times 10^9$/l
Red blood cells		
Male	4.5–6.5	$\times 10^{12}$/l
Female	3.8–5.8	$\times 10^{12}$/l
Haemoglobin: male*	130–170	g/l
Haemoglobin: female*	116–165	g/l
Packed cell volume (PCV)		
Male	0.40–0.54	l/l
Female	0.37–0.49	l/l
Mean cell volume (MCV)*	80.0–97.0	fl
Mean cell haemoglobin (MCH)	27.0–32.0	pg
Mean cell haemoglobin concentration (MCHC)	31.0–35.0	g/dl
Red cell distribution width (RDW)	11.5–15.0	–
Platelets*	150–400	$\times 10^9$/l
Erythrocyte sedimentation rate (ESR)		
Male*	<5	mm/hr
Female*	<7	mm/hr
Plasma viscosity	1.50–1.72	cp
Reticulocytes	0.2–2.0	%
Serum vitamin B_{12}	160–600	ng/l
Serum folate	2.0–10.0	µg/l
Red cell folate	125–600	µg/l
Ferritin		
Male	20–300	µg/l
Female premenopausal	12–250	µg/l
Female postmenopausal	20–300	µg/l
Haemoglobin (Hb) Hb_{A2}	1.8–3.5	%
HbF	0.2–1.0	%
Glucose-6-phosphate dehydrogenase	4.6–13.5	IU/g haemoglobin
Prothrombin time (PT)*	12.0–16.0	sec
Activated partial thromboplastin time (APTT)	21.0–27.5	sec
Fibrinogen	2.0–4.0	g/l
Fibrin degradation products (FDP) (D-dimer)	<0.5	mg/l
Bleeding time (adults)	1.6–8.0	min

*Values that you would be expected to know.

Table 2 Normal reference ranges for biochemistry

Index	Range	Value
Sodium*	132–144	mmol/l
Potassium*	3.5–5.0	mmol/l
Chloride	95–108	mmol/l
Bicarbonate*	24–30	mmol/l
Urea*	2.7–7.5	mmol/l
Creatinine*	50–120	µmol/l
Glucose		
Fasting	3.2–6.0	mmol/l
Random	3.3–9.2	mmol/l
Bilirubin	1–20	µmol/l
Calcium*	2.10–2.65	mmol/l
Phosphate*	0.70–1.40	mmol/l
Total protein	60–80	g/l
Albumin	33–49	g/l
Globulin	21–38	g/l
Urate		
Female	<0.38	mmol/l
Male	<0.42	mmol/l
Blood gases		
pH*	7.38–7.42	
P_{CO_2}*	4.5–6.0 (34–45)	kPa (mmHg)
P_{O_2}*	12–14.7 (90–110)	kPa (mmHg)
Base excess*	−2 to +2	
Enzymes		
Alkaline phosphatase (ALP) (adult)	25–110	IU/l
Amylase	10–87	IU/l
Aspartate aminotransferase (AST)	5–45	IU/l
Alanine aminotransferase (ALT)	5–45	IU/l
Gamma-glutamyl transferase (GGT)	<65	IU/l
Creatine kinase (CK)	<150	IU/l
Phosphokinase (CPK)		
Lactate dehydrogenase (LDH)	200–500	IU/l
Cerebrospinal fluid		
Protein*	0.25–0.75	g/l
Glucose* (depends on blood sugar)	2.5–5.5	mmol/l
Hormones		
Thyroxine (T_4)	50–150	nmol/l
Triiodothyronine (T_3)	1.1–2.8	nmol/l
Thyroid-stimulating hormone (TSH)	0.5–5.0	mU/l
Cortisol (morning 07:00–09:00 hr)	200–650	nmol/l
(night 22:00–24:00 hr)	60–250	nmol/l
Urine free cortisol	<300	nmol/24 hr
Lipids		
Total cholesterol		
Satisfactory	<5.2	mmol/l
Borderline	5.2–6.5	mmol/l
Unsatisfactory	>6.5	mmol/l
Fasting triglycerides	0.3–2.0	mmol/l
Iron	12–30	µmol/l
Total iron-binding capacity (TIBC)	45–70	µmol/l

*Values that you would be expected to know.

Cardiovascular disease

1.1 Background

Learning objectives

You should:

- be able to take with absolute confidence a history from a patient with chest pain or other major symptom of cardiovascular disease and construct a differential diagnosis
- be able to interpret the chest radiograph and electrocardiograph (ECG)
- know the place of echocardiography, exercise testing, coronary angiography and the investigations used in particular cardiovascular diseases (described below under diagnoses) and when to request them
- be competent at performing cardio-pulmonary resuscitation.

Case Study

A woman with factor V Leiden deficiency has had a haemodynamically significant pulmonary embolism. It is unusually easy to hear the splitting of her second heart sound because the acute pulmonary hypertension delays and accentuates the pulmonary component of the second heart sound.

Cardiovascular disease is the most common cause of death in the western world and a major preventable cause of chronic ill-health. It will impinge on whichever branch of medicine you choose and may dominate your practice. If you become a general practitioner, cardiovascular disease will present some of the commonest emergencies you have to treat. As an anaesthetist, you will have to decide whether patients with it can safely be anaesthetised. As a surgeon, you will have to exclude it as a cause of abdominal pain. Cardiovascular diseases are ubiquitous, so they figure large in the 'core' knowledge and skills of the medical graduate.

Anatomy

You need a knowledge of the surface anatomy of the heart, as seen from the front, to interpret physical signs, chest radiographs and electrocardiographs (Fig. 1). The heart has a triangular projection and lies mostly behind the sternum. The base of the triangle is parallel and slightly to the right of the right sternal border. The apex is in the interspace between the left fifth and sixth ribs in the mid-clavicular line. The right heart border is formed by the right atrium. The left border is composed of the left atrial appendage superiorly and left ventricle inferiorly. The anterior surface is composed, from right to left, of the right atrium, right ventricle, interventricular septum and left ventricle. The left atrium is at the back of the heart and, seen laterally, forms the upper posterior heart border. The lower border is formed by the left ventricle. The anterior heart border in a lateral projection is formed by the right ventricle (as illustrated under chest radiography in Fig. 4 below). The anatomy of the coronary circulation is described on pages 11–13.

Physiology

Cardiac output is maintained by:

- electrical impulse generation and propagation
- cyclical myocardial contraction
- an intact valvular system.

Impulse generation

The cardiac impulse is generated by cyclical depolarisation of the sino-atrial (SA) node, a specialised area close to the junction of the superior vena cava and right atrium. The impulse spreads rapidly through the right and left atria to reach the atrio-ventricular (AV) node. The ventricles are isolated electrically from the atria by the annulus fibrosus. The impulse is conducted by the His bundle, which leads

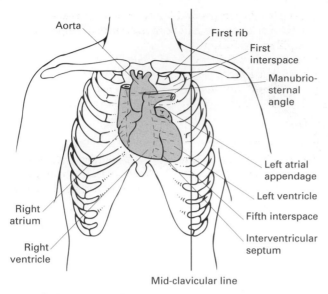

Fig. 1 Surface anatomy of the heart as seen from the front.

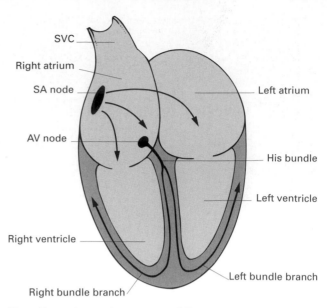

Fig. 2 The cardiac conducting system. SVC, superior vena cava; SA, sino-atrial; AV, atrio-ventricular.

into the right and left bundle branches, activating the right and left ventricles, respectively. The anatomy of impulse propagation is summarised in Figure 2. Spontaneous, rhythmic depolarisation is not unique to the SA node. It can arise lower in the conducting system. The lower in the conducting system the impulse arises, the slower the rate (e.g. atrium 60 beats/min, AV node 50 beats/min, ventricle 30 beats/min). The rate of ventricular contraction is governed by the most rapidly depolarising focus in the heart. Lower and slower pacemakers are overridden by impulses from above. Impulses can arise in diseased myocardium, often at a very fast rate (see dysrhythmias, p. 26). Impulses may pass through myocardial tissue when the conducting tissues are blocked (bundle branch block, p. 11) or through abnormal accessory pathways (p. 11).

The cardiac cycle

Atrial depolarisation causes contraction of the right then the left atrium, corresponding to (though lagging behind) the P wave on the electrocardiograph. There is an electrical pause (the PR interval) as the wave of depolarisation passes through the AV node, then contraction of the left and right ventricles (corresponding electrically to the QRS complex). Rising ventricular pressures close the mitral and tricuspid valves then open the aortic and pulmonary valves. At the end of systole, repolarisation occurs (T wave) and the ventricles relax. When aortic and pulmonary artery pressures exceed left and right ventricular pressures, respectively, the valves close. Closure of the mitral and tricuspid valves is heard as the first heart sound at the start of ventricular systole, and aortic and pulmonary valve closure as the second sound at the end of it. Atrial systole is responsible for 10% of ventricular filling in the normal heart, the rest occurring passively; atrial systole may account for up to 30% of filling in the abnormal fibrotic heart. Each ventricle ejects about 80 ml blood with each cardiac cycle. The proportion of end-diastolic volume ejected in each cardiac cycle (the ejection fraction) ranges from 55 to 75%.

Cardiac output

Cardiac performance is determined by cardiac rate and stroke volume. Rate is controlled by the balance between sympathetic stimulation, which increases it, and parasympathetic (vagal) stimulation, which reduces it. Stroke volume depends on contractility and the 'afterload' or resistance against which the heart is pumping; this principally comprises the peripheral vascular resistance or, in the case of aortic or pulmonary stenosis, the degree of outflow obstruction.

Stroke volume is also influenced by 'preload', the combined effect of venous filling pressure and the atrial 'kick'. The way in which cardiac muscle responds to changes in preload is an important physiological concept, known as **Starling's law of the heart**, which states that the energy of contraction is proportional to the initial length of the muscle fibres. The heart responds to increased preload by an increased stroke volume up to a level of preload at which it is overwhelmed and decompensation occurs (Fig. 3). Sympathetic stimulation, acting on cardiac β_1-adrenoceptors, increases cardiac performance for a given level of preload. How this relates to the pathophysiology and management of heart failure is considered on page 21.

Coronary artery perfusion occurs during diastole. A very fast heart rate increases myocardial work and, by reducing the length of diastole, reduces delivery of oxygen to the myocardium, so it can precipitate ischaemia. Tachycardias can also reduce cardiac output by shortening the time for ventricular filling.

Maintenance of blood volume

This is discussed in Chapter 4, which emphasises the close interrelationship between cardiovascular, renal and fluid/electrolyte physiology. That relationship is central to clinical management.

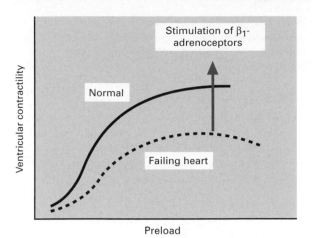

Fig. 3 The relationship between preload and cardiac contractility (Starling's relationship) and the effect of adrenergic stimulation.

Clinical assessment

History

The main symptoms of cardiovascular disease are:

- chest pain
- breathlessness
- ankle swelling
- fatigue
- palpitations
- syncope.

They result from impaired oxygen delivery to the myocardium (chest pain), brain (syncope) and all other tissues (fatigue), increased pulmonary and systemic venous pressure (breathlessness and ankle swelling) and abnormal cardiac rate and rhythm (palpitations). You should remember that chest pain may be caused by other cardiovascular problems: disease of the aorta (p. 51) and disease of adjacent structures including the chest wall, oesophagus, pleura, pulmonary circulation (pulmonary embolism/infarction, p. 49) and pericardium (pericarditis, p. 40).

Examination

Your examination should systematically test out the anatomy and physiology of the heart and circulation as described above and in Chapter 4. As with all other aspects of clinical examination, use all your senses in the order *look, feel, listen*.

Pulse rate and rhythm

Feel both radial pulses together and, if necessary, other pulses to measure the pulse rate and decide if the rhythm is fundamentally regular, perhaps with superimposed extrasystoles or dropped beats, or chaotic (atrial fibrillation).

Arterial circulation

The arterial circulation is assessed from:

- the blood pressure, measured first sitting or lying, then standing to detect postural hypotension caused by volume depletion, vasodilatation or autonomic neuropathy

- peripheral cyanosis and/or impaired capillary refill after blanching the nail beds, measures of impaired capillary perfusion
- the volume of the pulse, a crude way of assessing stroke volume
- the character of the carotid pulse, which may be abnormal in, for example, aortic valvular disease (p. 32).

Venous circulation

Venous circulation is assessed by examining the jugular venous pulse, auscultating the lung bases and testing for ankle and sacral oedema. There are several components to jugular venous examination:

- assessment of venous pressure as a sign of preload (p. 22)
- assessment of its response to respiration, discussed under pericardial effusions (p. 39)
- observation of the waveform, particularly important in detecting tricuspid incompetence.

Crackles at the lung bases may be a sign of pulmonary venous hypertension. Peripheral oedema indicates raised systemic venous pressure, fluid retention, a decreased serum albumin level or increased vascular permeability.

Heart and valves

The stethoscope allows you to detect:

- abnormalities of the first and second heart sounds
- added sounds as in, for example, valvular heart disease (p. 32), heart failure (p. 21) or pericarditis (p. 40).

Peripheral arterial system

You should remember to examine the abdominal aorta and carotid, femoral, popliteal, dorsalis pedis and posterior tibial pulses. Absence of pulses signifies arterial obstruction. Bruits are another sign of arterial obstruction but may also be caused by increased flow.

Stigmata of cardiovascular disease

Infective endocarditis (p. 37) is the classical cardiovascular disease in which non-cardiac signs are as important as cardiovascular examination in making the diagnosis. Some other diseases, discussed under valvular heart disease (p. 32), have important stigmata which should be picked up by observation or general examination.

Investigations

The chest radiograph

Echocardiography is a more sensitive and specific way of detecting structural and functional cardiovascular abnormalities than the chest radiograph but you are unlikely to be able to request one in the middle of the night and many patients can be managed without ever having one. Most relevant information can be obtained from a posteroanterior (PA) radiograph, but a lateral view can give extra information about individual chambers, particularly the left atrium. **Portable** films are taken anteroposterior (AP) and make the heart look larger than it is. Examine the radiograph systematically for:

- overall heart size
- changes in shape indicating disease of individual chambers
- calcification in valves (or the presence of prosthetic valves)
- abnormalities of the vessels, lung fields and costophrenic angles.

The main patterns that you should be able to recognise are summarised in Figure 4. The cardiovascular diagnosis you will most often make is heart failure. Several features shown in the figure deserve special mention:

- Increased pulmonary venous pressure causes dilatation of the upper lobe veins (>4 mm) and constriction of the lower lobe veins, termed 'upper lobe venous diversion'.
- You can assess heart size by measuring the ratio of the width of the heart to the width of the thorax, expressed as the cardiothoracic ratio: a ratio >50% signifies cardiomegaly (except on an AP radiograph).
- Septal ('Kerley') lines are caused by interstitial fluid; they are straight, often short (<1 cm), horizontal, peripheral and present first at the bases.

- Fluffy perihilar and more generalised shadowing signifies fluid in the alveolar spaces, i.e., *severe* pulmonary venous hypertension (or capillary leakage/exudation).

The ECG

If you are unclear about ECG interpretation, you should read one of the excellent concise texts devoted to the subject; this description is very much revision. No matter how experienced you are, you should read an ECG systematically looking for:

- the cardiac rate
- the rhythm
- the electrical axis
- ventricular hypertrophy
- abnormal PQRST configurations.

You should also check the calibration, normally printed at the head of the paper. A normal paper speed is 25 mm/s. One large square (5 mm) represents 200 µs and 1 small square (1 mm) represents 40 µs. 1 mV causes a vertical deflection of 1 cm.

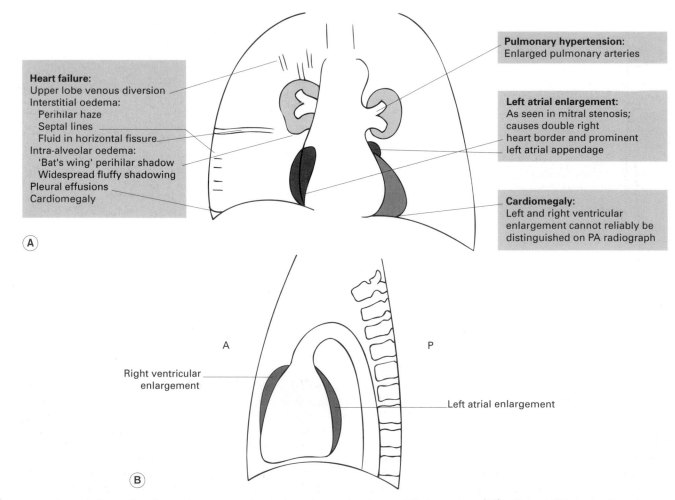

Fig. 4 Principal abnormalities that can be seen on a chest radiograph in cardiac disease. **A** Postero-anterior (PA) radiograph. **B** Lateral radiograph.

Rate, conduction and rhythm

Rate First check the QRS complexes to see if they are regular or irregular. If regular, divide the number of large squares between two consecutive R waves into 300 to give the rate. If irregular, divide the number of large squares between four R waves into 900. A normal rate is 60–100 beats/min or 5–3 large squares between two consecutive R waves.

Conduction Check for P waves as a sign that the impulses are arising within the atria. Next check the PR interval, which represents AV conduction. The PR interval (normal range 3–5 small squares) is short if the impulse is arising unusually close to the AV node or there is an electrical 'short-circuit' between the atria and ventricles ('accessory pathway'). The PR interval is lengthened by disease of the AV node or His bundle. Finally check the width of the QRS complexes; if they are three small squares in width or more, they are being propagated by slow electrical spread through muscle rather than the conducting tissues (bundle branch block or 'intraventricular conduction delay').

Rhythm Abnormalities are discussed under dysrhythmias (p. 26).

Axis

You cannot interpret ECGs without knowing from memory the vectors of each of the 12 leads, shown in Figure 5A. The highest voltage electrical activity in the normal ECG is left ventricular depolarisation, which spreads in a direction between −30° and 90° (the 'electrical axis'). This changes if ischaemic damage, hypertrophy or strain alter the net direction of depolarisation.

Axis deviation is detected by inspecting the R and S waves in leads aVL, I, II, aVF and III. Movement towards increasingly large R waves is movement towards the electrical axis.

Normal axis The R wave is larger than the S wave in I and II (i.e. the QRS complex is a predominantly positive deflection) and lead II is usually the tallest; S may be greater than R in lead III.

Right axis deviation The S wave is greater than the R wave (the RS complex is predominantly negative) in lead I.

Left axis deviation The S wave is greater than the R wave (the RS complex is predominantly negative) in lead II.

Ventricular hypertrophy

Muscle hypertrophy or strain causes increased electrical activity, as seen in the chest leads.

Left ventricular hypertrophy The sum of the downwards deflection in V1 or V2, whichever is the greater, and the upwards deflection in V5 or V6, whichever is the greater, is greater than 35 small squares. This may be accompanied by downsloping ST segments or T wave inversion in left-sided leads (strain pattern). There is usually left axis deviation.

Right ventricular hypertrophy The R wave is greater than the S wave in V1 and there is a deep S wave in V6 (in contrast to the normal situation shown in Fig. 5A). There is often a peaked P wave (right atrial hypertrophy) and right axis deviation in the limb leads.

The PQRST complex

Table 3 shows the normal PQRST configuration and a range of abnormal patterns, all of which you should be able to recognise. In diagnosing myocardial infarction, you should remember that it is normal to have a small Q wave in III; this disappears on deep inspiration. A Q wave must be at least 25% of the size of the R wave and 1 mm in width to be classified as 'pathological'.

1.2 Ischaemic heart disease

Case Study

The cardiology journal club discusses the implications for their work practices of a recent clinical trial showing that immediate angiographic intervention improves the prognosis of acute myocardial infarction.

Any disease process that disturbs the relationship between myocardial oxygen supply and demand can cause ischaemia. This may be:

- impaired coronary artery blood flow
  — coronary atherosclerosis
  — coronary artery spasm
  — occlusion of the coronary ostia by aortic dissection
  — tachycardia causing shortened diastole (p. 26)
- impaired oxygen delivery
  — hypoxia
  — anaemia
- increased cardiac work
  — any cause of increased afterload
  — tachycardia.

Ischaemia is often multifactorial. The term ischaemic heart disease (IHD) is used here to mean atherosclerotic coronary artery disease.

Coronary artery anatomy

Coronary artery anatomy is summarised in Figure 6. The right and left coronary arteries lead from the two coronary sinuses, which arise from the aorta above the aortic valve. The right coronary artery supplies the right atrium and ventricle, small parts of the interventricular septum and left ventricle and often the inferior wall. It supplies the SA node in 60% of patients and the AV node in 90%; consequently right coronary artery disease is prone to cause

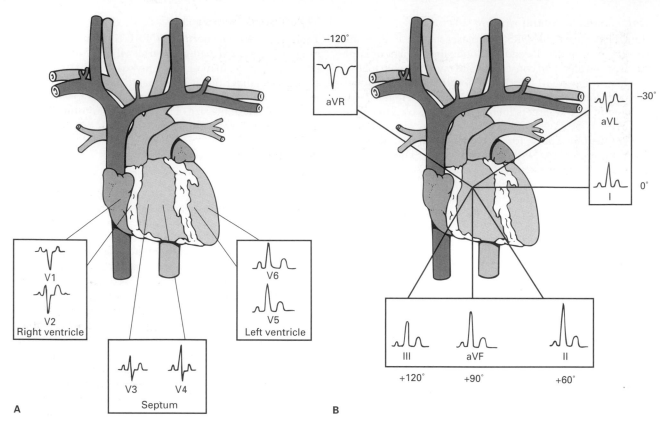

Fig. 5 The vectors of the chest leads for an ECG. **A** The chest leads are arranged radially across the precordium. **B** The other six leads are calculated from values given by leads on the arms and legs. The electrical axis is the result of electrical activity during systole measured in the limb leads.

Table 3 Abnormalities of the PQRST complex in disease

	Pattern	Description	Comment
Disease states			
Myocardial ischaemia		Horizontal or downsloping ST segment depression; T wave inversion	May occur at rest or, more usually, on exertion
Myocardial infarction		Q wave; ST segment elevation; T wave inversion	Changes appear in the order ST elevation, T inversion, appearance of Q wave. They revert in the same order; T wave inversion sometimes permanent and Q waves always permanent
Bundle branch block		'M-shaped complexes'; width ≥3 small squares	Left bundle branch block (LBBB): M-shaped complexes in I, aVL and lateral chest leads. Right bundle branch block (RBBB): 'RSR'configuration in V1–V2
Pericarditis		'Dished' (upwardly concave) ST segments	Widespread but usually best seen in chest leads
Effect of digoxin		'Reverse tick' appearance	

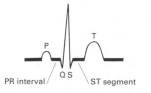

Normal PQRST complex (for comparison with others)

PR interval   Q S   ST segment

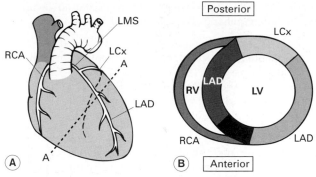

Fig. 6 Coronary artery anatomy. **A** Schematic. **B** Section across the heart (A–A) shows the approximate distribution of blood supply. The section marked in black is supplied by the RCA in many people. LAD, left anterior descending; LCx, left circumflex (dotted line shows its position at the back of the heart); LMS, left main stem; RCA, right coronary artery; RV, right ventricle; LV, left ventricle. (Source: Textbook of Medicine, ed. Souhami and Moxham, Churchill Livingstone, Edinburgh, 1997.)

sinus dysfunction and AV block. The left main coronary artery divides into its major **left anterior descending branch**, which supplies the anterior left ventricle and septum, and the **circumflex branch**, which supplies the posterior and inferior left ventricular wall. There is inter-individual variation in the territories of these vessels, which can influence clinical presentations.

Epidemiology

Risk factors

IHD is the single commonest cause of death in the developed world, accounting for 30% of male and 20% of female deaths in the UK. Knowledge of epidemiology is important for you as a clinician:

- to identify 'at-risk patients' and weigh differential diagnoses
- to practise preventive medicine.

The incidence of IHD:

- rises progressively with age
- is higher in men than women
- rises sharply at the menopause
- is higher in patients with a positive family history.

The 'big three' remediable risk factors are:

- hyperlipidaemia (p. 312)
- smoking
- hypertension.

The Framingham study showed that coronary risk varies fivefold across the cholesterol distribution in the normal population. Likewise, there are 'dose–effect' relationships between coronary risk and smoking and hypertension. These risk factors are additive. Diabetes is an important risk factor (p. 314). This disease affects 2% of the whole population and 10% of elderly people. It is 2–3 times as prevalent in Asian as Caucasian people and its prevalence is rising. Chronic kidney disease (p. 177) is another important risk factor.

Weaker risk factors include:

- obesity
- type A personality
- inactivity
- plasma homocysteine concentration.

High levels of coagulation factors (e.g. fibrinogen) and inflammatory makers (C-reactive protein) are associated with an increased coronary risk but are not used in routine clinical practice.

Prevention

Cardiovascular prevention is an important growth area in medicine. An increase in body mass index of 1 kg/m² in an otherwise healthy young to middle-aged adult increases the risk of cardiovascular mortality by 10%; from this the value of healthy eating is self-evident. Likewise, aerobic exercise reduces cardiovascular risk, as does a moderate alcohol intake (the current UK recommendation is less than 14 units per week in women, and less than 21 in men). Discouraging young people from starting smoking is an important public health issue and smoking cessation rates may be increased by nicotine replacement or bupropion therapy. Powerful evidence that lowering plasma cholesterol with statins is effective in primary prevention (preventing cardiovascular disease in people not yet affected) has been provided by clinical trials, leading to an ongoing debate about the level of plasma cholesterol, and cardiovascular risk, at which statins should be prescribed for primary prevention. Even modest lowering of plasma cholesterol, and lowering within the 'normal' range, is highly effective in secondary prevention (preventing recurrent or worsening IHD). Angiotensin-converting enzyme (ACE) inhibitor treatment in patients at high cardiovascular risk, particularly those with diabetes or established IHD, improves mortality. An important practical point is that patients at the highest absolute risk benefit most from treatment. Therefore, a middle-aged smoker who has had a myocardial infarct will benefit greatly, whereas the benefits in an otherwise healthy young person with raised serum cholesterol may be slight. Because so many people stand to benefit, there are important cost-effectiveness arguments about exactly who should and should not receive statin therapy. Secondary prevention will be considered in more detail under 'myocardial infarction' (p. 17).

Pathophysiology

Coronary artery stenosis and thrombosis, the causes of angina and myocardial infarction, are caused by atherosclerosis. Atherosclerotic plaques are composed of free lipid within the intima associated with smooth muscle cell and macrophage proliferation, fibrosis, and hyperplasia of the overlying endothelium. Shearing forces created by blood flow and/or contraction of the arterial wall cause fissure or rupture of the atherosclerotic plaque, exposing thrombogenic material within the plaque. Platelet thrombi form at the site of plaque rupture. These may embolise into the distal coronary artery, cause thrombotic occlusion of the artery or resolve. Despite re-endothelialisation, the lesion may progress and stenose the artery. These events cause the various clinical manifestations of IHD and provide the basis for prevention and treatment. Both angina and myocardial infarction are caused by myocardial hypoxia, but only in myocardial infarction is there muscle necrosis.

Stable angina

Angina may be caused by:

- a fixed stenosis (>50%) of one or more coronary arteries
- coronary artery spasm
- diseases other than IHD, e.g. aortic stenosis.

Clinical presentation

Symptoms

Typical angina is an exercise-related, pressing precordial chest pain, radiating to the jaw and left arm and relieved by nitrates. It is often worse when exercising in cold air. Sometimes, angina is experienced as 'breathlessness' (resulting from transient left ventricular dysfunction) rather than pain. Anginal pain may come on when lying down at night (decubitus angina, caused by increased venous return in patients with incipient heart failure) or at rest (fixed coronary atheromatous disease or coronary artery spasm). Coronary ischaemia may be painless (silent ischaemia — particularly common in people with diabetes), detected by cardiographic monitoring.

Important differential diagnoses are:

- gastro-oesophageal reflux and oesophageal spasm (p. 121)
- peptic ulcer and cholecystitis
- aortic dissection (p. 51) and pericarditis (p. 40)
- hyperventilation, air-swallowing and other psychosomatic disorders.

There is also a syndrome of uncertain cause (reflected by its name, **syndrome X**) in which patients with angiographically normal coronary arteries experience typical angina.

Signs

You should examine patients carefully and keep in mind the cardiovascular and systemic diseases that can disturb the balance of oxygen supply and demand (e.g. dissecting thoracic aneurysm, aortic stenosis, anaemia). Look for risk factors such as hypertension. Patients with IHD may have signs of heart failure or peripheral vascular disease, but many will have no abnormal signs at all.

Investigations

ECG

The resting ECG may show ST segment or T wave changes suggestive of ischaemia, or evidence of unsuspected previous myocardial infarction or hypertension, but it is often normal. It is most likely to be abnormal if recorded 'in pain'.

Exercise testing

Exercise can be used to provoke symptomatic or asymptomatic ECG changes that are absent at rest. After recording a baseline ECG, the patient is exercised on a treadmill or bicycle ergometer and the work load serially increased under medical supervision with resuscitation facilities immediately to hand. The following are criteria for a positive response:

- horizontal or downsloping ST segment depression >2 mm
- typical ischaemic symptoms
- dysrhythmias (e.g. ventricular tachycardia)
- fall in blood pressure.

The result is expressed as a *probability* of IHD, recognising that some patients with IHD have negative tests and that minor ST segment changes may develop in patients without IHD (false negative and false positive, respectively).

Exercise testing is contraindicated immediately after acute myocardial infarction and in uncontrolled hypertension, severe aortic stenosis and unstable angina.

The test must stop immediately if:

- the patient develops severe ischaemic symptoms or cannot tolerate the test
- the systolic blood pressure falls >10 mmHg
- there is ST segment depression >3 mm
- an arrhythmia develops.

Indications for exercise testing include assessment of:

- severity of IHD, e.g. after myocardial infarction
- chest pain, if the diagnosis is unclear from the history and resting ECG
- a patient's capacity to exercise
- prognosis, e.g. to decide on the safety of returning to work
- response to treatment.

Other investigations

ST segment changes can be 'captured' by monitoring patients with unstable angina (see Acute coronary syndrome, p. 16) in the coronary care unit or, out of hospital, by ambulatory ECG monitoring. ST changes may occur with pain or 'silently'. Isotope scintigraphy may be used; a myocardial perfusion (usually technetium) scan performed at rest and after myocardial stress (provoked by exercise or pharmacologically) can detect areas of impaired myocardial perfusion. Conventional echocardiography cannot directly assess the coronary circulation but can exclude valvular lesions as the cause of chest pain in patients with murmurs (aortic stenosis or mitral valve prolapse) and may be performed in angina to assess left ventricular function and detect abnormalities of ventricular wall motion caused by IHD. Dobutamine stress echocardiography assesses ventricular wall motion at rest and during pharmacological stress. It is as effective as isotope myocardial perfusion scanning in identifying areas of myocardial ischaemia.

Coronary angiography

Imaging the coronary arteries after injection of radiographic contrast medium into them is the 'gold standard' investigation to detect atherosclerotic disease of the coronary arteries. Indications are:

- investigation of chest pain of uncertain aetiology
- assessment of severity of IHD in patients with positive exercise tests.

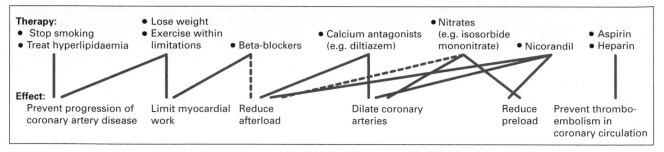

Fig. 7 The medical treatment of angina. Dotted lines indicate minor effects.

Coronary angiography can reliably assess the severity of coronary atherosclerosis and exclude its presence but cannot absolutely exclude ischaemia as the cause of chest pain. Myocardial perfusion scanning may be diagnostic of coronary ischaemia in patients with normal coronary arteries (syndrome X).

Management

The goals of management are to:

- prevent progression of coronary artery disease and optimise life expectancy
- relieve symptoms.

To achieve the first, you should advise smokers to stop and prescribe aspirin, a statin and usually an ACE inhibitor. Life expectancy can also be improved by coronary revascularisation (angioplasty or bypass graft) in selected cases. Other aspects of secondary prevention are discussed under Acute coronary syndrome (p. 16). Figure 7 summarises the treatments which relieve symptoms. Beta-blockers are cardioprotective and can be expected to reduce mortality as well as relieve symptoms.

Patients with angina should be told that it does not necessarily herald an early, sudden death and warned that situations that increase oxygen demand (anxiety, hurrying, cold weather, anger, etc.) may bring on symptoms. The four main classes of drug used to treat angina have additive effects and are prescribed stepwise. Some patients with mild angina are reluctant to take maintenance therapy and prefer to use sublingual nitrate as needed. Beyond that, the choice is likely to be:

- **first step**: beta-blocker, if not contraindicated
- **second and third steps**: calcium antagonist then nitrate
- **fourth step**: nicorandil
- **finally**: revascularisation if symptoms uncontrolled; earlier if a strongly positive exercise test.

Aspirin

Unless it is contraindicated by allergy, intolerance or active peptic ulceration, all patients should have aspirin (75 or 150 mg daily) to prevent future myocardial infarction. Its mode of action is described on page 281. Clopidogrel (75 mg daily) should be used in patients who are hypersensitive to aspirin.

Diet

Obesity increases cardiac work and is a risk factor for disease progression. Obese patients should be encouraged to lose weight; a diet low in animal fat may help to improve their lipid profile.

Beta-blockers

Beta-blockers are competitive antagonists of adrenaline (epinephrine) and noradrenaline (norepinephrine) at β-adrenoceptors. There are two types of receptor: β_1 and β_2. Beta-blockers may be 'selective' to β-adrenoceptors in the heart (β_1-blockers) or non-selective, in which case bronchial receptors are blocked as well and bronchospasm can result. Atenolol and metoprolol are commonly used cardioselective beta-blockers; propranolol is non-selective. Beta-blockade reduces the rate and contractility of the heart, reduces cardiac work and limits the heart rate during exercise.

A cardioselective beta-blocker such as metoprolol is often used as first-line treatment for angina, particularly if the patient is also hypertensive or has had a myocardial infarct.

The two main side-effects/contraindications are inherent in their mode of action; the negative inotropic effect of beta-blockers can precipitate or worsen heart failure if started in an inappropriately high dose (but note that if used carefully they can improve symptoms and prognosis of patients with heart failure) and blockade of β_2-adrenoceptors precipitates bronchospasm in patients with obstructive airways disease, so they are contraindicated in asthma. They may also cause peripheral vasoconstriction; for most patients, that just means cold hands, but these drugs can worsen intermittent claudication or cause gangrene in those with peripheral vascular disease.

Calcium antagonists

There are many drugs that are calcium antagonists; all block calcium channels but they have different tissue specificities and, therefore, different actions. The dihydropyridines (including nifedipine, nicardipine, nimodipine and amlodipine) principally vasodilate peripheral arterioles and the coronary arteries, lowering blood pressure, reducing afterload and relieving coronary artery spasm. A reflex sinus tachycardia can also result. Verapamil impedes the transport of calcium across myocardial smooth muscle cells, including the conducting tissues, prolonging the action potential and refractory period and having a negative inotropic effect. It is often used as an antiarrhythmic though it is also an effective antihypertensive drug. Diltiazem has similar cardiac effects but is less negatively inotropic.

All drugs in the class are effective antianginals and antihypertensives. Diltiazem is often used as the first-choice calcium antagonist. Side-effects include negative inotropy, sinus bradycardia and atrioventricular block. Other 'class' effects result from vasodilatation; they include headache, flushing, hypotension and ankle swelling.

Nitrates

Nitrates work directly on vascular smooth muscle, with three main effects:

- venodilatation, reducing preload and cardiac work
- peripheral arterial vasodilatation, reducing afterload
- coronary artery vasodilatation.

A commonly used drug is glyceryl trinitrate, dissolved under the tongue or sprayed under it. It is used either to prevent pain or to give acute relief. Long-acting oral nitrates (usually isosorbide mononitrate) is given to patients who need glyceryl trinitrate more than occasionally. Tolerance develops, so any patient on maintenance nitrate must have a daily nitrate-free interval of at least 6 hours.

Headache, palpitations and dizziness — direct results of vasodilatation — are the main side-effects. They are usually transient but may be intolerable.

Nicorandil

Nicorandil has a dual mode of action, leading to relaxation of vascular smooth muscle. Its potassium channel-opening action causes coronary and peripheral vasodilatation, and its nitrate activity causes venodilatation. It therefore relieves angina by reducing preload and afterload and relieving coronary artery spasm.

Nicorandil has vasodilator side-effects, as described under Nitrates and Calcium antagonists above, and is contraindicated in severe heart failure and hypotension.

Coronary revascularisation

Referral for coronary angiography with a view to percutaneous coronary angioplasty (PTCA), usually followed by insertion of a stent (see below), or coronary artery bypass grafting (CABG) is indicated in:

- angina occurring in the period after a myocardial infarct
- unstable angina
- severe IHD, even if controlled medically, to improve life expectancy
- stable angina uncontrolled with medical therapy.

The survival advantage is greatest in patients with severe coronary artery disease (left main stem or triple artery disease). The risks may outweigh any likely benefits in patients who are grossly obese or continue to smoke despite the presence of IHD. Old people benefit as much from revascularisation as the young, so age is not in itself a contraindication, particularly for angioplasty.

PTCA and stenting is less invasive than CABG, meaning that it can be performed in patients who are unfit for CABG and in acute myocardial infarction when major surgery has an unacceptably high mortality. It is also increasingly taking the place of CABG in less severe coronary artery disease, such as single or limited stenoses. Up to 20% of patients treated by PTCA and stenting need repeat procedures due to restenosis at the site of the PTCA. The use of stents coated with drugs to reduce restenosis shows promise, with re-stenosis rates as low as 1% reported, though evidence of long-term safety is needed.

Effective as it may be in improving symptoms, there is currently no evidence that PTCA and stenting improves prognosis in stable IHD, unlike CABG, for which such evidence exists. There is, however, good evidence that PTCA and stenting can improve the prognosis in acute coronary syndromes. Overall, the higher acceptability of a less invasive procedure is progressively shifting the choice away from CABG.

Acute coronary syndrome (ACS)

The advent of highly sensitive and specific markers of myocardial damage and of the ability to reduce risk with a variety of drugs and percutaneous coronary interventions has revolutionised the diagnosis and management of ischaemic heart disease in recent years. ACS can be thought of as a spectrum of increasing myocardial damage and mortality risk, including:

- unstable angina
- non-ST elevation myocardial infarction (NSTEMI)
- ST elevation myocardial infarction.

The first two are discussed together here because it can take 12 hours for the rise in cardiac troponin that distinguishes between them to become apparent, so they are managed in the same way acutely. ST elevation myocardial infarction is discussed separately.

Clinical presentation

Presentations include:

- new-onset angina
- rest angina, usually of > 20 min duration
- increasing severity of angina: longer in duration, occurring after lesser exertion, or responding less well to therapy than previously.

Unstable angina

This is diagnosed when a patient has:

- typical ischaemic chest pain
- and/or ECG changes: ST segment depression, transient ST elevation, and/or new T wave inversion
- no elevation of cardiac troponin or creatinine kinase after 12 hours.

NSTEMI

This term is used when the patient has:

- typical ischaemic chest pain
- a rise in cardiac troponin or creatinine kinase, signifying cardiac damage
- no Q waves, which are usually associated with ST segment elevation and indicate myocardial infarction.

Pathophysiology of ACS

ACS is caused by rupture of an atheromatous plaque with platelet thrombo-embolism in the coronary circulation. Even in NSTEMI, coronary angiography does not usually show coronary artery occlusion. That high rate of spontaneous reperfusion explains why NSTEMI has a better prognosis than acute myocardial infarction.

Management of ACS

The patient is admitted to a coronary care unit for close observation of haemodynamic state and pain relief. Treatment consists of:

- antithrombotic measures
  - aspirin 300 mg, unless hypersensitive
  - clopidogrel, unless urgent percutaneous coronary intervention is likely, in which case the combination of aspirin and clopidogrel increases the risks of major bleeding
  - Glycoprotein IIb/IIIa inhibitor if clopidogrel is contraindicated
  - heparin, particularly if there is left ventricular thrombus or atrial fibrillation
- nitrate sublingually and/or by infusion
- morphine as needed for pain
- beta-blocker therapy
- intravenous potassium and/or magnesium to correct electrolyte abnormalities
- statin therapy, e.g. atorvastatin
- an ACE inhibitor

On present evidence, thrombolytic therapy should not be given routinely for acute coronary syndrome because of the high rate of spontaneous reperfusion and a lack of clinical trial evidence of its benefit.

The decision as to whether a patient should have a percutaneous coronary intervention depends on an estimate of risk. Risk factors include:

- ST segment depression
- the degree of rise in cardiac troponin
- haemodynamic instability
- persistent pain
- cardiac dysrhythmias such as ventricular tachycardia.

The precise indication for intervention depends on local policy and resources. When angiography is not performed, the patient should have an exercise tolerance test (to assess the degree of coronary artery stenosis) and echocardiogram (to assess left ventricular function) before discharge.

Myocardial infarction

Pathology

Angiography has shown that myocardial infarction is caused by coronary artery occlusion in at least 90% of patients. The effects of coronary occlusion can be predicted from the coronary anatomy (Fig. 6), although you should remember that coronary anatomy and the sites of stenoses vary from individual to individual. Occlusion of the left anterior descending artery causes lateral, anterior or septal infarction, and this may be very extensive. Right coronary artery occlusion causes right ventricular and inferior infarcts, which tend to be smaller and may involve part of the septum, including the AV node. Posterior infarction is caused by occlusion of the distal circumflex artery. 'Subendocardial' infarction is the term given to a diffuse and concentric pattern of myocardial damage not caused by a localised coronary artery occlusion. It may occur in diffuse coronary artery disease, in association with increased ventricular wall thickness or pressure, or in conditions of reduced coronary artery perfusion or generalised hypoxia.

Clinical presentation

Diagnosis is based upon:

- history and signs
- ECG
- cardiac enzymes
- other circumstantial evidence.

History and signs

The pain of myocardial infarction differs from angina in two ways:

- duration, usually lasting > 15 min and often several hours
- lack of association with exercise and lack of relief from nitrates.

The pain varies from mild 'indigestion' to excruciating pain. It may be accompanied by a sense of impending death (angor animi). There may be breathlessness and/or palpitations. The presentation may be with syncope caused by a dysrhythmia. About 50% of patients have a previous history of angina or myocardial infarction and many of the remainder have obvious risk factors such as hypertension or cigarette smoking.

Sweating and pallor are common. There may be a bradycardia (resulting from increased vagal tone, typically in inferior infarction) or tachycardia. Blood pressure is usually normal or low. There may be basal crackles and a third or fourth heart sound, indicative of left ventricular failure. The jugular venous pressure is not usually raised at presentation; if it is, and particularly if there are no signs of left ventricular failure, think of **right ventricular infarction**.

Investigations

ECG

The patterns of injury and order in which they develop were discussed on page 11 and shown in Table 3. Examples are given in the self-assessment section. It follows from Figure 5 that:

- inferior infarction causes changes in leads II, III and aVF
- anterior infarction is seen across the anterior chest leads V1–4 (termed septal if confined to leads V3–4)
- lateral infarction is seen in I, aVL and V5–6
- posterior infarction is the subtlest change: a dominant R wave in lead V1, often associated with ST depression in the anterior leads.

One

'Hyperacute T waves' (increased height with a dramatic peaked appearance) are the earliest sign of full-thickness myocardial infarction but are seen in only a minority of patients. The order of development of other changes is summarised in Table 3. The ST segment changes usually normalise within 1 week of infarction. T wave changes may be permanent or revert later. Q wave changes are usually permanent. The ECG signs of non-Q wave infarction are ST segment depression and T wave inversion.

Release of cardiac enzymes

A variety of enzymes are released into blood after acute ischaemic myocardial damage; however, the mainstay of diagnosis and assessment of prognosis is now cardiac troponin. As discussed under Acute coronary syndrome (p. 16), an increased troponin concentration may first be detected 4 hours after myocardial damage and the level cannot be confidently declared normal until 12 hours have elapsed; it remains raised for up to 12 days. A specific isoenzyme of creatinine kinase (CK-MB) was, until recently, widely used as a marker of myocardial damage. It rises and falls faster than cardiac troponin and can be useful for detecting myocardial damage in patients whose pain recurs within the time it takes for cardiac troponin to normalise. A raised cardiac troponin in end-stage renal failure and other disorders such as pulmonary embolism can lead to an incorrect diagnosis of ACS.

The rise in markers of cardiac muscle damage is proportional to the amount of necrotic cardiac muscle and gives a rough guide to severity. A firm diagnosis is based on the combination of a diagnostic rise in cardiac troponin, typical symptoms and/or ECG changes.

Other circumstantial evidence

There is often a small rise in temperature at about 12 hours, a rise in erythrocyte sedimentation rate (ESR) and a neutrophil leucocytosis. These are non-specific signs of tissue necrosis. More specific evidence is the development of heart failure, dysrhythmias or pericarditis.

Immediate management

Faced with a patient with suspected acute myocardial infarction, your immediate responsibilities are to:

- give aspirin (300 mg as an immediate dose, repeated at a dose of 75–150 mg once daily) *on suspicion* of acute myocardial infarction
- give high-concentration oxygen to correct any hypoxia caused by left ventricular failure
- site a venous cannula
- record an ECG
- take a rapid history
- assess the cardiac rhythm, and arterial and venous circulations (p. 191)
- relieve pain with diamorphine and an antiemetic (e.g. metoclopramide or prochlorperazine)
- give thrombolytic therapy with the shortest possible 'door-to-needle' time if there is definite ST segment elevation or (suspected) new LBBB
- take blood for urea, creatinine and electrolytes (particularly potassium) and cardiac enzymes
- arrange admission to a coronary care unit.

The reason for checking potassium is that catecholamines secreted in response to myocardial infarction drive potassium into cells. The patient may already be hypokalaemic as a result of previous diuretic therapy. Hypokalaemia predisposes to cardiac dysrhythmias, so you need to prescribe potassium supplements to maintain plasma potassium ≥3.5 mmol/l. Plasma urea and creatinine are measured to detect pre-existing renal failure, and as a baseline in case renal function deteriorates acutely.

You must also:

- ensure adequate pain relief with opiates and antianginals
- consider i.v. beta-blocker therapy
- identify and treat heart failure.

These are discussed in more detail under Complications below.

Thrombolysis

The use of drugs that break down fibrin can restore flow in the occluded artery in about two-thirds of patients. There are two main types of drug: *streptokinase*, which works by activating free plasminogen, and tissue plasminogen activator (TPA-alteplase, reteplase, tenecteplase, etc.), which activates plasminogen bound to fibrin. Streptokinase is a foreign, antigenic protein; there is a risk of anaphylaxis if it is repeated. TPA is non-antigenic. Both drugs are given by i.v. infusion. Streptokinase is much cheaper and is used as treatment of first choice. It may cause hypotension. TPA is indicated in patients who have previously received streptokinase and in patients who become hypotensive during streptokinase therapy.

Contraindications to thrombolysis include:

- recent history of haemorrhage
- trauma, surgery, recent childbirth or vascular injury
- active peptic ulceration
- recent history of stroke, particularly haemorrhagic
- uncontrolled hypertension, liver disease or varices
- active proliferative diabetic retinopathy at risk of bleeding
- pregnancy (fetal death may result).

The main side-effect of thrombolysis is bleeding and this may cause acute haemorrhagic stroke. More than 10% of patients admitted to coronary care units have diabetes and they have twice the mortality of other patients. They must not be denied thrombolytic therapy because of ill-founded concerns about retinal haemorrhage.

Aspirin and thrombolytic therapy, given appropriately, together reduce the acute mortality of myocardial infarction by over 30%.

Invasive management

In some centres, immediate angiography is performed with a view to primary angioplasty if the patient presents very early.

Subsequent management

Patients should continue to receive aspirin (unless there is a contraindication); many will need further analgesia or nitrate therapy and some will receive diuretic therapy for heart failure. More specific management details are considered under the headings of Complications, Postinfarction prophylaxis and Rehabilitation.

Complications

There is a high risk of ventricular fibrillation during the first 4–6 hours. Patients often respond well to resuscitation and have an excellent prognosis.

Complications developing later are more ominous. Bad prognostic signs are:

- hypotension or marked left ventricular failure
- extensive or progressive ECG changes
- acute hyperglycaemia or history of diabetes
- rise in blood urea
- greater age.

Dysrhythmias

Dysrhythmias may occur early after fibrinolytic therapy, when they are caused by reperfusion of ischaemic myocardium (reperfusion dysrhythmias). They have a benign prognosis and should not be treated unless the patient is haemodynamically compromised. Dysrhythmias are covered in detail below (p. 26). Common dysrhythmias specific to acute myocardial infarction are:

Ventricular ectopic beats, tachycardia (VT) and fibrillation (VF) Isolated ventricular ectopics are of little significance. Ectopics that are multifocal, come in runs or occur close upon the previous complex (R on T) may precede VF. They can be suppressed by intravenous lidocaine and magnesium sulphate but this does not prevent VF; consequently they should not be treated unless there is haemodynamic compromise.

Sinus tachycardia This may be caused by heart failure or anxiety. There is no specific treatment.

Sinus bradycardia This occurs early and results from increased vagal tone. It can be treated with atropine if symptomatic.

Atrial fibrillation This is a bad prognostic sign because it signifies severe myocardial damage. It requires cardioversion if it causes acute haemodynamic compromise. Otherwise, the treatment is beta-blockade or digoxin. Anticoagulation is essential to reduce the risk of embolism from the fibrillating atrium.

Supraventricular tachycardia

Complete heart block There are two quite distinct situations. Patients with **inferior myocardial infarcts** may develop oedema of the AV node, which causes first-degree, then second-degree, and then third-degree (complete) heart block. Complete block is usually transient with a satisfactory idioventricular rate (p. 27) because the escape pacemaker is relatively high in the conducting system. Such patients do not usually require pacing. Patients with **anterior infarcts** may develop 'bifascicular block' (an ECG diagnosis based on right bundle branch block with left axis deviation), which can progress to complete heart block and signifies widespread myocardial damage with interruption of the conduction pathways below the His bundle. If complete heart block occurs, it causes profound bradycardia and hypotension and may not resolve spontaneously.

Heart failure

Left ventricular dysfunction may cause 'forwards failure' — hypotension, renal impairment, impaired capillary perfusion — and 'backwards failure' — pulmonary oedema (p. 22). Treatment is with diuretics and nitrates, orally or i.v. Provided the patient is not hypotensive (systolic < 100 mmHg), an oral ACE inhibitor (e.g. lisinopril) should be started without delay. A specific beta-blocker (bisoprolol, carvedilol or metoprolol) is added later, once heart failure is controlled, and increased to the highest dose a patient can tolerate.

Right heart failure may occur secondary to left ventricular dysfunction, in which case the treatment is as above. If it develops without signs of left ventricular failure, right ventricular infarction should be suspected and the treatment is the exact opposite: infusion of colloid to increase right ventricular filling pressure. Diuretic therapy worsens cardiac output in this situation, as do nitrates.

Cardiogenic shock is caused by severe left ventricular dysfunction. There is:

- hypotension
- poor capillary perfusion: cold, cyanosed nail beds with delayed capillary refill
- poor cerebral perfusion: impairment of consciousness
- impaired renal perfusion: renal failure.

Oxygen, a nitrate infusion and a diuretic are given to relieve breathlessness. Dobutamine (an inotropic agent) is infused to optimise left ventricular performance. Dopamine may also be infused in low dose to improve renal perfusion. A pulmonary artery catheter may be inserted to monitor the haemodynamic response. The mortality is up to 90% despite treatment. In the setting of acute myocardial infarction, cardiogenic shock is an indication for urgent angiography with a view to revascularisation.

Unremitting pain

The pain of myocardial infarction usually settles within hours and requires just one or two doses of opiate, but there are patients in whom anginal pain continues. Opiates should be given as needed, nitrate infused or given orally, and a beta-blocker and/or calcium antagonist given. Heart failure and dysrhythmias should be controlled because they worsen angina and oxygen should be given. If pain continues and/or there are new ST segment changes on the ECG, the patient needs coronary angiography with a view to revascularisation (see Acute coronary syndrome above).

Pericarditis

Pericarditis can occur about 48 hours after full-thickness myocardial infarction. The pain (p. 40) is recognisably different from that of the infarct and usually transient. Anticoagulants should be withheld because there is a risk of haemorrhage into the pericardial space.

Septal rupture

An acute ventricular septal defect is a rare result of ischaemic septal damage. There is acute haemodynamic deterioration and a pansystolic murmur, often accompanied by a thrill. The only effective treatment is surgery.

One

Ruptured papillary muscle

Rupture of a papillary muscle can vary in severity from mild mitral valve prolapse to florid mitral incompetence. If mild, it is managed medically. If severe, the treatment is valve replacement, which has a high mortality.

Left ventricular aneurysm and cardiac rupture

Full-thickness myocardial infarction causes softening and dyskinesia (impaired contraction) of the ventricular wall, which heals by fibrosis. If the dyskinetic area is large, the healing area of infarction may form an aneurysm which is non-contractile and, paradoxically, enlarges during systole. There is likely to be mural thrombus (see below). Left ventricular aneurysms are associated with:

• persistent and severe left ventricular dysfunction
• a dyskinetic 'feel' to the cardiac apex on examination
• dysrhythmias
• a high risk of arterial thrombo-embolism
• persistent (>1 week) ST segment elevation on the ECG.

Diagnosis is by echocardiography. Some left ventricular aneurysms can be treated surgically.

The area of softening may rupture before it has become fibrotic. This usually causes sudden death a week or more after infarction (there is pulseless electrical activity — complexes on the ECG with no cardiac output), though occasionally the rupture may be walled off by thrombus, resulting in a pseudoaneurysm.

Mural thrombus

Even without aneurysm formation, thrombus can form on the endocardial surface after full-thickness infarction, particularly if the left ventricle is contracting poorly. The thrombus may embolise to the brain, limbs or mesenteric circulation. Full-thickness infarction, poor left ventricular performance and aneurysm formation are indications for prophylactic anticoagulation. The thrombus may be demonstrated by contrast echocardiography.

Venous thrombo-embolism

Myocardial infarction causes:

• recumbency
• reduced cardiac output
• increased synthesis of coagulation factors, as a response to acute illness.

All these predispose to deep venous thrombosis and pulmonary embolism, classically 10 or more days after the infarct. Management is discussed on page 48. You should encourage patients to keep their legs mobile in bed and avoid unnecessarily long recumbency and you should prescribe prophylactic heparin. Patients with poor cardiac output or evidence of venous thrombosis should be fully anticoagulated.

Post-infarction prophylaxis

Prophylaxis is summarised in Box 1. Most of the treatments have been tested in clinical trials and shown to

---

Box 1: An approach to improving prognosis and preventing complications after myocardial infarction

Immediate
• Fibrinolysis
• Consider i.v. beta-blocker
• Aspirin — continue indefinitely — and clopidogrel for 14 days
• Lipid measurement — start a statin
• Heparin — prophylactic use if patient is likely to remain in bed for 3 days or more
• Primary angiography with a view to revascularisation in centres that provide that service

First 24–48 hours
• ACE inhibitor (ramipril or perindopril; lisinopril if left ventricular ejection fraction (LVEF) < 35%) — if full-thickness anterior MI or any evidence of left ventricular failure (LVF) (unless hypotensive); continue indefinitely
• Beta-blocker — if controlled LVF (unless asthmatic etc.); continue indefinitely

Rest of hospital stay
• Full anticoagulation — if severe LV dysfunction or dysrhythmias
• Coronary risk factors — identify and discuss, e.g. smoking, inactivity
• Consider omega III fatty acids

After discharge
• Cardiac rehabilitation — encourage physical activity, advise about diet, smoking, alcohol
• Hyperlipidaemia — monitor response to statin; screen other family members
• Exercise text — refer for angiography with a view to revascularisation if positive
• ACE inhibitors and/or beta-blockers — ensure these are being taken
• Consider eplerenone (aldosterone antagonist) if there are signs of heart failure and an LVEF < 40%.

---

improve survival, but not in all of their possible permutations, leaving an element of choice to the clinician. The indications for and contraindications to thrombolytics, aspirin and anticoagulants have already been discussed; hyperlipidaemia is discussed on page 312, exercise testing on page 14 and cardiac rehabilitation below. Diuretics, nitrates and calcium antagonists are given for specific indications but have no general role in improving life expectancy.

Beta-blockers

Beta-blockers have been proven to reduce coronary mortality if given intravenously on admission and, in a separate trial, orally for up to 5 years afterwards. Policies differ about i.v. use. Any patient without a contraindication such as asthma should be given a beta-blocker as soon as it is clear they are not developing hypotension or heart failure, particularly if their LVEF is reduced. The dose should be titrated up to the highest the patient can tolerate. If they develop heart failure, a beta-blocker should be given once it is controlled.

ACE inhibitors

ACE inhibitors are also of proven value in left ventricular dysfunction and are most effective if introduced early. Assessment of left ventricular function by echocardiography is desirable. Failing that, a practical policy is to start a small dose of a short-acting ACE inhibitor in any patient who has left ventricular failure (LVF) and is not hypotensive and in all patients with anterior infarcts, because they are likely to have left ventricular dysfunction. ACE inhibitor therapy is now very routine. Perindopril is the drug of choice for younger people, ramipril for people aged over 55 years.

Plasma lipids

The stress of myocardial infarction increases plasma lipids within about 24 hours; as a result they should be measured either immediately or 3 months later. Since statins improve prognosis even with 'normal' serum cholesterol, lipid measurements are more to monitor response than to decide on treatment, because that should be routine. There is clinical trial evidence that aggressive treatment with atorvastatin is particular beneficial.

Cardiac rehabilitation

Patients with uncomplicated myocardial infarction are usually only kept in bed for as long as they are acutely ill; they are then allowed to return gradually to normal mobility during a hospital stay of 4–5 days. Sensitive management by medical and nursing staff alleviates anxiety and helps the patient come to terms with their diagnosis. Investigations and treatment choices should be discussed and the diagnosis and its implications carefully explained, with plenty of opportunity to ask questions. Patients should be supplied with written material appropriate to their diagnosis and level of interest and given a chance to discuss their future plans and prospects, ideally by introducing them to the cardiac rehabilitation team while they are still in hospital.

After discharge, cardiac rehabilitation can improve the outcome of myocardial infarction in physical as well as psychosocial terms. It consists of supervised exercise training, education and counselling. Important points to discuss are:

- resumption of sexual activity
- return to work (a time of difficulty, particularly in patients who are self-employed or have manual jobs)
- physical activity.

1.3 Heart failure

Learning objectives

You should:
- have a clear understanding of the pathophysiology of heart failure and the range of disease processes that can cause it
- be competent at diagnosing heart failure from the symptoms, signs and chest radiograph
- understand its treatment and how that relates to the pathophysiological mechanisms and long-term prognosis.

Case Study

A patient with alcoholic cardiomyopathy is admitted for the third time in as many months with severe breathlessness and oedema. He is switched from oral to intravenous furosemide and started on digoxin. There is discussion about whether he could be given a beta-blocker despite his mild asthma.

Heart failure is common. The overall prevalence is about 1%, rising to over 10% in old people. Together with IHD it is a leading cause of acute hospital admission. It has a high mortality; the overall 5-year survival is about 50% and severe heart failure has a prognosis as bad as that of disseminated cancer. Its symptoms have a major impact on quality of life. On the positive side, recent clinical trials have shown that the prognosis can be improved by both traditional and new drugs.

Definitions

Getting to grips with some terms used to describe heart failure will help you understand the range of clinical manifestations. First, remember that 'heart failure' is not a precise diagnosis in itself but the common end-product of a range of pathological processes. Good clinical practice is to base treatment on as precise a *pathological* diagnosis as possible.

Low-output versus high-output heart failure

Heart failure can be defined as failure to maintain a cardiac output sufficient to meet the needs of the tissues despite an adequate filling pressure (excluding haemorrhagic shock and volume depletion). It may be caused by 'pump failure' (low-output heart failure) or increased demand (high-output heart failure), as in anaemia (p. 22).

Left versus right heart failure

Pure failure of one side of the heart is unusual because:

- disease processes do not usually affect just one chamber
- left heart failure increases pulmonary venous pressure and leads to right heart failure.

Pure right heart failure resulting from pulmonary hypertension or right ventricular infarction is a notable exception. However, symptoms and signs may be *predominantly* right- or left-sided. Right heart failure causes symptoms and signs of *systemic* venous congestion whereas left ventricular failure causes *pulmonary* venous congestion.

Biventricular failure is a better term than congestive cardiac failure to describe a combination of the two.

Forwards versus backwards failure

Forwards and backwards describe the effects of a reduced cardiac output on the arterial and venous circulations respectively. The relationship of forwards and backwards failure to the symptoms of heart failure is discussed below and Figure 8 shows how these terms relate to the signs.

Severity and chronicity

Heart failure ranges from asymptomatic systolic dysfunction to a disease causing intolerable symptoms. It may be chronic or, as when caused by a cardiac dysrhythmia, transient and completely reversible.

Pathophysiology of heart failure

The earliest effect of impaired cardiac contractility is failure to increase cardiac output in response to exercise, experienced by the patient as exertional dyspnoea. Eventually the failing heart cannot maintain an adequate stroke volume at rest and venous pressure rises. At first, the Starling effect (p. 8) restores contractility at the cost of cardiac dilatation. As contractility progressively fails, venous pressures rise and pulmonary and systemic oedema result.

A reduced cardiac output reduces the *effective* arterial volume and triggers compensatory mechanisms, including activation of the renin–angiotensin–aldosterone system and secretion of catecholamines and arginine vasopressin (antidiuretic hormone; p. 295). Hyperaldosteronism causes salt and water retention, expanding the blood volume, further increasing venous pressure and causing oedema. Catecholamine secretion tends to restore cardiac output by increasing contractility and heart rate but also increases peripheral vascular resistance (afterload). Increased venous pressure increases secretion of natriuretic peptides but insufficiently to counteract the combined sodium-retaining effects of venous hypertension and secondary hyperaldosteronism.

Think of heart failure as a vicious circle in which these compensatory mechanisms initially maintain cardiac output but later become part of the disease process. Since contractility cannot usually be corrected, the treatment of heart failure (Fig. 9 below) is directed primarily at those compensatory mechanisms.

Causes of heart failure

IHD is the most common cause, but only one of many. Others include:

- decreased myocardial contractility
  - heart muscle disease, e.g. alcoholic cardiomyopathy
- altered cardiac rhythm
  - tachycardia
  - bradycardia
- increased arterial resistance
  - systemic hypertension
  - pulmonary hypertension
- increased blood volume
  - overtransfusion
  - renal failure

- valvular lesions
  - outflow resistance, e.g. aortic stenosis
  - increased flow, e.g. mitral regurgitation
- compromised cardiac filling
  - constrictive pericarditis
  - pericardial effusion
- increased demand (high-output cardiac failure)
  - anaemia
  - thyrotoxicosis
  - left to right shunt.

There is often more than one cause.

Clinical presentation

Symptoms and signs

This section integrates symptoms and signs and lists them according to the underlying mechanisms (Fig. 8):

- increased venous pressure
- reduced cardiac output
- failing heart.

Increased venous pressure

Symptoms

Breathlessness Increased pulmonary venous pressure causes alveolar oedema, which impairs gas exchange and reduces the compliance of the lungs. Dyspnoea occurs only after exertion in mild heart failure and at rest in more severe failure. Lying flat increases venous return and makes breathlessness worse (orthopnoea). There may be severe nocturnal episodes of left ventricular failure (paroxysmal nocturnal dyspnoea).

Cough This may be unproductive or productive of white frothy sputum, sometimes pink-tinged or frankly blood-stained.

Wheeze Heart failure may cause airway narrowing with wheeze (cardiac asthma) indistinguishable from the wheeze of obstructive airways disease.

Signs of left ventricular failure

Basal crackles Crackles that do not disappear after coughing may be a sign of pulmonary oedema.

Signs of right ventricular failure

Oedema Fluid collects first in the most dependent parts of the body, usually the ankles, and spreads proximally. Press firmly over the medial aspect of the shin just proximal to the ankle for a few seconds to detect it. *Sacral* oedema may be more prominent in bedbound patients. Severe right heart failure causes ascites and pleural effusions by the same mechanism as ankle swelling.

Hepatomegaly

Raised jugular venous pressure This is covered in detail on page 194. Look for pulsation behind sternomastoid, observe how it varies with respiration and, if necessary, accentuate it by pressing briefly over the liver to increase venous return (hepato-jugular reflux).

Reduced effective arterial volume

Symptoms

Dizziness and syncope These are caused by impaired cerebral perfusion, worse on standing and often exacerbated by diuretic and vasodilator therapy.

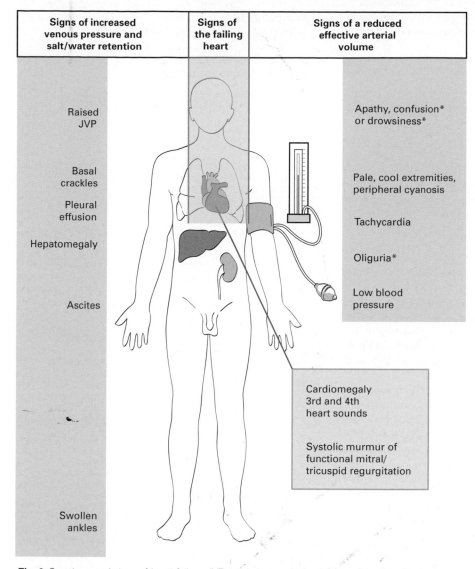

Signs of increased venous pressure and salt/water retention	Signs of the failing heart	Signs of a reduced effective arterial volume

Raised JVP

Basal crackles

Pleural effusion

Hepatomegaly

Ascites

Swollen ankles

Apathy, confusion* or drowsiness*

Pale, cool extremities, peripheral cyanosis

Tachycardia

Oliguria*

Low blood pressure

Cardiomegaly 3rd and 4th heart sounds

Systolic murmur of functional mitral/ tricuspid regurgitation

Fig. 8 Symptoms and signs of heart failure. JVP, jugular venous pulse. * Signs of cardiogenic shock.

Fatigue

Signs

Low blood pressure This results in pale, cool extremities with peripheral cyanosis.

Tachycardia This results from sympathetic activation.

Failing heart

Signs

Cardiomegaly Cardiac dilatation is fundamental to the pathophysiology of heart failure (p. 22). The apex beat is displaced. If you place the heel of your hand over the sternum and your fingers over the apex, you will feel right ventricular dilatation under the heel and left ventricular dilatation under the fingers.

Added sounds (gallop rhythm) The third heart sound is caused by diastolic filling of a diseased and non-compliant ventricle and the fourth sound by atrial contraction. Both are pathological in older adults, but a third sound may be heard in fit young people. They are heard best at the apex with the bell of the stethoscope. To understand what a third heart sound is like, say 'Kentucky' repeatedly without pausing; for a fourth heart sound, say 'Tennessee'. If there is a tachycardia, you may not be able to distinguish between them. Both may be present.

Pansystolic murmur Cardiac dilatation stretches the mitral and tricuspid valve rings so you may also hear a pansystolic murmur as an *effect* of heart failure.

Investigations

It is usually possible to diagnose heart failure from the history, examination and chest radiograph (p. 10). An echocardiogram is much more sensitive and specific than the radiograph for confirming the diagnosis and identifying its cause. A radionuclide scan, which measures ventricular size in systole and diastole, is more accurate than the echocardiogram at measuring the ejection fraction. The choice of other investigations is guided by a thorough history and examination. An ECG may show signs of underlying IHD or point to other diagnoses. Do not forget to exclude systemic diseases such as alcoholism, anaemia and thyrotoxicosis.

Clinical syndromes

There are two main clinical presentations of heart failure, which are different enough to be described separately:

- acute left ventricular failure
- chronic biventricular failure.

Pure right heart failure may also occur (p. 21).

Acute left ventricular failure

Acute left ventricular failure is caused by:

- acute myocardial infarction (p. 17)
- chronic IHD
- fluid overload, e.g. renal failure (p. 179)
- valve failure, e.g. infective endocarditis (p. 38).

The patient is sitting bolt upright, gasping for breath and often coughing up profuse pink, frothy sputum. There is a tachycardia, third and/or fourth heart sounds and bibasal pulmonary crackles. The chest radiographic appearances are as shown on page 10. Immediate management is shown in the emergency box. Loop diuretics are the mainstay of treatment but a nitrate by bolus injection or infusion has been shown to be at least as effective without causing more hypotension. A loop diuretic and a nitrate may be used together.

Patients with severe left ventricular failure often respond gratifyingly well. Their acute attack may have been triggered by acute myocardial infarction so cardiac enzymes should be measured. Once the patient has recovered, assess the cause of heart failure to decide on further management.

Chronic biventricular failure

Heart failure is all too often overlooked or treated inappropriately with antibiotics or bronchodilators. None of its symptoms (p. 23) clearly distinguishes it from chronic airflow limitation; even orthopnoea is not specific to heart failure. The distinction depends on a full history, physical examination and a chest radiograph. Patients may, of course, have both cardiac and pulmonary disease.

Management

You should aim to:

- relieve symptoms
- optimise the long-term prognosis.

A stepwise approach to management is outlined in Figure 9; treatment includes drugs and changes to lifestyle; ultimately it can include transplantation. The modes of action of the drugs are summarised in Figure 10.

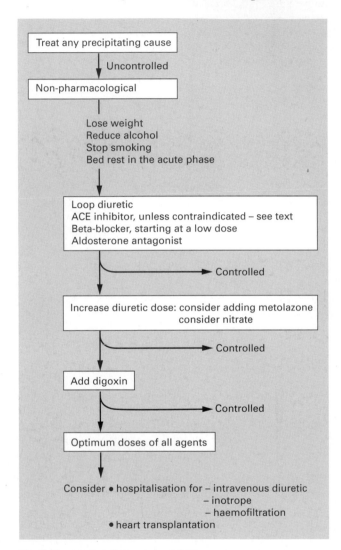

Fig. 9 Management of chronic heart failure.

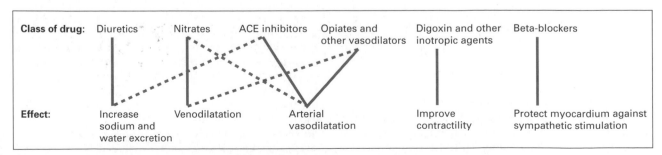

Fig. 10 The modes of action of drugs used in heart failure. Dotted lines indicate minor effects. ACE, angiotension-converting enzyme.

Non-pharmacological treatments

Diet Obesity increases cardiac work. Overweight patients should be advised to diet and hyperlipidaemic patients treated to prevent progression of coronary artery disease.

Abstinence from alcohol Excessive alcohol impairs contractility and may cause permanent heart muscle damage (cardiomyopathy).

Bed rest This improves heart failure in the short term, although in the longer term patients should be advised to remain active.

Limitation of salt and fluid intake Thirst is common and may exacerbate heart failure.

Stopping smoking

Drug treatment

Figure 9 summarises an approach to drug use.

Clinical Box: Emergency treatment: management of acute left ventricular failure

- Give 100% oxygen, unless there is a possibility that the diagnosis is exacerbation of chronic airflow limitation rather than LVF
- Do an ECG to exclude acute myocardial infarction or dysrhythmia
- Give diamorphine or morphine with an antiemetic (e.g. prochlorperazine)
- Give furosemide 40–80 mg i.v.; repeat and increase dose as necessary

  Depending upon response:
- Start a nitrate infusion unless the patient is hypotensive
- Consider inotrope infusion (dobutamine) if severely hypotensive
- Admit to coronary or intensive care unit
- Repeat diamorphine as needed
- Consider ventilation for intractable pulmonary oedema

Diuretics A loop diuretic (furosemide or bumetanide) is usually the first-line treatment. Hypokalaemia may occur so the diet should include plenty of potassium (e.g. from fruit). Thiazides are an alternative first-line treatment and work synergistically with a loop diuretic in severe heart failure. Metolazone is the most effective thiazide in that context. Potassium-sparing diuretics (e.g. amiloride) are relatively ineffective on their own but may be given in combination with a loop diuretic or thiazide if hypokalaemia is a problem. Electrolytes should be checked several weeks after starting treatment and potassium supplements or combination therapy given as necessary.

ACE inhibitors ACE inhibitors act:

- as vasodilators, by reducing the synthesis of angiotensin II, a potent vasoconstrictor
- as mild diuretics, by reducing aldosterone synthesis
- on the tissues to inhibit cardiac hypertrophy in hypertension.

They relieve symptoms, retard the progression of heart failure and improve mortality. An ACE inhibitor (e.g. lisinopril, ramipril) should be given (with a diuretic) unless there are contraindications. These are:

- likelihood of pregnancy, because they can cause fetal anomalies
- renal artery stenosis (p. 187)
- low blood pressure (e.g. < 100 mmHg systolic), because they can exacerbate hypotension
- severe aortic or mitral stenosis, because they may cause syncope.

Patients with heart failure may have a precipitous fall in blood pressure when given an ACE inhibitor; this may be a 'first-dose' or sustained effect. You should observe the following precautions:

- In mild heart failure, omit diuretics for 24–48 hours before starting the ACE inhibitor.
- In patients with low blood pressure or severe heart failure
  — start with a small dose
  — start treatment recumbent in hospital and monitor blood pressure closely after the start of treatment.

Blood pressure, renal function and electrolytes should be monitored after starting ACE inhibitors to detect hyperkalaemia (a direct effect of ACE inhibition) or worsened renal function.

Other vasodilators Patients who cannot tolerate ACE inhibitors (e.g. because of intractable cough) or do not respond to them (black people) can be treated with other vasodilators such as candesartan (an angiotensin receptor antagonist), hydralazine or prazosin, which act predominantly by reducing afterload. Nitrates may be used to reduce preload but their long-term benefit is limited by tolerance.

Beta-blockers Although they can precipitate heart failure when started in high doses, carvedilol, bisoprolol and metoprolol have been shown in large trials to improve the symptoms and prognosis for survival of patients with heart failure. They act by protecting the myocardium against sympathetic stimulation. A small initial fall in ejection fraction is followed by a sustained rise.

Aldosterone antagonists Spironolactone and eplerenone, competitive inhibitors of the effect of aldosterone on its receptor, have been shown in trials to improve survival in severe, chronic heart failure.

Digoxin Digoxin is both an inotropic and an antidysrhythmic agent of proven value in reducing symptoms and the need for hospitalisation in heart failure associated with both atrial fibrillation and sinus rhythm. It can be given together with diuretics and ACE inhibitors or other vasodilators. Hypokalaemia potentiates digoxin and may cause toxicity.

Biventricular pacing

This can improve symptoms and prognosis in some patients with left ventricular dyssynchrony on the echocardiogram and broad LBBB on the ECG.

Cardiac transplantation

Cardiac transplantation relieves the symptoms of heart failure and has a 5-year survival of up to 70%. It is reserved for younger patients (< 60 years) with end-stage disease and a proven poor physiological response to exercise. The indications include:

- IHD
- cardiomyopathies
- intractable ventricular tachydysrhythmias
- congenital heart disease
- cardiac tumours.

If there is significant pulmonary vascular disease, combined heart–lung transplantation is required. This is technically more demanding and has a lower survival.

1.4 Dysrhythmias

Learning objectives

You should:

- understand how to recognise and treat the common dysrhythmias
- be alert to the clinical presentations of dysrhythmias
- understand how to diagnose them from the ECG
- be prepared to manage dysrhythmic emergencies
- know how to manage cardiac arrest
- have a good understanding of atrial fibrillation and its complications and treatment.

Case Study

A patient with a pulse rate of 168 beats/min is at first thought to be in ventricular tachycardia but an old ECG shows that the QRS complex had the same configuration when he was recently discharged and had a pulse rate of 80 beats/min. He is in atrial fibrillation and the broad QRS complexes are due to bundle branch block.

You must be ready to manage cardiac dysrhythmias from your first day as a house officer. One per cent of the general population and 10% of old people are in atrial fibrillation. Supraventricular tachycardia is a not infrequent acute medical emergency. You must be ready to treat ventricular fibrillation or complete heart block causing sudden collapse after acute myocardial infarction.

Causes of dysrhythmias

Many different sites within the heart can act as pacemakers. An ectopic pacemaker with a faster rate of depolarisation can override the SA node. If impulse generation or conduction fails, a slower pacemaker lower down the conducting system will take over (p. 8). Dysrhythmias can be of the following types:

- slow rate or missed beats
  - increased vagal stimulation of the SA node (sinus bradycardia)
  - slow, erratic or absent impulse generation in the SA node
    - impaired AV conduction (heart block)
- fast rate or extra beats
  - increased adrenergic stimulation of the SA node (sinus tachycardia)
  - impulse generation from an ectopic site
  - totally disorganised impulse generation from within the myocardium (atrial or ventricular fibrillation).

Dysrhythmias may arise:

- spontaneously
- as a result of heart disease
  - IHD
  - cardiomyopathy (p. 41)
- as a result of systemic disease, e.g. thyrotoxicosis
- as an *effect* of therapy with antidysrhythmic drugs, particularly digoxin.

Remember that dysrhythmias may be precipitated or exacerbated by hypokalaemia; this is particularly important because of the association of hypokalaemia with diuretic therapy for heart disease and the stress of acute myocardial infarction (p. 17). Hypoxia and acidaemia are other precipitants.

Re-entry

Impulses normally propagate through the atria, conducting tissue and ventricles in an orderly manner, followed by a refractory period before the tissues are receptive to the next impulse. Electrical circuits in diseased myocardium can allow impulses to go round in circles and repeatedly re-activate the myocardium at a greatly increased rate. Re-entrant dysrhythmias include atrioventricular re-entrant tachycardia, atrial flutter, atrial fibrillation and sustained monomorphic ventricular tachycardia.

Re-entrant circuits can also be formed by congenital accessory pathways which carry impulses between the atria and ventricles faster than the His bundle. The impulse passes down the accessory pathway, back up the His bundle and round in circles, setting up a tachycardia. Ectopic impulses are propagated backwards as well as forwards through the conducting system so that, depending on the site of the ectopic pacemaker, atrial contraction may occur before, simultaneously with, or after ventricular contraction. On the ECG, this determines the timing of the P wave in relation to the QRS complex. Retrograde conduction causes inversion of the P wave.

Clinical presentation

Both bradycardias and tachycardias can cause syncope and heart failure, by reducing heart rate and compromising ventricular filling, respectively. A fast heart rate can also cause angina (p. 13) and palpitations. Dysrhythmias may be a chance ECG finding.

Symptoms

The word 'palpitations' means different things to different people. The challenge is to get a clear description of what the patient actually experiences. Key features are the speed and regularity of the heart beat during the attack, its duration, precipitating and relieving factors, and associated symptoms. The state of ventricular function can modify symptoms. Thus, a patient with severe ventricular disease may have no palpitations during a dysrhythmia that would cause intolerable palpitations in someone with good myocardial contractility. Poor ventricular function can cause intolerable left ventricular failure or syncope during a dysrhythmia that would cause little more than fluttering in the chest in a patient with a healthy myocardium.

Signs

A pulse rate < 60 or > 100 beats/min or an irregular cardiac rhythm constitutes a dysrhythmia. If the rhythm is irregular, you have to decide if it is chaotic (atrial fibrillation) or added/missed beats are superimposed on a fundamentally regular rhythm. A pulse rate > 140 beats/min at rest is unlikely to be a sinus tachycardia unless there is a very severe and obvious systemic illness causing it. Profound bradycardia (< 40/min) is strongly suggestive of complete heart block.

Investigations

For most patients, the ECG is the only way of diagnosing the dysrhythmia, and is the 'gold standard' for all patients. If you do not see the patient during an attack, you may be able to 'catch one' by hospital monitoring or on an ambulatory ECG. You should examine the ECG systematically for:

- the presence of P waves
- their rate and rhythm
- their relationship to the QRS complexes
- the ventricular (QRS) rate and rhythm
- the shape of the QRS complex.

You may need to use a piece of blank card to mark out the position of P waves and check their regularity. Examples of ECGs are shown in the self-assessment section.

The spectrum of dysrhythmias

These are the important dysrhythmias, classified by the nature of the pulse. Unless otherwise stated, the pulse is regular.

- cardiac arrest (no pulse)
  — asystole
  — electromechanical dissociation (EMD)
  — ventricular fibrillation
- bradycardias (slow pulse)
  — complete heart block
  — sinus bradycardia, as in the sick sinus syndrome
- dropped beats
  — second-degree heart block (pulse regularly irregular)
- extrasystoles (single extra beats)
  — supraventricular (regularly irregular)
  — ventricular (regularly irregular)
- tachycardias (fast pulse)
  — sinus tachycardia
  — atrial fibrillation (irregularly irregular)
  — atrial tachycardia
  — atrial flutter
  — junctional (AV nodal) tachycardia

— accessory pathway tachycardia
— accelerated idioventricular rhythm
— ventricular tachycardia.

Each type is discussed in more detail below.

Cardiac arrest

The patient is collapsed and pulseless. First, you should establish an airway and start cardiopulmonary resuscitation. (If you are unclear about how to do so, request (re)training urgently.) Once an ECG is available, it will show:

- asystole: no QRS complexes
- Pulseless electrical activity (PEA): QRS complexes but no palpable pulse
- ventricular fibrillation or tachycardia.

There are nationally agreed management guidelines, summarised in Figure 11, and you should not join a cardiac arrest team until you know them. Lidocaine or another antidysrhythmic drug is given to stabilise the ventricular rhythm after ventricular fibrillation or tachycardia and/or for ventricular dysrhythmias resistant to DC shock. Emergency pacing is often required for bradycardias. Arterial blood gases should be checked as soon as possible in all patients and i.v. 4.2% or 8.4% bicarbonate given to correct the lactic acidosis that may result from anaerobic metabolism. Asystole and PEA have an appalling (< 10%) prognosis for successful resuscitation unless there is a rapidly treatable cause such as cardiac tamponade.

Bradycardias and dropped beats

Heart block

The SA node depolarises regularly but AV conduction is abnormal or absent.

First-degree heart block

There is prolongation of the PR interval to > 5 small squares (0.2 s) in every complex because of delayed conduction in the AV node.

Second-degree heart block

There are two broad subtypes

- Wenckebach phenomenon: the PR interval lengthens progressively until a beat is missed.
- Dropped beats: some P waves are not followed by a QRS complex; the beats may be dropped randomly or regularly, e.g. two-to-one or three-to-one (total to conducted).

Third-degree (complete) heart block

AV conduction is completely blocked so that the atria (P waves) and ventricles (QRS complexes) are dissociated. The rate of the P waves is faster than the QRS rate, which is determined by the level of the block in the conducting system (p. 18). A 'junctional' (high) pacemaker may produce a satisfactory ventricular rate (e.g. 50 beats/min). A lower block, as after anterior myocardial infarction (p. 19), will cause a catastrophically slow ventricular rate (20 beats/min) with broad QRS complexes (≥ 3 small squares) because the impulse spreads in a disorganised

One

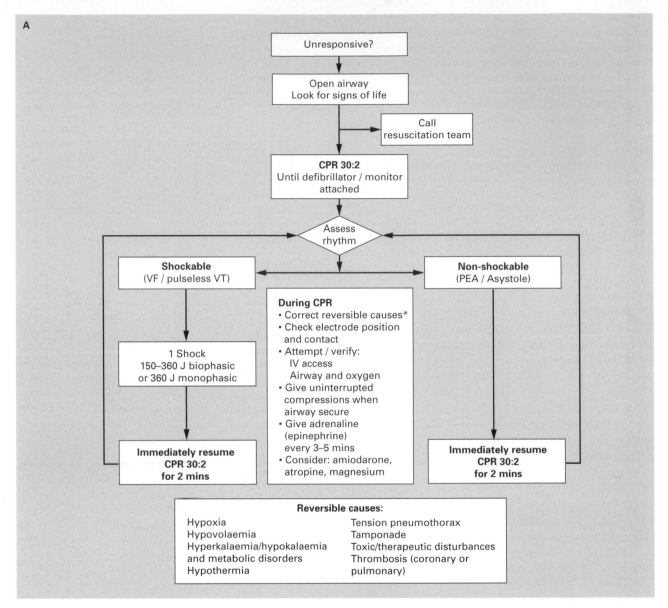

A

Unresponsive?

Open airway
Look for signs of life

Call
resuscitation team

CPR 30:2
Until defibrillator / monitor
attached

Assess
rhythm

Shockable
(VF / pulseless VT)

Non-shockable
(PEA / Asystole)

During CPR
• Correct reversible causes*
• Check electrode position
  and contact
• Attempt / verify:
  IV access
  Airway and oxygen
• Give uninterrupted
  compressions when
  airway secure
• Give adrenaline
  (epinephrine)
  every 3–5 mins
• Consider: amiodarone,
  atropine, magnesium

1 Shock
150–360 J biophasic
or 360 J monophasic

**Immediately resume
CPR 30:2
for 2 mins**

**Immediately resume
CPR 30:2
for 2 mins**

Reversible causes:

Hypoxia	Tension pneumothorax
Hypovolaemia	Tamponade
Hyperkalaemia/hypokalaemia	Toxic/therapeutic disturbances
and metabolic disorders	Thrombosis (coronary or
Hypothermia	pulmonary)

Fig. 11 Management guidelines. **A** Flow diagram of resuscitation procedures (based on the recommendations of the UK Resuscitation Council). ABC, airway, breathing, circulation; AF, atrial fibrillation; AV, atrio-ventricular; CPR, cardio-pulmonary resuscitation; PEA, pulseless electrical activity; PSVT, paroxysmal supraventricular tachycardia; VF, ventricular fibrillation; VT, ventricular tachycardia.

way through the myocardium rather than through conducting tissue.

Heart block may result from, in order of frequency:

• ischaemia or fibrosis of the conducting system
• drugs, e.g. digoxin, calcium antagonists
• congenital causes; despite complete heart block, there is often a satisfactory ventricular rate and no symptoms.

Sinus bradycardia

The heart rate is < 60 beats/min but P waves are present and each is followed by a QRST complex after a normal PR interval. This is common in athletes, patients on beta-blockers and soon after acute myocardial infarction. Less common causes are untreated hypothyroidism, obstructive jaundice and raised intracranial pressure.

Sick sinus syndrome

The P waves are slow or erratic owing to disease of the SA node, but conduction is normal. There are also tachycardias (tachy-brady syndrome). The cause is ischaemia or degeneration of the SA node.

Clinical presentation and management of bradycardias

First- and second-degree block are asymptomatic, although in second-degree block the dropped beats can be felt in the pulse. Sinus bradycardia may cause hypotension and syncope after acute myocardial infarction. Severe bradycardia caused by complete heart block or sinus arrest presents with syncope which may be intermittent (Stokes–Adams attacks). If bradycardia persists, it may also cause heart failure.

You should assess a bradycardic patient as follows.

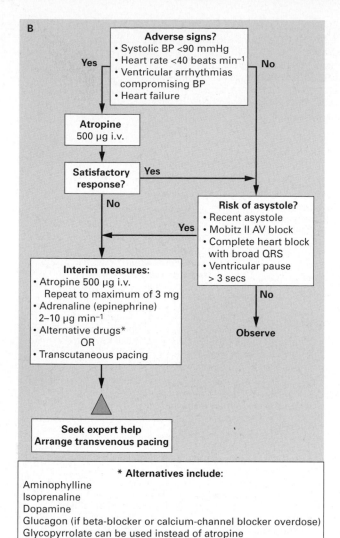

B

Adverse signs?
- Systolic BP <90 mmHg
- Heart rate <40 beats min⁻¹
- Ventricular arrhythmias compromising BP
- Heart failure

Yes / No

Atropine
500 µg i.v.

Satisfactory response? — Yes

No

Risk of asystole?
- Recent asystole
- Mobitz II AV block
- Complete heart block with broad QRS
- Ventricular pause > 3 secs

Yes / No

Interim measures:
- Atropine 500 µg i.v. Repeat to maximum of 3 mg
- Adrenaline (epinephrine) 2–10 µg min⁻¹
- Alternative drugs*
  OR
- Transcutaneous pacing

Observe

Seek expert help
Arrange transvenous pacing

* Alternatives include:
Aminophylline
Isoprenaline
Dopamine
Glucagon (if beta-blocker or calcium-channel blocker overdose)
Glycopyrrolate can be used instead of atropine

Fig. 11 cont'd B Algorithm for the management of bradycardia, including rates inappropriately slow for the patient's haemodynamic state (reproduced with permission of the UK Resuscitation Council).

Is the bradycardia causing hypotension or heart failure?

If not, no immediate action is needed. If so, give atropine immediately. This will treat sinus bradycardia and improve some forms of second- and third-degree heart block by reducing vagal tone on the AV node. If the patient is collapsed and/or does not respond to atropine, call for senior help with a view to emergency pacing. Intravenous isoprenaline (β_1-agonist) is a poor second-best emergency measure.

Is the bradycardia a warning sign?

For example, it could signal heart block after myocardial infarction — call for senior help if you suspect this.

Is there a drug or other disease causing the bradycardia?

Intermittent bradycardias causing syncopal attacks or persistent, symptomatic complete heart block are indications for permanent pacing.

Figure 11B summarises the management of bradycarida, as recommended by the UK Resuscitation Council.

Extrasystoles and tachycardias

Extrasystoles are single extra beats. They most commonly occur in normal people with normal hearts and are benign. A tachycardia is a heart rate > 100 beats/min that is inappropriate to the patient's haemodynamic state.

Supraventricular extrasystoles

Supraventricular extrasystoles arise in the atrium or AV node and have the same QRS configuration as normally timed impulses. Depending on their origin, they may have a relatively normal P wave, one which follows the QRS complex or none at all. They are benign and need no treatment.

Ventricular extrasystoles

Ventricular extrasystoles are more sinister because they signify automaticity within the ventricles, which may predispose to malignant arrhythmias. Particularly if they are multifocal (arising from several different sites within the ventricles, as shown by multiple different QRS configurations) they are a sign of underlying ventricular disease, often with a bad prognosis. Antidysrhythmic drugs may themselves provoke dysrhythmias and clinical trials have shown them to do more harm than good when given for asymptomatic ventricular extrasystoles.

Sinus tachycardia

Sinus tachycardia is an adrenergically mediated, physiological response to exercise, volume depletion, anxiety or disease. The PQRST complexes are normal and the rate rarely exceeds 140 beats/min at rest. Treatment is aimed solely at the underlying disease, except in thyrotoxicosis (p. 297) and phaeochromocytoma (p. 311), when adrenergic blockers may be needed.

Other tachycardias

A sustained tachycardia > 140 beats/min is usually pathological, although pathological tachycardias may have ventricular rates < 140/min. Having excluded a sinus tachycardia, the task is to distinguish supraventricular from ventricular tachycardias because the management differs. This depends on ECG interpretation. Figure 11C presents the UK Resuscitation Council recommendations for the management of tachycardia. Figure 12 leads you through the ECG interpretation of tachycardias.

There are three key steps:

- Is it a *narrow complex* (QRS < 3 small squares) or *broad complex* tachycardia?
- Are there P waves?
- Are the complexes completely irregular?

Narrow and broad complex tachycardias

A narrow complex tachycardia must be 'supraventricular' (arising in the atrium or AV node) because the narrowness of the complexes indicates that they were propagated through the His–Purkinje system. A broad complex tachycardia is *probably* arising in the ventricle, its breadth being

One

C

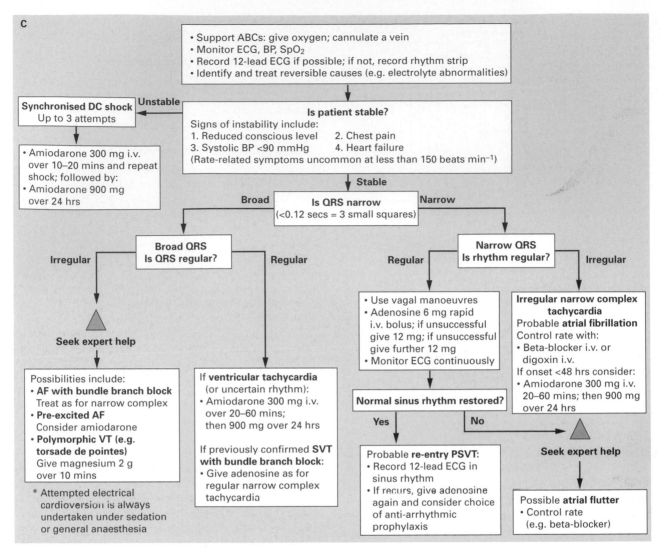

Fig. 11 cont'd C Algorithm for the management of tachycardia with a pulse (reproduced with permission of the UK Resuscitation Council).

caused by slow propagation through ventricular muscle. However, the complexes may be broad in a supraventricular tachycardia if there is 'aberrant conduction' (bundle branch block).

P waves

The presence of P waves may help to identify a broad complex tachycardia as supraventricular. The shape of the P waves and relationship to the QRS complexes is also important. In an atrial tachycardia, the P waves precede the QRS complex. If they are absent, immediately before or after the QRS complex, it is a nodal tachycardia. In atrial fibrillation, fibrillation waves may be seen every 1–2 small squares. In atrial flutter, there are 'saw-tooth waves' at a rate of about 300/min (1 large square between them).

Regularity

If the complexes are completely irregular, the diagnosis is atrial fibrillation.

Other clues

Other ways of identifying a broad complex tachycardia as supraventricular are:

- If ECGs during the dysrhythmia and in sinus rhythm are available for comparison, the QRS configuration will be unchanged in a supraventricular tachycardia with bundle branch block and changed in ventricular tachycardia.
- Very broad complexes (> 4 small squares) usually indicate a ventricular tachycardia.

You may be able to cause atrial activity (P waves) to show by performing carotid sinus massage (see below), which will slow the ventricular rate if the rhythm is supraventricular.

Management of ventricular tachycardias

The management of ventricular tachycardia and fibrillation has been considered in Figures 11A and C. If the patient is collapsed, the treatment is DC shock. Recurrent ventricular tachycardia or sustained tachycardia not requiring immediate cardioversion may be treated with drugs such as amiodarone (which prolongs the duration of the action potential). The best treatment for severe recurrent ventricular dysrhythmias — for example, those associated with IHD — is an implantable defibrillator,

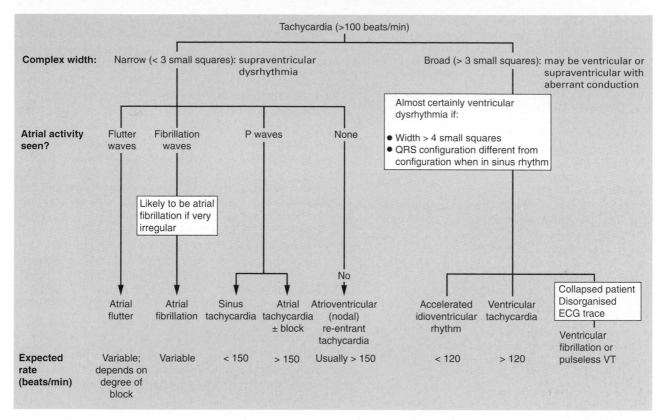

Fig. 12 Diagnosis of tachycardias.

which prolongs survival more effectively than drug therapy.

Management of supraventricular tachycardias

If there is severe cardiovascular compromise, urgent cardioversion is needed. A DC shock is given, synchronised to the QRS complex to avoid precipitating ventricular fibrillation. Otherwise, the following treatments are given in the order indicated.

Vagal stimulation The Valsalva manoeuvre may restore sinus rhythm or at least slow AV conduction enough to show P waves on the ECG and aid diagnosis.

Adenosine This transiently induces complete heart block and may correct junctional tachycardia. Like vagal stimulation, it may transiently reveal P waves.

Verapamil This impedes the transport of calcium across myocardial smooth muscle cells, prolonging the action potential and refractory period. Given i.v., it may restore sinus rhythm. It must never be given to patients taking beta-blockers (because the combination can cause asystole) or if there is a suspicion of ventricular tachycardia.

Beta-blocker or digoxin Unless emergency cardioversion is needed (see above), a beta-blocker (or calcium channel-blocker) is used to control fast atrial fibrillation. Digoxin can also be used. It is rapidly absorbed and can be given orally as a loading dose, or 'titrated' against the heart rate. It may be used for other refractory dysrhythmias. Before use, check that the patient is not already taking it because it can *cause* dysrhythmias: classically atrial tachycardia with two-to-one block.

Amiodarone This has a long half-life and is given i.v. for refractory supraventricular dysrhythmias including atrial fibrillation.

Atrial pacing and cardioversion Atrial pacing 'takes over' impulse generation from the ectopic focus as a temporary measure to restore sinus rhythm. Resistant dysrhythmias are treated by cardioversion. You should remember that patients who are digoxin-toxic (particularly if hypokalaemic) may develop asystole or malignant dysrhythmias after cardioversion. The treatment is to stop digoxin, correct hypokalaemia and give digoxin-specific antibodies for severe, resistant toxicity.

Supraventricular tachycardia associated with Wolff–Parkinson–White syndrome

This tachycardia is caused by a congenital accessory conducting pathway between the atria and ventricles (Re-entry, p. 26). There is a short PR interval (< 3 small squares) and slurred upstroke to the R wave (delta wave). Supraventricular tachycardias may occur and can be terminated by adenosine or verapamil. Atrial fibrillation may also occur. Destruction of the accessory pathway by radiofrequency ablation may be needed as a long-term solution.

Atrial fibrillation

Atrial fibrillation is the commonest dysrhythmia. It can be intermittent ('paroxysmal') or sustained. Apart from the fibrillation waves, there is an irregular QRS rhythm caused by the haphazard transmission of atrial impulses to the ventricles. Cardiac output is impaired by loss of atrial systole (p. 8) and varies with the length of diastole, causing variability in blood pressure and strength of the peripheral pulses. The heart rate can only reliably be measured at the cardiac apex or on an ECG.

Causes

Any condition that causes atrial dilatation, such as mitral stenosis, heart muscle disease, hypertension and ischaemia, can cause atrial fibrillation. Pericarditis and systemic diseases including thyrotoxicosis and alcohol abuse are other causes. There may be no obvious cause ('lone atrial fibrillation').

Effects

Reduction of cardiac output causes dyspnoea and lethargy and may precipitate heart failure (p. 21). Uncontrolled atrial fibrillation causes palpitations, ischaemic chest pain and syncope. Intracardiac thrombus can form in the dilated atrium leading to stroke, particularly in patients with associated valvular disease. The risk is low in young people with lone atrial fibrillation but increases with:

- age
- coincident heart disease
- instability of the rhythm: conversion between atrial fibrillation and sinus rhythm may dislodge atrial thrombus.

Management

The priorities of treatment are to control the ventricular rate and prevent thrombo-embolism.

Traditionally, digoxin has been used to slow the ventricular rate by increasing the degree of atrioventricular (AV) block and reducing the number of atrial impulses propagated to the ventricles. Beta-blockers and calcium antagonists are now used more often, in preference, or adjunctively to digoxin. Patients with atrial fibrillation of less than 12 months' duration and no underlying cause may be cardioverted. Flecainide, sotalol or amiodarone (which prolong the duration of the action potential) is used to prevent paroxysmal atrial fibrillation; amiodarone is the more effective.

Patients under 60 years of age with lone atrial fibrillation have such a low risk of stroke that anticoagulation is not needed, although aspirin is advisable. Low-intensity (International Normalised Ratio (INR) 2–3, p. 282) chronic anticoagulation with warfarin is indicated for older people and those with diabetes, hypertension, a history of left heart failure or non-haemorrhagic stroke unless they have a contraindication.

1.5 Valvular and congenital heart disease

Case Study

A medical student is pretty sure he has diagnosed mixed aortic valve disease but his registrar points out that a mid-systolic murmur is commonly heard in patients with aortic regurgitation, whether or not they have aortic stenosis, because of increased flow across the valve. The blood pressure of 210/80 mmHg makes aortic stenosis unlikely but there is little doubt about the aortic regurgitation.

The bedside differential diagnosis of rheumatic and congenital heart disease is less important in an era when echocardiography is freely available but you must still be able to *detect* valvular heart disease and identify common lesions. The spectrum of disease is shifting away from rheumatic disease towards endocarditis, a complication of i.v. drug abuse, and the valvular lesions of cardiac ischaemia and old age.

Clinical presentation

Symptoms and signs

Valvular heart disease impairs cardiac output and increases pulmonary and systemic venous pressure; as a result, the symptoms are no different from those of other cardiac diseases (p. 9).

To understand murmurs, orientate your thinking around ventricular contraction. Incompetence of one of the AV valves causes back-flow into the atrium from the moment the valve should have shut, heard as a pansystolic murmur. A ventricular septal defect also causes a pansystolic murmur. Stenosis of the aortic or pulmonary valve causes a murmur that is loudest when blood flow is at its greatest, mid- to late systole. Mitral or tricuspid stenosis causes a low-pitched rumbling murmur that is loudest when blood is flowing into the ventricle in mid-diastole. Aortic or pulmonary incompetence causes a leak back across the valve early in diastole when the pressure differential is greatest, heard as a high-pitched 'whiff'. Thrills are palpable murmurs, most often felt with systolic murmurs. Apart from the character and timing of the murmur, there are three other features which help you in your diagnosis:

- the position (and radiation)
- relationship to respiration
- presence of other cardiovascular signs.

The physical signs of valvular heart disease are summarised in Table 4. Remember that:

- mitral murmurs are heard best at the apex
- aortic and pulmonary stenotic murmurs are usually heard best at the upper right and left sternal edges, respectively
- other common murmurs (e.g. aortic and tricuspid regurgitation) are often heard best at the left sternal border.

The relationship with respiration is easy to remember. During inspiration, blood is drawn into the lungs. This increases flow through the right side of the heart and

Table 4 The physical signs of valvular heart disease: common murmurs

	Character	Best heard	Radiation	Associated signs
Systolic				
Mitral regurgitation		Apex	Left axilla	
Mitral prolapse		Apex	Left axilla and back	
Ventricular septal defect		Lower LSE	Whole precordium	
Tricuspid regurgitation		Lower LSE		Giant V waves in jugular venous pulse; pulsatile hepatomegaly
Aortic stenosis		Upper RSE	Carotids and apex	Plateau pulse; narrow pulse pressure
Diastolic				
Mitral stenosis		Apex	Left axilla	Malar flush; parasternal heave; tapping apex
Aortic regurgitation		Lower LSE		Collapsing pulse; wide pulse pressure; mid-systolic flow murmur.

LSE, left sternal edge; RSE, right sternal edge; OS, opening snap; IPSA, presystolic accentuation if in sinus rhythm.

reduces flow on the left side. The situation is reversed on expiration. Thus, inspiration makes tricuspid and pulmonary murmurs louder. However, *any* murmur may be louder on expiration. A safe rule is that a murmur that increases on inspiration is likely to be right-sided. Other features, including radiation and the associated signs, are summarised in Table 4. For more detail, you are referred to a textbook of bedside diagnosis.

Causes of valvular heart disease

In the developed world, the causes of valvular heart disease are, in approximate order of frequency:

- degenerative disease
- secondary to disease of the heart and aorta: dilatation of supporting structures causes incompetence by stretching the valve
- rheumatic heart disease, usually affecting the mitral valve alone or mitral and aortic valves
- congenital, including 'floppy mitral valve' (p. 34)
- infective endocarditis, affecting the mitral (most common), aortic, tricuspid and pulmonary (least common) valves.

Mitral valve disease

You should be familiar with three mitral lesions:

- stenosis
- regurgitation
- prolapse.

Mitral stenosis

Mitral stenosis is almost invariably rheumatic, is the commonest lesion of rheumatic heart disease and is more common in women than men. There is thickening, fusion and eventually calcification and immobility of the valve cusps, which narrow the orifice and increase left atrial pressure. The principal effects of mitral stenosis are **left atrial hypertrophy** and **pulmonary venous hypertension** leading, eventually, to right ventricular failure.

Symptoms and signs

The symptoms of pulmonary venous hypertension and right heart failure are described on page 22. Haemoptysis is a common symptom of mitral stenosis. There may be palpitations resulting from atrial fibrillation. The signs are shown in Table 4. The loud first heart sound and opening snap (caused by increased left atrial pressure) are only heard if the valve is mobile and are lost as it becomes increasingly calcified.

Investigations

The heart is usually of normal size on a chest radiograph but the following abnormal signs may be seen, in approximate order of frequency:

- left atrial hypertrophy: 'double shadow' to the right heart border
- enlargement of the pulmonary artery, pulmonary venous engorgement and septal lines (as described for left ventricular failure, p. 10)
- calcification of the mitral valve ring.

One

Echocardiography is needed to confirm the diagnosis and estimate severity. The gradient across the mitral valve and the valve area can be measured and signs of pulmonary hypertension identified.

Complications

Atrial fibrillation, caused by left atrial enlargement (p. 31), is almost invariable in significant mitral stenosis. **Stroke and other forms of arterial thrombo-embolism** result from stasis of blood in the enlarged, fibrillating left atrium. **Pulmonary embolism** may result from reduced cardiac output and venous stasis. An abrupt increase in pulmonary venous pressure, as when the patient goes into atrial fibrillation, can cause overt **pulmonary oedema** but subacute symptoms are more common. Alveolar oedema predisposes to **infection**.

Management

Management of mitral stenosis comprises long-term anticoagulation to prevent thrombo-embolism, antibiotic prophylaxis against endocarditis (p. 38), diuretics for pulmonary oedema and right heart failure, and digoxin for atrial fibrillation. Antibiotics may be needed for chest infections.

Surgery is indicated for pulmonary hypertension (which progresses irreversibly if surgery is delayed) and uncontrolled symptoms. The options are valvotomy (closed or open), balloon valvuloplasty, and valve replacement, which is needed if the valve is calcified and/or there is significant mitral regurgitation.

Mitral regurgitation

The common causes of mitral regurgitation, in approximate order of frequency, are:

- secondary to left ventricular dilatation, as in left heart failure
- secondary to papillary muscle dysfunction or ruptured chordae tendineae
- rheumatic
- bacterial endocarditis.

Mitral regurgitation may develop acutely as a result of papillary muscle rupture after myocardial infarction (p. 20).

As the valve becomes incompetent, the regurgitated blood is accommodated by dilatation of the left atrium. There is pulmonary hypertension but it is less severe than in mitral stenosis because the atrium is able to empty during diastole. The left ventricle enlarges to accommodate the increased stroke volume but may eventually fail. These adaptive changes cannot occur in *acute* mitral regurgitation so there is left ventricular failure.

Symptoms and signs

There are no specific symptoms. The signs reflect the systolic flow across the valve, increased stroke volume and, if present, left and right ventricular failure. The murmur is described in Table 4. There may be left ventricular enlargement, a soft first heart sound because of non-apposition of the mitral valve cusps, and a third heart sound from increased diastolic inflow to the left ventricle.

Investigations

The chest radiograph may show enlargement of the left ventricle and atrium, pulmonary oedema and valve calci-

fication. The ECG may show left ventricular hypertrophy (p. 11) and atrial fibrillation. Echo Doppler examination may show an enlarged left atrium and ventricle, with flow from the ventricle into the atrium during systole. If the valve is rheumatic, the cusps will be thickened and the chordae shortened.

Complications

Complications are heart failure, infective endocarditis and atrial fibrillation. This is less common than in mitral stenosis because the left atrium is less dilated.

Management

All patients should be advised about antibiotic prophylaxis against endocarditis (p. 38). Uncomplicated mitral regurgitation can be left untreated and observed for the development of left ventricular dysfunction, which is treated with diuretics and ACE inhibitors, or dysrhythmias. Surgery is indicated for poorly controlled symptoms and left ventricular dysfunction/enlargement.

Mitral valve prolapse

Mitral valve prolapse can be congenital or acquired.

- Congenital: primary mitral valve prolapse ('floppy mitral valve') is caused by degeneration of the chordae resulting in prolapse of the valve cusps. It affects 2–3% of the population, particularly young adult women. Mitral valve prolapse may also be associated with rare inherited disorders of collagen, e.g. Marfan's syndrome.
- Acquired: this is usually a result of ischaemic papillary muscle dysfunction.

This discussion concentrates on primary mitral valve prolapse.

There is mitral regurgitation caused by late systolic prolapse of the valve cusps into the left atrium. The regurgitation varies from trivial to severe.

Symptoms and signs

Patients are usually asymptomatic initially but may present with anginal or atypical chest pain or other complications (noted below). The signs are summarised in Table 4. There may be a mid-systolic 'click' in some cases.

Investigations

The diagnosis is made by echocardiography.

Complications

Mitral valve prolapse is often an innocent, chance finding. Uncommonly, there may be myxomatous degeneration of the valve cusp causing arterial thrombo-embolism, notably strokes. Ventricular or supraventricular tachydysrhythmias may occur.

Management

Antibiotic prophylaxis against endocarditis is indicated if there is significant mitral regurgitation. Thrombo-embolic complications are treated by anticoagulation. Often these valves are surgically repairable.

Aortic valve disease

You need to know about two lesions:

- aortic stenosis
- aortic incompetence.

Aortic stenosis

Aortic stenosis may be rheumatic or congenital. If it is rheumatic, the mitral valve is likely to be affected as well. Congenital aortic stenosis is usually associated with a bicuspid aortic valve. Other causes are congenital supravalvular or subvalvular stenosis resulting from malformation of the aorta and left ventricle, respectively.

Fusion of the valve cusps causes left ventricular outflow obstruction, compensatory myocardial hypertrophy and increased cardiac work. Cardiac output is limited and cannot rise in response to exercise. Coronary perfusion is impaired and myocardial ischaemia results. Ultimately, the left ventricle cannot overcome the outflow resistance and left ventricular failure occurs.

Symptoms and signs

You must be alert to the diagnosis of aortic stenosis because it may be asymptomatic until too late a stage in its natural history for good surgical results. It is easy to misattribute the symptoms to other diseases. The symptoms are:

- **dyspnoea**, at first exercise-related but later occurring at rest
- **orthopnoea** and **paroxysmal nocturnal dyspnoea** resulting from left ventricular failure
- **angina**, which is caused by the imbalance between myocardial work and coronary perfusion and may occur without coronary artery disease
- **exertional syncope**, a sinister symptom of severely limited cardiac output, which presages sudden death.

A crucial point is that the intensity of the murmur (Table 4) is a poor guide to the severity of stenosis. You need to distinguish aortic sclerosis, a degenerative and innocent condition which is common in old people, from aortic stenosis. Sclerosis causes a loud murmur but has little haemodynamic effect, whereas the murmur of tight aortic stenosis may be inaudible because flow across the valve is severely limited. Other signs (absent in aortic sclerosis) are a slow-rising, low-volume carotid pulse, narrow pulse pressure (systolic minus diastolic) and thrusting apex beat, which is not displaced unless there is left ventricular failure. A thrill may be felt in the aortic area or over the carotid arteries. The aortic component of the second heart sound may be soft because of impaired valve mobility, and there may be a fourth heart sound.

Investigations

The chest radiograph may be normal or show:

- prominence of the left ventricle
- cardiac enlargement if there is left ventricular failure
- prominence of the ascending aorta because of 'post-stenotic dilatation'
- calcification of the valve.

The ECG shows LBBB or left ventricular hypertrophy and strain (p. 11). Echocardiography demonstrates the dis-ordered anatomy of the valve, the gradient across it and the degree of left ventricular hypertrophy and dilatation.

Complications

These include **left ventricular failure** (a serious sign of decompensation), **dysrhythmias** which are triggered by exertion, presumably because of myocardial ischaemia, and may cause sudden death, **systemic embolism** from the diseased valve and **infective endocarditis**.

Management

Antibiotic prophylaxis should be recommended and patients advised against strenuous activity. **Vasodilators should not be given** because they increase the risk of syncope. Beta-blockers can be used for angina. Heart failure is treated with diuretics. Symptomatic aortic stenosis requires early surgical replacement. A modified Bruce exercise tolerance test can help decide on surgery in severe asymptomatic aortic stenosis.

Aortic regurgitation

Aortic regurgitation can have acute and chronic causes (Table 5). There is back-flow of blood into the left ventricle during diastole, which is accommodated by dilatation of the left ventricle and an increased stroke volume. If the disease progresses slowly, the left ventricle can adapt to remarkably severe regurgitation. The cardiovascular system is 'hyperdynamic' because blood is passing to and fro across the valve. The pulse pressure is wide. Myocardial ischaemia occurs because the increased stroke volume increases myocardial work and the low diastolic pressure impairs coronary perfusion.

Symptoms and signs

Patients may be dyspnoeic and aware of a 'pounding heart beat'. The signs (Table 4) are:

- hyperdynamic circulation: a collapsing pulse, wide pulse pressure, aortic systolic flow murmur and visible, palpable or audible pulsation in the arterial or capillary circulation
- left ventricular dilatation: a displaced, heaving apex
- regurgitation: an early diastolic murmur heard best on expiration, with the patient leaning forwards, in the third left interspace with the diaphragm of the stethoscope. The aortic component of the second heart

Table 5 Causes of aortic regurgitation

	Acute	Chronic
Dilatation of valve ring	Aortic dissection	Idiopathic: severe, prolonged hypertension Syphilitic aortitis Inherited disorder of collagen, e.g. Marfan's syndrome
Diseased valve cusps	Infective endocarditis	Congenital: bicuspid aortic valve Acquired: rheumatic heart disease

sound is absent because of non-apposition of the cusps.

Significant aortic regurgitation will be accompanied by a systolic flow murmur. To decide if the diagnosis is pure aortic incompetence or mixed aortic valve disease, you must distinguish this from the mid-systolic murmur of aortic stenosis. Only diagnose aortic stenosis if the pulse pressure is not widened.

Investigations

There is cardiomegaly and possibly calcification of the valve on the chest radiograph, and left ventricular hypertrophy and strain on the ECG. An echo Doppler examination shows the abnormal valvular anatomy, left ventricular dilatation and regurgitant jet.

Complications

Dilatation and ischaemia of the left ventricle cause left ventricular failure and secondary right ventricular failure. There is atrial fibrillation in about 20% of patients and angina, particularly if there is coincident coronary artery disease.

Management

This consists of antibiotic prophylaxis (p. 39), treatment of heart failure and dysrhythmias, and early surgical referral. Once there is heart failure, left ventricular function is unlikely to recover.

Right heart valvular disease

Right heart valvular disease is less common than left heart disease because both infective endocarditis and rheumatic disease affect the left side more than the right. It may be congenital or, more commonly, secondary to left heart disease or pulmonary arterial disease.

If the lesion is secondary to left heart disease, there will be both left and right heart failure. If it is primary, there will only be symptoms and signs of systemic venous hypertension and a reduced cardiac output. You can work out from first principles the *cardiac* signs of right-sided valvular disease if you know how to palpate for right ventricular hypertrophy; the signs are similar to the analogous left-sided lesion but get louder on inspiration. The only lesion you will commonly encounter is tricuspid regurgitation resulting from pulmonary hypertension (see p. 46 for causes). You should consult a reference textbook for other lesions.

Tricuspid regurgitation

The pathognomonic feature is transmission of right ventricular systolic pressure into the systemic venous system. There are giant V waves in the jugular venous pulse, pulsatile hepatomegaly and signs of right ventricular failure. Other signs include a parasternal heave of right ventricular dilatation, pansystolic murmur at the left sternal edge (Table 4), third heart sound and (often) atrial fibrillation. The diagnosis is made by recognising pulsatile venous hypertension.

Treatment is primarily aimed at underlying left heart failure or pulmonary disease. The systemic venous pressure often cannot be normalised so care is needed with diuretic therapy. If you aim for a normal jugular venous pressure, there is a danger that you will cause volume depletion.

Congenital heart disease

Some congenital lesions have been described above. Others that are rare or do not present in adulthood are not discussed in this book. Several which might be seen in adults are described briefly.

Atrial septal defect

Atrial septal defect (ASD) may be diagnosed for the first time in adult life. The septal defect allows blood to flow from the left to the right atrium. There is compensatory right ventricular enlargement and increased output. A sustained increase in pulmonary vascular flow causes pulmonary hypertension. Exceptionally, this increases right heart pressure to a level where the flow across the defect reverses and the patient becomes cyanosed from right-to-left shunting of deoxygenated blood. At that stage, the problem is irreversible, even with surgery.

An ASD may present with dyspnoea or fatigue, respiratory infections secondary to increased pulmonary blood flow, palpitations from atrial fibrillation or heart failure. The physical signs, resulting from increased right ventricular flow, are:

- right ventricular hypertrophy
- splitting of the second heart sound that does not vary with respiration ('fixed'), and a loud pulmonary second sound
- an ejection systolic murmur caused by increased flow across the pulmonary valve
- a tricuspid diastolic flow murmur.

The chest radiograph shows pulmonary plethora, enlargement of the pulmonary arteries and cardiomegaly. The ECG shows RBBB. The diagnosis is confirmed by echocardiography.

Antibiotic prophylaxis is not necessary for isolated ASD. Significant defects should be closed surgically before pulmonary hypertension develops.

Ventricular septal defect

Small ventricular septal defects (VSDs) may not be diagnosed until adulthood. There is flow from the left to the right ventricle in systole. Cardiac output is limited and patients may experience dyspnoea and fatigue. As with ASDs, pulmonary hypertension and right-to-left shunting may occur. Small defects may be associated with loud murmurs; therefore, the intensity of the murmur is a poor guide to the seriousness of the lesion. With larger defects, the murmur may become softer with time as right and left ventricular pressures equalise as a result of pulmonary hypertension.

Apart from the murmur (Table 4), there is biventricular dilatation. The chest radiograph shows prominence of the pulmonary arteries and cardiomegaly.

Antibiotic prophylaxis is essential and haemodynamically significant defects should be closed before pulmonary hypertension develops.

Coarctation of the aorta

In aortic coarctation, there is narrowing of the aorta distal to the arch and the origin of the main arteries. It is commonly associated with a congenitally bicuspid aortic valve, which predisposes to aortic stenosis. Coarctation is more common in males than females and may be associated with Turner's syndrome. Obstruction to blood flow by the coarct causes the blood pressure in the lower half of the body to be low, delays the lower body pulse wave, impairs renal perfusion and causes compensatory hypertension in the upper body.

Patients may present with (upper body) hypertension, left ventricular failure or hypertensive subarachnoid haemorrhage. Other physical signs include radiofemoral delay, a mid-systolic murmur caused by blood flow across the coarct and left ventricular hypertrophy. The chest radiograph shows dilatation of the aorta, left ventricular hypertrophy and rib notching (caused by collateral arteries bypassing the coarct).

The diagnosis is confirmed by echocardiography and computed tomography (CT) or magnetic resonance (MR) scanning or aortography. Treatment is by balloon dilatation or surgical resection. The longer the patient has been hypertensive, the less the likelihood that surgery will be curative, so it should be performed without delay.

1.6 Infective endocarditis

Learning objectives

You should:
- be able to distinguish between the different forms of infective endocarditis and the diagnostic and therapeutic approach to each
- know the indications for prophylaxis of infective endocarditis and where to find current information on appropriate regimens.

Case Study

A 57-year-old man is admitted for investigation of weight loss and raised inflammatory markers. The admitting doctor notes a soft systolic murmur in the aortic area, which has not been noted before, and another doctor hears a faint early diastolic murmur at the left sternal edge. Low-grade fever is observed. The patient admits to being breathless when he lies flat. The medical team are not sure if they should request transthoracic or transoesophageal echocardiography to look for vegetations.

Infective endocarditis is infection of one or more of the heart valves or other endocardial structures. It is relatively uncommon and can be hard to diagnose, but it is treatable and potentially fatal if it is not diagnosed. The case fatality rate has not fallen in recent years, as it tends to affect the increasing elderly population.

Predisposing cardiac defects

Predisposing defects include:

- prosthetic valves
- congenital heart disease, especially ventricular septal defect, bicuspid aortic valve
- rheumatic heart disease
- degenerative valve disease, e.g. calcified mitral annulus.

About 30% of patients, particularly i.v. drug abusers, have no underlying valve defect. Some cardiac defects, including ASD and mitral valve prolapse without regurgitation, carry virtually no risk of endocarditis.

Microbiological diagnosis of endocarditis

The cardinal microbiological feature is *persistent* bacteraemia. To confirm this, you should take at least three cultures at different times (e.g. separated by 1–3 hours). If the patient has recently received antibiotics, cultures may need to be drawn over 2–3 days.

The important microbial causes of endocarditis, together with features specific to individual organisms, are shown in Table 6. Most patients (around 80%) have positive blood cultures. False-negative cultures occur in patients previously treated with antibiotics, if bacteraemia is below the level of detection or the organism is non-culturable (e.g. *Coxiella burnetii*, causing Q fever). The rare bacteria grow slowly and blood cultures may take 10–20 days to become positive. Most laboratories discard blood cultures after 7 days so it is important to speak to your local

Table 6 Microbial causes of infective endocarditis (IE) in approximate order of frequency

Organism	Particular features
Viridans group streptococci	Archetypal subacute IE
Staphylococcus aureus	Acute IE with rapid valve destruction; common in drug abusers, and then often on tricuspid valve
Enterococcus faecalis	Variable course, may be fulminant; difficult to treat successfully
Streptococcus bovis	Usually subacute, may be associated with colonic carcinoma
Staphylococcus epidermidis	Particularly associated with prosthetic valves, often subacute
Candida spp.	One cause of culture-negative IE; with large vegetations, surgery indicated
Rare bacteria	Unusual causes of subacute IE with slow-growing (1–3 weeks) organisms, very responsive to treatment
Q fever endocarditis (*Coxiella burnetii*)	Always culture-negative; subacute IE with positive serology; difficult to treat

microbiologist if you are seriously considering the diagnosis of endocarditis.

Clinical presentation

The clinical features of endocarditis depend on whether it is acute, subacute or associated with a prosthetic valve.

Acute endocarditis

The patient may present with acute pulmonary oedema or biventricular failure and is almost always febrile and seriously ill. A loud murmur is usually apparent unless severe aortic incompetence has resulted from perforation or rupture of the valve leaflets. The systemic features of subacute infective endocarditis are absent (see below). A regurgitant murmur is much more likely to represent endocarditis than an aortic systolic or mitral diastolic murmur. In staphylococcal endocarditis, Janeway lesions are common (see below).

The white cell count is usually elevated. Blood cultures are usually positive within 12–48 hours.

Subacute infective endocarditis

Subacute bacterial endocarditis (SBE) can be a difficult diagnosis. About 30% of patients present with a stroke, transient ischaemic attack or peripheral embolic episode. Most are chronically ill with few distinctive features. Weight loss, malaise, fatigue and anorexia are typical. Patients may report rigors but often do not report febrile episodes; they are usually febrile on hospital admission. Vascular phenomena, mostly caused by immune complex deposition, are relatively common but may only be found by repeated examination. These are:

- petechiae, without marked thrombocytopenia
- splinter haemorrhages of the nails
- conjunctival haemorrhages
- Roth's spots in the fundi (small 'bull's eye' haemorrhagic lesions)
- Osler's nodes (tender, erythematous lesions of the finger or toe pads)
- Janeway lesions (non-painful vasculitic lesions)
- glomerulonephritis (with red cells, casts and proteinuria)
- finger clubbing
- splenomegaly.

A murmur is usually heard and may change; for example, a regurgitant murmur may worsen. As with acute endocarditis, a regurgitant murmur is more specific than a simple flow murmur.

Many other abnormalities may accompany SBE. Oral hygiene may be poor or there may be a history of dental extraction without prophylaxis. Other portals of entry may be apparent such as skin sepsis, clinical features suggesting a large bowel cancer, signs of i.v. drug abuse, evidence of exposure to a likely source of Q fever or prior bacteraemia.

Often the white cell count is raised, usually the patient has a normochromic, normocytic anaemia and the ESR or plasma viscosity is almost always elevated. However, these laboratory features are non-specific. A positive rheumatoid factor is commonly associated with vascular phenomena.

Prosthetic valve endocarditis

Prosthetic valve endocarditis occurs in two forms:

- early (up to 2 months after surgery)
- late (≥2 months after surgery).

Early infections are probably acquired during surgery whereas late infections are either acquired after discharge from hospital or caused by organisms of 'low pathogenicity' such as *Staphylococcus epidermidis*. Clinically, these infections range in severity from fulminant to chronic. You will find the diagnosis difficult, especially if you do not take blood cultures prior to treatment or in cases caused by unusual organisms. A new regurgitant murmur or valve dysfunction should raise the question of endocarditis.

Investigations

Echocardiography

Echocardiography is often helpful in diagnosis. Three features are useful. These are regurgitation, the presence of vegetations and a periannular abscess (Table 7). Valve thickening is not specific enough to confirm the diagnosis. Transthoracic scans have about a 65% sensitivity for vegetations; therefore, a negative scan does not rule out the diagnosis. Transoesophageal echocardiography is considerably more sensitive (95%) than the transthoracic technique, although more difficult. Echocardiography is also important in helping decide whether or not surgical intervention is indicated.

Management

Once blood cultures have been obtained, you should start empirical treatment if the diagnosis is strongly suspected and the patient is acutely ill. Acute endocarditis on a native or prosthetic valve is rapidly fatal unless urgently treated. Do not wait for blood culture results or take more than three sets when the patient is ill.

Table 7 Typical abnormalities on echocardiography of infective endocarditis

Acute	Subacute	Prosthetic
Regurgitant valve	Small or large vegetations on left side of heart	Periannular abscess
Periannular abscess	Regurgitant valve	Regurgitant valve
Tricuspid vegetation (i.v. drug abusers)		Improperly functioning valve
Small vegetations		

Table 8 Initial antibiotic treatment of infective endocarditis

Type	Antibiotic regimen
Acute endocarditis	
Native valve	Ampicillin + flucloxacillin + gentamicin*
Prosthetic valve	Vancomycin + ceftazidime + gentamicin*
Subacute endocarditis	Ampicillin + gentamicin*

*Some units prefer other aminoglycosides such as netilmicin.

Antibiotic treatment

Empirical treatment regimens are shown in Table 8. Culture results will determine the best therapy and appropriate duration. You will be guided in this by a microbiologist.

The duration of antibiotic therapy varies. The shortest courses are for *viridans* streptococci (2–4 weeks). Fully 6 weeks of i.v. therapy are required for staphylococcal and enterococcal endocarditis as they are difficult to cure. Longer courses of therapy (months) are required for fungal and Q fever endocarditis and even then these are difficult or impossible to cure.

Supervising treatment

During the treatment of endocarditis, you must be constantly searching for signs of worsening valvular disease by listening for new regurgitant murmurs and by repeating echocardiography. Persistent or recurrent fever is quite common and represents one or more of:

- worsening endocarditis with myocardial abscess formation
- drug fever, often with eosinophilia or skin rash
- another complication, such as urinary tract infection, deep vein thrombosis or splenic or liver abscess, etc.

Surgery

Valve replacement is indicated in the following circumstances:

- large vegetation (e.g. ≥ 1 cm) still present after 2 weeks of medical therapy (to prevent stroke or peripheral embolus)
- persistent fever, without another cause
- recurrent emboli in spite of appropriate antibiotics
- myocardial (periannular) abscess, especially if near conducting system and if fever persists
- heart block
- severe valvular dysfunction leading to cardiac failure
- fungal endocarditis (if possible)
- prosthetic valve endocarditis.

Prevention of endocarditis

Good dental hygiene Regular dental checks are the most important means of prevention in at-risk individuals. You should stress this to your patients.

Antibiotic prophylaxis of endocarditis Antibiotic prophylaxis is indicated for the following valvular or vascular defects:

- any prosthetic valve or arterial dacron graft (higher risk)
- prior infective endocarditis (higher risk)
- all congenital heart disease except ASD
- any acquired valve defect
- rheumatic valve disease
- mitral valve prolapse, but only if the valve is regurgitant
- hypertrophic obstructive cardiomyopathy.

Procedures that justify antibiotic prophylaxis include dental work that leads to bleeding of the gums and upper respiratory tract surgery. Obstetric, gynaecological, genitourinary and gastrointestinal surgery (including oesophageal dilatation) justify prophylaxis only in higher-risk patients. Current guidelines on which procedures require prophylaxis and the recommended antibiotics are available from many sources, including the British Heart Foundation and the *British National Formulary*. The antibiotic should be given 1 hour before the procedure.

1.7 Pericardial and heart muscle disease

Learning objectives

You should:
- be able to recognise pericarditis and construct an appropriate differential diagnosis
- be able to recognise cardiac tamponade and understand how to manage a pericardial effusion
- understand how to recognise myocarditis and other heart muscle diseases.

Case Study

A 17-year-old schoolboy is brought to accident and emergency agitated and short of breath, having been perfectly well 3 days ago. He is febrile (38.2°C), has a respiratory rate of 30 breaths/min, a tachycardia of 124 beats/min and a BP of 87/50 mmHg. He has a gallop rhythm and raised jugular venous pulse but his chest is clear. His ECG shows a sinus tachycardia with numerous atrial ectopics and generally low-voltage deflections. Viral myocarditis is suspected.

The pericardium is a fibrous sac surrounding the heart. There is a potential space between it and the heart. Pericarditis is inflammation of the pericardium, usually causing an accumulation of fluid in the pericardial sac. Large pericardial effusions can obstruct cardiac filling (tamponade).

Pericardial disease causes characteristic symptoms and signs. The pain is described as sharp or burning, often radiating to the back and relieved by leaning forwards. It is similar to the pain of pleurisy and the two types of pain may coexist. Pericardial inflammation causes a distinctive 'friction rub', which is distinguished from a murmur by its 'scratchy' character, making it sound 'close to your

Box 2: The causes of pericarditis

Infections
- Purulent (e.g. bacterial — especially pneumococcal)
- Tuberculous
- Viral
- Other infections, e.g. *Aspergillus*, amoebic, etc.

Inflammatory
- Full-thickness myocardial infarction
- Autoimmune disease, e.g. systemic lupus erythematosus (SLE)
- Contiguous inflammatory process (e.g. pulmonary infection)

Malignant
- For example, bronchogenic carcinoma with direct spread, Hodgkin's disease

Other
- Uraemic pericarditis
- Postoperative pericarditis

ears'. It may be there one minute, gone the next and present in both systole and diastole. Pericardial rubs are very positional. If you suspect pericarditis, listen to the heart with the patient lying flat, at 45°C, sitting up and lying on the left side.

Pericarditis

Causes

There are many causes of pericarditis (Box 2). In young people in the UK, viral pericarditis is by far the most common cause. Systemic lupus erythematosus (SLE, p. 353) is a rare cause and pericarditis can be a complication of tuberculosis and Hodgkin's disease. In older patients, a full-thickness myocardial infarct, or bronchogenic or breast carcinoma is more common. Tumour, infection and uraemia may also present with effusions.

Viral pericarditis

Young and middle-aged, otherwise healthy adults are most often affected by viral pericarditis. The presentation is sudden, with typical pericardial pain (see above), dysrhythmias and/or breathlessness. The pain may be severe enough to require morphine. Sometimes there is a recent personal or family history of a viral illness.

There is a characteristic pattern of ST segment elevation across the chest leads of the ECG (Table 3). An echocardiogram may reveal pericardial fluid. The disease resolves spontaneously over 3–10 days. Most cases are caused by viruses, such as Coxsackie virus.

Purulent pericarditis

Although purulent pericarditis is uncommon, it is fatal if not recognised and treated. It presents with:

- features of bacterial infection (fever, night sweats, chills)

- chest symptoms (dyspnoea, cough and chest pain)
- hypotension.

It is not immediately distinguishable from a chest infection but there is usually a pericardial or pleural rub and signs of tamponade. An echocardiogram reveals an effusion and the diagnosis is established by aspirating pericardial fluid (pericardiocentesis). The fluid is examined in the same way as pleural fluid.

Cardiac tamponade

Large pericardial effusions can obstruct blood flow through the heart. The patient is breathless and lying still with a sinus tachycardia (typically >125/min). The heart sounds are quiet. The jugular venous pressure (JVP) is greatly raised. Unlike the raised JVP of heart failure, this *rises* on inspiration (Kussmaul's sign). The absence of signs of left ventricular failure (no crackles or wheeze on auscultation of the chest) helps differentiate tamponade from left ventricular failure. In severe cases, the systolic blood pressure falls > 10 mmHg on inspiration and peripheral pulses disappear completely, reappearing on expiration. This is because cardiac filling is limited by external compression and the inspiratory fall in intrathoracic pressure critically causes cardiac output to drop. Confusingly, both the inspiratory *rise* in JVP and the *fall* in blood pressure are termed 'paradoxical'. Only the rise in JVP is truly paradoxical; the fall in blood pressure is an exaggeration of normal physiology.

If the patient is moribund with severe hypotension and other features of cardiac tamponade, a long (e.g. lumbar puncture) needle should be inserted into the pericardium alongside the xiphisternum as an emergency procedure. You may have to do this yourself, although you should get senior help quickly.

Constrictive pericarditis

In chronic pericarditis (particularly tuberculous) the continuous inflammatory process leads to pericardial fibrosis. The pericardium becomes calcified and visible on a chest radiograph or CT scan. As fibrosis usually leads to tissue contraction, the pericardium becomes too small for the heart leading to cardiac failure. These patients benefit substantially from pericardiectomy.

Myocarditis

Myocarditis is infection of the myocardium leading to cardiac dysfunction. It may be associated with pericarditis.

Causes

Most cases are caused by viruses such as Coxsackie virus. Myocarditis may also be caused, rarely, by Epstein–Barr virus (glandular fever), a paramyxovirus (mumps) or rubella virus. In patients with acquired immunodeficiency syndrome (AIDS) and cardiac transplant recipients, *Toxoplasma* myocarditis is a problem. Rare instances of myocardial dysfunction are caused by dermatomyositis and poisons such as ethylene glycol (antifreeze). A few bacterial toxins also reduce myocardial contractility substantially, in particular streptococcal toxins in the context of severe streptococcal disease (see p. 411).

Clinical presentation

Viral myocarditis varies in severity from an ECG abnormality in a patient with a viral illness to a fulminating illness causing heart failure and death in 5–10 days despite intensive care. It is characterised by fever, chest pain (which may be pericardial in character), dyspnoea and cardiac dysrhythmias. Signs include tachycardia, a third heart sound, a friction rub (if there is pericardial involvement) and evidence of heart failure.

Investigations

There may be cardiomegaly and signs of heart failure on the chest radiograph, non-specific ST segment and T wave changes on the ECG, and raised cardiac enzyme levels indicative of myocardial damage. Echocardiography shows cardiac enlargement and impaired contractility. Endomyocardial biopsy is not often performed because it is of little value.

Management

Management consists of strict bed rest, treatment of dysrhythmias and anticoagulation if there is significant heart failure. The likelihood is complete recovery, although patients may die in the acute phase or progress to chronic disease. Cardiac transplantation may have to be considered.

Cardiomyopathy

This is a broad pathological term which covers many individual diseases. It is subclassified into:

- **dilated cardiomyopathy**, in which the primary problem is poor contractility leading to dilatation, usually of both sides of the heart, increased filling pressures and reduced cardiac output
- **hypertrophic cardiomyopathy**, in which there is hypertrophy of the myocardium, reducing the size of the cardiac chambers and sometimes obstructing cardiac outflow; contractility is maintained or increased
- **restrictive cardiomyopathy**, in which systolic contraction may be preserved but there is poor compliance of the wall, usually because of an infiltrative process, which impedes inflow and reduces stroke volume.

A feature that the various heart muscle diseases have in common is an increased risk of thrombo-embolism and dysrhythmias. The mainstays of treatment, together with the management of heart failure, are anticoagulant and antidysrhythmic therapy. Most cardiomyopathies are rare diseases. You should consult a reference textbook for more details.

Cardiac tumours

The neoplastic disease of the heart that you are most likely to encounter is external invasion by a malignant tumour such as carcinoma of the bronchus. This can cause tamponade, dysrhythmias and other cardiac complications. *Primary* tumours are rare and usually benign. One which deserves mention is **cardiac myxoma**. This is a gelatinous,

polypoid lesion that usually develops in the left atrium and can obstruct the mitral valve, simulating mitral stenosis. There are three features to cardiac myxoma:

- **Systemic.** Patients are systemically unwell and have a high ESR and finger clubbing. These are reactions—presumed immunological—to the tumour tissue.
- **Thrombo-embolism.** The tumour provides a focus on which intracardiac clot can form and from which it can embolise.
- **Haemodynamic.** The tumour prolapses through the mitral valve during diastole. This can cause left heart failure and pulmonary hypertension. Prolapse of the tumour can be heard as a diastolic 'plop' at about the time of a third heart sound. There may be a mid-diastolic and/or systolic murmur.

Left atrial myxomas are rare but should be considered in a patient with an unidentified source of arterial emboli. Right atrial myxomas are even rarer and cause pulmonary rather than systemic embolism. The diagnosis is made by echocardiography and treatment is surgical.

1.8 Hypertension

Learning objectives

You should:
- understand how hypertension is defined
- be aware of its causes and the risk factors for it
- understand when and how to treat it.

Case Study

Persistent hypokalaemia in a newly presenting hypertensive man on no treatment leads to the finding of a 1.3 cm aldosterone-secreting adrenal tumour but adrenal surgery fails to cure his hypertension.

Essential hypertension is a condition of uncertain aetiology in which peripheral vascular resistance is increased and blood pressure 'reset' to a higher level. Hypertension may also be secondary (Box 3) to diseases which:

- increase blood volume by reducing sodium and water excretion
- increase peripheral vascular resistance.

The endocrine causes of hypertension listed in Box 3 are discussed in Chapter 7, renal artery stenosis in Chapter 4 and coarctation of the aorta on pages 36–37.

Whatever its cause, high blood pressure thickens the arterial media and intima and accelerates atherosclerosis. In the kidney, this arterial damage can cause a vicious circle of worsening renal function, sodium/water retention and hypertension by impairing glomerular perfusion and causing secondary aldosteronism (p. 310). Another

---

Box 3: Causes of secondary hypertension

Sodium/water retention
- Renal failure of any cause

- Increased glucocorticoid
  - Steroid therapy
  - Cushing's syndrome

Other vascular diseases
- Coarctation of the aorta

Drugs
- Non-steroidal anti-inflammatory drugs (NSAIDs)

- Oral contraceptives

- Sympathomimetics

Increased aldosterone
- Renal artery stenosis

- Primary aldosteronism (Conn's syndrome)

Increased catecholamine secretion
- Phaeochromocytoma

Neurogenic
- Raised intracranial pressure

---

important pathological feature is left ventricular hypertrophy caused by the increased cardiac load of hypertension. In the severest ('accelerated' or 'malignant') hypertension, there is fibrinoid necrosis in the arterioles and loss of capillary autoregulation, leading to widespread haemorrhage, ischaemia and tissue necrosis, clinically important in the eyes, kidneys and brain (p. 46).

Epidemiology

Systolic and diastolic blood pressure are normally distributed. The distribution varies from population to population and is higher in blacks than whites. Blood pressure increases with age. Pulse pressure also increases so that the systolic pressure increases disproportionately to the diastolic. There is no clear cut-off which defines 'abnormal' blood pressure. With increasing systolic and diastolic pressure, there is a progressive increase in the risk of stroke and cardiovascular disease. The British Hypertension Society defines a blood pressure over 139/89 mmHg as abnormal; further, it recognises three grades of hypertension:

- **Grade 1:** 140–159/90–99 mmHg
- **Grade 2:** 160–179/100–109 mmHg
- **Grade 3:** ≥180/≥110 mmHg.

Further, it recognizes 'isolated systolic hypertension' as:

- **Grade 1:** 140–159/<90 mmHg
- **Grade 2:** ≥160/<90 mmHg.

Risk factors for hypertension are:

- a positive family history
- obesity
- alcohol abuse

- non-insulin-dependent diabetes (50% of patients are hypertensive)
- high salt intake (more a 'population' than an 'individual' risk factor)
- inactivity
- environmental stress.

Only 5–10% of cases of hypertension are secondary, but the possibility must always be considered, particularly in patients below the age of 40 who have a low prevalence of essential hypertension.

Complications

Cardiac complications
These are:

- left ventricular hypertrophy, an effect of a sustained increase in cardiac work; this may lead to left ventricular failure, particularly if complicated by IHD
- IHD (p. 11), for which hypertension is one of the three main risk factors
- atrial fibrillation (p. 31).

Cerebrovascular disease
Hypertension is strongly associated with stroke because it:

- causes cerebral atherosclerosis and predisposes to cerebral thrombosis
- directly causes intracerebral haemorrhage through its effects on the cerebral vasculature
- increases the risk of subarachnoid haemorrhage.

Renal disease
The chicken/egg relationship between hypertension and renal disease has been mentioned above and is discussed in more detail in Chapter 4.

Retinal disease
This includes retinal artery thrombosis and retinal vein thrombosis.

Aortic aneurysm and peripheral vascular disease
Aortic dissection results from cystic medial necrosis in the arterial wall and is an effect of hypertension.

Clinical approach

The diagnosis is made by opportunistic blood pressure measurement or screening high-risk patients (see risk factors above).

Blood pressure measurement
Blood pressure varies minute-to-minute, especially on sight of a doctor ('white coat hypertension'). It should be measured under as relaxed conditions as possible, repeated after a few minutes if high and (unless *very* high) repeated days or weeks apart before a decision is made to treat.

Important points of technique are to:

- measure blood pressure sitting; repeat it standing if the patient is old, has risk factors for orthostatic hypotension or a history of it

- use a large cuff if the patient has a fat arm; a normal cuff will over-read
- raise pressure in the sphygmomanometer 20 mmHg above the palpated systolic blood pressure before lowering it so that you are not caught out by the 'auscultatory gap'
- lower the column of mercury in the sphygmomanometer at a rate of 2 mm per heart beat to ensure accuracy and read to the nearest 2 mmHg. Because mercury is an environmental health risk, aneroid sphygmomanometers and semi-automated devices are taking the place of traditional sphygmomanometers.

History

Having established that the blood pressure is high, consider the following.

Why is it high? Ask about family history of hypertension, history of renal disease, prolonged enuresis in childhood or urinary infection. Take a careful alcohol and drug history. Be alert to the triad of headache, sweating and palpitations. These are the symptoms of phaeochromocytoma, an uncommon cause of hypertension but all too often diagnosed in the post-mortem room rather than the clinic.

Is there target organ damage? Take a careful cardiovascular history, with particular attention to angina and previous strokes or transient ischaemic attacks.

How high is the patient's cardiovascular risk? Ask about diabetes, smoking and family history of IHD.

Examination

Your examination should answer the same three questions: Why? Is there target organ damage? How high is the risk?

General appearance Uncommon though it is, Cushing's disease will only be diagnosed by an alert clinician who spots the characteristic appearance. Remember, also, the more common association between hypertension and obesity; measure the patient's body mass index. Take note of breathlessness.

Retinal examination Sustained hypertension causes atherosclerotic changes in the retinal arterioles (irregularity, increased light reflex and attenuation of the veins at arterio-venous crossings — nipping). Similar changes occur with age. It is now clear that these changes cannot be interpreted precisely enough to be used as an index of hypertensive tissue damage, particularly given the better information available from investigations (see below). However, *severe* hypertension can cause quite specific changes:

- cotton wool spots, signs of retinal ischaemia
- flame haemorrhages, caused by vessel rupture and extravasation of blood into superficial nerve fibre layers
- papilloedema or swelling of the optic disc, a sign of cerebral oedema; loss of venous pulsation at the optic disc is the most specific manifestation.

Papilloedema is an imprecise sign but to be taken very seriously as evidence of accelerated hypertension (p. 46)

if unequivocally present. Cotton wool spots and haemorrhages are easier to identify and always a sign of serious microvascular disease.

Heart Examine carefully for atrial fibrillation or other dysrhythmia, left ventricular hypertrophy and signs of heart failure. The aortic component of the second heart sound may be loud, reflecting increased pressure on the valve.

Kidneys Even if renal disease is present, the kidneys are more likely to be small than large but there is a chance you might feel an enlarged hydronephrotic or polycystic kidney.

Peripheral vascular system Examine for:

- radio-femoral delay: uncommon though coarcts may be, they will only be diagnosed at a treatable stage if alert clinicians routinely check this sign in new hypertensives, particularly young people
- signs of a thoracic or abdominal aneurysm: inequality of the blood pressure in the two arms with signs of aortic valve dysfunction and a pulsatile abdominal mass, respectively
- renal or aortic bruits and signs of peripheral vascular disease: pointers to renal artery stenosis.

Investigations

Ambulatory blood pressure (ABP) monitoring is now widely used to:
- confirm the diagnosis of hypertension
- assess severity
- monitor the response to treatment.

It is particularly useful in white coat hypertension, but mean daytime pressure (and mean home blood pressure measurements) are, on average, 10/5 mmHg lower than office measurements and must be interpreted in that light.

Other investigations are used to answer the same three questions as the history and examination.

Mandatory tests

Test urine Test for proteinuria as a sign of primary renal disease or hypertensive nephropathy. Examine the urine under the microscope for cells and casts and culture it if there is proteinuria or other evidence of renal disease.

Measure serum creatinine and electrolytes These are to detect underlying renal disease and Conn's syndrome (p. 310). Conn's is rare but easily diagnosed and, unlike essential hypertension, curable; it will only be detected if every new case of hypertension is screened by measuring serum potassium *before a drug is prescribed*.

ECG Look for signs of left ventricular hypertrophy and strain or IHD, both of which constitute target organ damage and strengthen the case for treatment.

Chest radiograph This is to exclude cardiac hypertrophy, left ventricular failure and rib notching caused by coarctation of the aorta.

Fasting glucose and lipids Diabetes and hyperlipidaemia are associated with hypertension and increase the risk of cardiovascular disease. They increase the likely benefits of treatment.

Other optional tests

These may be indicated in individual cases.

Echocardiography This is more sensitive than either the ECG or chest radiograph for left ventricular hypertrophy and dysfunction. Arguably, it should be done in every patient.

Renal ultrasound scan and i.v. urography Examination of the renal tract is indicated if the history, physical examination or urinalysis point to renal disease. Ultrasound is the first-line test.

Management

When to treat hypertension

If the blood pressure is very high (>120 mmHg diastolic) more than transiently, there is an imminent risk of stroke and you should treat without delay. You should remember, however, that:

- high blood pressure can be an *effect* of raised intracranial pressure: for example, after acute stroke
- the cerebral circulation adapts to sustained hypertension by 'autoregulation', an upwards shift of the range of blood pressures over which cerebral circulation is unaffected by a drop in blood pressure. Lowering blood pressure too far and too fast in a patient with severe, sustained hypertension can abruptly lower perfusion and cause cerebral ischaemia.

Blood pressure must, therefore, be lowered cautiously and with consideration of its likely causes and complications, even in the severest cases. The management of hypertensive emergencies is considered on page 46. In most cases, you are treating a well patient to prevent strokes, heart attacks, heart failure, renal failure and death in the distant future. You need to understand the 'pros and cons' of treatment and explain them to the patient.

Clinical trials have consistently shown that treating hypertension is more effective at preventing strokes than heart attacks. For a blood pressure reduction of 5–6 mmHg diastolic over 5 years, you can expect a 40% reduction in the risk of stroke and a 15% reduction in coronary risk. These are *relative* risks, so the benefit to an individual depends on his/her absolute risk. That risk increases with age, the presence of other risk factors (e.g. smoking and hyperlipidaemia), the presence of established complications and the level of blood pressure. Therefore, more than 500 patient-years of treatment are needed to prevent one stroke in a group of 50-year-olds compared with 300 patient-years in 70-year-olds. Given the inconvenience and possible side-effects of treatment, it is clear that patients must be well informed to help them to make the decision. The treatment recommendations of the British Hypertension Society are summarised in Figure 13.

Isolated systolic hypertension is rather easily catered for by the recommendation that, when systolic and diasto-

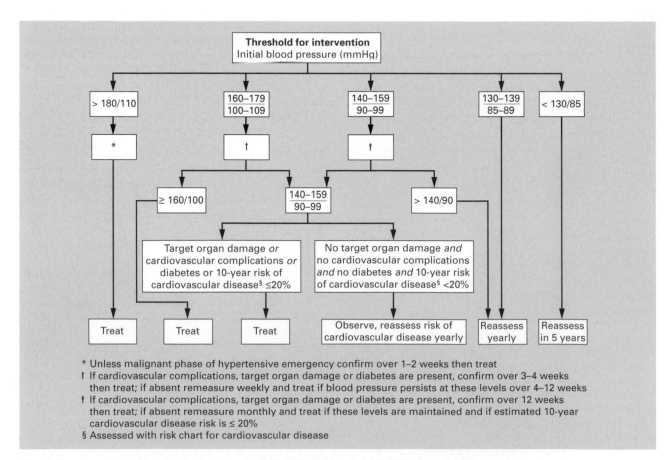

Fig. 13 The management of hypertension based on the British Hypertension Society's 2004 recommendations.

lic blood pressure fall into different categories, the higher value should be taken for classification.

Treatment

The aim of treatment is to achieve a blood pressure as near normal as possible, certainly <150/90. A more acceptable level of control is ≤140/85 and a stricter target of ≤130/85 is recommended for people with diabetes, renal disease, or established cardiovascular disease.

Non-pharmacological treatment

Non-drug treatments can be introduced at borderline levels of hypertension and as part of a general 'healthy living' policy. These are to:

- aim for 'ideal' body weight
- drink alcohol in moderation
- avoid added salt in cooking or at the table
- take regular exercise
- eat at least five portions/day of fresh fruit and vegetables
- reduce the intake of total and saturated fat.

These alone can lower blood pressure enough to avoid drug treatment and should be coupled with general lifestyle advice to reduce cardiovascular risk, particularly to stop smoking.

Drug treatment

Once-daily treatment is convenient and improves compliance. Side-effects, even if they seem trivial to you, are a significant disadvantage in the treatment of an asymptomatic disease. The presence of target organ disease, other cardiovascular risk factors and contraindications all influence choice. Drugs act in different ways to achieve their antihypertensive results and can be used synergistically. This narrative explains the 'ABCD' approach advocated by the British Hypertension Society, first introducing the drugs, and then showing the order in which they are introduced and the way they can usefully be combined.

ACE inhibitors These generally have fewer side-effects than other antihypertensives. ACE inhibitors may be used as monotherapy in moderate hypertension and are strongly indicated in hypertensive patients with heart failure and/or IHD or increased cardiovascular risk, in whom they improve life expectancy. They have an important role in the management of *severe* hypertension. They act synergistically with loop diuretics. They may precipitate acute renal failure in renovascular disease (p. 187). Their other main side-effect is cough, which affects up to 20% of patients.

Angiotensin receptor antagonists Because these are newer drugs, their place is less well established than ACE inhibitors. They have similar effects, are well tolerated and do not cause cough.

Beta-blockers These are proven effective for both mild and severe hypertension. They are cardioprotective and relieve angina. They improve survival after myocardial infarction, and improve both symptoms and survival in heart failure. However, they are contraindicated in asthma, may worsen intermittent claudication and can cause erectile dysfunction.

Calcium antagonists Long-acting drugs (e.g. amlodipine) are usually chosen as first-line calcium antagonists. They relieve angina but must be used cautiously in heart failure because of their negative inotropic effect. Ankle swelling is a common side-effect.

Diuretics

Thiazides In low dose (e.g. bendroflumethiazide 2.5 mg daily) these are a proven effective first-line therapy for mild hypertension, particularly in elderly people. Erectile dysfunction is their main side-effect. In high doses (which are no more effective at lowering blood pressure than low doses) they can cause gout, diabetes and hypokalaemia.

Loop diuretics These are less effective than thiazides in essential hypertension but more effective in salt-retaining states (e.g. renal failure). They are indicated in hypertensive heart failure. They are particularly effective in combination with ACE inhibitors.

Other antihypertensive drugs

Alpha-blockers Newer agents like doxazosin are better tolerated than older members of the class. They are usually used as second-line agents for more severe hypertension, often in combination with other drugs. They may be used as first-line therapy in men with prostatism, which they relieve.

The 'ABCD' approach This use of antihypertensive drugs, which is soundly based on theory and research evidence and easy to remember, is illustrated in Figure 14. Essential hypertension can be categorised into 'high-renin' and 'low-renin' subtypes. Younger people (age less than 55) are more likely to have high-renin hypertension. Older people and black people are more likely to have low-renin hypertension. So, drugs that inhibit the renin–angiotensin

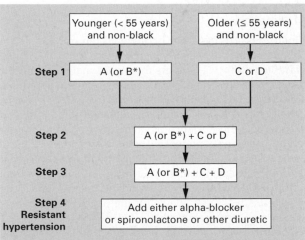

A: ACE inhibitor or angiotensin receptor blocker
B: Beta-blocker
C: Calcium channel blocker
D: Diuretic (thiazide and thiazide-like)

* Combination therapy involving B and D may induce more new onset diabetes compared with other combination therapies

Fig. 14 Recommendations for combining blood pressure-lowering drugs. (Adapted from: Brown, Cruickshank, Dominiczak, et al., Better blood pressure control: how to combine drugs. J Hum Hypertens 2003; 17: 81–86.)

system (A or B) are a logical first choice in younger people, and the C and D drugs (which do not inhibit it) are the first-line choice in older and black people. An ACE inhibitor tends to be chosen in preference to a beta-blocker because a B + D combination is prone to precipitate diabetes when the 'D' is a thiazide diuretic. So, the patient progresses from one drug of either class to one drug from each class, then increasing numbers of drugs in combination, as shown in Figure 14. Many patients receiving antihypertensive therapy for primary prevention, and all patients receiving it for secondary prevention, will receive an aspirin and a statin as well.

Accelerated ('malignant') hypertension

Clinical presentation

Accelerated hypertension is rare in the days of widespread screening for hypertension and effective, well-tolerated drugs. The clinical signs are diastolic blood pressure often >140 mmHg, **proteinuria**, resulting from fibrinoid necrosis in the renal vasculature, **retinal haemorrhages** and **exudates**, caused by similar changes in the retinal microcirculation, and **papilloedema**, caused by cerebral oedema. There may be left ventricular failure from cardiac overload. Unlike mild – moderate hypertension, accelerated hypertension may be symptomatic, even before major complications develop. The symptoms include:

- visual disturbance
- headache
- breathlessness.

Patients may present with impaired consciousness, focal neurological signs or fits (hypertensive encephalopathy) and are at high risk of cerebral haemorrhage. They may develop acute renal failure.

Management

Blood pressure must not be lowered too quickly or too far. The aim is to reduce it to no lower than 100 mmHg diastolic within 12–24 hours then to normalise it with the usual treatments over 2 or 3 days. The patient should be admitted to hospital for bed rest. Oral treatment should be used, if possible; for example, sublingual nifedipine and an oral beta-blocker such as atenolol or any other commonly used antihypertensive such as amlodipine. If the patient is seriously ill (encephalopathy or left ventricular failure), treatment is usually with an i.v. infusion of sodium nitroprusside or labetalol (a combined alpha- and beta-blocker). Always ask yourself if the patient could have a phaeochromocytoma. If one is suspected, the first-line treatment is an infusion of phentolamine (an alpha-blocker). If you see severe hypertension with major neurological signs, ask yourself if the patient could have hypertension *secondary* to an intracranial haemorrhage and arrange an urgent CT scan.

Hypertension in pregnancy

Mild–moderate hypertension is a common complication of pregnancy, usually treated with methyldopa, nifedipine, oral labetalol or another beta-blocker. ACE inhibitors increase the risk of congenital malformations and are con-traindicated. Hypertension may be a sign of pre-eclampsia, other signs of which are proteinuria, oedema and hyperuricaemia. Severe hypertension associated with pre-eclampsia necessitates delivery.

1.9 Pulmonary vessel disease

Learning objectives

You should:

- understand the range of causes
- be able to work out from simple physiological principles the symptoms, signs, radiological and electrocardiographic features
- understand the principles of treatment.

Case Study

An elderly woman who has severe chronic obstructive pulmonary disease caused by heavy smoking is extremely breathless and oedematous. She has the parasternal heave of right ventricular hypertrophy and very prominent V waves in her jugular venous pulse. She has cor pulmonale and perhaps tricuspid regurgitation due to pulmonary hypertension.

Causes of pulmonary hypertension

Pulmonary hypertension may be caused by left heart disease transmitted through the pulmonary vein and capillaries or by disease of the pulmonary circulation itself (Box 4). While *acute* left heart failure causes pulmonary oedema, there are adaptive changes to *chronic* pulmonary venous hypertension which minimise pulmonary oedema and transmit pressure into the pulmonary arteries. This is

---

Box 4: Some causes of pulmonary hypertension

Acute
- Pulmonary embolism
- Left ventricular failure

Chronic
- Increased pulmonary venous pressure
  - Left ventricular failure
  - Mitral incompetence or stenosis
- Increased flow
  - Atrial or ventricular septal defect
  - Patent ductus arteriosus
- Pulmonary arterial disease
  - Recurrent pulmonary embolism
  - Autoimmune disease
  - Primary pulmonary hypertension
- Secondary to parenchymal lung disease
  - Chronic obstructive pulmonary disease
  - Pulmonary fibrosis; sarcoidosis
- Secondary to hypoxia
  - Alveolar hypoventilation

well exemplified by mitral stenosis (p. 33). Disease of the pulmonary circulation is usually secondary to lung disease. This may be direct obliteration of the pulmonary vascular bed or a reflex vasoconstriction to hypoxia. An extreme example of the latter is alveolar hypoventilation associated with gross obesity (Pickwickian syndrome) in which there is diminished alveolar ventilation, hypoxia and secondary pulmonary hypertension. Cor pulmonale describes right heart failure secondary to chronic airflow limitation. Pulmonary hypertension may be secondary to increased flow, as in chronic left-to-right shunting of blood. *Primary* pulmonary hypertension is a rare disease of unknown aetiology, chiefly affecting young women.

It follows from the pathophysiology that:

- pulmonary venous hypertension or left-to-right shunts should be corrected as early as possible, before irreversible changes have occurred
- hypoxic vasoconstriction may be a reversible factor at all stages in the natural history of pulmonary hypertension and oxygen therapy has an important place in treatment.

Clinical presentation

The symptoms and signs result from 'forwards' and 'backwards' heart failure. They include dyspnoea, chest pain, lassitude and syncope. Signs include the parasternal heave of right ventricular hypertrophy and a loud pulmonary second heart sound. There may be the pansystolic murmur of functional tricuspid regurgitation (from right ventricular dilatation) and the early diastolic murmur of pulmonary regurgitation (secondary to increased pulmonary artery pressure).

Investigations

The chest radiograph shows enlargement of the pulmonary arteries at the hila with reduced peripheral vascular lung markings (pruning). On the ECG, there is a tall and peaked P wave in lead II (P pulmonale, caused by right atrial hypertrophy) and signs of right heart hypertrophy and strain; a dominant R wave in V1, T wave changes in leads V1–3 and right axis deviation. Blood gases should always be checked to detect hypoxia. Other relevant investigations include radionuclide lung scanning to detect pulmonary embolism, CT pulmonary angiography, echocardiography, pulmonary function tests, right heart catheterisation with pulmonary angiography and lung biopsy.

Management

The principles of management are:

- Correct any underlying cause. For mitral stenosis and other structural cardiac diseases, that means surgery.
- Avoid hypoxia. That often means domiciliary oxygen therapy.
- Treat heart failure. This relieves breathlessness and, in the case of left heart failure, directly relieves pulmonary hypertension. Diuretics must not be overused because an adequate right heart filling pressure is essential to maintain cardiac output.

- Consider anticoagulation. Pulmonary embolism may be the primary cause of pulmonary hypertension. It may also result from a reduced cardiac output and exacerbate pulmonary hypertension of some other cause.

Bosentan (an endothelin receptor antagonist) or intravenous or aerosolised epoprostenol (prostacyclin, a potent vasodilator) reduces pulmonary artery pressure and improves exercise capacity in patients with primary pulmonary hypertension. Patients with a right-to-left shunt caused by an ASD, VSD or patent ductus, or young women with intractable primary pulmonary hypertension, have a 50% 5-year survival expectancy with a heart–lung transplant.

1.10 Venous thrombo-embolism

Learning objectives

You should:
- have a clear understanding of venous and arterial thrombo-embolism and how to recognise them
- understand the causes, in terms of Virchow's triad
- understand how to investigate and treat a deep venous thrombosis or pulmonary embolism.

Case Study

A 26-year-old single parent presents to the emergency admissions unit with pleuritic-type chest pain, which came on after carrying a heavy shopping bag. She has had no previous ill health, has no other symptoms or signs, and her vital signs are normal. She is on the pill. Having assessed the clinical probability of a pulmonary embolism, the doctor requests a D-dimer measurement, which is not raised. She is told she has definitely not had a pulmonary embolism and sent home with paracetamol but no follow-up.

It is important to distinguish clearly between **venous** and **arterial** thrombo-embolism. The lungs provide such an effective filter that the venous and arterial systems are separate from the point of view of thrombo-embolism (except in the rare case of patent foramen ovale or ASD, when there may be paradoxical embolus transfer from the right to the left circulation). It is a good intellectual discipline to use the rather cumbersome terms 'venous thrombo-embolism' and 'arterial thrombo-embolism'.

Deep venous thrombosis

Keep in mind Virchow's triad, the three factors that predispose to thrombosis:

- stasis
- increased coagulability of blood
- disease of the blood vessel wall.

Diseases which cause venous thrombosis may do so by more than one of these mechanisms. A patient convalescing after surgery is both immobile and hypercoagulable. A tumour can increase blood coagulability, compress the vessel wall and cause stasis. The reason *in situ* thrombosis is more common in veins than in arteries is that blood flows slower in veins. An important point in relation to the first member of the triad is that, whatever its cause, venous thrombosis *causes* stasis and so tends to propagate. An important predisposing factor in women is oestrogen, either during pregnancy or in the form of the contraceptive pill. Other risk factors are increasing age, obesity and cigarette smoking. Thrombophilia is discussed on page 284.

Deep venous thrombosis (DVT) is common and often 'silent'. It has been shown, for example, that one-third of patients develop venous thromboses after acute myocardial infarction and over 80% of old people develop them after hip fractures. A DVT may be the presenting feature of malignant disease. An understanding of the natural history and causes is valuable both in making the diagnosis and in deciding whether or not there is underlying cancer. The peak time for the development of a DVT is a week or more after an acute insult. A swollen leg the day after a fracture is unlikely to be caused by a DVT but it is very likely to be caused by one when it occurs after a week or more. By the same logic, a DVT 2 weeks after a long air flight or a broken leg in an otherwise healthy young person is probably the result of immobility while the same problem developing out of the blue in a middle-aged person with no history of immobility should be considered to be the presentation of an occult tumour until proven otherwise. Thrombo-embolism that recurs or responds poorly to anticoagulation is a particularly sinister sign.

Only leg vein thrombosis is discussed here because it is the commonest and potentially the most serious form of venous thrombosis but remember that thromboses may occur in other sites, including the axillary and renal veins. The principles of diagnosis and management are similar whatever the site.

Clinical presentation

The symptoms of DVT of the leg are:

- pain
- swelling
- heaviness or a bursting sensation in the affected limb.

  The signs are:

- swelling and 'turgor' (heaviness to palpation)
- mild cyanosis or reddening
- tenderness over the affected veins
- increased warmth
- dilated superficial veins.

Your ability to detect swelling can be improved by measuring limb girth above and below the knee. Asymmetry >1 cm can be taken as significant. Although the whole leg may feel painful, tenderness is often localised to the affected vein. In calf vein thrombosis, there is tenderness over the back of gastrocnemius. Femoral vein thrombosis may cause tenderness over the antero-medial aspect

of the thigh. However, physical signs have serious limitations:

- pelvic vein thromboses may occur with no symptoms or signs at all; the DVT of a fatal pulmonary embolism may be clinically 'silent'
- involvement is often more extensive than the clinical signs suggest
- compared with venography, physical signs are unreliable in diagnosing DVT.

Differential diagnosis

DVTs have to be distinguished from superficial thrombophlebitis and cellulitis. Thrombophlebitis is inflammation in a superficial vein (often varicose) with secondary thrombosis; it is tender, palpable as a hard 'knot' and often visibly inflamed and red. It is treated with nonsteroidal analgesia. Cellulitis, like DVT, causes diffuse swelling and pain. Features that favour a diagnosis of cellulitis are:

- no localised tenderness over veins
- more reddening in cellulitis, sometimes with a clear demarcation line
- obvious portal of entry and spread of infection from it.

A ruptured popliteal cyst is another condition that mimics DVT; it usually occurs in patients with rheumatoid arthritis or other joint disease and can be diagnosed by arthrography. DVT can complicate all of these diagnoses.

The most important point is that clinical examination is unreliable in the diagnosis of DVT and confirmatory investigations are needed.

Diagnosis

This first step is to assess the clinical probability, using the criteria shown in Table 9.

A second step is to measure D-dimer, a split product of fibrin that is very sensitive (bound to be positive if the patient has a DVT) but not very specific (high false-positive rate). If the clinical probability is low and D-dimer is not raised, DVT has virtually been excluded. Patients with a moderate or high probability of DVT should first be investigated by ultrasound scanning (measuring D-dimer in such patients is as likely to confuse as help). A positive ultrasound confirms the diagnosis. If the clinical probability is high and the scan is negative, venography may be performed. Alternatively, the scan may be repeated after several days. If the clinical probability is high, anticoagulants should be continued while investigations are under way.

Management

Patients who are immobile or have cardiovascular disease should have *prophylactic* heparin (p. 283) and/or compression stockings, which divert blood flow into the deep veins. In established DVT, the aims are to:

- relieve pain and swelling
- prevent further propagation of the clot
- prevent pulmonary embolism

Table 9 Pretest probability of deep vein thrombosis (Wells score)*

Clinical feature	Score
Active cancer (treatment ongoing or within the previous 6 months or palliative)	1
Paralysis, paresis/or recent plaster immobilisation of the lower extremities	1
Recently bedridden for more than 3 days or major surgery, within 4 weeks	1
Localised tenderness along the distribution of the deep venous system	1
Entire leg swollen	1
Calf swelling by more than 3 cm when compared to the asymptomatic leg (measured below tibial tuberosity)	1
Pitting oedema (greater in the symptomatic leg)	1
Collateral superficial veins (non-varicose)	1
Alterative diagnosis as likely as or more likely than that of DVT	−2

High probability   = 3 or greater
Moderate probability = 1 or 2
Low probability   = 0 or less

Modification This clinical model has been modified to take one other clinical feature into account: a previously documented DVT is given the score of 1. Using this modified scoring system, DVT is either likely or unlikely, as follows:

DVT likely   = 2 or greater
DVT unlikely = 1 or less

*Adapted from Wells PS, Anderson DR, Bormanis J et al. 1997 Lancet 350:1795 and Wells PS, Anderson DR, Rodger M et al. 2003 N Engl J Med 349:1227.

- allow healing and minimise the chances of permanent venous damage
- prevent recurrence.

Established DVT is treated by anticoagulation unless there are strong contraindications. Immediate treatment is with low molecular weight heparin (LMWH), which is continued for 5 days to prevent propagation and initiate healing. Warfarin is introduced once the clinical diagnosis is certain. Bed rest elevation of the limb and compression stockings relieve swelling.

Anticoagulants are continued for 4–6 weeks when DVT complicates short periods of immobility, 6 months in cases of spontaneous DVT and life-long for recurrent DVT or in patients with proven thrombophilia. Anticoagulation is discussed on page 283.

Complications

There may be permanent damage to the veins, resulting in a 'post-phlebitic limb', which is permanently swollen, uncomfortable and prone to cellulitis and further episodes of thrombosis. Even without that complication, thrombosis may recur, particularly at times of illness or immobility. Pulmonary embolism is the most serious complication.

Pulmonary embolism

Pulmonary emboli usually come from the iliac, femoral or distal leg veins but may arise elsewhere in the venous system or right side of the heart. Risk factors and causes are as for DVT. Pulmonary embolism, like DVT, may be clinically 'silent' and found post mortem. Individual small pulmonary emboli are not haemodynamically significant but a large embolism or multiple small emboli cause pulmonary hypertension, which may become chronic (p. 46).

Pulmonary embolism is a dynamic situation. Emboli are quickly removed by the fibrinolytic system; unless the patient succumbs to the initial event, the threat is from further embolism. Anticoagulation, the mainstay of treatment, works by limiting the formation of new clot in the deep veins. Fibrinolytic therapy is not given for anything but massive pulmonary embolism because there is a risk of dislodging further emboli and the endogenous fibrinolytic system is effective at removing blood clot.

Embolism and infarction

An important conceptual point is the distinction between pulmonary embolism and infarction. Emboli may cause infarction of the affected lung if there is severe and lasting ischaemia but not if the embolus is small, dissolution is rapid and/or there is an adequate collateral blood supply from the bronchial arterial system. Clinically, embolism can be inferred from its cardiovascular effects, and infarction from its effects on the lungs, chiefly pleurisy if the infarct extends out to the pleural surface.

Clinical presentation

Dyspnoea is the most frequent presenting symptom and tachypnoea the most frequent sign. A typical history of pulmonary embolism is a sudden onset of tight chest pain and dyspnoea, often followed by haemoptysis. However, pulmonary emboli can be asymptomatic or present purely with breathlessness or right heart failure. There may be syncope caused by an abrupt reduction in cardiac output. If there is pulmonary infarction, the pain may change in character, becoming sharp and related to respiration. Pleurisy may be the sole presenting symptom. Patients may present with infection in an area of infarcted lung. Often, the circumstances give a clue to the diagnosis, e.g. recent immobility or treatment with the contraceptive pill.

On examination, there is tachypnoea and tachycardia, and there may be cyanosis, a pleural rub and signs of an effusion. There may be a parasternal heave, increased splitting of the second heart sound and a raised jugular venous pressure. The patient may or may not have signs of a DVT.

Massive pulmonary embolism presents as an emergency with collapse, severe dyspnoea, hypotension, pallor, cyanosis, tachycardia and signs of right heart strain or failure.

Investigations

The **chest radiograph** is usually normal but may show oligaemia (reduced lung markings in the affected area), consolidation, loss of volume and a raised hemidiaphragm, a pleural effusion and one or more linear opacities representing areas of atelectasis. The most frequent **ECG** change is T wave inversion in the anterior chest leads. There may also be signs of right ventricular strain, seen as right axis deviation, RBBB or an 'SI, QIII, TIII pattern' (S wave in lead I, Q wave in lead III and T wave inversion in lead III). The **blood gases** usually show hypoxia with a reduced partial pressure of carbon dioxide (Pco_2). A more specific investigation is a **ventilation : perfusion radionuclide scan**. A technetium isotope is given intravenously to detect areas of non-perfusion; labelled xenon is inhaled to demonstrate non-aerated lung. Areas that are aerated but not perfused suggest embolism. Infarction may affect aeration as well as perfusion, but pulmonary emboli are often multiple, so it is usually possible to demonstrate some areas of ventilation : perfusion mismatch in addition to 'matched' defects corresponding to areas of infarction. Ventilation : perfusion scanning is a very sensitive test for pulmonary embolism but can produce false-positive results. With the availability of fast, high-resolution imaging, CT pulmonary angiography is becoming the definitive way of confirming a suspected diagnosis of pulmonary embolism. It is the emergency investigation of choice to confirm a suspected massive pulmonary embolism.

Diagnosis

This description assumes that CT pulmonary angiography, isotope ventilation and perfusion lung scanning, and a D-dimer assay with good sensitivity and specificity are readily available. Figure 15 summarises British Thoracic Society recommendations. First comes an assessment of clinical probability using the criteria in Table 10. A low or intermediate clinical probability and negative D-dimer virtually rule out pulmonary embolism. If there is an intermediate probability with a raised D-dimer, or a high probability, further imaging is needed. In patients with a normal chest radiograph and no active cardiorespiratory disease, that should be an isotope scan, otherwise a CT pulmonary angiogram.

Management

Apart from analgesia and oxygen, the treatment is anticoagulation, as described for DVT. Massive pulmonary

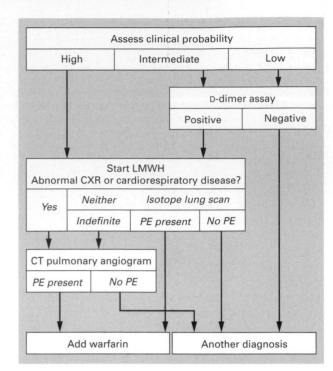

Fig. 15 Diagnostic algorithm for pulmonary embolism. CT, computed tomography; CXR, chest X-ray; LMWH, low molecular weight heparin; PE, pulmonary embolism. (Reproduced with permission, British Thoracic Society.)

Table 10 Modified Wells criteria: clinical assessment for pulmonary embolism (PE)*

Clinical feature	Score
Clinical symptoms of DVT	3.0
Other diagnosis less likely than PE	3.0
Heart rate >100	1.5
Immobilisation or surgery in the previous 4 weeks	1.5
Previous DVT/PE	1.5
Haemoptysis	1.0
Malignancy	1.0

High probability = >6.0
Moderate probability = 2.0–6.0
Low probability = <2.0

*Data from Wells PS et al. 2001 Ann Intern Med 135:98.

embolism is treated with intravenous tissue plasminogen activator. It is tempting to treat right heart failure in pulmonary embolism with diuretics, but that is inappropriate because a high filling pressure is needed to maintain right heart output. If there is severe hypotension, inotropic support may be given.

1.11 Arterial disease

Learning objectives

You should:
- understand the causes and clinical presentations of aortic aneurysms at their various sites.

Case Study

A 69-year-old man is admitted with agonising central chest pain radiating up to the right side of his neck and through to his back. His blood pressure is 170/94 mmHg. His ECG shows no acute ischaemic changes but a chest radiograph shows a widened mediastinum and his blood pressure cannot be found in the right arm. He is admitted to coronary care and his blood pressure is controlled with intravenous nitroprusside. His family are given a very guarded prognosis.

Diseased arteries can expand and rupture or narrow and occlude. They may be occluded by disease in their wall, thrombosis on a diseased wall or embolism from elsewhere in the arterial system. The arterial wall may, itself, be a source of emboli. The causes of arterial disease are atheroma, other degenerative processes and inflammation (vasculitis). There are many causes of inflammation, including infection and autoimmunity. Arteritis is considered under the individual diseases (Chapter 10). You are referred to a textbook of surgery for information about occlusive peripheral arterial disease. Thoracic and abdominal aneurysms may present to you as emergencies so they are discussed briefly here.

Thoracic aortic aneurysm

Atheroma is by far the most common cause of thoracic aortic aneurysm. Syphilis, once common as a cause of aortic incompetence and aneurysm, is now rare. Arteritides of the aorta are also a rare cause. Aneurysms may develop in patients with Marfan's syndrome, a congenital disorder of collagen whose other stigmata are a high, arched palate, 'spidery', long fingers, tall stature and dislocated lenses. Atheromatous aneurysms occur most often in middle-aged or elderly men and are strongly associated with hypertension and generalised arterial disease. They involve the ascending aorta, arch and descending aorta in roughly equal proportions. They may:

- expand, be painful and have pressure effects
- dissect
- rupture.

Expanding thoracic aneurysm

An expanding aneurysm may be found by chance on a chest radiograph, or it may stretch the aortic valve ring and present with pain or pressure symptoms of aortic incompetence. The pain is central or to one side of the chest and radiates to the back. Pressure symptoms include:

- dysphagia
- hoarseness
- dyspnoea
- superior vena caval obstruction.

The most important radiographic sign is widening of the mediastinum. Further investigation is by transthoracic or transoesophageal echocardiography, MR or CT scanning.

Surgery for acute dissection has an extremely high mortality and rupture is terminal so early diagnosis and elective surgery give the best prognosis. Marfan's syndrome causes thoracic aortic aneurysms in young people and is an important indication for elective surgery. Elderly patients may be unfit for surgery.

Ruptured thoracic aneurysm

A ruptured thoracic aneurysm presents with sudden death or collapse associated with chest pain and shock. It is untreatable.

Dissecting thoracic aneurysm

Dissection occurs when there is a breach in the intima and blood tracks into the media. It may arise in the ascending or descending thoracic aorta.

Clinical presentation

Dissection is an uncommon cause of chest pain and can be difficult to diagnose but you must consider it because to give fibrinolytic therapy for a presumed myocardial infarct may kill your patient. The problem is made more difficult by the fact that a dissecting aneurysm can occlude a coronary ostium and actually present with myocardial ischaemia. Depending on its location in the aorta, the pain is felt in the centre or to one side of the anterior chest, radiating to the back, neck and arms. The patient may describe a sudden tearing sensation and the pain may be excruciating.

About 50% of patients with a dissection are hypertensive at the time of presentation. They may have a difference of systolic blood pressure >20 mmHg between the two arms because of occlusion of the subclavian arteries. There may be signs of spinal or carotid artery occlusion. Aortic regurgitation may develop as a result of stretching of the valve ring or pericarditis as a result of blood tracking into the pericardial sac.

Investigations

The chest radiograph may show mediastinal widening, a left-sided pleural effusion or enlargement of the aortic knuckle. The ECG may be normal or non-specifically abnormal, or show signs of acute myocardial ischaemia. Transoesophageal echocardiography is the investigation of choice to confirm the diagnosis and locate the intimal tear. CT or MR scanning may also be used.

Management and prognosis

Pain should be controlled. The mortality during acute aortic dissection is 1% per hour. It can be reduced by lowering blood pressure to <110 mmHg systolic with i.v. labetalol or nitroprusside. If the ascending aorta is involved, immediate surgery is indicated. Dissection of the descending aorta is treated by strict bed rest and blood pressure control because surgery has a higher mortality than medical management.

Abdominal aortic aneurysm

Abdominal aortic aneurysm is the most common aneurysm encountered in clinical practice. The causes are similar and the mechanisms which lead to symptoms and signs are analogous to thoracic aortic aneurysm.

Clinical presentation

The cardinal symptom is abdominal pain radiating to the back and the cardinal sign a pulsatile abdominal mass. Sometimes the mass may be found by chance on physical examination. It is important to distinguish between tender and non-tender pulsatile masses because tenderness is a sign of impending rupture. Apart from pain, an expanding aneurysm may present with complications, including obstruction of a ureter (caused by an inflammatory reac-

tion to the aneurysm) or embolism into the peripheral arterial system. Rupture presents with pain and hypotension together with the tender abdominal mass. There may be involvement of the renal arteries causing renal failure and involvement of the distal arteries causing leg ischaemia.

Investigations

Ultrasound, CT or magnetic resonance imaging are first-line investigations. Small aneurysms are unlikely to rupture but those over 5 cm are at high risk.

Management

Risk factors, including hypertension, should be treated. Small aneurysms are observed by serial scanning to detect expansion and impending rupture. High-risk aneurysms should be treated surgically before they rupture. Emergency surgery has a better outlook than for thoracic aneurysms but still carries a high mortality.

Self-assessment: questions

Multiple choice questions

Any or all of each set of five statements may be true or false. Choose your answers and see the reasoning behind the correct answer on pages 63–68.

1. The anatomy of the heart:
   a. If you stand on the patient's right side with your right hand across the sternum and cardiac apex, the left ventricle lies under the sternum
   b. On a postero-anterior (PA) chest radiograph, the left heart border is mostly formed by the left ventricle
   c. On an ECG, disease of the interventricular septum causes changes in chest leads V3–4
   d. When examining the heart, the cardiac apex is the point where the heart beat can be felt most strongly
   e. Occlusion of the left anterior descending coronary artery causes infarction of the anterior wall of the left ventricle and interventricular septum

2. Cardiac physiology/physical examination:
   a. Bedside examination of the jugular venous pressure gives an estimate of cardiac preload
   b. A pulse rate <30 beats/min is probably a sinus bradycardia
   c. Heart rates >160 beats/min are usually initiated by a pacemaker other than the SA node
   d. The mitral and tricuspid components of the second heart sound can usually be heard as two separate sounds during inspiration
   e. An increased pulse pressure (systolic–diastolic BP) does not necessarily signify an increased stroke volume

3. The ECG:
   a. The T wave corresponds to atrial contraction
   b. If the S wave is greater than the R wave in lead I, there is right axis deviation
   c. If the S wave is greater than the R wave in lead II, there is left axis deviation
   d. ST segment depression may be a sign of cardiac ischaemia
   e. A tall R wave in V1 may be a sign of right ventricular hypertrophy

4. Pericardial disease:
   a. A normal heart size on chest radiography rules out pericardial disease
   b. In tamponade, crackles at the lung bases and peripheral oedema are usual
   c. A low-voltage ECG is a clue to the presence of a large pericardial effusion
   d. Hard-to-hear heart sounds are typical of a large pericardial effusion
   e. Almost all cases of purulent pericarditis have a pericardial friction rub

5. In a patient with a raised jugular venous pulse:
   a. A further increase on expiration is characteristic of pericardial tamponade
   b. Giant V waves suggest tricuspid stenosis
   c. Facial engorgement and lack of pulsation in the jugular venous pressure are characteristic of superior vena caval obstruction
   d. The cause could be pulmonary embolism
   e. Diuretic therapy is indicated, whatever the cause

6. The following are true of valvular/congenital heart disease:
   a. Mitral stenosis is usually caused by rheumatic heart disease
   b. An indication for surgery in mitral stenosis is worsening pulmonary hypertension
   c. A patient with rheumatic aortic valve disease is likely also to have mitral valve disease
   d. Coarctation of the aorta may be associated with a chromosomal abnormality
   e. Angiotensin-converting enzyme (ACE) inhibitors are the treatment of choice for dyspnoea caused by aortic stenosis

7. In acute dissection of the thoracic aorta:
   a. The operative mortality is about 30%
   b. Spinal cord ischaemia may occur
   c. Hypertension should be treated aggressively
   d. Acute aortic stenosis may occur
   e. The patient may develop myocardial ischaemia

8. Heart failure:
   a. ACE inhibitor therapy is reserved for patients whose symptoms are uncontrolled by large doses of diuretics
   b. May be caused by alcohol abuse
   c. Previous tuberculous pericarditis could cause it
   d. The presence of a wheeze discriminates asthma from heart failure
   e. A suspected diagnosis of heart failure in a 23-year-old woman is supported by hearing a third heart sound

9. Hypertension:
   a. Treatment is of no proven benefit in patients over the age of 70 years
   b. The symptoms of phaeochromocytoma include headache, sweating and palpitations
   c. Oral treatment producing a fall in diastolic blood pressure of 20 mmHg over 24 hours might be regarded as successful treatment of accelerated hypertension

d. ACE inhibitors are the drugs of choice for hypertension in pregnancy

e. Addison's disease should be considered a possible cause in a hypertensive patient with hirsutism

10. In ischaemic heart disease:

a. Prevalence is increased in chronic renal failure

b. Untreated hypothyroidism predisposes to it

c. Polycythaemia may precipitate myocardial ischaemia

d. An alcohol intake of 18 units per week in a man increases the risk of ischaemic heart disease

e. A high plasma fibrinogen reduces the risk

11. Cardiac dysrhythmias:

a. Digoxin toxicity may cause supraventricular tachycardia

b. A patient with a completely irregular pulse of 180 beats/min is likely to be in atrial fibrillation

c. Complete heart block may be asymptomatic

d. Digoxin is effective in preventing paroxysms of atrial fibrillation

e. A QRS width less than 3 small squares on the ECG indicates that a tachycardia is supraventricular

Single best answer multiple choice questions

For each numbered question, only one of the options lettered a–e is correct.

1. A 65-year-old woman is admitted comatose with a right hemiparesis. Her blood pressure is 170/106 mmHg. Her blood glucose is 12 mmol/l. You examine her fundi through an ophthalmoscope and find retinopathy. Which of the following features is most suggestive that she has established diabetes rather than stress hyperglycaemia?

a. Cotton wool spots

b. Arterio-venous nipping

c. Flame haemorrhages

d. New vessels

e. Hard exudates

2. In the treatment of hypertension, ACE inhibitors:

a. Cause ankle swelling in over 5% of patients

b. Work synergistically with loop diuretics to lower blood pressure

c. Given intravenously, are the treatment of choice for a hypertensive crisis

d. Are contraindicated in patients with renal failure

e. Worsen blood glucose control in people with diabetes

3. In a hypertensive 50-year-old man presenting with angina:

a. Lipid-lowering treatment is indicated if the plasma cholesterol is ≥5 mmol/l

b. Clopidogrel is the most appropriate first-line antiplatelet agent

c. Left access deviation on the ECG is an indication for echocardiography

d. Ramipril (or an alternative ACE inhibitor) reduces mortality risk

e. A beta-blocker should be avoided if the patient also has heart failure

4. In endocarditis:

a. It is important to take blood cultures over at least a 24-hour period to make the diagnosis

b. Transthoracic echocardiography is a sensitive means of making or confirming the diagnosis

c. Most patients with *Staphylococcus aureus* bacteraemia have endocarditis

d. Viral endocarditis leads to valvular abnormality

e. In patients with a new stroke or transient ischaemic attack (TIA), endocarditis must be considered even if the patient is afebrile

5. In the treatment of endocarditis:

a. Intravenous antibiotics for 6 weeks are necessary to cure *viridans* type streptococcal endocarditis

b. Staphylococcal endocarditis on the tricuspid valve in a drug addict is treated with flucloxacillin and valve replacement

c. Replacement of an infected prosthetic valve usually leaves the new valve infected

d. Combination antibiotic therapy is almost always appropriate for endocarditis

e. If gentamicin is used for treatment, it should not be used for more than 2 weeks

Extended matched questions

EMQ 1

Theme: Drugs/treatments

Options

1. Protamine
2. Intravenous furosemide
3. Phenytoin
4. Digoxin
5. Labetalol
6. Unfractionated heparin
7. Cardioversion
8. Enalapril
9. Etacrynic acid
10. Warfarin
11. Low molecular weight heparin
12. Lidocaine
13. Adenosine

14. Sodium bicarbonate

15. Aminophylline

16. Temporary cardiac pacing

17. Aspirin

18. Fresh frozen plasma

19. Atropine

20. Alteplase

For each of the following patients that a house officer might be called to see, select the best treatment (more than one may be correct). Each item can be used once, more than once or not at all.

A. A 65-year-old man with hypertension and ischaemic heart disease taking aspirin, atenolol and ramipril who is having episodes of ischaemic chest pain at rest and after minimal exertion.

B. A 58-year-old woman convalescent from pneumonia whose only drug therapy is amoxicillin and who has developed a regular, narrow complex tachycardia, rate 180 beats/min.

C. A healthy, teetotal 70-year-old man newly found to have atrial fibrillation with a ventricular rate of 82 beats/min.

D. A 50-year-old woman with an acute inferior myocardial infarct who has had aspirin and streptokinase; she feels extremely faint and has a blood pressure of 88/60 mmHg, 40 beats/min.

E. A 78-year-old woman with severe congestive cardiac failure in sinus rhythm with no ankle oedema or basal crackles. She is taking oral furosemide, spironolactone, ramipril and low-dose bisoprolol and has been admitted for the third time in 2 months with dyspnoea and lethargy.

EMQ 2

Theme: Drugs/investigations
Options
1. Transoesophageal echocardiogram
2. Cardiac troponin estimation
3. Exercise ECG
4. D-dimer estimation
5. Ventilation : perfusion lung scan
6. Transthoracic echocardiogram
7. Pulmonary angiogram
8. 24-hour ECG tape
9. Coronary angiography
10. Exercise thallium scan
11. Thoracic computed tomographic (CT) scan
12. Venogram
13. Ambulatory blood pressure monitoring
14. Resting 12-lead ECG
15. Chest radiograph
16. Magnetic resonance (MR) scan
17. Doppler leg scan

For each of the following patients that a house officer might be called to see, select the best investigation (more than one may be correct). Each item can be used once, more than once or not at all.

A. A 30-year-old woman on the contraceptive pill who has a swollen right leg, with tenderness over the antero-medial aspect of the thigh.

B. A 22-year-old female i.v. drug abuser with a systolic murmur, positive blood cultures and a low-grade fever.

C. A 70-year-old man with widespread arterial disease suspected of having a dissecting thoracic aneurysm.

D. A 29-year-old athlete who has developed agonising, central chest pain relieved by leaning forwards 5 days after an upper respiratory infection.

E. A 58-year-old woman who smokes heavily and takes isosorbide, aspirin, atenolol and amlodipine, presenting to casualty after a family argument with a pressing central chest pain and non-specific T wave changes on the ECG.

EMQ 3

Theme: Myocardial infarction
Options
1. Observe but take no specific action
2. Say there is >80% chance of complete recovery
3. Say there is <50% chance of survival
4. Increase dose of loop diuretic
5. Discontinue loop diuretic
6. Add thiazide diuretic
7. Give sodium nitroprusside
8. Give intravenous lidocaine
9. Give intravenous amiodarone
10. Give intravenous digoxin
11. Give intravenous flecainide
12. Cardiovert

For each of the following problems a junior doctor might be asked to advise on in a patient who has had a myocardial infarct, select the best course of action (more than one may be correct). Each item can be used once, more than once or not at all.

A. A patient with a raised jugular venous pressure who is on intravenous loop diuretics and becoming increasingly hypotensive

B. A patient who had streptokinase 2 hours ago and is haemodynamically stable, but has developed ventricular dysrhythmias

C. The wife of a patient whose intraventricular septum has ruptured, who is asking for information about the prognosis

D. A nurse asks for lidocaine to be prescribed prophylactically to a patient recovering uneventfully from an ST segment elevation myocardial infarction to prevent dysrhythmias

Objective structural clinical examination (OSCE) stations

OSCE 1

This is a 5-minute station for peripheral vascular examination with a middle-aged 'real' patient on a couch.

Examiner: Mr Jones, here, is complaining of pain in his left calf when he walks 50 yards, relieved by rest. Please examine his legs for signs of peripheral arterial disease.

OSCE 2

This is a 10-minute station in a finals OSCE. An elderly man is lying on a bed undressed below the waist. Both legs are swollen, one more than the other.

Examiner: What explanations can you think of for the appearance of Mr Taylor's legs?

Examiner: Please examine him to gather information that will help decide which of your explanations is correct.

OSCE 3

A patient of yours is being considered for a renal transplant. The surgeon wishes to know if he has ischaemic heart disease. How would you tell?

Case history questions

Case history 1

A 58-year-old woman presents with biventricular failure. She admits to drinking a bottle of sherry and smoking 20 cigarettes per day. Echocardiography reveals a dilated, poorly contracting left ventricle.

1. Suggest two causes for her heart failure.
2. Name two complications of her cardiac disease which might develop.

It is suggested she should have anticoagulation therapy.

3. List two contraindications either suggested by her history or which you might identify on a more detailed history/examination.

Case history 2

A 68-year-old man has had difficulty managing his garden for some time because of breathlessness. Recently, he has not only been breathless when he exerts himself but he has noticed precordial tightness radiating to the neck and left arm. He has used his wife's bronchodilator spray but it hasn't helped at all. On one occasion 2 weeks ago he found himself lying on the lawn after attempting to mow it. He has been brought up to the emergency department after a particularly severe attack of pain. His blood pressure is 106/82 mmHg, pulse 80 beats/min sinus rhythm, the apex beat has a thrusting character and he has a soft mid-systolic murmur. His chest radiograph shows cardiomegaly and his ECG shows an R wave in V5 of 35 mm. He is not receiving any treatment.

1. Suggest a differential diagnosis.
2. How would you investigate him?

Key features questions

1. A 75-year-old woman attends her general practice for a health check. Her blood pressure is 152/98 mmHg. She attends twice more over the next 3 weeks, and the average of the three measurements is 150/96 mmHg. Her husband is disabled following a stroke and she finds caring for him and looking after the house very stressful. She is not able to get out much and takes little exercise. She tends to eat convenience foods high in both fat and salt. Both her elder sisters died of ischaemic heart disease. Her body mass index is 31. Her estimated glomerular filtration rate is 80 ml/min (serum creatinine 80 μmol/l). She does not smoke. Her serum cholesterol is 6.4 mmol/l. On the ECG, the sum of the downwards deflection in V2 and the upwards deflection in V5 is 36 mm with T wave inversion in leads I and aVL. A random blood glucose level is 6.6 mmol/l. Her son, who is a paramedic, has found the British Hypertension Society recommendations for the treatment of blood pressure on the Internet. She is not keen to have drug treatment and she and her son have together concluded she does not need it.

a. Which factors, present in this woman's case, should lead to a different interpretation of the BHS guidelines, favouring treatment?

1. Impaired glucose tolerance
2. Diabetes
3. Her serum cholesterol
4. Renal impairment
5. Her age
6. Her gender
7. The fact that her high blood pressure was found by chance
8. Family history of ischaemic heart disease
9. High salt intake

10. High saturated fat intake
11. Obesity
12. Left ventricular hypertrophy
13. Right ventricular hypertrophy
14. Left ventricular strain
15. Right ventricular strain
16. First-degree heart block
17. Left ventricular failure
18. Inactivity
19. Environmental stress
20. Her husband's dependence on her

b. What drug(s) would it be appropriate to prescribe as first-line monotherapy for her hypertension?

1. Amiloride
2. Bendroflumethiazide
3. Spironolactone
4. Bumetanide
5. Furosemide
6. Atenolol
7. Bisoprolol
8. Carvedilol
9. Terazocin
10. Doxasocin
11. Prazocin
12. Amlodipine
13. Verapamil
14. Nifedipine
15. Lisinopril
16. Ramipril
17. Irbesartan
18. Losartan
19. Atorvastatin
20. Simvastatin
21. Rosuvastatin

2. A 32-year-old woman is involved in a road traffic accident and experiences a blow to the right side of the chest and extensive bruising of her right leg. She is in such pain that she is bedbound for a week afterwards. When she begins to mobilise, she notices that her whole right leg is larger than her left. She has pain in the right side of the chest which catches her when she breathes. The antero-medial aspect of her right thigh is tender below the inguinal region.

Which of the following would be appropriate immediate actions?

1. Prescribing aspirin
2. Prescribing clopidogrel
3. Prescribing low molecular weight heparin
4. Prescribing streptokinase
5. Prescribing tissue plasminogen activator (tPA)
6. Prescribing warfarin
7. Measuring plasma fibrinogen
8. Measuring D-dimer
9. Measuring plasma plasminogen
10. Measuring fibrin degradation products
11. Recommending anti-embolism stockings
12. Requesting a ventilation : perfusion lung scan
13. Requesting an ultrasound scan of the leg veins
14. CT pulmonary angiography
15. Angiography with a pulmonary catheter, left in place afterwards for streptokinase infusion

Single key features question

A young man of mixed race is admitted with fever, tachycardia and anxiety. He reports dealing in heroin and has been a user for more than 5 years. On direct questioning he mentions that he has a tender area in his left groin and has been tested for hepatitis and AIDS. Examination reveals a 2 cm tender left groin swelling, tattoos and old venous injection track marks on his arms. He has hepatomegaly and a loud systolic murmur over his precordium, loudest at the right sternal edge.

You suspect the diagnosis of left groin abscess, tricuspid endocarditis and hepatitis C. Which features lead you to these diagnoses? How would you manage him?

Data interpretation questions

1. Each of the following signs is strongly suggestive of a cardiovascular diagnosis; what is the diagnosis and what is the cause/mechanism of the sign?
   a. Splinter haemorrhages
   b. Absent A wave in the jugular venous pulse
   c. Septal lines on a chest radiograph
   d. M-shaped QRS complex >3 small squares on the ECG
   e. A mid-systolic click and late systolic murmur
   f. Unmatched perfusion defect on a ventilation: perfusion lung scan
   g. Diastolic opening snap
   h. Pulsatile hepatomegaly
   i. Collapsing pulse
   j. Rib notching on chest radiograph

2. What cardiac rhythm is shown in each of the short rhythm strips given in Figure 16A–N?

3. Interpret the 12-lead ECGs given in Figure 17.

4. The two traces shown in Figure 18 were taken from a patient in a coronary care unit. At the time of the first (Fig. 18A) she was free of pain. The second (Fig. 18B) was taken after she complained of chest pain. Interpret the first ECG. What new changes are shown in the second?

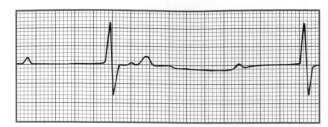

Fig. 16E

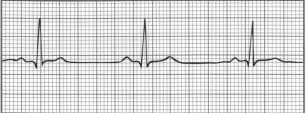

Fig. 16A

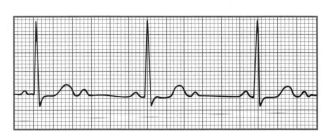

Fig. 16F

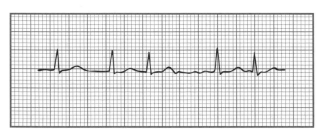

Fig. 16B

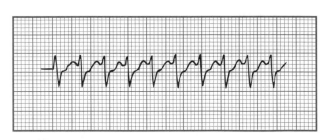

Fig. 16G

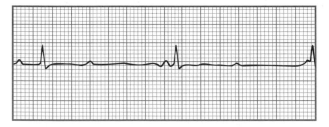

Fig. 16C

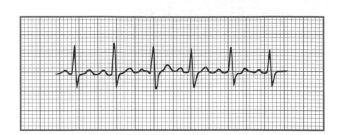

Fig. 16H

Fig. 16D

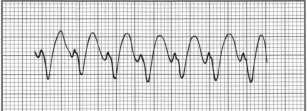

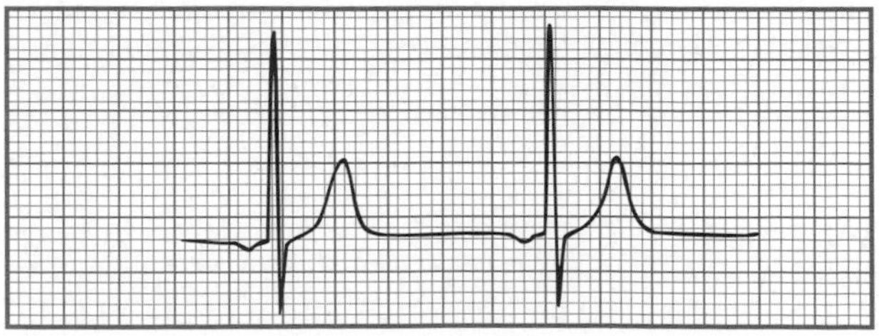

Fig. 16I

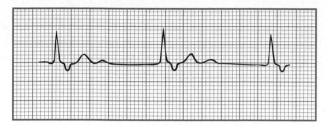

Fig. 16J

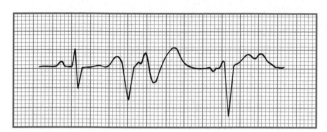

Fig. 16K

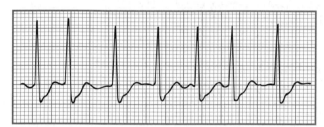

Fig. 16L

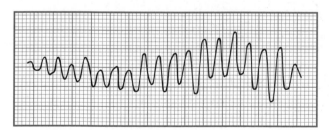

Fig. 16M

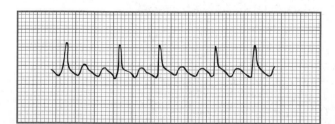

Fig. 16N

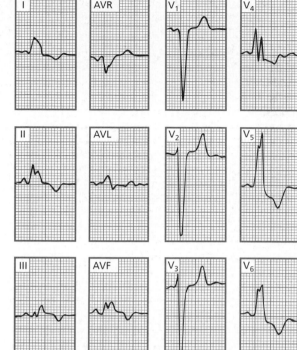

Fig. 17A

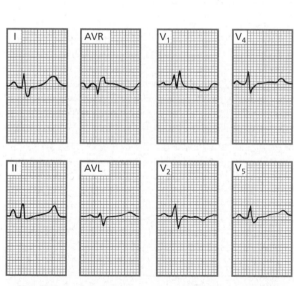

Fig. 17B

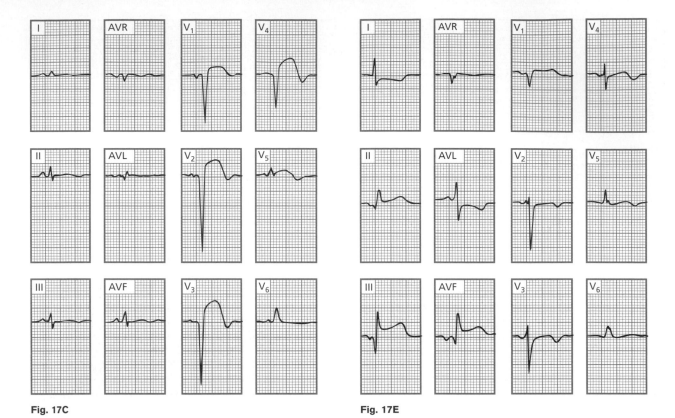

Fig. 17C

Fig. 17E

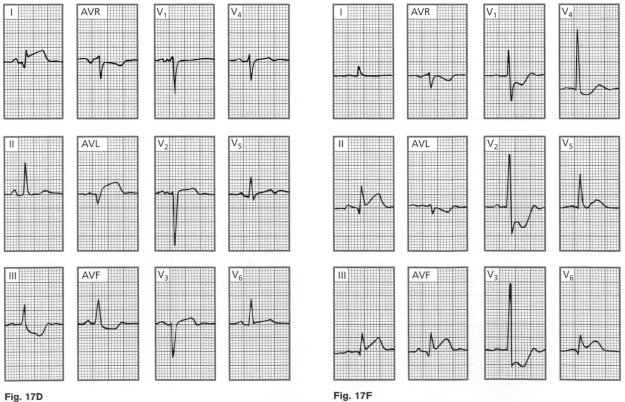

Fig. 17D

Fig. 17F

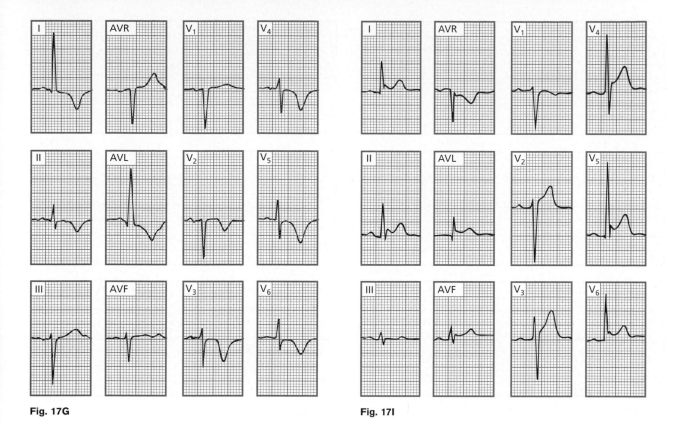

Fig. 17G

Fig. 17I

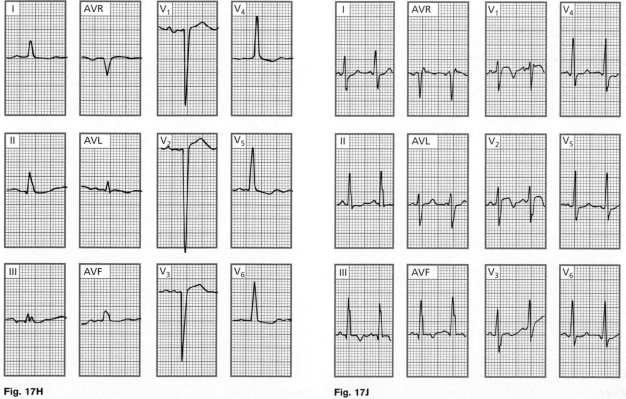

Fig. 17H

Fig. 17J

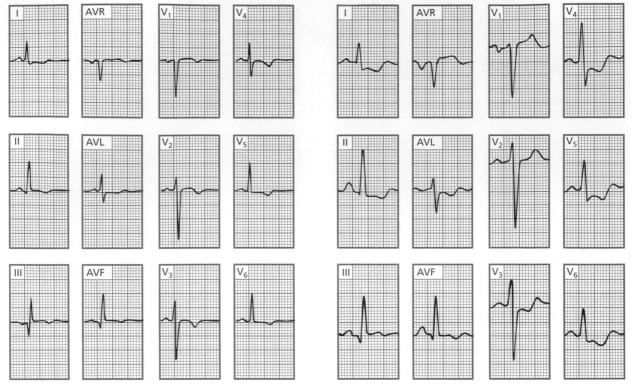

Fig. 18A

Fig. 18B

Self-assessment: answers

Multiple choice answers

1. a. **False.** The *right* ventricle presses against the sternum; the left ventricle constitutes the apex and is felt under the fingers.

   b. **True.**

   c. **True.**

   d. **False.** The apex is the downmost, outermost point at which pulsation can be felt, not the point of maximum impulse.

   e. **True.** Anterior myocardial infarction is caused by disease of the left anterior descending artery.

2. a. **True.**

   b. **False.** Parasympathetic slowing of the sino-atrial (SA) node would not be expected to cause such a slow pulse rate. The likely explanation is conducting tissue disease with an 'idioventricular' pacemaker relatively low in the conducting system, i.e. complete heart block.

   c. **True.** This is faster than would be expected for a sinus tachycardia.

   d. **False.** This is nonsensical because the mitral and tricuspid sounds make up the *first* heart sound.

   e. **True.** Lack of compliance of the arterial walls is a feature of ageing. Old people may have a high pulse pressure despite a normal or reduced stroke volume.

3. a. **False.** See Table 3.

   b. **True.**

   c. **True.**

   d. **True.** It may also be a digoxin effect.

   e. **True.**

4. a. **False.**

   b. **False.** Rare; the clues to cardiac tamponade are: (i) raised jugular venous pressure, (ii) quiet heart sounds, (iii) absence of chest signs, (iv) pulsus paradoxus.

   c. **True.**

   d. **True.**

   e. **False.** About 50% have a rub, which is one reason why the diagnosis is difficult.

5. a. **False.** It is normal for the jugular venous pressure to rise on expiration; Kussmaul's sign of pericarditis is for it to rise on *inspiration*.

   b. **False.** This is a sign of tricuspid incompetence.

   c. **True.**

   d. **True.** Pulmonary embolism may cause acute right heart failure.

   e. **False.** In some situations, e.g. right ventricular infarction and acute pulmonary embolism,

diuretic therapy worsens cardiac output by reducing the abnormally high filling pressure.

6. a. **True.**

   b. **True.**

   c. **True.**

   d. **True.** Turner's syndrome, 45X0.

   e. **False.** Because the cardiac output is fixed and cannot rise with exercise, vasodilator therapy is dangerous.

7. a. **False.** It is much higher.

   b. **True.**

   c. **True.** Nitroprusside or labetalol infusion is a recommended treatment.

   d. **False.** Aortic *regurgitation* may occur.

   e. **True.** The coronary ostia may be occluded by the dissection.

8. a. **False.** An ACE inhibitor is indicated early in almost every patient with heart failure because it improves life expectancy.

   b. **True.** Alcoholic cardiomyopathy.

   c. **True.** Tuberculosis may cause constrictive pericarditis in later years although, since this causes extrinsic compression of the heart, some people may not call it 'heart failure'.

   d. **False.** Wheeze may occur as a result of heart failure alone (cardiac asthma).

   e. **False.** Third heart sounds may be heard in healthy young people.

9. a. **False.** There is well proven benefit, particularly in the prevention of stroke.

   b. **True.**

   c. **True.**

   d. **False.** ACE inhibitors are teratogenic and, therefore, are contraindicated in pregnancy.

   e. **False.** Cushing's syndrome, not Addison's disease.

10. a. **True.**

    b. **True.** Hypothyroidism causes hypercholesterolaemia and atherosclerosis.

    c. **True.** By increasing blood viscosity and impairing blood flow.

    d. **False.**

    e. **False.**

11. a. **True.** Typically, paroxysmal atrial tachycardia.

    b. **True.**

    c. **True.** Particularly congenital complete heart block.

d. **False.** Digoxin slows the ventricular rate during paroxysms of atrial fibrillation but does not prevent them; sotalol or amiodarone may prevent them.

e. **True.**

Single best answer multiple choice answers

1. **d is correct.** It is possible for a person who is not diabetic to become hyperglycaemic because the acute stress of a stroke causes large amounts of adrenaline (epinephrine) to be released. It is also possible for a person to become hypertensive because of the 'space-occupying' effect of an intracranial haemorrhage. Of course, hypertension and diabetes are risk factors for stroke. So both hypertension and hyperglycaemia have a 'chicken and egg' relationship with acute stroke. Examining the fundi can give important evidence as to which of those disorders antedated the stroke. Unfortunately, both diabetes and hypertension cause stroke by affecting small blood vessels, so their retinal appearances are similar. Arterio-venous nipping is a feature of hypertensive retinopathy. Hard exudates, flame haemorrhages and cotton wool spots are features of both diabetic and hypertensive retinopathy. The correct answer is **new vessels**, because they are specific to diabetic retinopathy.

2. **b is correct.** Particularly in hypertensive patients who are volume-expanded, a loop diuretic is a useful adjunct to an ACE inhibitor. a is incorrect because ACE inhibitors are mildly diuretic. c is incorrect because oral therapy or intravenous labetalol would be appropriate treatments for a hypertensive crisis. d is incorrect because ACE inhibitors are beneficial in many cases of renal failure, though they can worsen renal failure in patients with renovascular disease. e is incorrect because ACE inhibitors increase insulin sensitivity and are more likely to cause hypoglycaemia than hyperglycaemia.

3. **d is correct.** a is incorrect because the threshold for prescribing a statin is much lower in secondary than primary prevention. b is incorrect because aspirin would be a more appropriate choice. c is incorrect because left axis deviation is likely to be due to hypertension in this situation and is not an indication for echocardiography. e is incorrect because beta-blockers improve the prognosis in patients with heart failure; whilst it would be appropriate to control the heart failure first, a beta-blocker should be given to such a patient in due course.

4. **e is correct.** About 10% of patients with subacute bacterial endocarditis (SBE) present with a TIA or stroke and so this diagnosis should always be considered. About 10–20% of patients with SBE have little or no fever. a is incorrect. Three sets

taken separately over a maximum of 12 hours (and preferably less if the patient is acutely ill) are necessary. b is incorrect — transthoracic echocardiography is specific but not sensitive. Transoesophageal echocardiography is better. c is incorrect. Older, hospitalised patients are less likely to have endocarditis than younger patients from the community. d is incorrect because viruses have not been reported to cause endocarditis alone.

5. **d is correct.** For two reasons; first, the selected combinations are usually additive or synergistic. Second, to prevent the development of resistance. a is incorrect because *viridans* organisms are usually exquisitely susceptible to penicillin and gentamicin and 2 weeks of therapy suffices. b is incorrect; although flucloxacillin (with gentamicin or rifampicin) is the medical treatment of choice but valve replacement is not appropriate. Insertion of a prosthetic heart valve into a drug addict is very likely to lead to prosthetic valve endocarditis subsequently because of their continuing habit. c is incorrect. Once appropriate antimicrobial treatment is given, infection is rarely a problem. e is also incorrect. Toxicity (deafness, loss of balance and/or renal impairment) is more common if treatment is given for more than 2 weeks and so blood level monitoring is even more important.

Extended matched answers

EMQ 1

A. **11.** Heparin therapy is indicated in this situation; although low molecular weight heparin costs more than unfractionated heparin, it has been shown in clinical trials to be more effective and avoids the cost of laboratory monitoring.

B. **13.** As a house officer, you should call for senior help and probably admit the patient to a coronary care unit, but intravenous adenosine ('medical cardioversion') is usually the first-line therapy.

C. **10.** There are no obvious contraindications to warfarin, which reduces the risk of stroke caused by cerebral embolism.

D. **19.** She has a symptomatic bradycardia, which is likely to resolve spontaneously but should — in the short term — be treated with intravenous atropine.

E. **4.** Digoxin has been shown to relieve the symptoms of chronic congestive cardiac failure and reduce the hospital admission rate.

EMQ 2

A. **17 or 12.** D-dimer might be considered appropriate, but she has such a high pre-test probability of DVT that she should proceed directly to an ultrasound scan without D-dimer measurement. Venography would also be informative but is only indicated if the ultrasound scan is inconclusive.

B. **1.** Direct visualization of the heart valves may reveal vegetations; echocardiography is more informative by the transoesophageal than the transthoracic route.

C. **1.** Again, transoesophageal echocardiography is the investigation of choice. MR or CT scan may also be used.

D. **14.** The history strongly suggests acute pericarditis. In the first instance, a 12-lead ECG should be performed. Extensive upwardly concave ST segments would support the diagnosis.

E. **2.** The important diagnosis not to miss here is myocardial infarction, given that she has a history suggestive of angina and is taking a number of antianginal drugs. Cardiac troponin is a sensitive investigation, which allows you to exclude a diagnosis of myocardial infarction.

EMQ 3

A. **5.** Raised jugular venous pressure after acute myocardial infarction suggests a right ventricular infarct. The management is to maintain a good filling pressure to the right ventricle. Diuretics can worsen it, so (apparently paradoxically) diuretic therapy can have an adverse effect in this situation.

B. **1.** 'Reperfusion dysrhythmias' in a haemodynamically stable patient early after acute myocardial infarction do not need to be treated.

C. **3.** The prognosis is poor in this situation.

D. **1.** There is no indication for 'routine' antidysrhythmic therapy.

Responses to OSCE stations

OSCE 1

Although the patient's symptoms are in the left leg, you should examine them both. He may have arterial disease in both legs; perhaps his left leg stops him walking far enough to get pain in the right one. Alternatively, he may have only one affected leg, in which case a comparison of the two sides will be informative. You should expose both legs up to the level of the groin, covering his genitalia with a blanket if he is not wearing pants.

Inspection Comment on surgical scars (e.g. from previous bypass surgery), signs of established ischaemia or ulceration, skin changes, or the rather atrophic, hairless legs of peripheral vascular disease.

Palpation Examine the feet carefully, including under the heel and between the toes, for signs of ulcers. If a dressing is present, indicate to the examiner that you would like to look underneath it. Test for capillary refill by pressing on a nail bed for a moment or two and observing the length of time for colour to return (usually ≤2 s). Feel the femoral, popliteal, dorsalis pedis and posterior tibial pulses of both feet. Also, listen over the femoral arteries for bruits.

Buerger's manoeuvre Ischaemic limbs quickly become pale when elevated to 45°. When the limb is then lowered, reddening and cyanosis may occur.

OSCE 2

a. Swollen legs may be caused by:

- cellulitis
- raised venous pressure, systemically or locally
- lymphoedema
- hypoalbuminaemia.

This man has a process affecting both legs so think first of a disease process which is systemic or proximal to the legs. It could be heart failure, lymphoedema, hypoalbuminaemia or vena caval compression or thrombosis; but why is the swelling asymmetrical? Perhaps he has dual pathology. Patients with bilateral swollen legs for those reasons may develop a secondary venous thrombosis or cellulitis within one leg. The patient could also have bilateral deep vein thromboses (DVTs) or bilateral cellulitis affecting one leg more than the other.

b. You should examine the legs for the signs of DVT and cellulitis (Ch. 10); look for signs of heart failure (Fig. 8). Do a careful abdominal examination and say you would proceed to a rectal examination because lymphoedema, caval compression/thrombosis and bilateral DVTs could be caused by abdominal malignancy. Although you were not directly asked this, it would show that you are thinking through the problem logically if you state that you would like to know the patient's plasma albumin.

OSCE 3

You should structure your answer and, ideally, show your depth of knowledge by indicating the weight of each piece of information.

History History of myocardial infarction and symptoms of angina or heart failure; suggestive of ischaemic heart disease (IHD) if present but unable to exclude IHD.

Examination Signs of heart failure might indicate underlying IHD and signs of peripheral vascular disease would be presumptive evidence of widespread arterial disease, but physical examination is relatively insensitive for IHD.

Investigations Resting ECG may show evidence of old myocardial infarction or ischaemia; informative if abnormal but relatively insensitive.

Ambulatory ECG may show 'silent' ischaemic changes at rest or precipitated by exertion.

Exercise ECG is much more sensitive than the resting ECG but lacks the sensitivity and specificity of coronary angiography.

Coronary angiogram is the 'gold standard', both sensitive and specific for IHD.

A myocardial perfusion scan at rest and after stress is a sensitive investigation to detect areas of impaired coronary perfusion.

Case history answers

Case history 1

1. Most likely causes are alcoholic cardiomyopathy and ischaemic heart disease. Possible causes are hypertension and valvular heart disease.

2. The most likely complications are arterial thrombo-embolism and dysrhythmias.

3. Likelihood of continued drinking, which could cause dangerously unstable anticoagulation. Peptic ulcer and/or oesophageal varices are likely in view of severe alcohol abuse.

Case history 2

1. The history and signs strongly suggest aortic stenosis; he has exertional dyspnoea, angina and syncope. His pulse pressure is narrow and he has left ventricular hypertrophy. He may have ischaemic heart disease (IHD). He is not hypertensive so an aortic aneurysm is unlikely. You should exclude anaemia.

2. He needs an urgent echocardiogram. If the diagnosis of tight aortic stenosis is confirmed, he needs referral to a cardiac surgeon urgently. If not, he should be investigated for IHD.

Key features answers

1a. **3, 8, 12, 14 are correct**. You cannot diagnose impaired glucose tolerance or diabetes on her random blood glucose level. Many features of her history increase the risk of hypertension but are not, in themselves, indications for therapy. The strongest argument in favour of treatment is that she has high cardiovascular risk by virtue of:

- high serum cholesterol
- family history of ischaemic heart disease.

The ECG is compatible with left ventricular hypertrophy and strain, which is evidence of target organ damage and a further indication for treatment.

1b. **2, 12, 13 and 14 are correct**. According to the 'A, B, C, D' approach, appropriate first-line monotherapy for an older hypertensive patient would be a thiazide diuretic or calcium antagonist. Amlodipine would be suitable, as would delayed-release preparations of nifedipine or verapamil.

2. **3, 11 and 13 are correct**. She has a high clinical probability of deep vein thrombosis (DVT) so D-dimer should not be measured. She should be heparinised pending an ultrasound scan of the affected leg. It would be reasonable to recommend anti-embolism stockings to increase blood flow in the affected calf and reduce oedema. Since she is very likely to have a positive scan of her leg veins, it is unnecessary to perform a lung scan because knowing she has had a pulmonary embolism will not change the management if (as is likely) a DVT is diagnosed.

Single key features answer

Tricuspid endocarditis = fever and murmur of tricuspid incompetence. It is a common problem in intravenous drug addicts. Is the hepatomegaly pulsatile? Does he have giant J waves in his jugular venous pulse? (Go back and examine him!)

Groin abscess = fever and tender groin swelling. Does he have femoral thrombophlebitis as well? Is there any swelling of his left leg or oedema? (Go back and examine him!)

Hepatitis C = long history of intravenous drug abuse, history of being tested and hepatomegaly. However, hepatomegaly may be due to tricuspid incompetence. He needs testing for hepatitis C virus (HCV) RNA as well as HCV antibodies.

Investigations include

- blood culture (two or three samples at different times), ECG, chest radiograph, urea and electrolytes (to manage antibiotics), full blood count
- aspiration of groin abscess for aerobic and anaerobic culture
- hepatitis BsAg, hepatitis C antibody (and liver function tests) and possibly HIV
- echocardiogram (urgent)
- label all blood specimens 'high risk'.

Management depends on status:

- Cardiac status poor and left-sided lesions: commence antibiotics immediately after taking blood cultures and consider transfer to regional cardiothoracic unit immediately.
- Cardiac status reasonable and left-sided lesion: commence antibiotics after taking blood cultures and arrange urgent echocardiogram.
- Right-sided lesion: clinically, commence antibiotics immediately after blood cultures taken and monitor carefully to check no other complications of sepsis and you have not missed a left-sided lesion.

You will probably need a central line. Give ampicillin 2 g 4-hourly, flucloxacillin 2 g 4-hourly and gentamicin 1.5 mg/kg 12-hourly (or equivalent) if renal function normal. Add metronidazole orally for groin abscess. The drugs and dosages may need to be altered when the results of cultures are known. Surgical referral is not necessary unless left-sided endocarditis occurs. After appropriate counselling, an HIV test would be appropriate.

Data interpretation answers

1. a. Infective endocarditis. Caused by a small vessel vasculitis.

   b. This indicates loss of atrial contraction, typically seen in atrial fibrillation.

c. Pulmonary venous hypertension. Caused by interstitial oedema.

d. Bundle branch block or intraventricular conduction delay. The width of the complex indicates that the impulse has spread slowly through ventricular muscle rather than conducting tissues.

e. Mitral valve prolapse. Caused by the valve cusps sliding over one another during systole and prolapsing back into the left atrium.

f. Pulmonary embolism. Signifies non-perfusion of an aerated segment of lung.

g. Mitral stenosis. Caused by high left atrial pressure and the opening of a stenotic mitral value in early diastole; this sign is lost when the value is calcified and immobile.

h. Tricuspid incompetence. Pressure is transmitted back into the venous system from the right ventricle through the incompetent valve.

i. Aortic regurgitation. Incompetence of the valve causes a low diastolic pressure and increased stroke volume causes a high systolic pressure; the increased pulse pressure is felt as a collapsing pulse.

j. Coarctation of the aorta. Caused by collateral intercostal vessels bypassing the coarct.

2. A. Sinus bradycardia, rate 52/min. Each QRS complex is preceded by a P wave with a normal PR interval.

B. Atrial fibrillation, rate 105/min. The QRS complexes are completely irregular; fine fibrillation waves can be seen between the third and fourth complexes.

C. Complete heart block with junctional escape rhythm. The ventricular rate is 42 beats/min. P waves can be seen at a rate of 75/min; the fifth P wave can just be seen before the upstroke of the R wave. The atria and ventricles are beating independently of one another. The complexes are less than three small squares in width indicating that ventricular depolarisation is propagating through the normal conducting pathways. The ventricular rate, though slow, is not catastrophically slow. Contrast this with Figure 16E.

D. Broad complex tachycardia (>3 small squares), rate 166/min. On this rhythm strip alone, you cannot distinguish between ventricular and supraventricular tachycardia (see text).

E. Complete heart block with left ventricular escape rhythm. The ventricular rate is 29/min; P waves can be seen at a rate of 53/min, again completely independent of the ventricular complexes. The complexes are broader than in Figure 16C, confirming their origin within the ventricles.

F. Sinus tachycardia, rate 143/min. P waves are clearly visible before each QRS complex.

G. Second-degree (Mobitz type) heart block, rate 52/min. Each QRS is preceded by a P wave with a normal PR interval but for every conducted P wave there is one which is not conducted. Contrast this with Figure 16C in which the atria and ventricles are completely dissociated.

H. Supraventricular tachycardia, rate 250/min. The fact that it is a narrow complex tachycardia (<3 small squares) indicates that it is supraventricular. It is absolutely regular, excluding atrial fibrillation.

I. (High) junctional rhythm, rate 56/min. There are small P waves at the same interval before each QRS complex. The PR interval is short and the P waves are inverted. The impulse is arising in the region of the atrioventricular (AV) node, spreading backwards through the atrium (hence the inverted P wave) and causing atrial depolarisation just ahead of ventricular depolarisation.

J. (Low) junctional rhythm. Similar to Figure 16I but the inverted P waves are coming between the R and the T wave. The site of impulse generation is closer to the ventricle than the atrium and the order of depolarisation is reversed.

K. Multifocal ventricular ectopic beats. There is a sinus beat followed by two bizarre, broad complexes (their breadth indicating that they arise within the ventricle) which differ from one another in shape, showing that they arise from different foci. The configuration of the P wave and the electrical axis of the fourth complex have changed from the first beat but the complex is of supraventricular origin.

L. Fast atrial fibrillation, rate 140/min. Narrow complexes with an irregular rhythm are diagnostic of atrial fibrillation. The faster the rate, the harder it may be to detect the irregularity. Mark out the complexes with a piece of paper and slide it along the rhythm strip to detect irregularity.

M. Ventricular fibrillation. Broad, rapid, disorganised impulses are diagnostic of ventricular fibrillation.

N. Atrial flutter with variable block, rate 113/min. This is a narrow complex tachycardia with obvious flutter waves. The timing of the QRS complexes is irregular because of variable conduction of the flutter impulse.

3. A Left bundle branch block. There are P waves and a normal PR interval but the QRS complex is >3 small squares because of slow spread through the ventricular muscle. M-shaped complexes in the lateral chest leads are the characteristic of *left* bundle branch block.

B. Right bundle branch block. Like Figure 17A, a sinus rhythm, but in this case the M-shaped complexes are in V1. The right-sided chest leads are normally predominantly negative; in this case, most of the deflection is in a positive direction.

C. Acute anterior myocardial infarct. There are Q waves (indicating full thickness infarction), ST segment elevation and T wave inversion in leads V1–5, characteristic of anterior infarction. ST segment elevation usually does not persist more than a few days, showing that it is a recent event. Note also that the T waves are flat or inverted in the lateral (I, aVL) and inferior (II, III, aVF) leads, suggesting widespread ischaemia.

D. Acute lateral infarct. There are Q waves and ST segment elevation in leads I and aVL. There is also some ST segment elevation in the anterior chest leads. There is ST segment *depression* in leads III and aVF. Misleadingly termed 'reciprocal ST segment depression', this is a sign of ischaemia extending beyond the area which has actually infarcted.

E. Acute inferior infarct. There are Q waves in III and aVF, and ST segment elevation in II, III and aVF. Reciprocal ST segment depression is seen in I and aVL. There is T wave inversion in V2–5, suggesting widespread ischaemia. Note also the short PR interval and inverted P waves suggesting a junctional rhythm.

F. Inferior infarct with posterior and lateral extension. The changes of inferior infarction are similar to Figure 17E, including reciprocal ST depression in the anterior chest leads. There is ST elevation in V6, indicating lateral extension. Note that V1 is predominantly positive, without the M-shaped complex of right bundle branch block. This is the appearance of posterior infarction.

G. Subendocardial (non-Q wave) infarct. There is deep T wave inversion in V2–6, I, aVL and II but no Q waves. This suggests extensive partial thickness (subendocardial) myocardial infarction.

H. Left ventricular hypertrophy. The maximum downwards deflection is in V2 (37 small squares). The maximum upwards deflection is in V5 (15 small squares). The sum (52 small squares) is very much increased. There are widespread downsloping ST segments. There are also Q waves across the septal leads (V1–3), suggesting a previous myocardial infarct.

I. Pericarditis. There is ST segment elevation in leads I, II, aVL and V2–6. The shape of the ST segment ('dished' or upwardly concave), seen well in V4–6 (contrast with ECG C), is characteristic of pericarditis, as is the wide distribution of the ST segment elevation.

J. There is a sinus tachycardia (115/min) with T wave inversion in V1–3, an S wave in lead I and a Q wave and T wave inversion in lead III ('SI, QIII, TIII'). These changes result from acute right ventricular strain; pulmonary embolism is a likely cause.

4. The first ECG (Fig. 18A) shows an inferior myocardial infarct. There are Q waves and T wave inversion in III and aVF. There is also T wave inversion in V1–6 compatible with anterior ischaemia. The second ECG (Fig. 18B) shows myocardial ischaemia. ST segment depression has developed in V3–6, I and aVL. This is characteristic of ischaemia. Her chest pain is probably caused by unstable angina, an indication for urgent angiography with a view to revascularisation.

Respiratory disease

2.1 Clinical aspects

Learning objectives

You should be able to:

- describe how the important principles of respiratory anatomy and physiology are affected in the common respiratory diseases
- interpret the common respiratory symptoms and signs and construct a differential diagnosis based on probabilities
- describe how you would use investigations in respiratory medicine appropriately for the clinical problem
- set out the principles of management of the common respiratory diseases and the immediate treatment of the common respiratory emergencies.

Case Study

John has been troubled by periods of wheezing over many years, often with an irritating cough following a cold. Mostly, he finds that if he uses his brown inhaler regularly, then he only needs the blue one occasionally or if his chest is bad. Recently, he has become worried because of coughing up yellow 'plugs' and his wheezing has been worse.

Anatomy

You must know the important anatomy of the respiratory tract as this influences the ways in which clinical problems present or diseases develop.

The right main bronchus divides into the upper and intermediate bronchi, with the latter dividing into the **middle** and lower lobe bronchi.

On the left side, the main bronchus divides into the upper and lower lobe bronchi. The **lingular** branch of the upper lobe bronchus is sometimes affected by bronchiectasis (p. 79). All bronchi divide into segmental and subsegmental branches until the acinus is reached, in which a terminal bronchus subdivides into bronchioles supplying alveoli.

The divisions of the major bronchi are linked to the lobes of the lungs. The left lung is divided into upper and lower lobes by the **oblique** fissure, which runs from the fourth vertebra to the sixth costochondral junction anteriorly. The right lung is subdivided into upper, middle and lower lobes by the addition of the **horizontal** fissure, which begins at the oblique fissure in the mid-axillary line running anteriorly to the sternal end of the fourth costochondral cartilage.

Diaphragm

The diaphragm is a muscular sheet with a central tendon on which the pericardium sits; hence the cardiac shadow on a chest radiograph is narrowed and elongated when the patient inspires (diaphragm *descends*) and is broadened when the person *expires*. Cardiomegaly may, therefore, be erroneously diagnosed on a radiograph if the patient fails to breathe in adequately. Conversely, cardiac enlargement may be missed in hyperinflation. The nerve supply to the diaphragm is the phrenic nerve (C3, 4, 5). Paralysis causes *paradoxical* movement, i.e. on inspiration, the diaphragm on that side ascends (instead of descending).

Interpretation of examination and radiographic findings

In any patient with a possible respiratory (or cardiac) problem, a chest radiograph is a useful investigation. You need to be able to relate the anatomical relationships to your clinical findings or radiographic abnormalities. Important points to note are:

- If possible, you should always request posteroanterior (PA) films. AP (portable) films may give a false impression of cardiomegaly.
- Abnormalities posteriorly on clinical examination point to pathology in the lower lobes.
- You should describe masses on PA radiographs as being in the upper, mid- or lower zones (*not lobes*).

- A lateral radiograph will help to localise an abnormality.
- Upper lobe collapse causes *tracheal* deviation.
- Lower lobe collapse causes *mediastinal* shift and the *left* lower lobe collapses behind the heart.
- The right *middle* lobe collapses as a triangle adjacent to the right heart with loss of the border.

Pulmonary vasculature and lymphatics

The divisions of the pulmonary arteries follow those of the bronchi to the lung parenchyma. The pulmonary venules eventually drain into the four pulmonary veins. In heart failure, 'upper lobe diversion' is reported on radiographs, meaning that the upper lobe veins are visible and distended (p. 9).

In pulmonary hypertension, the peripheral arteries become narrowed. On a radiograph, this is seen as 'pruning' of the pulmonary arteries, with little flow to the periphery (oligaemia). In a large pulmonary embolus, blocking one of the large arteries may limit the oligaemia to one zone of the radiograph.

The lungs have an extensive lymphatic network that may be infiltrated by cancer cells, causing blockage. Usually the lymph channels are not visible on a radiograph, but in **lymphangitis carcinomatosis** they can be seen as fine lines adjacent to the peripheral lung borders — **Kerley B lines**. The lymphatic network drains into the **thoracic duct**, which runs posteriorly to the root of the neck. *Trauma* and *malignancy* may cause blockage of the duct and leakage of lymph into the pleural space — **chylothorax**.

Pulmonary physiology

The main function of the lungs is gas exchange and to achieve this efficiently there needs to be:

- adequate ventilation of the alveoli
- matching between ventilation ($\dot{V}$) and perfusion ($\dot{Q}$)
- adequate diffusion of gases between the alveoli and the capillary bed
- carriage of gases in the blood.

Other functions of the lungs include the modification of drugs and hormones (e.g. conversion of angiotensin I) and the provision of a physical and immunological (e.g. cilia, macrophages, immunoglobulin A, neutrophil elastase and α_1-antitrypsin) barrier to noxious agents, including pathogens.

Ventilation

Mechanics

Inspiration is an active process whereas expiration depends mainly on passive elastic recoil. The ribs move up and out (think of a bucket handle) and the diaphragm descends. As resistance to airflow increases (*obstruction*, as in chronic bronchitis and emphysema), the accessory muscles and the abdominal musculature are utilised.

Conditions which affect these structures may interfere with ventilation. For example:

- respiratory muscle weakness: Guillain–Barré syndrome

- diaphragmatic weakness: phrenic nerve palsy
- thoracic spine and rib disorders: kyphoscoliosis.

When ventilation is impaired, the cardinal abnormality is a raised partial pressure of carbon dioxide in an arterial blood sample (Pa_{CO_2}).

Control

The respiratory centre in the brainstem controls respiration. Neurogenic stimuli (pain, anxiety, volition) may affect respiration. The major function of the centre is to match respiration with metabolic needs, maintaining:

- Pa_{O_2} 11–13 kPa (80–100 mmHg)
- Pa_{CO_2} 4.8–6.0 kPa (35–45 mmHg)
- pH   7.35–7.44
- bicarbonate   22–30 mmol/l.

where Pa is arterial partial pressure.

These values are maintained, at rest, by a pulmonary blood flow of 5 l/min and a ventilation of 6 l/min. In any single breath, the tidal volume ($\approx$500 ml) can be divided into alveolar ventilation and dead-space ventilation; the latter is where no gas transfer takes place. In health, this is predominantly in the large airways ($\approx$150 ml), but pulmonary emboli, for example, can cause an increase in dead-space ventilation.

There are strong chemical stimuli (Pa_{O_2} and H^+) to breathe via the carotid and aortic bodies and the respiratory centre in the medulla. The most potent stimulus to ventilation is an increase in Pa_{CO_2}. In patients with chronic obstructive pulmonary disease (COPD), sensitivity to changes in Pa_{CO_2} can be lost such that reliance is placed on *hypoxic* drive (Pa_{O_2} < 8 kPa (60 mm Hg)). Correction with high inspired oxygen can then be dangerous (p. 89).

An increase in H^+ concentration (acidosis) stimulates ventilation, as in **Kussmaul's** respiration seen in **metabolic acidosis** (p. 198). The respiratory centre can be depressed (e.g. opiates, sedatives) or stimulated (e.g. aspirin) by drugs. Other stimuli include pulmonary embolism and sepsis.

Match of ventilation and perfusion

There is a wide variation in matching between alveolar ventilation ($\dot{V}A$) and perfusion ($\dot{Q}$) within the lungs. Towards the apices, ventilation tends to dominate, with the reverse being true towards the lung bases. Where there is perfusion without ventilation, **shunting** occurs, producing **hypoxaemia**, which is the hallmark of $\dot{V}/\dot{Q}$ mismatching. Normally, where ventilation is inadequate, the local control of blood flow causes vasoconstriction of arterioles. In diseases affecting the lung parenchyma, e.g. fibrosing alveolitis, this control breaks down and perfusion still occurs, causing hypoxia. It can also occur in atelectasis or collapse. In certain non-respiratory conditions such as sepsis or chronic liver disease, pulmonary arterioles can open up, again bypassing the alveoli and causing a shunt (and hence hypoxia).

In contrast to the change in blood-flow mechanisms causing hypoxia, increases in Pa_{CO_2} tend to occur where global (mechanical) ventilation is inadequate, e.g. in respiratory muscle weakness.

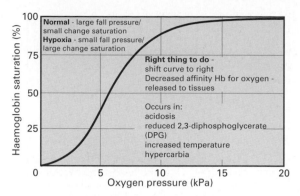

Fig. 19 Haemoglobin (Hb) dissociation curve and the variables that affect it.

The $\dot{V}/\dot{Q}$ match is used in the diagnosis of pulmonary emboli (p. 49). A ventilation:perfusion scan can show areas of the lung which are being ventilated but not perfused. Multiple defects are often seen in areas remote from a chest radiograph abnormality or the side with the pleuritic pain. However, there are significant limitations in the usefulness of $\dot{V}/\dot{Q}$ scans in diagnosis, particularly in COPD, where there is marked $\dot{V}/\dot{Q}$ mismatching. Computed tomography (CT) techniques (p. 50) are being used more and more in the diagnosis of pulmonary emboli.

Oxygen transport

Oxygen is carried within the blood predominantly as oxyhaemoglobin. The shape of the dissociation curve is sigmoid and its position can be shifted by change in other variables (Fig. 19). This ability is important as it can facilitate the transfer of oxygen to the tissues. Furthermore, the steepness of the middle part of the curve ensures that at Po_2 of ≤ 5.3 kPa (40 mmHg), as it is in the tissues, the haemoglobin readily gives up its oxygen. You need to be aware of the shape of the curve because of the widespread use of oxygen saturation monitors as a proxy for Pao_2. Whilst the arterial partial pressure is varying at the top part of the curve, the oxygen saturation will not change very much. However, on the steep part of the curve, a small change in saturation can indicate a large fall in Pao_2. A common pitfall is to equate the two measurements, but a saturation of 80% may indicate a Pao_2 of only 8 kPa (60 mm Hg).

Common symptoms

Breathlessness

Breathlessness is a subjective description of the sensation experienced by the patient. It does not equate completely with dyspnoea, which is difficulty with breathing deduced from your observations, nor is it tachypnoea (rapid rate of breathing).

You should clarify how much the patient is limited by shortness of breath. Two patients may answer 'quite a lot' meaning for one the inability to climb the stairs without stopping, for the other being unable to complete his daily 2–3 mile stroll. The onset of breathlessness may give a clue to the underlying pathological process. A smoker who has had worsening exercise tolerance over many years is likely to have chronic bronchitis and emphysema. If, however, the

same person has experienced a rapid deterioration coupled with general malaise and a productive cough, the problem is probably an acute infective exacerbation of his COPD.

Any variation in breathlessness needs to be assessed. How long have patients experienced breathlessness? How does it vary with time? What affects their breathing? For example, asthmatic patients may be worse in the summer or when they wake ('morning dipping').

Wheeze

Wheezing is a frequent symptom of patients with airflow obstruction. As with breathlessness, diurnal or seasonal variation would suggest asthma. Heart failure may present with wheezing — 'cardiac asthma'. A further consideration is whether the patient is not actually describing wheezing, but rather inspiratory stridor implying extrathoracic airflow obstruction.

Cough

Either in association with breathlessness or on its own, cough is an important symptom. In most people, it is simply caused by a recent infection. Some infections, such as *Mycoplasma*, can cause a prolonged dry cough (<4 weeks), but persistence may reflect bronchial hyperactivity resulting from asthma. You should initiate basic investigations (e.g. chest radiograph, peak expiratory flow rate (PEFR) measurement spirometry) in any patient with a persistent cough.

A productive cough is commonly seen in smokers, with the production of clear mucoid sputum. In patients with infection, the sputum colour changes to yellow or green and increases in volume. In patients with bronchopulmonary aspergillosis, yellow mucus plugs may be expectorated. Bronchiectasis is typically associated with a large volume of sputum that is frequently coloured, implying infection.

A chest radiograph should be requested in any smoker with a recent onset of a persistent cough.

Haemoptysis

Coughing up blood is a frightening symptom. Your framework for management is:

- Confirm that the problem is haemoptysis and not haematemesis or bleeding from the nasopharynx.
- Investigate thoroughly to exclude the possibility of a bronchial carcinoma; being a smoker will increase the likelihood of this.
- Consider other possible causes: for example, dry bronchiectasis (p. 79). Other causes are rupture of a small bronchial vein during a coughing bout (particularly in severe airflow obstruction) and pulmonary infarction.

Any current or ex-smoker, over 40 years, with haemoptysis should have a fibreoptic bronchoscopy and CT scan of the thorax even if the chest radiograph is normal.

Chest (non-anginal) pain

Chest pain is a common symptom. As with haemoptysis it is useful to have a framework:

Two

- Is it pleuritic? Sharp pain, worse on inspiration or coughing.
- Is it caused by a rib fracture? Sudden onset (prolonged coughing in a patient with chronic bronchitis); history of trauma; pain is worse on movement but may be increased by breathing/coughing; localised chest wall tenderness.
- Is it musculoskeletal? Very common; history similar to rib fracture but often lacking definite onset; strong relationship to movement; not particularly worsened by inspiration; often diagnosis by exclusion.
- Other causes? For example, herpes zoster can present with severe chest wall pain and is often misdiagnosed until the characteristic rash appears (pericardial pain is covered on p. 39, gastro-oesophageal reflux disease (GORD) on p. 121).

Respiratory investigations

Imaging

Plain radiographs have been considered above. CT is very useful in:

- diagnosis and staging of primary and secondary tumours
- detecting pulmonary infiltration, e.g. tumour
- assessing diffuse parenchymal lung disease
- assessing mediastinal masses including percutaneous lung biopsies
- CT-pulmonary angiography in the diagnosis of pulmonary emboli.

Magnetic resonance imaging (MRI) is now being increasingly used. Radioisotope scanning (ventilation:perfusion) is used in the diagnosis of pulmonary embolism (p. 49).

Respiratory function

For most patients, very simple tests are all that is required to assess respiratory function. **Peak expiratory flow rate** (PEFR) is a standard test for airflow obstruction; low values can also be obtained with poor technique or respiratory muscle weakness (e.g. in myasthenia gravis, p. 244). Normal or increased values may be seen in restrictive lung disease. Its principal use is in monitoring airflow obstruction at home or in hospital. You should be able to demonstrate the technique of measuring PEFR to the patient:

1. Hold the PEFR meter and take a deep breath in.
2. Place the mouthpiece in the mouth and wrap your lips around it.
3. Breathe out *as hard and as fast as you can.*

Ask the patient to repeat the measurement three times and record the best value.

The PEFR is dependent on age, height and gender. You should always interpret a test result by comparing it with the predicted value or (if monitoring airflow obstruction) with the patient's best value. There is a *diurnal* variation in bronchomotor tone, with it being greatest in the early hours of the morning (i.e. bronchoconstriction). In asthma, this variation is often exaggerated, producing **morning dipping** which can be severe (p. 94).

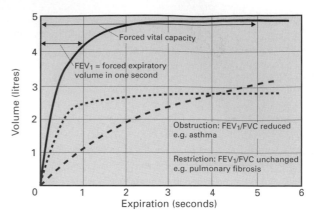

Fig. 20 Spirometric traces showing normal FEV_1 and FVC and those in obstructive and restrictive defects.

Spirometry provides more information, giving measurement of **forced expiratory volume in one second** (FEV_1) and **forced vital capacity** (FVC). Normal values are again dependent on age, height and gender. There is also a correction factor for race (10% reduction for patients of Indian subcontinent origin). Different traces are obtained depending on the pathophysiology present (Fig. 20).

Transfer factor is a measure of gas transfer in the alveoli. In most patients, reduction reflects $\dot{V}/\dot{Q}$ mismatching. For example, in pulmonary fibrosis the cause of hypoxia is not difficulty of oxygen passing across a thickened alveolar–capillary barrier, but the distortion of the pulmonary architecture such that part of the lungs are being perfused and not adequately ventilated. In patients with an increased amount of functioning haemoglobin in the lungs (polycythaemia, p. 273), shunts or fresh haemorrhage, transfer factor may be increased. The predominant use for measurement of transfer factor is as a surrogate marker for lung pathology.

Fibreoptic bronchoscopy

Fibreoptic bronchoscopy may be of use in:

- visualising and taking biopsies, brushings and washings (cytology) of possible endobronchial malignancies
- culture of secretions, brushings and washings for microbiological diagnosis (particularly for tuberculosis (p. 79) and *Pneumocystis jirovecii (carinii)* infection (p. 9); however, induced sputum (nebulised saline) has largely superseded this indication)
- **transbronchial biopsy** for diffuse parenchymal disease, e.g. sarcoid or extrinsic allergic alveolitis
- **broncho-alveolar lavage** for parenchymal disease; usually the cells in the washings are predominantly macrophages: in sarcoidosis, increased lymphocytes are found (T helper cells); in fibrosing alveolitis, there is an increase in polymorphs in active disease.

Pleural aspiration and biopsy

See page 97.

Blood gas analysis

In all patients with suspected respiratory disease oxygen saturation should be measured. In some respiratory conditions, blood gas analysis should be undertaken (e.g. airflow obstruction). In certain circumstances — for example, acute asthma — it is negligent not to do so if the oxygen saturation breathing air is <92%. Normal values are given in Table 2.

Interpretation of the results is important as further action will be based on this. Patients with acute $\dot{V}/\dot{Q}$ mismatching (e.g. acute asthma, penumonia) are hypoxic, with a respiratory alkalosis. This is type 1 respiratory failure (remember type 1: *low* $Paco_2$). If the mismatching continues, then renal excretion of bicarbonate over several hours/days will compensate (respiratory alkalosis with *compensatory* metabolic acidosis).

Patients with ventilatory failure (e.g. respiratory muscle weakness as in Guillain–Barré syndrome) are both hypoxic and hypercarbic, with a respiratory acidosis. This is type 2 respiratory failure (remember type 2: *high* $Paco_2$). In this, the kidney will retain bicarbonate and excrete H^+ to compensate (respiratory acidosis with *compensatory* metabolic alkalosis). Acid–base disturbances are discussed on page 197. Later in this chapter, there is discussion of the patterns of blood gas abnormalities found with specific respiratory diseases.

Microbiological investigations

Sputum examination, blood culture and serology are the most important tests for infection, which are discussed in detail under each disease.

Common drugs

Bronchodilators

The β-adrenoceptor agonists

Beta-agonists work, predominantly, by direct stimulation of β_2-adrenoceptors located in the airways. The primary consequence of this stimulation is smooth muscle relaxation.

The β-agonists are divided into short- and long-acting drugs, with the duration of action being 4 hours for the former and approximately 12 hours for the latter. Examples of short-acting drugs are salbutamol and terbutaline. Examples of long-acting drugs are salmeterol and formoterol. Short-acting drugs are usually used on an 'as-required' basis to treat acute symptoms of airflow obstruction, while long-acting drugs are used regularly, twice a day, to control symptoms.

The preferred route of administration is by inhalation, although tablet and nebuliser preparations are available. Metered-dose inhalers (MDI) are the most commonly prescribed device, although patients often cannot use them. Explanation about the reasons for using the device and objective measurements of inhaler technique are essential components of inhaler prescription. The basic technique for an MDI is:

1. Remove the cap
2. Shake the inhaler
3. Fully expire
4. Place inhaler in mouth and 'fire' at the start of inspiration
5. Continue to full inspiration
6. Hold breath, then repeat if prescribed.

If the patient finds this difficult, spacer systems or dry powder systems (e.g. accuhalers, turbohalers) should be tried (e.g volumatic, nebuhaler). Occasionally, oral administration is necessary, but large doses must be used to produce the same effects on airway smooth muscle, in which case toxic side-effects (tremor, anxiety and palpitations) may occur. In severe chronic asthma, home nebuliser therapy can be effective.

Anticholinergics

There is a cholinergic nerve supply to the bronchial tree, stimulation of which causes bronchoconstriction. Both short-acting (ipratropium and oxitropium) and long-acting (tiotropium) anticholinergics are available. They have a place in the management of some patients with COPD but their value in chronic asthma is small. They are poorly absorbed orally and are given as an MDI or, in severe cases, home nebuliser. In acute severe asthma, ipratropium is given in combination with β_2-agonists.

Theophyllines

Theophyllines have a complex mechanism of action. A primary effect is antagonism of intracellular phosphodiesterase, thereby preventing the breakdown of cyclic adenosine monophosphate (cAMP). As with β-adrenoceptor stimulation, this promotes smooth muscle relaxation. Oral theophyllines are available in a variety of forms. Monitoring of blood levels is advisable and prescription should specify a brand as different makes of theophylline have differing bioavailability. Side-effects include gastrointestinal (nausea, abdominal pain), cardiac (palpitations, arrhythmia) and central nervous system (insomnia, anxiety and, occasionally, convulsions) symptoms. Overdose may cause convulsions and dysrhythmias.

Prophylaxis and anti-inflammatory drugs

Corticosteroids

Corticosteroids work by suppressing the inflammatory response. Inhaled fluorinated corticosteroids (beclometasone, fluticasone, budesonide) should be administered on a regular basis to patients who have reversible airflow limitation *and* who require bronchodilators more than three times a week or who have had acute exacerbations in the last 2 years. One problem you will encounter is oropharyngeal candidiasis with dysphonia. Oral corticosteroids should be reserved for patients with chronic asthma unresponsive to maximum inhaled combined treatment. The dose of prednisolone should be kept, where possible, to under 10 mg to reduce adrenal suppression and long-term problems such as osteoporosis and cataracts. The patient should be monitored for hypertension and diabetes. If oral corticosteroids are prescribed for more than 3 months, a bisphosphonate should be given to prevent osteoporosis. Inhaled and oral steroids can be combined.

Corticosteroids are used in other respiratory conditions, such as vasculitis or sarcoidosis. Again, the dose of prednisolone should be kept to a minimum to decrease the risk of side-effects. The use of other immunosuppressive drugs is considered in the relevant sections.

Leukotriene antagonists

Leukotriene antagonists (LTAs) are used as an adjunctive oral prophylactic treatment for mild-to-moderate asthma. Leukotrienes are formed by the breakdown of arachidonic acid and are important inflammatory mediators (C_4, D_4 and E_4) in asthma. Two products, montelukast and zafirlukast, bind to the leukotriene D_4 receptor and block the production of some leukotrienes, benefiting some patients with asthma as an add-on treatment with inhaled cortico-steroids and a short-acting β_2-agonist (step 3, British guidelines, p. 92). Patients with aspirin-sensitive asthma are particularly likely to benefit from this treatment. Side-effects of LTAs include nausea, abdominal pain, headache and rashes.

Sodium cromoglicate

A primary action of sodium cromoglicate is to stabilise the mast cell preventing histamine release. It is occasionally used as prophylaxis in young people with asthma and/or atopy and is administered as a dry powder inhaler. There are no major side-effects.

Antitussives

You should always consider why the patient has a cough; is there an underlying mechanism that can be treated: for example, left ventricular failure or asthma? The consequences of suppressing a cough should also be considered; would it cause the pooling of secretions and a hypostatic pneumonia?

Many proprietary antitussives work predominantly by the soothing nature of the liquid carrier. For this reason 'simple linctus' is the most appropriate starting point for a mild irritative cough. Opioids are the best cough suppressants, working both on lung and central brain receptors. Codeine or pholcodine elixir are reasonable first-line treatments; use morphine if there is another indication (e.g. pain).

Antibiotics

Antibiotics are discussed on page 429.

2.2 Infective disorders

Learning objectives

You should be able to:
- describe the classification of pneumonia and other forms of respiratory infection
- set out the major causes of respiratory infection and their treatment
- write down the clinical presentation and appropriate investigations for respiratory tract infection
- discuss which patients require specialised advice and/or procedures
- describe the diagnosis of tuberculosis and its management.

Case Study

An 84-year-old woman, who still plays golf most weeks, presents with a 48-hour history of increasing confusion. Vital signs are normal, except for a respiratory rate of 28 breaths/minute and a sinus tachycardia of 110 beats/minute. On examination she is disorientated in time but not person or place, is well nourished and has coarse crackles and bronchial breathing at her left base. Her daughter reports that she had the 'flu jab' 2 months ago and the 'pneumonia jab' last winter.

Classification of infective disorders

Pneumonia and respiratory infection are classified as follows:

Pneumonia

This is an acute, presumed infective, respiratory illness typified by fever, cough, dyspnoea and a new infiltrate on a chest radiograph. The term bronchopneumonia is subsumed under pneumonia and implies the production of purulent sputum in addition to the above features. Lobar pneumonia refers to infection located in one circumscribed area of the lung with sharp edges radiologically and is most likely caused by *Streptococcus pneumoniae* infection. Pneumonia may be community- or hospital-acquired. One variant of the latter is ventilator-associated pneumonia.

Atypical pneumonia

This term is used with two imprecise meanings:
- erythromycin- (e.g. mycoplasma) or tetracycline-responsive (e.g. Q fever) pneumonia, including *Legionella* pneumonia
- non-bacterial pneumonia (which includes viruses, *Mycoplasma*, etc. but excludes *Legionella* spp.).

Often atypical pneumonia presents with extrapulmonary manifestations such as headache, abnormal hepatic function, diarrhoea, etc.

Aspiration pneumonia

Following vomiting or reflux, gastric contents may enter the lungs leading to both an infective and a chemical (acidic) pneumonia. This is common in alcoholics, patients with stroke and neuromuscular disorders such as motor neurone disease and those with impaired mental function.

Pneumonitis

This is an imprecise term meaning a new diffuse pulmonary process, which may or may not be infective. It implies fine bilateral shadows on the chest radiograph. Infections are typically caused by viruses such as adenovirus, or cytomegalovirus in immunocompromised patients.

Acute bronchitis

This is an acute infection of the bronchial tree characterised by a productive cough usually with mucopurulent sputum, with or without fever, with no new chest radiograph abnormalities. It is usually caused by bacteria that cause pneumonia.

Acute tracheitis or tracheobronchitis

In this typically viral infection (e.g. parainfluenza), the patient complains of a painful rasping cough, with pain in the anterior chest, commonly without fever. The chest radiograph is usually normal. It must be distinguished from stridor caused by a foreign body and bacterial epiglottitis.

Community-acquired pneumonia

Epidemiology

Community-acquired pneumonia is increasingly common with increasing age and is also more common in debilitated patients. Mortality varies between 6 and 20%.

Pathophysiology

The vast majority of pneumonias follow microscopic aspiration of bacteria from the nasopharynx, throat and oesophagus. Radioisotope tracer studies of normal adults have shown that 45% aspirate during sleep. Pneumonia develops when enough bacteria enter the trachea, reproduce and cause bronchial and/or parenchymal infection. The implication is that the bacterial flora of the nasopharynx and throat determines the causative organism.

Causes of pneumonia and clinical syndrome

There are many different causes of pneumonia (Table 11). However, some are more common in the community, others in hospital.

Pneumococcal and Haemophilus pneumonia

Pneumococcal pneumonia is the most common community-acquired pneumonia (50–80%), partly because *Streptococcus pneumoniae* is a frequent inhabitant of the nasopharynx. Many cases occur in young or middle-aged adults, but elderly people, those with chronic chest disease, alcoholics and patients with acquired immunodeficiency syndrome (AIDS) are at higher risk. Smoking is a risk factor for bacteraemic pneumococcal infection.

Although a frequent pathogen in patients with COPD, *Haemophilus influenzae* is an uncommon cause of pneumonia.

Clinical presentation Onset is usually abrupt in lobar pneumonia, but bronchopneumonia may be more gradual in onset. Other features include:

- fever: usually high and almost always present
- shaking chills or rigors: initially common but rigors imply bacteraemia as well as pneumonia
- cough: virtually universal and usually productive
- pleuritic chest pain: common
- dyspnoea: usual
- an acute confusional state: common, particularly in elderly patients
- headache: unusual (cf. atypical pneumonia).

The clinical signs of pneumococcal (lobar) pneumonia represent the archetype for all bacterial pneumonias. The signs include:

- pyrexia and toxic appearance (flushed and distressed)
- raised respiratory rate and use of accessory muscles of respiration
- central cyanosis (if severe)
- unilateral (or bilateral) crackles over affected lung area, usually with bronchial breathing
- pleural rub (occasional)
- labial herpes simplex reactivation
- confusion (poor prognosis).

Table 11 Aetiology of bacterial pneumonia

Aetiological agent	Community-acquired			Hospital- or community-acquired	
	Bronchopneumonia	Lobar	Approximate frequency in UK (%)	Aspiration	Hospital-acquired/ ventilator pneumonia[a]
Streptococcus pneumoniae	+++	+++	60–75	+	+
Haemophilus spp.	+	±	5	+	+
Legionella spp.	+	+	2–5	–	+
Staphylococcus aureus	±	+	1	+	+
Gram-negative organisms	±	+	<1	+	++
Anaerobes	±	–	<1	++	+
Mycoplasma	±	+	5–18	–	–
Chlamydophila spp.[b]	+	+	>5	–	–
Coxiella burnetii	+	+	<1	–	–

[a] Usually a bronchopneumonia in pattern, occasionally lobar.
[b] *Chlamydophila* spp. includes *C. trachomatis* (pneumonitis in babies), *C. pneumoniae* (adults) and *C. psittaci* (adults, related to bird exposure).

Two

75

Table 12 Investigations in pneumonia

Test	Reason
Chest radiograph	For type and extent of involvement (if >1 lobe affected, the prognosis is poor)
Blood gases	To determine oxygen therapy (PO_2 <8 kPa (60 mmHg) is poor prognosis)
Blood count	May help with initial differential diagnosis
Blood culture	To isolate relevant bacteria
Urea and electrolytes	Hyponatraemia is typical of *Legionella* infection; urea > 7 mmol/l has poor prognosis
Liver function tests	Often abnormal in atypical pneumonia
Serum for serology (baseline)	For later aetiological diagnosis (first specimen is often positive for influenza)
Sputum for microbiology (Gram stain and culture)	For diagnostic purposes, especially if very ill or hospital-acquired infection
Pneumococcal antigen (sputum and urine)	To diagnose pneumococcal pneumonia
Legionella antigen (urine)	To diagnose *Legionella* infection

Investigations The investigations required to manage patients are listed in Table 12.

Management You should administer high concentrations of humidified oxygen. Tracheal aspiration and physiotherapy in patients with sputum production are important general measures. Despite the rising incidence of low-level penicillin resistance, i.v. penicillin and ampicillin are effective for ill (e.g. hospitalised) patients with pneumonia. Third-generation cephalosporins (e.g. cefotaxime or ceftriaxone) are also effective. The older quinolones (ciprofloxacin or norfloxacin) are not active against *S. pneumoniae* but the newer ones are. Macrolides are a reasonable first choice in the community but there is increasing resistance (10–15%).

Prognosis Pneumococcal pneumonia carries a 5% mortality rate but if patients need admission to an intensive care unit, this approaches 75%. Several factors are predictive of high mortality regardless of age in community-acquired pneumonia. These are:

- respiratory rate > 30/min
- diastolic blood pressure < 60 mmHg
- serum urea > 7 mmol/l.

Complications The most common complication is respiratory failure. Indications for ventilation include a rising PCO_2, a low PO_2 (e.g. ≤70 mmHg (9 kPa)) on oxygen or an exhausted patient. Other complications include empyema, pericarditis, meningitis, endocarditis, arthritis or bacterial peritonitis. You should carefully examine and investigate any patient with a persistent fever despite antibiotics.

Patients who are asplenic, including sickle cell anaemia patients, are at risk of overwhelming pneumococcal infections (mortality >60%). Immunisation and lifelong antibiotics are appropriate prophylactic measures (p. 264, 382).

Prevention Patients with chronic respiratory disease and those about to undergo splenectomy should be immunised with pneumococcal vaccine. Pneumococcal vaccine is now routinely offered to elderly people in the UK.

Staphylococcal pneumonia

Staphylococcal pneumonia occurs usually as a superinfection following influenza and has a high mortality. Patients rapidly become extremely ill with respiratory failure, high fever and general features of sepsis. A Gram stain of sputum or tracheal aspirate will show Gram-positive cocci in clusters, usually intracellularly, and this alone is enough evidence in a very ill patient to treat with maximal antistaphylococcal antibiotics (e.g. flucloxacillin 2 g 4-hourly or linezolid for meticillin-resistant *Staph. aureus* (MRSA), Ch. 10).

Legionnaire's disease (infection with **Legionella**)

Legionella can be found in hot water systems of all types, including showers, especially large ones such as those in hotels and hospitals.

Legionnaire's disease accounts for 1–15% of community-acquired cases and 1–5% of hospital-acquired cases of pneumonia. Chronic chest disease and smoking, together with increasing age, are the greatest risk factors, although immunosuppression is important. In hospital-acquired cases, surgery is an important risk, especially transplant surgery.

Clinical presentation Disease varies in severity from a mild cough and fever to a multisystem disease with severe pneumonia and unconsciousness. The symptoms are often misleadingly vague with malaise, headache, myalgia and anorexia. Important clinical features are:

- cough (often mild) and minimally productive
- chest pain (non-specific)
- high fever (usually)
- diarrhoea
- change in mental status (in severe cases).

Investigations Multiple laboratory abnormalities are common, but only hyponatraemia is useful in distinguishing legionnaire's disease from other pneumonias. Chest radiograph abnormalities are often more marked than you would suspect from examination. A pleural effusion is common. Progression of radiological findings despite appropriate antibiotics is typical. Culture of the organism is possible but requires specialised techniques. Immunofluorescence on sputum or urine is a useful rapid diagnostic procedure. The urine may contain *Legionella* antigen (75%). Convalescent serology is the usual diagnostic method.

Management Effective treatment is high-dose ciprofloxacin, or other quinolones, or clarithromycin. Clinical data suggest that the quinolones are superior. A delay in starting treatment is the most important factor leading to a poor outcome. Mortality in the UK is about 20%.

Mycoplasma *pneumonia*

Mycoplasma pneumonia is the archetypal atypical pneumonia with constitutional features (fever, malaise and headache) preceding respiratory symptoms. It is most common in the 5–20-year age group and tends to occur in 4-yearly cycles. It may affect whole families concurrently.

Clinical presentation The cough is usually nonproductive, although haemoptysis (usually mild) is sometimes seen. *Mycoplasma* may cause tracheobronchitis and/or pharyngitis (sore throat and retrosternal chest pain). Fever is usually moderate (37.5–38.0°C).

Management Tetracycline and macrolides are effective therapy.

Complications These include:

- myringitis — inflammation of the eardrum (15%)
- maculopapular skin rashes (15%)
- meningoencephalitis and other neurological problems (≤10%).

Up to half of patients develop cold haemagglutinins (cross-reaction with the I antigen of red cells) after 10 days of illness.

Chlamydial pneumonia

Chlamydophila pneumoniae is a common cause worldwide of upper respiratory tract infection, usually presenting with cough with a higher frequency of sore throat, hoarseness and sinusitis. Reinfection is common, so a molecular diagnosis or a rise in antibody titre is required for confirmation.

Complications include (rarely):

- Guillain–Barré syndrome
- myocarditis
- meningoencephalitis
- synovitis.

Treatment is with macrolides such as azithromycin or doxycycline.

Influenza

Influenza is caused by RNA influenza viruses A and B. It is a common infection, especially in winter, and individuals may suffer from it multiple times in their life because of the remarkable antigenic variation of the viruses. As influenza affects birds and animals, there is a significant risk of new strains developing to which few are immune, leading to an epidemic or pandemic. The incubation period is 1–3 days. Only immunisation or antiviral prophylaxis with amantadine reduces attack rates, apart from segregation of infectious individuals. Treatment with neuraminidase inhibitors, oseltamivir and zanamivir, is partially effective and may reduce transmission.

Clinical presentation Influenza is distinctive in its more severe forms. The onset is abrupt. Systemic symptoms of feverishness, chills, headaches, myalgia, malaise and anorexia predominate. Painful movement of the eye muscles, together with a burning sensation in the eyes and tearing, can create an impression of photophobia. A dry cough and clear nasal discharge are typical. The patient appears toxic and flushed with watery reddened eyes. The throat may be reddened and small lymph nodes are often palpable in the neck. The illness usually lasts 3–10 days.

Severe influenza Influenza outbreaks lead to increased deaths from 'pneumonia' among elderly people. This probably results from secondary bacterial pneumonia complicating influenza. If infected with *Staph. aureus*, there is a high mortality. In unusual circumstances, a primary influenzal pneumonia can occur in young people and this has a high mortality. Severe influenza is more common in pregnancy and in those with cardiovascular disease.

Prevention Influenza A infection can be prevented by immunisation. Different strains circulate each year and so new vaccines are prepared and should be given annually. Indications for vaccination are chronic pulmonary, cardiac or renal disease, immunosuppression, diabetes mellitus, age over 65 years and healthcare workers.

Other viruses

In adults, other viral causes of pneumonia are uncommon. Adenoviruses are perhaps the most common, together with measles. In immunocompromised patients, viral pneumonia, especially caused by cytomegalovirus, is relatively common and often life-threatening. In 2003 a new corona virus infection, called severe acute respiratory syndrome (SARS) occurred but has now receded.

Hospital-acquired pneumonia

Hospital-acquired pneumonia is a common cause of death. It particularly affects elderly people, those with chronic chest disease, ventilated patients and those who have had major abdominal or thoracic surgery (splinting of the diaphragm).

Pathogenesis

Hospital-acquired pneumonia is usually caused by Gram-negative organisms (Table 11). A number of factors influence this. The use of broad-spectrum antibiotics given for other infections changes the flora of the nasopharynx to a predominantly Gram-negative one. This alteration also occurs without antibiotics in ill patients; particularly those with nasogastric or endotracheal tubes. A further factor is the use of histamine H_2 receptor antagonists, which increases stomach pH significantly. This allows the proliferation of Gram-negative bacteria in the stomach.

Clinical presentation

The symptoms are similar to those of community-acquired pneumonia. Lobar pneumonia is rare and, apart from legionnaire's disease, atypical pneumonia is very rare.

Management

Antibiotic management should be directed to Gram-negative pathogens. Typical choices are cefotaxime, a carbapenem, or ceftazidime if *Pseudomonas* spp. is suspected.

Aspiration pneumonia

Aspiration pneumonia is a relatively common problem in hospital. In a sense, all pneumonias are aspiration pneumonias (see above), but the term implies a sudden, large-volume inhalation of gastric or pharyngeal contents.

Clinically, it is similar to other pneumonias and varies substantially in severity. Involvement of the superior or basilar segment of either lower lobe or the posterior segment of the upper lobes suggests the diagnosis.

The management is the same as for community-acquired pneumonia except for one point. Anaerobes are more commonly implicated and you should use metronidazole or another antibiotic with good anti-anaerobic activity (e.g. a carbapenem).

Pneumonia in the immunocompromised patient

Pneumonia, pneumonitis or respiratory infection in the immunocompromised patient includes all the above considerations for community- and hospital-acquired pneumonia, but has some additional distinctive features. The key points are:

- Any new respiratory symptom or new radiological infiltrate must be urgently investigated; for example, the time from first cough to death with cytomegalovirus pneumonitis or *Aspergillus* pneumonia is typically 5–7 days.
- Important organisms to consider include *Pneumocystis, Pseudomonas, Aspergillus* and other fungi, *Nocardia,* cytomegalovirus and *Mycobacterium tuberculosis*. It is, therefore, *much* more important to reach an aetiological diagnosis in an immunocompromised patient than in one with a community-acquired pneumonia.
- Helpful investigations (if done rapidly) include CT scanning of the chest, bronchoscopy and broncho-alveolar lavage, and percutaneous lung biopsy.
- Empirical treatment is virtually always appropriate, based on an educated guess, but with modification following the results of specific investigations.
- Expert advice is essential.

Lung abscess

Some pneumonias will develop into a lung abscess, particularly following aspiration. Typical causative organisms are *Staph. aureus*, anaerobes, *Klebsiella pneumoniae* and fungal infections such as *Aspergillus*. On chest radiographs and CT scan, you will see a large circular lesion with cavitation and an air/fluid level. Management consists of long-term (e.g. 2–4 months) antibiotics or antifungals with postural drainage, and occasionally surgery.

Tuberculosis

Learning objectives

You should be able to:
- describe how to diagnose pulmonary and extrapulmonary tuberculosis
- discuss the limitations of diagnostic tests
- discuss the implications of a positive or negative tuberculin skin and blood interferon test for tuberculosis
- write down how tuberculosis is transmitted and how to interrupt transmission
- describe the principles of management of tuberculosis, including the importance of resistance.

Case Study

A 53-year-old professional man attends the rapid access clinic because of productive cough and weight loss. He is a smoker and had whooping cough as a child. His maternal grandmother and her sister both had tuberculosis in their twenties. He reports night sweats but no fever. His chest X-ray shows left apical shadowing without cavitation and his acid-fast bacilli (AFB) sputum smear is negative.

Microbiology

Tuberculosis is caused by *Mycobacterium tuberculosis*. Infection can also be caused by so-called atypical mycobacteria (Table 13). Pulmonary infections with atypical mycobacteria are similar to those caused by *M. tuberculosis* (classical tuberculosis) but are much rarer and in general more resistant to treatment.

Epidemiology

Approximately a third of the world's population are currently infected with *M. tuberculosis*. In the developed world, tuberculosis rates are rising as a result of two major factors: AIDS and deteriorating social conditions in the inner cities. Primary infection can occur at any age, commonly in childhood in the underdeveloped world. In the UK, the majority of cases occur in adults originating from the Indian subcontinent. People particularly at risk include:

- the very old
- immunocompromised patients (especially with AIDS)
- homeless and displaced persons
- alcoholics.

The vast majority of infections are acquired by droplet inhalation from an infected person who coughs. It follows that the most infectious group of patients is those with cavitary pulmonary tuberculosis with sputum containing visible acid-fast bacilli (smear-positive) who are coughing; this group is followed by those whose sputum is culture-positive but smear-negative (much less infectious). *Patients who do not cough are essentially non-infectious.*

Table 13 Important 'atypical' mycobacteria

Species	Characteristic infection
M. kansasii, M. xenopi *M. malmoense*	Similar to classical TB
M. avium intracellulare	Disseminated infection: AIDS Pulmonary disease like TB Neck lymphadenopathy
M. chelonae, M. fortuitium	Skin and catheter infections
M. marinum	Fish tank granuloma (skin)
M. ulcerans	Buruli ulcer (skin, topical)
M. leprae	Leprosy

The risk of a contact acquiring tuberculosis depends on the closeness of the contact and on the infectiousness of the patient.

Clinical presentation

Patients with pulmonary tuberculosis present with:

- a chronic, mildly productive cough
- fever (often present but not always) and night sweats
- weight loss.

Investigations

A simple chest radiograph is virtually always abnormal; the only exceptions are patients with miliary tuberculosis. Usually, the chest radiograph shows asymmetrical upper lobe infiltrates with cavitation. Sometimes the apex of the lower lobe is affected instead.

The essential diagnostic test is sputum collection for microscopy and culture of *Mycobacteria* (acid-fast bacilli). You should obtain three sputum samples, preferably early in the morning and on separate days. If these are negative or the presentation is atypical in any way, a bronchoscopy (with washings or brushings) is appropriate to verify the diagnosis. Sputum after bronchoscopy is useful.

Skin testing

Tuberculin skin tests were developed to detect infection with *M. tuberculosis*. There is very little cross-reactivity with other atypical mycobacteria. Skin testing is used for four reasons:

1. population surveys for the prevalence of exposure to *M. tuberculosis*
2. to assess whether contacts of a patient with tuberculosis are themselves infected
3. as a diagnostic aid for tuberculosis
4. to determine if a person is latently infected.

An alternative test is a blood test for interferon-gamma production with tuberculosis antigens. A positive test indicates infection or latency.

A tuberculin skin test result is not foolproof. An immunocompromised patient will often have a false-negative response or an inappropriately mild response, which may be misleading. This is also true in some patients with miliary tuberculosis, sarcoidosis or malnourished patients. By comparison, a florid positive response (grade 3 or 4) implies not simply prior exposure to *M. tuberculosis* but also disease.

Management

It is essential to treat tuberculosis with multiple drugs because of resistant organisms. At present in the UK, 10% of clinical isolates show frank resistance to one first-line drug and about 4% have resistance to two or more drugs. Patients infected with isoniazid- *and* rifampicin-resistant *M. tuberculosis* are defined as having multi-drug resistant tuberculosis (MDR TB). Recently described are extensively drug-resistant *M. tuberculosis* (XDR-TB) in which isolates are resistant to rifampicin, ixoniazid and ≥3 classes of second line agents. Generally rifampicin, isoniazid, pyrazi-

namide and ethambutol are used together. As isoniazid can cause pellagra (mixed peripheral neuropathy and hyperpigmentation), pyridoxine (vitamin B_6) is generally given to prevent this.

In patients with susceptible organisms who respond to therapy promptly (e.g. in 1–4 weeks) and who are not immunocompromised, 6 months of therapy is appropriate. After 2 months of treatment, pyrazinamide (and ethambutol) can be stopped, leaving the patient on rifampicin and isoniazid for the last 4 months of therapy. Assuming the patient is compliant (which is a major problem in some), the relapse rate following a 6-month course is less than 3%. Much higher relapse rates are seen in those who only complete 2–4 months of therapy.

Expert advice should be sought for infections caused by MDR TB, XDR-TB or atypical mycobacterial infections. MDR TB XDR-TB patients have to be cared for in special facilities in the UK.

Prognosis

The outcome from tuberculosis depends in part on how early treatment is initiated and how ill the patient is. In the UK, 500–750 people die each year of or with tuberculosis. The mortality rate is around 10–15%.

Chronic pulmonary and bronchial sepsis

Cavities in the lung or dilatation and deformity of the bronchi provide friendly environments for bacteria and fungi to live, almost in harmony with the patient. Cavities are caused by tuberculosis, sarcoidosis, lung cysts, ankylosing spondylitis and a few other unusual lung pathologies. These cavities usually communicate with the bronchial tree and so organisms can get in and pus can get out.

Aspergilloma

Cavities in the lung can become infected with *Aspergillus*. This airborne fungus is breathed in, reproduces and causes a fungus ball (aspergilloma). Invasion of the cavity wall or formation of new cavities signifies chronic cavitary pulmonary aspergillosis. Productive cough, haemoptysis and weight loss are typical. Precipitating antibody (precipitins) to *Aspergillus* is usually found in serum. Treatment is long-term with itraconazole or voriconazole.

Bronchiectasis

Literally this term means dilatation of the bronchi. There are many causes of bronchiectasis:

- congenital or genetic, e.g. cystic fibrosis
- childhood infection, e.g. whooping cough
- bronchial obstruction, e.g. overlooked foreign body
- allergic disease, e.g. allergic bronchopulmonary aspergillosis
- autoimmune disease, e.g. primary biliary cirrhosis.

Clinical presentation

In clinical terms, bronchiectasis occurs in 'wet' or 'dry' forms.

Dry bronchiectasis Dry bronchiectasis is usually asymptomatic. It may be identified on a chest radiograph as curly or ring shadows in the lung. The commonest presentation is haemoptysis. Often the patients are young or middle-aged and unheralded haemoptysis leads to immediate suspicion of cancer. However, bronchoscopy is usually normal and the diagnosis can be confirmed, if necessary, with a high-quality CT scan of the chest.

Wet bronchiectasis Wet bronchiectasis is quite different in its manifestations. These patients present with chronic productive cough. The sputum volume is large and it is grossly purulent. Despite this large amount of purulent material, fever is usually absent. Symptoms are most marked in the morning. Clubbing is usual when the disease is chronic and well established. Coexisting sinusitis is also common. Bacteriology shows the same organisms that cause pneumonia, although *Pseudomonas aeruginosa* may appear later in antibiotic-treated patients. Bronchiectasis is a common presentation of hypogammaglobulinaemia (Ch. 9).

Management

The principles of management of bronchiectasis are:

- exclude immune defects
- antibiotics for exacerbations (with occasional admissions for i.v. antibiotics)
- physiotherapy with postural drainage.

Occasionally only one lobe is involved and respiratory function is good; in these patients surgical resection is feasible. Cor pulmonale from pulmonary fibrosis and brain abscess are occasional complications.

2.3 Tumours

Learning objectives

You should be able to:

- write down the importance of bronchial carcinoma in the community
- describe the different pathological types of lung cancer, how they differ in their presentation and progression and the aetiological variation
- discuss the principles of investigation, management and treatment
- state how other tumours can affect the respiratory system.

Case Study

Vera is very upset and frightened as she has just been told that she has lung cancer. From what she can remember, the specialist said that it was an 'aggressive' sort that had spread and that she would need several courses of drugs to shrink it, but they might not work. The doctor has also explained that her blood chemistry was affected and that the tumour was blocking one of the 'big veins'.

Bronchial carcinoma

Bronchial carcinoma is the most common malignancy in the UK in males and is second to breast cancer in females. The male to female ratio is 3–4:1. The incidence has pla-

teaued in males (or is even descreasing) but is still rising in females because of changing smoking habits. It is more common in urban areas and is associated with atmospheric pollution. In the UK, there are around 40 000 new cases of lung cancer each year. Currently around 65% of these are in men and about 40% of all cases are in people over 75 years of age. It is uncommon to find anyone under 40 years of age with lung cancer but it does occur.

Aetiology

The vast majority of cases (90%) are related to smoking (up to 20-fold higher than non-smokers) and linked to duration and intensity of exposure (expressed as pack-years). If a person stops smoking, the risk decreases, but is never as low as in lifelong non-smokers. Passive smoking increases the risk for non-smokers. Tumours associated with occupation/chemical exposure are usually adenocarcinomas, though these are still associated with cigarette smoking. Asbestos, particularly in smokers, (see below) and radon are aetiological factors in a *small* number of tumours.

Pathology

Lung cancer is an epithelial carcinoma, generally occurring in the mucosa of the bronchi but occasionally in the parenchyma. Most tumours (80%) arise in the main lobar or segmental bronchi.

Four major carcinoma cell types account for over 95% of primary lung cancers:

- squamous cell carcinoma
- adenocarcinoma
- undifferentiated large cell carcinoma
- small cell carcinoma.

Squamous carcinoma, adenocarcinoma and large cell carcinoma are often all grouped under the term non-small cell lung cancer. These histologies are classified together because, when localised, all have the potential for cure with surgical resection. By contrast, small cell carcinoma has almost always metastasised by the time of presentation and so is not amenable to curative surgery.

Non-small cell (squamous) carcinoma

The commonest tumour is the squamous carcinoma, which accounts for just under half of all primary malignancies. Squamous metaplasia leads to carcinoma-in-situ and then to invasive carcinoma, ranging from well-differentiated to poorly differentiated. The tumour is usually central in origin and frequently cavitates. If peripheral, it may invade the chest wall. Distant metastasis occurs frequently. Squamous cell carcinomas commonly cause hypercalcaemia through either bone destruction or production of parathyroid hormone-related peptide (PTHrP).

Adenocarcinoma

Adenocarcinomas account for approximately 10% of lung cancers. They occur peripherally or in areas of lung scarring. The tumours are seen in non-smokers as well as smokers (where it is associated with the *RAS* oncogenes). The risk is increased by asbestos exposure. Cavitation is *not* a feature. If the tumours are biopsied, the differentiation from a primary adenocarcinoma arising elsewhere may be difficult (e.g. gastrointestinal tract). Local invasion, notably of the pleural space, is a dominant feature. The prognosis is usually worse than squamous cell carcinomas.

Large cell carcinoma

Large cell carcinomas are undifferentiated tumours that account for approximately one-quarter of all lung cancers. They tend to arise centrally, metastasise early and carry a poor prognosis when compared with squamous cell tumours.

Small cell carcinoma

Small cell (oat cell) carcinomas arise from the amine precursor uptake decarboxylase (APUD) system. Neurosecretory granules are frequently seen and these tumours secrete peptides with hormonal activity, e.g. antidiuretic hormone (ADH) or adrenocorticotrophic hormone (ACTH). They arise centrally and are rapidly growing with early dissemination. The tumour is associated with both activation of oncogenes (e.g. *myc*) and inactivation of tumour suppressor genes (e.g. retinoblastoma [*RB*] tumour suppressor gene). Small cell carcinomas constitute around 30% of lung tumours.

Clinical presentation

Generally, if you suspect a patient might have a bronchial carcinoma, you should take a detailed smoking and occupational history. For specific symptoms and signs a useful framework is:

- local problems (chest wall, lung, etc.)
- distant problems
- non-metastatic manifestations.

Local symptoms

Visualising the chest contents enables you to deduce the possible symptoms and signs of local invasion, but many patients have coexistent COPD. The most common presentation of bronchial carcinoma is with persistent cough or breathlessness. Alternatively, infection may be the first manifestation with signs of collapse/consolidation and there may be superadded cavitation. Your suspicions should be raised if infection is slow to clear or recurs. Chest pain may occur, often ill-defined or pleuritic in nature, and associated with an effusion. Local invasion of the chest wall, ribs and/or vertebra are seen in some patients with severe unremitting pain.

Occasionally haemoptysis may be the first symptom, with endobronchial erosion into blood vessels. There are other benign causes of haemoptysis, but you must always take the symptom seriously and investigate it adequately.

Apical tumours may infiltrate the lower portion of the brachial plexus (C7, 8, T1), causing pain along the medial border of the hand and arm together with weakness of the muscles of the hand, including the thenar and hypothenar eminences (**Pancoast's syndrome**). A **Horner's syndrome** may also occur as a result of damage to the sympathetic outflow through T1. The subclavian veins may be infiltrated, causing thrombosis.

A central tumour with hilar involvement can obstruct the superior vena cava, presenting with facial fullness/ swelling, headache and dilated chest wall veins. Central tumours can also damage the phrenic nerve producing an elevated diaphragm with paradoxical movement (elevation on inspiration).

Urgent specialist referral is needed for:

- persistent haemoptysis in a smoker
- signs of superior vena caval obstruction
- stridor (tracheal narrowing).

Distant symptoms

The first manifestation of a bronchial carcinoma may be a distant metastasis. Secondary disease may become apparent in the brain (fits, hemiparesis, etc.), bone (pain, pathological fracture), liver (hepatomegaly), lymph nodes or elsewhere. Small cell carcinomas are more likely to present with distant metastases, but they are seen with all tumours.

Non-metastatic manifestation of malignancy

It is often forgotten that symptoms such as anorexia and weight loss may be classified as 'non-metastatic', i.e. general effects of malignancy. Quite often bronchial carcinoma presents in this way, particularly small cell carcinoma.

The classical **paraneoplastic** syndromes are shown in Figure 21.

Investigations

The main principles you should adopt are:

- If lung cancer is suspected, refer to a multidisciplinary lung cancer team.
- Try to achieve a histological diagnosis.

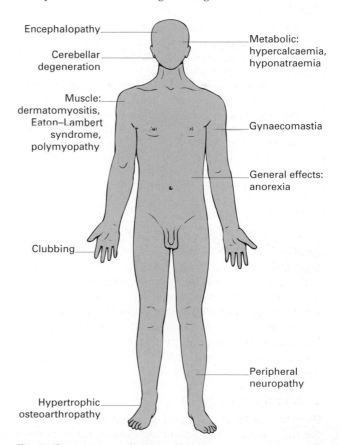

Encephalopathy

Cerebellar degeneration

Muscle: dermatomyositis, Eaton–Lambert syndrome, polymyopathy

Clubbing

Hypertrophic osteoarthropathy

Metabolic: hypercalcaemia, hyponatraemia

Gynaecomastia

General effects: anorexia

Peripheral neuropathy

Fig. 21 Classical paraneoplastic syndromes.

Two

- If curative treatment appears feasible, then attempt to stage the tumour accurately.

The main investigations are radiology and bronchoscopy.

Radiology
If an abnormality is seen on a plain PA radiograph a lateral film should be taken. Sometimes, the diagnosis is suspected because of an abnormality on a film done for another purpose (e.g. preoperatively). Some worrying appearances on a chest radiograph are:

- irregular pulmonary mass, possibly with cavitation
- partial or complete collapse of a lobe
- a hilar mass
- a pleural effusion, often combined with the above.

Many abnormalities are highly suggestive of a malignant process (such as sequential enlargement of a mass) but are not absolutely diagnostic. You should *always* try to obtain previous films to compare with the most recent one. A CT scan is very helpful both in diagnosis and staging.

Bronchoscopy
This is the single most useful investigation, allowing visualisation of an endobronchial tumour that is centrally located (i.e. in the major bronchi) as well as biopsy, brushings or lavage for malignant cells.

Other techniques
If pleural disease is present, then fluid may be aspirated (exudate may be bloodstained, see Table 16) and pleural biopsies taken, preferably under direct vision (thorascopy). Peripheral or even central masses may be sampled by percutaneous needle biopsy under ultrasound or CT guidance. Mediastinoscopy may be used in mediastinal disease. There is no place for routine sputum cytology because of the difficulty in obtaining adequate samples and the high false-negative rate. More recently, positron emission tomography (PET) scanning (F18 fluorodeoxyglucose uptake) has proved useful for staging disease.

Management
A staging system based on the tumour, node and metastases stage (TNM) is used to determine the management and prognosis of non-small cell carcinoma (Tables 14 and 15). The TNM system is not useful for small cell carcinoma because most tumours have already metastasised by the time of presentation. Consequently, small cell carcinoma is classified only as 'limited' or 'extensive' depending on its spread inside and outside the chest.

The use of the different modalities of treatment according to cell type is shown in Table 16.

Table 14 Staging of non-small cell lung cancer using the tumour (T), node (N) and metastases (M) system (TNM)

Level	Definition
Tumour	
T1	Tumour <3 cm in diameter, lobar or distal
T2	Tumour >3 cm in diameter or invades visceral pleura or lobar collapse to hilum
T3	Tumour any size with direct extension to chest wall, diaphragm, trachea or mediastinal pleura <2 cm carina
T4	Tumour any size, invades mediastinal structures, vertebrae or carina, or causes a malignant effusion
Node	
N1	Nodal metastases in ipsilateral hilum
N2	Nodal metastases in ipsilateral mediastinum, subcarinal
N3	Nodal metastases in contralateral hilum, mediastinum and/or supraclavicular fossa
Metastasis	
M	Distant metastases

Table 15 Staging based on TNM

Stage	Components
I	T1 or T2
II	T1 or T2 + N1
IIIa	T3 + N1 or N2, or T1 + T2 + N2
IIIb	T4 + any N or any T + N3
IV	Any T or N + M

Table 16 Treatment of bronchial carcinoma

Type	Radiotherapy	Surgery	Chemotherapy
Non-small cell (squamous)	Curative 20% 5-year survival, Used in palliation	25% 5-year survival, higher in confined disease	Limited response
Large cell, undifferentiated	Palliation	Less benefit compared with squamous cell	Limited response
Adenocarcinoma	Poor response, some palliation	Poor survival	Poor response
Small cell (oat)	Used in reducing tumour bulk	Used in debulking	Good response relative to no treatment; median survival <1 year

Surgery

Unfortunately, only 20–30% of patients are fit for surgery but resection may cure a small percentage of these (25%, 5 years). Your assessment of the patient's fitness and suitability for surgery should include several factors.

What is the cell type? Non-small cell carcinoma may be amenable to surgery. In addition, debulking operations are occasionally carried out on small cell tumours as an adjuvant to chemotherapy.

Is the tumour confined to the lung? Staging is very important. Evidence of metastases precludes surgery (plain radiographs, CT or ultrasound scanning may demonstrate dissemination). Non-metastatic manifestations are not a contraindication; these may respond to resection.

Is the tumour technically resectable? A tumour that is located close to the carina or involving more than one lobe is unsuitable for surgery.

What is the patient's lung function? An FEV_1 of <1.5 l militates against a successful outcome.

What are the patient's quality of life and general health like? Concomitant disease — for example, coronary artery disease — increases the operative risks. The use of scales such as the Karnofsky or WHO (Zubrad) is important in quantifying performance status, which impacts on tolerance of intensive treatment.

Radiotherapy

Radiotherapy is mainly used in palliation, but some patients with non-resectable squamous cell carcinoma achieve long remission after treatment. Intraluminal radiotherapy can be of help in bulky endobronchial disease that is causing obstruction. Haemoptysis, bone metastases and superior vena caval (SVC) obstruction often respond well. In high doses, radiation pneumonitis may occur and, in the long term, progressive fibrosis can develop with breathlessness. Radiotherapy combined with chemotherapy is used in small cell carcinoma.

Chemotherapy

Chemotherapy has improved the outlook in small cell carcinoma, with a median survival of 2 months without treatment and approaching a year with combination (platinum-based, e.g. carboplatin, cisplatin) chemotherapy. Some patients achieve much longer remission. Combination (including a platinum agent) and single-agent therapy can also give some remission in non-small cell carcinoma.

Prognosis

Prognosis in lung cancer is affected by a number of factors (Box 5).

Non-small cell lung cancer

The prognosis for non-small cell carcinoma depends largely on the stage of the disease and hence whether the cancer can be surgically resected. The prognosis for patients in stage I can be quite good. The 5-year survival after surgery for patients with a small T1 N0 tumour is 70–80%. With a larger, T2 tumour, the 5-year survival is 60–70%. By contrast, if surgery is not possible, the cure rate is only 10–30%.

It is important to be aware that patients who have undergone surgical resection are likely to live long enough

---

> **Box 5:** Prognostic factors in lung cancer
>
> - Cell type (non-small cell versus small cell)
> - Stage
> - Performance status
> - Weight loss
> - Large tumour
> - Genetic alterations (e.g. activation or overexpression of the oncogenes *c-myc*, *k-ras*, inactivation of the tumour suppressor genes retinoblastoma, *p53* or the gene on 3p)
> - Autocrine growth factors (e.g. bombesin, epidermal growth factor receptor (EGFR), Erb-B2 (Her-2 neu))

to be at significant risk for the development of a second lung cancer.

The most common presentation for stage II non-small cell carcinoma involves N1 disease (hilar involvement). The 5-year survival for this stage is significantly lower than that for stage I: approximately 30–50%.

Stage III, or locally advanced, disease encompasses a wide range of patients — both operable (IIIA) and inoperable (IIIB) but prognosis for both groups is poor (few patients will live longer than 1 year).

Small cell lung cancer

Without treatment, small cell lung cancer has the most aggressive clinical course of any type of lung cancer, with median survival from diagnosis of only 2–4 months. Even with treatment the overall survival at 5 years is only 5–10%. It is much more likely to have metastasised at the time of presentation than non-small cell carcinoma and surgical resection is rarely effective. However, it is much more responsive to combination chemotherapy and irradiation. Use of chemotherapy, together with other treatments, improves survival by at least four- to fivefold, if referral is rapid and early. Furthermore, about 20% of patients remain disease-free for over 2 years from the start of chemotherapy.

Patients with limited disease (about 40% at the time of diagnosis) can expect a median survival time of 16–24 months with current forms of treatment, whereas patients with extensive disease have a median survival of 6–12 months.

Palliative care

All patients should have access to a multidisciplinary lung cancer team (including a nurse specialist) to coordinate their management and support. Patients throughout their illness need psychological support and access to counselling. Help for your patients can be provided by the MacMillan nurses (some of whom are involved in multidisciplinary palliative care teams) and, outside of hospital, the hospices or local patient support groups as well as community MacMillan nurses and the primary care team.

You must always be alert to the patient becoming depressed and, if so, involve the psychiatry services. As the disease progresses, re-evaluation of treatment goals is required, allowing the switch to palliation to be made at the appropriate time. At any stage, radiotherapy and occasionally single-agent chemotherapy may be helpful in alleviating symptoms. Pain, breathlessness, haemoptysis, etc. may all require specific intervention.

Other tumours

Alveolar cell carcinoma

Alveolar cell carcinoma is a very rare slowly growing tumour that is not related to smoking. It often arises in areas of damaged lungs and the characteristic histological appearance is of malignant cells growing along bronchi. It can have a single focus or may be multifocal. Presentation is usually with breathlessness; occasionally large volumes of sputum are produced (**bronchorrhoea**). A chest radiograph may show single or multiple areas of 'consolidation' with an **air bronchogram**, meaning that the surrounding lung is opaque (non-aerated) and is outlining the air-filled bronchi. Pleural effusions occasionally occur. Diagnosis can be difficult; sputum cytology may be positive, but differentiation from adenocarcinoma may not be possible. Needle or surgical biopsy may be required. Surgical resection in the early stages gives good results but lymphatic involvement is common.

Bronchial adenoma

Bronchial adenomas are uncommon tumours with low-grade malignancy. The majority arise from the APUD cell line (carcinoid), like small cell carcinomas. Most present in young adults, with an equal sex incidence. As endobronchial tumours, they produce local effects — airway obstruction, collapse and distal infection. Common presentations are with a cough, haemoptysis, unilateral wheeze or recurrent non-resolving infection. Occasionally the carcinoid syndrome may occur. Metastatic spread is rare. The tumour is *not* usually visible on a chest radiograph, though there may be collapse. CT scanning is the best way of imaging these tumours. Most can be diagnosed on bronchoscopy. Surgical resection is curative with a good prognosis.

Metastatic disease

The lung is the site of metastases in many carcinomas, with lymphangitis carcinomatosis (see below), multiple or single secondaries, pleural deposits and associated effusions. Single or multiple metastases, particularly from certain tumours (e.g. hypernephroma), may have a 'cannon ball' appearance, implying a smooth rounded opacity as opposed to the ill-defined border of a primary bronchial cancer with streaky shadowing.

Lymphomas can affect the lung with diffuse infiltration, blockage of the thoracic duct (chylothorax) or mediastinal lymph node enlargement.

CT scanning is the best imaging modality.

Solitary pulmonary nodule

An important differential diagnosis is the solitary pulmonary nodule that has been picked up as part of 'routine' investigation. Approximately 40% represent a malignant process (the majority being bronchial carcinomas; the next commonest are metastatic deposits). However, most are benign: for example, either infective (tuberculous) or non-infective (Wegener's) granulomas. The larger the lesion, the more likely it is to be malignant.

Your ability to trace previous radiographs will greatly help in determining the probability of a malignant process. A CT scan may show other metastases and delineate the nodule better. As nodules are parenchymal, bronchoscopy is usually unhelpful but PET scanning is showing promise. A fine needle biopsy is of much greater value but surgical resection is often required to establish the diagnosis.

Lymphangitis carcinomatosis

In lymphangitis carcinomatosis, malignant cells grow along the lymphatic channels of the lungs. Bronchial carcinoma can disseminate via this route, but other tumours may be responsible, notably breast (in females, always look for both breast shadows on a chest radiograph), stomach and pancreas.

Patients usually present with intense breathlessness and a dry cough. Physical signs may be absent, or there may be a few fine basal crackles. A chest radiograph may be normal or may show streaky fine basal shadowing with Kerley B lines. A CT scan is usually helpful (p. 70). There is no specific treatment; opiates may help the breathlessness.

2.4 Airflow obstruction

Leading objectives

You should be able to:

- diagnose and assess the severity of airflow obstruction
- discuss the importance of looking for reversibility of airflow obstruction in terms of treatment
- plan management both as an emergency and in the long term
- describe the importance of asthma in terms of prevalence, morbidity and mortality
- set out how to diagnose, assess and treat acute asthma
- discuss the principles of long-term management in the community.

Case Study

Sam works in a laboratory and is worried that the 'fumes' are affecting his chest. Over the last year, he has been bothered by episodes of wheezing and cough, which seemed to have been much worse when he was at work, though sometimes they seem to be triggered when he plays football on a Sunday morning. He decided to seek some help when his chest flared up again soon after he had been away on holiday.

The diagnosis of airflow obstruction is based on:

- reduced peak expiratory flow
- FEV_1 < 80% predicted
- reduced FEV_1: FVC ratio (<70%).

The history and clinical findings are central in deciding the cause and the main possibilities are:

- COPD (chronic bronchitis and emphysema)
- chronic asthma
- bronchiectasis (p. 79).

Chronic obstructive pulmonary disease

The National Institute for Clinical Excellence (NICE) and British Thoracic Society (BTS) guidelines have a working definition of COPD. It is characterised by airflow obstruction that is usually progressive, is not fully reversible and does not change markedly over several months. The disease is predominantly caused by smoking. In practice, the diagnosis of COPD requires the presence of objective evidence of airflow obstruction (usually involving measurement of FEV_1 and FVC using a spirometer) that does not return to normal with treatment. Usually there is a history of chronic progressing respiratory symptoms, and the patient is, or has been, a heavy smoker. Family history may be important for the rare patient with α_1-antitrypsin deficiency (onset at young age). Your examination findings will be a mixture of the signs set out in Figure 22. The main differential diagnoses are compared in Table 17.

Chronic bronchitis

Pathologically in chronic bronchitis, there is an increase in bronchial wall thickness with hyperplasia and hypertrophy of the mucous glands. The excess mucus secretion and wall thickening produces airflow limitation. *Clinically*, the definition requires a history of at least 2 years of a productive cough on most days for a minimum of 3 months of each year, but the overarching term COPD is usually used.

Emphysema

Emphysema commonly accompanies chronic bronchitis, but these do *not* always occur together. Emphysema is a *pathological* diagnosis characterised by destruction of the acinus. The commonest type is **centrilobular**, affecting the proximal part of the acinus and associated with cigarette smoking. It is seen predominantly in the upper part of the lung. You should be aware of the panacinar type which

Pink puffer	Blue bloater
High respiratory drive	Low respiratory drive
Hypoxic	Hypoxic
Hypocarbic	Hypercarbic
Desaturates on exercise	Right heart failure (oedema)
Type 1 respiratory failure	Type 2 respiratory failure

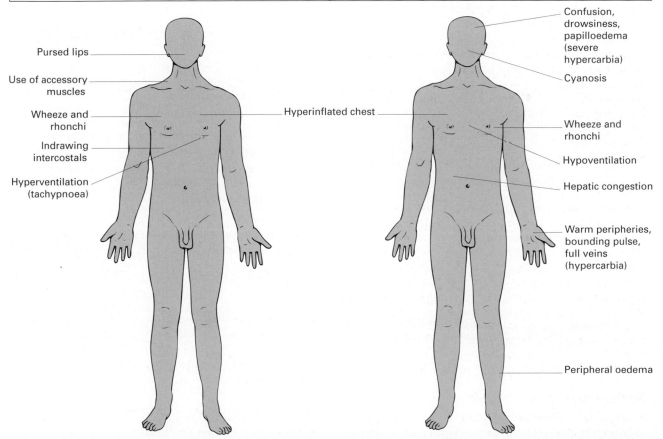

Fig. 22 The signs of chronic obstructive pulmonary disease. The 'pink puffer' and 'blue bloater' are two ends of a spectrum. Patients may move from type 1 to type 2 respiratory failure and any patient with severe airflow obstruction may develop cor pulmonale.

Table 17 Comparison of the three main aetiological types of chronic airflow obstruction

	Chronic obstructive pulmonary disease	Chronic asthma	Bronchiectasis
Smoking	+++	+/ −	+/−
Diurnal variation	+/−	+++	+/−
Cough	++	+/ −	+++
Sputum	Mucoid/purulent	Mucoid/scanty	Purulent/mucoid
Wheeze	++	+++	+
Crackles (crepitations)	−	−	+++ localised
Clubbing	−	−	++
Reversibility (>15%)	+/−	++	+/−
Night-time waking with wheeze or breathlessness	−	++	+/−

Table 18 Medical Research Council dyspnoea scale

Grade	Degree of breathlessness related to activities
1	Not troubled by breathlessness except on strenuous exercise
2	Short of breath when hurrying or walking up a slight hill
3	Walks slower than contemporaries on level ground because of breathlessness, or has to stop for breath when walking at own pace
4	Stops for breath after walking about 100 m or after a few minutes on level ground
5	Too breathless to leave the house, or breathless when dressing or undressing

occurs in association with α_1-**antitrypsin deficiency**. It is inherited as an autosomal recessive (1 : 5000 population) disease and homozygotes (ZZ, normal is MM) may develop severe emphysema with progression to respiratory failure in the fourth and fifth decades. Cigarette smoking, by activating proteases, exacerbates this. The disease predominantly affects the *lower* zones (cf. the common centrilobular type in the upper lobes). Panacinar emphysema is also seen in cigarette smokers.

Prevalence and aetiology

The major association of COPD is with cigarette smoking. There is a clear relationship between the exposure to cigarette smoking, expressed as *pack-years* (number of cigarettes per day divided by 20 and multiplied by years smoking), and the risk of death. Other interlinked associations of COPD include:

- male sex
- living in urban areas
- low social class
- air pollution
- occupation: coal miners.

In women, there is a rising prevalence of COPD that is almost certainly a *cohort* effect related to smoking habits of different generations.

There is large international variation in the prevalence of COPD. In the UK, the highest rates are seen in the northwest. Fortunately, there is some decrease in the incidence, which probably relates to changing smoking habits, including low-tar brands, and less atmospheric pollution.

Clinical presentation

Symptoms

It is important to realise that by the time symptoms occur significant airflow obstruction may be present. The hallmark of COPD is a 'smoker's cough' with clear mucoid sputum and gradually increasing breathlessness over many years. The Medical Research Council (MRC) dyspnoea scale is useful for quantifying the breathlessness (Table 18). People often complain of 'colds going onto the chest', with infective exacerbations, particularly during the winter months, associated with purulent (green/yellow) sputum. Patients may complain that their symptoms are worsened by:

- cold weather
- pollution (poor air quality)
- fog
- waking up (*but you should always consider chronic asthma if there is marked diurnal variation*).

Signs

The signs that may appear on examination are shown in Figure 22. The symptoms and signs cannot be used to predict accurately whether the pathological changes are predominantly emphysema or chronic bronchitis, which is why the term COPD is used. There is no single diagnostic test for COPD and diagnosis is based on a mixture of history, examination and investigations.

Investigations

The main investigations are:

- **Body mass index (BMI).** A low BMI is predictive of a worse outcome.
- **Chest radiograph.** This may show hyperinflation, upper zone bullae (lower zone in α_1-antitrypsin deficiency) and evidence of pulmonary hypertension (prominent pulmonary conus, pruning of pulmonary vasculature).
- **Haemoglobin level.** This may be increased (secondary erthyrocytosis).
- **Electrocardiogram.** 'P' pulmonale, right ventricular hypertrophy.
- **Lung function tests.** These will show reduced PEFR, low FEV_1, normal or reduced FVC, low FEV_1/FVC ratio (Fig. 20). Increased or normal total lung capacity, and reduced or normal transfer factor (depends on degree of emphysema) may also be seen.
- **Blood gases.** These may be:
  — normal
  — hypoxia with low $Paco_2$ (high respiratory drive: pink puffer)
  — hypoxia with high $Paco_2$ (low respiratory drive: blue bloater).

Other investigations include:

- α_1-**antitrypsin:** if early onset, little smoking or family history
- **CT scan chest:** any abnormalities on chest radiograph. Symptoms not in keeping with airflow obstruction.

Management

Once the diagnosis of COPD is established and its severity assessed, then the aims of management are:

- preventing progression of the condition
- relieving symptoms
- treating and reducing exacerbations

Central to the management of any chronic disease is the maintenance of a positive attitude to the condition. At present, there are only two interventions that have been shown to reduce mortality in patients with COPD: smoking cessation and long-term oxygen therapy (LTOT) in patients who develop hypoxic cor pulmonale. Other treatment modalities are concerned with improving symptoms and health status.

All patients with COPD who continue to smoke should be vigorously encouraged to stop. Success in this has been shown to be associated with advice from doctors, and brief structured interventions from nurses, individual and

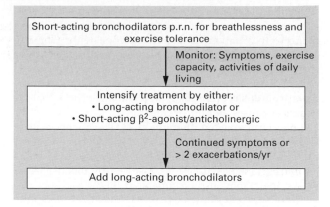

Fig. 23 A schema for the use of inhaled bronchodilators in COPD.

group therapy. Unless there are contraindications, all patients should be offered pharmacological support (e.g. bupropion or nicotine replacement therapy).

Symptom control

NICE and the BTS have produced guidelines for therapy (see http://www.nice.org.uk and http://www.britthoracic.org.uk which give a clear, logical approach to managing patients with COPD.

Inhaled bronchodilators Figure 23 provides a diagrammatic schema for increasing the intensity of inhaled therapy, starting with short-acting β_2-agonists such as salbutamol and proceeding to use of long-acting β_2-agonists (e.g. salmeterol) or anticholinergics (e.g. ipratropium or tiotropium — long-acting).

Inhaled corticosteroids These should be used in combination with other therapies. You need to be aware that tests of reversibility using oral steroids do **not** predict the response to inhaled corticosteroids. They should be prescribed in patients with significant COPD ($FEV_1 < 50\%$ predicted), who have frequent exacerbations requiring antibiotics or oral steroids. The goal is to reduce the number of exacerbations and the worsening of the disease. Oral steroids should be avoided if possible as maintenance therapy. If used, then it should be in the lowest dose acceptable to the patient and prophylaxis should be prescribed for osteoporosis.

Theophyllines If inhaled bronchodilators do not produce sufficient benefit or they cannot be tolerated, then oral theophyllines can be used, but plasma concentrations have to be measured and care taken to avoid drug interactions (particularly in elderly patients with comorbidities and altered phamacokinetics). You need to be aware that both macrolide (e.g. erythromycin) or fluoroquinolone (e.g. ciprofloxacin) antibiotics can increase the plasma levels of theophyllines.

Combined therapy The NICE/BTS guidelines indicate that patients who are symptomatic on monotherapy can benefit (symptoms, activities of daily living, lung function and exercise capacity) from combined therapy with:

- β_2-agonist and anticholinergic
- β_2-agonist and theophylline
- anticholinergic and theophylline
- long-acting beta$_2$-agonist and inhaled corticosteroid.

Delivery systems You should ensure that all your patients receive training in the use of their bronchodilator therapy. If a patient is unable to cope with a breath-actuated device (e.g. standard meter-dose inhaler), then a spacer should be tried. Nebuliser therapy is used in patients with severe symptoms, not helped by maximum therapy. If this is prescribed, then you must check that the nebuliser causes an improvement.

Long-term oxygen therapy (LTOT) Patients with a Pao_2 of less than 7.3 kPa (55 mm Hg) should be considered for LTOT. Other patients with a Pao_2 of up to 8 kPa (60 mm Hg) (stable disease as assessed by blood gases 3 weeks apart) may also be suitable if they have other evidence of severe disease such as erythrocytosis, nocturnal hypoxaemia, pulmonary hypertension or pulmonary oedema. The long-term benefits of LTOT are only seen if the therapy is used for at least 15 hours each day and is supplied using oxygen concentrators.

Intermittent oxygen therapy Portable oxygen can be used for patients who are able to leave their home. It can be of benefit (symptoms, walking distance) to those patients with significant further desaturation on exercise. It can also be prescribed ('short-burst' therapy) for patients with episodes of severe breathlessness.

Vaccination All patients with COPD should be advised to have pneumococcal and influenza (annual) vaccination. In addition, patients may benefit from antiviral (e.g. zanamivir or oseltamivir) therapy at the start of an influenza-like illness.

Pulmonary rehabilitation

Pulmonary rehabilitation comprises a structured multi-disciplinary programme of non-pharmacological treatment and general support. The programme is multidimensional comprising participation in exercise, smoking cessation advice, nutritional assessment, advice on benefit entitlements, and overviews of COPD and treatment options. The aim is to empower patients to take greater interest in, and control over, their condition. Most programmes last for 6–8 weeks and are based in secondary care units.

Exacerbations of COPD

You need to know how to assess and manage a patient with an exacerbation of COPD. Most will present with an acute worsening of their breathlessness or cough with increased sputum production and change in colour (yellow or green). A key question is whether a patient needs to be admitted to hospital and Table 19 illustrates the different profiles. Hospital-at-home schemes (and also assisted discharge schemes) are effective multiprofessional approaches to managing suitable patients.

If a patient is admitted to hospital, then you need to arrange for a number of investigations:

- chest radiograph: excludes a pneumothorax and assesses any coexistent heart failure and also pulmonary infiltrates suggestive of pneumonia
- arterial blood gases (respiratory failure — see below): remember to record the FIO_2

Table 19 Important factors in deciding whether a patient with an exacerbation of COPD should be admitted for treatment*

Factor	Treat at home	Treat in hospital
Able to cope at home	Yes	No
Breathlessness	Mild	Severe
General condition	Good	Poor/deteriorating
Level of activity	Good	Poor/confined to bed
Cyanosis	No	Yes
Worsening peripheral oedema	No	Yes
Level of consciousness	Normal	Impaired
Already receiving LTOT	No	Yes
Social circumstances	Good	Living alone/not coping
Acute confusion	No	Yes
Rapid rate of onset	No	Yes
Significant comorbidity (especially cardiac disease and insulin-dependent diabetes)	No	Yes
$Sao_2 < 90\%$	No	Yes
Changes on the chest radiograph	No	Present
Arterial pH level	≥7.35	<7.35
Arterial Pao_2	≥7 kPa (52 mm Hg)	<7 kPa (52 mm Hg)

*Adapted from NICE guidelines: http://www.nice.org.uk/page.aspx?o=guidelines.completed. LTOT, long-term oxygen therapy.

- monitoring oxygen saturation
- full blood count (raised white cell count) and urea and electrolytes (salt and water depletion)
- sputum culture: if purulent
- blood cultures: if patient is pyrexial
- ECG: atrial arrhythmias
- measurement of theophylline levels if prescribed.

The mainstay of treatment is the use of increased doses of short-acting bronchodilators (e.g. salbutamol, ipratropium). Mostly, this is done using nebulisers (take care with use of oxygen as the driving gas — worsening respiratory hypercapnia and acidosis). You should prescribe oral corticosteroids (e.g. prednisolone 30 mg) for 7–14 days. Theophyllines are used if the patient does not respond to nebulised bronchodilators.

In addition, patients with evidence of infection (more purulent sputum, consolidation on chest radiograph, raised C-reactive protein, leucocytosis or pyrexia) should be prescribed suitable antibiotics: an aminopenicillin (e.g. amoxicillin), a macrolide (clarithromycin) or a tetracycline. Cephalosporins (e.g. cefuroxime) are often used but there is an increased risk of antibiotic-associated diarrhoea (*Clostridium difficile*).

Respiratory failure

Blood gas analysis is discussed on page 73. Patients with a high respiratory drive (pink puffers) may have type 1 respiratory failure with hypoxia and a low $Paco_2$ at rest. When the airflow limitation is not severe, the signs may appear only on exercise.

Blue bloaters with a low respiratory drive may develop type 2 respiratory failure with hypoxia and high $Paco_2$. If the patient is stable, the pH will be normal because retention of bicarbonate will have compensated for the rise in $Paco_2$. In acute deterioration, this compensation will not have had time to occur and the pH will be low (respiratory acidosis).

Your major aims of management of acute respiratory failure are:

- treat the underlying cause
- improve arterial and tissue oxygenation (oxygen saturation >90%)
- avoid further deterioration of acidosis (pH < 7.35).

You should always treat heart failure (p. 31) and correct any hypovolaemia as it will help the delivery of oxygen to the tissues and correction of local acidosis. Other problems may also require specific intervention, e.g. infection or a pneumothorax. Any sedatives should be discontinued.

The principal treatment of respiratory failure is controlled oxygen therapy to maintain the oxygen saturation above 90% without worsening respiratory acidosis. In patients with acute type 2 respiratory failure, correction of the hypoxia may reduce respiratory drive with worsening hypercarbia and acidosis, but this risk has been overemphasised in the past. Clinical signs of rising $Paco_2$ are drowsiness, warm peripheries, dilated veins and a bounding pulse. Controlled oxygen therapy and the increasing use of nasal intermittent positive pressure ventilation (NIPPV) have improved outcome in acute treatment,

which should be considered in any patient with a pH of <7.35. A few patients with persistent hypercapnia can benefit from domicillary NIPPV. Mechanical ventilation may be indicated if severe acidosis is present (pH < 7.25).

Cor pulmonale

Cor pulmonale means heart failure developing secondary to lung disease. It is most commonly seen with COPD because of its high prevalence in the UK. In the early stages, pulmonary hypertension occurs with consequent right ventricular and right atrial hypertrophy. Eventually the heart fails with marked fluid retention, giving peripheral oedema, an elevated jugular venous pressure and worsening breathlessness. Although the load is predominantly on the right side of the heart, you should remember that both ventricles eventually fail. Other than management of the lung disease, diuretics are the mainstay of treatment.

Other problems

Patients can be severely compromised by even small **pneumothoraces** (p. 98). A **pulmonary embolus** may also occur in *immobile* patients (p. 49).

Prognosis

Patients with severe COPD and cor pulmonale have a markedly reduced life expectancy. Patients are also at risk of developing other smoking-related diseases, notably carcinoma of the bronchus (p. 82) and ischaemic heart disease (p. 11).

Asthma

The diagnosis of asthma is not easy, but the International Consensus Report describes it as:

A chronic inflammatory disorder of the airways. In susceptible individuals, inflammatory symptoms are usually associated with widespread, but variable airflow obstruction and an increase in airway response to a variety of stimuli. Obstruction is often reversible, either spontaneously or with treatment.

This description incorporates all the key features of asthma from which you can deduce the symptoms and signs. Asthma is a common condition that causes considerable morbidity and results in approximately 1500 deaths per year in the UK.

Epidemiology

Between 12 and 15% of children have attacks of wheezing typical of asthma. In adults the prevalence is around 5%. There is some geographical variation and the prevalence is increasing.

Occupational asthma is an important cause of work-related disease. For example, workers in the polyurethane industry (toluene diisocyanate) or in textiles (cotton; byssinosis) may be affected. The hallmark of occupational disease is work-related symptoms.

Aspirin-sensitive asthma (ASA) is a metabolic disorder in which individuals suffer acute asthma on exposure to aspirin or non-steroidal anti-inflammatory drugs

Two

(NSAIDs). These individuals are thought to have variant metabolic pathways for the breakdown of arachidonic acid.

Pathophysiology

The common factor in asthmatics is bronchial hyper-reactivity, which can be demonstrated by provocation testing. Asthmatics broncho-constrict at much lower concentrations of the stimulus (e.g. methacholine, histamine) than normal subjects. Many factors may initiate an asthmatic attack:

- irritants: smoke, paint, chemicals
- exercise (cold, dry air)
- respiratory infections
- airborne allergens, e.g. dog hair, moulds
- drugs: aspirin, beta-blockers.

Pathophysiology of atopic asthma

In atopy, the increased production of IgE is consequent upon a disproportionate response of T-helper lymphocytes type 2 (TH2) over the TH1 type. The trigger for this response is exposure to environmental antigens. The immunoglobulin E (IgE) produced binds to mast cells in the bronchial mucosa where subsequent antigens react with mast cell IgE to cause the cell to degranulate and release a host of inflammatory proteins. Consequent upon this a two-phase reaction takes place in the airway.

The acute phase response Vascular leakage and smooth muscle contraction are the predominant features. These usually clear within 1–2 hours. Substances released from mast cells in the acute response include:

- histamine (vascular permeability)
- tryptase and chymase (protease enzymes that promote tissue degradation)
- leukotrienes (smooth muscle contraction and vascular permeability)
- platelet activating factor (vascular permeability)
- chemokines and cytokines (facilitate the late response).

The late response This is characterised by eosinophilic and lymphocytic infiltration of the bronchial mucosa. It usually starts up to 6 hours after the acute phase and may persist for 24 hours. The response is orchestrated by a number of mediators:

- interleukin 5 (IL5): recruitment of eosinophils
- eosinophilic breakdown products (e.g. eosinophilic cationic protein) which promote bronchial inflammation
- TH2 lymphocytes: production of cytokines.

The long-term structural consequences of the release of these proteins for the airway are:

- loss of surface epithelium
- increased basement membrane thickness
- marked increase in smooth muscle mass
- marked local inflammatory cell infiltrate
- increased vascular permeability
- remodelling of the airways.

Clinical presentation

Symptoms

The diagnosis of asthma is a clinical one as there is no definitive diagnostic test. The predominant symptoms of asthma are shortness of breath, wheeze, chest tightness and cough. Commonly, the symptoms are much worse in the night and early morning (diurnal variation). There may be seasonal variation, with attacks coinciding with high pollen counts. Cough may be the only problem and, if so, you may miss the underlying diagnosis. If the cough is productive of mucus plugs, you should consider allergic bronchopulmonary aspergillosis (p. 93). Triggers to attacks should be sought, including home environment and work. In some patients, particularly where the asthma has developed later in life, there may be little variation in symptoms, with chronic shortness of breath and wheeze. Many of these patients are allergic to moulds and have severe asthma with fungal sensitisation (SAFS).

Signs

The signs depend on the severity of the asthma and its chronicity. You will often see patients in an acute attack, where observation will show the patient to be distressed, centrally cyanosed, tachypnoeic and using their accessory muscles. Tachycardia is usually present; this may partly reflect the overuse of β_2-agonists. Usually, you will find widespread inspiratory and expiratory wheezes.

Features of severe asthma include:

- PEFR 33–50% best or predicted
- subject cannot complete sentences in one breath
- respiratory rate ≥25 breaths/min
- pulse >110 beats/min.

It is important to be able to assess the severity of an attack (see the emergency box).

Inability to speak This should not *substitute* for measuring the peak flow, but its presence should alert you.

Disturbance of conscious level This implies muscle fatigue, profound hypoxia and a rising carbon dioxide level.

A silent chest Where the asthma is severe, mucus plugging compounds the airflow obstruction and the breath sounds diminish and disappear.

Life-threatening features These are:

- PEFR <33% best or predicted
- silent chest — feeble respiratory effort
- bradycardia or hypotension
- exhaustion, confusion or coma
- $Spo_2 < 92\%$ or $Pao_2 < 8$ kPa (60 mm Hg)
- normal $Paco_2$ (4.6–6.0 kPa (34–45 mm Hg)).

Response to signs If any of the above signs is present or if you are worried then you **must** ask for help with a view to immediate intervention and admission to intensive care. Remember that deaths in asthmatics in hospital are associated with *inadequate assessment* (no chest radiograph, no blood gases) and *poor treatment* (no steroids, discharge from casualty emergency room, slow response).

Clinical Box: Emergency treatment: acute asthma (bronchoconstriction)

Assess severity quickly

- Measure peak expiratory flow rate (severe: <35% best or predicted, may be unrecordable)
- Life-threatening features
  - Silent chest, cyanosis, poor respiratory effort
  - Bradycardia, arrhythmia, hypotension
  - Exhaustion, confusion, coma
- Take a detailed history when appropriate
- Oximetry (severe: saturation <92%)
- Take arterial sample for blood gas analysis (severe: PaO_2 < 8 kPa (60 mmHg); $PaCO_2$ > 4.6 kPa (34 mmHg)

Management

- If moderate/severe (PEF 33–75%)
  - Give high-flow oxygen
  - Give nebulised β_2-agonist (5 mg salbutamol)
  - Give steroids (200 mg hydrocortisone or 50 mg prednisolone)
- If features of a life-threatening attack present
  - Obtain senior/ICU help immediately
  - Add ipratropium bromide 500 µg to nebuliser
  - Continuous salbutamol nebuliser (5–10 mg/hr)
  - Consider i.v. magnesium sulphate 1.2–2.0 g over 20 mins

Investigations

- Request a chest radiograph: particularly to exclude pneumothorax

Reassess frequently; ask for help early

Diagnosis

In order to make the diagnosis of asthma you need to demonstrate a variation in airflow obstruction of at least 15%. A history of episodic wheeze, shortness of breath and cough makes the diagnosis more straightforward; it is much more difficult in chronic asthma where there may be little variation in symptoms over time and no obvious triggers. You need a high index of suspicion, backed up by measurement of airflow limitation and reversibility. The last may require a 1–2 week trial of corticosteroids.

Wheeze does not necessarily indicate asthma; other common medical conditions should be considered, particularly heart failure and pulmonary emboli. Obstruction either from tumour or foreign body may occasionally be the cause. Other rare conditions may cause airflow obstruction, e.g. eosinophilic syndromes (p. 93) (tropical eosinophilia and Churg–Strauss syndrome). Carcinoid syndrome may present with wheeze.

Investigations

You should know how to assess a patient with either acute or chronic asthma. Spirometry (FEV_1, FVC) may show a reduced ratio, though in many people it is normal between attacks. The patient should be encouraged to monitor their disease by symptom diaries linked to peak flow recording. More detailed lung function may show hyperinflation

with increased total lung capacity and residual volume. Transfer factor is normal. Blood gas analysis is commonly normal, though hypoxaemia is sometimes found in severe asthmatics even between attacks.

A chest radiograph is often normal, though it can show hyperinflation and, occasionally, atelectasis (segmental/lobar) or lung collapse caused by mucus plugging, particularly in severe disease.

In young subjects, mild blood eosinophilia may be seen in association with atopy (hay fever, eczema). Skin tests to common allergens commonly show multiple reactions (Ch. 9).

Management

Emergency treatment is outlined in the box on this page.

Studies of asthma deaths have demonstrated a number of important factors:

- most deaths in patients with chronic severe disease
- excessive use of β_2-agonist rather than steroids
- inadequate monitoring of the severity of the asthma including lack of follow-up, delayed referral and under-use of written management plans.

Acute asthma (status asthmaticus)

The patient usually presents with progressive deterioration over several hours or days, sometimes associated with a definite trigger such as a chest infection or ingestion of aspirin (or another NSAID). Occasionally *brittle* asthma is present, when the onset is abrupt and life-threatening. The clinical signs in acute asthma are given above. The key to management is proper assessment. You *must* perform the following investigations on all patients in the accident and emergency department:

- PEFR
- pulse oximetry
- blood gases (if oxygen saturation is <92%)
- chest radiograph.

In a severe attack PEFR is grossly reduced (<100 l/min) and may be unrecordable. Chest radiograph shows hyperinflation. Atelectasis and/or collapse caused by mucus plugging may be seen. Evidence of infection may be present. A **pneumothorax** must be excluded on a chest radiograph; even small ones may compromise patients with airflow obstruction.

Blood gases commonly show hypoxaemia with hypocarbia and alkalosis, reflecting increased respiratory drive. In severe airflow limitation, **normocarbia** is a bad sign, signalling failing alveolar ventilation. You must continue to monitor the patient's condition, documenting improvement or worsening of the airflow obstruction.

You should ensure that a high concentration of oxygen (>60%) is administered to all patients on arrival; hypercarbia will *not* occur. A β_2-agonist, such as salbutamol (2.5–5 mg), should be administered via a nebuliser and can be repeated 3–6-hourly or can be given continuously. Nebulised ipratropium bromide can be used. In all cases of asthma that require admission, corticosteroids should be given as a bolus of hydrocortisone i.v. (3–6 mg/kg) followed by oral prednisolone 40–50 mg in divided doses (or 100 mg hydrocortisone 6-hourly). In a patient who responds and is not usually on maintenance oral steroids, prednisolone can be stopped after 5 days and replaced by inhaled steroid therapy.

In patients with acute severe asthma who do not respond to the initial bronchodilator therapy, intravenous magnesium sulphate (1.2–2 g over 20 mins) can be given in consultation with senior medical staff. Aminophylline is only rarely used and again is only administered under the direction of senior staff. A bolus of 5 mg/kg is given over 30 mins followed by an infusion of 0.5 mg/kg/hr. If a patient is already on oral theophyllines, blood levels must be measured before a bolus is give.

Supportive therapy is essential. Fluid intake must be maintained and dehydration corrected. Appropriate antibiotics are prescribed *if* there is evidence of infection (p. 429). Sedation *must* be avoided.

A small percentage of patients will continue to deteriorate. You must seek expert help urgently. Worrying signs are exhaustion, with disturbance of consciousness and blood gas analysis showing respiratory alkalosis being replaced by worsening hypoxia, hypercarbia and acidosis, as alveolar ventilation decreases and fails. Early intervention with intubation and mechanical ventilation is mandatory.

Monitoring treatment
- Repeat measures of PEFR 15–30 minutes after starting treatment.
- Ensure oximetry shows saturations ≥92% (if saturation <92% then measure arterial blood gases).
- Measure heart rate.
- Monitor serum potassium and blood glucose.
- Transfer patient to intensive care unit in the event of:
  — deteriorating PEFR
  — worsening or persisting hypoxia, or hypercarbia
  — fall in pH or rising H^+ concentration
  — exhaustion, feeble respirations
  — confusion or drowsiness
  — coma or respiratory arrest.

Chronic asthma

Patients with chronic asthma should be seen regularly either as hospital outpatients or in specialist clinics in primary care. Proactive review is of proven benefit. Severe asthmatics are often given open access to a specialist service. *Education* is an important principle, with the person being encouraged to monitor their disease, and to understand its basis and the use of various treatments and delivery systems.

Drug treatment in chronic asthma The aims of management in chronic asthma are to:

- minimise asthma symptoms during the night and day
- ensure no limitation on physical activity
- maintain lung function at the best possible at all times (aim for normal)
- prevent exacerbations
- ensure minimal need for reliever medication.

The overall goals are to:

- prevent the development of permanently abnormal lung function
- reduce the risk of death from an acute attack

- achieve the best possible quality of life for a patient with asthma.

Two types of drugs are used:

- **relievers**: β2-agonists, theophylline, anticholinergics
- **preventers**: corticosteroids, cromones (cromoglicate), antileukotrienes, corticosteroid-sparing agents (methotrexate, ciclosporin).

A patient with anything but mild symptoms *must* receive regular prophylactic treatment; undue reliance should not be placed on symptomatic treatment. You need to have a clear grasp of these drugs (p. 73). A stepwise approach to treatment has been recommended by the BTS (Table 20).

For a patient following an acute attack, you should:

- stop oral steroids after 5 days, (or 5 days following recovery) and substitute inhaled steroids
- ensure that this is done in conjunction with the patient carefully monitoring their symptoms with an asthma action plan.

Self-management education One of the challenges is to incorporate the recommendations for the long-term

Table 20 A stepwise approach to treatment in chronic asthma as recommended by the British Thoracic Society

Step	Component
1	Short-acting β2-agonist drugs (salbutamol/terbutaline), 'as required' use only If needed more than once daily, go to step 2
2	Regular preventer medication First-line treatment should be inhaled corticosteroids (beclometasone/budesonide/fluticasone) Alternatives include inhaled cromones (sodium cromoglicate/nedocromil) or antileukotrienes (only zafirlukast currently licensed for use without concomitant inhaled steroids in the UK)
3	Increased preventer medication and/or addition of long-acting β-agonists (salmeterol/formoterol), theophylline (e.g. aminophylline) or antileukotrienes (zafirlukast/montelukast)
4	High-dose inhaled steroids and combinations of other step 3 drugs Although short-acting β2-agonists should be prescribed for 'as required' use only, many patients in this group require them regularly Anticholinergic agents may be tried (ipratropium/oxitropium)
5	All medications in step 4 with the addition of regular oral corticosteroids All patients in the higher groups should be referred for specialist assessment

Step down
An important but poorly adhered to aspect of asthma management
Once control has been achieved (3–6 months' duration) look to reduce medication
Do not stop inhaled steroid medication before other regular therapy

Table 21 Part of an asthma action plan for chronic asthma

Peak flow (% at best)	Symptoms	Action taken
80–100	None/infrequent	Continue inhaled steroids; step down if stable for 6 months; β_2-agonist for relief as required
60–80	Nocturnal symptoms; chronic cough; 'cold-like' symptoms; frequent use of β_2-agonist	Start inhaled steroids if not taking regularly; double existing dose of steroids; treat respiratory infection if evidence of one
40–60	Increasing breathlessness; limited activity; β_2-agonist every 2–3 hours	Start oral corticosteroids; contact doctor; attend A&E
<40	Breathless; difficulty talking; no response to β_2-agonist	Start oral corticosteroids; call ambulance or contact emergency doctor

treatment of asthma within the framework of a simple and practical management regime that can be undertaken by the asthmatic subjects. This has led to the development of personalised asthma action plans in which patients make changes to their treatment in response to the recognition of changes in the severity of their asthma, in accordance with predetermined guidelines. This system involves the integration of self-assessment and self-management, incorporating written guidelines for both the long-term treatment of asthma and the treatment of severe asthma attacks.

Since the requirements of individuals will vary considerably, no single plan is likely to be suitable for every patient. Certain features may need to be varied, depending on the needs of the patient for whom the plan is developed. However, plans must include:

- structured personalised education
- specific advice about monitoring asthma control
- actions to be taken if asthma worsens.

An example of a personalised asthma action plan is given in Table 21.

Complications

Apart from those discussed above, pneumothorax, together with lung collapse (mucus plugging), is the most important complication of acute asthma. You should always consider whether a pneumothorax has been excluded in a deteriorating asthmatic.

Pulmonary eosinophilia

Pulmonary eosinophilia is defined as a blood eosinophilia with pulmonary infiltrates, which are often transient and peripheral on the chest radiograph. Most patients are asymptomatic, but they can present with breathlessness and a cough.

In chronic asthma, the diagnosis of allergic bronchopulmonary aspergillosis should be borne in mind. Hypersensitivity to the fungus *Aspergillus fumigatus* (which is ubiquitous) develops. Patients usually have pre-existing asthma and present with a cough productive of green 'rubbery' plugs together with fever. Recurrent pulmonary infiltrates with a blood eosinophilia (if not on steroids) are the hallmarks. A chest radiograph may show shadowing

(often of the upper lobe). Patients have high IgE levels and positive precipitins to *Aspergillus*. Treatment is with oral corticosteroids in acute attacks and long term itraconazole.

Other causes of pulmonary eosinophilia

You should be aware of other forms of pulmonary eosinophilia which have a heterogeneous aetiology.

- drug-induced, e.g. sulphonamides, nitrofurantoin
- helminthic infection, e.g. *Ascaris lumbricoides* (Loeffler's syndrome)
- fungi, e.g. *Aspergillus, Candida*
- cryptogenic, e.g. eosinophilic pneumonia
- granulomatosis, e.g. Churg–Strauss syndrome.

2.5 Interstitial lung disease

Learning objectives

You should be able to:
- discuss how different disease processes can cause pulmonary fibrosis
- integrate the clinical features and investigations into a list of possible diagnoses
- list some of the rarer causes of the problems.

Case Study

The chest physicians have decided that they need to look further into the breathlessness that has been bothering Kenneth Mapfumo for several months. He has been under follow-up for a year after a routine chest radiograph was abnormal when he came to this country a year ago at the age of 29 years. He had not had any other problems apart from being given steroids for a 'red eye'.

Pulmonary fibrosis is a description of the final pathological effect of several different disease processes. It may be focal or diffuse. In the end stage, the latter is often described as *honeycomb*.

The preferred term for interstitial lung disease is diffuse parenchymal lung disease. You need a strategy for assessment, investigation and management of patients, but a key element is referral to a respiratory physician. Key aspects of assessment are:

- a detailed history including occupation, past medical history, travel, environment (including pets and hobbies), drugs and smoking
- a careful general and respiratory examination looking for evidence of systemic disease (e.g. pyrexia, skin involvement, joints).

Investigations

These should include:

- full blood count and eosinophil count (p. 265)
- C-reactive protein/ESR (general inflammatory markers)
- antinuclear antibody and rheumatoid factor
- urea and electrolytes (renal involvement)
- liver function tests (liver involvement)
- calcium (sarcoidosis).

Other tests (e.g. antineutrophil cytoplasmic antibody — ANCA) are dependent on the clinical picture.

Imaging

You should start by requesting a standard PA chest radiograph. If this suggests interstitial lung disease, then it is important to track down previous radiographs for comparison.

A high-resolution CT scan is the imaging investigation of choice, particularly in patients with suspected cryptogenic fibrosing alveolitis.

Pulmonary function

The minimum pulmonary function tests are spirometry and measurement of transfer factor. The latter, together with vital capacity, is used for disease monitoring. Remember that evidence of airflow obstruction does not exclude the diagnosis of interstitial lung disease (the two can coexist).

Biopsy

A lung biopsy is required where the diagnosis of interstitial lung disease is not clear. Occasionally, open lung biopsy is needed, but mostly transbronchial lung biopsies are sufficient.

Cryptogenic fibrosing alveolitis

Cryptogenic fibrosing alveolitis is a disease of unknown aetiology which typically occurs in middle age. It is more common in males. The pathological features are an inflammatory response within the alveoli. Polymorph leucocytes predominate in the broncho-alveolar washings. Subsequently, progressive fibrosis supervenes. A rare acute form (**Hamman–Rich syndrome**) occurs with rapid progression to death within a few months. More typically, patients present with a gradual onset of breathlessness and a dry cough. On examination, clubbing is common, and fine late inspiratory crackles are heard at the bases. Respiratory rate may be increased and cyanosis occurs in the end stage of

the disease. Pulmonary function shows a *restrictive* pattern (p. 72 and Fig. 20) and arterial hypoxia with a reduced $Paco_2$ (high respiratory drive) on blood gas analysis. The chest radiograph characteristically has *bilateral basal* shadowing with honeycombing. A high-resolution CT scan is the best imaging modality. Diagnosis is confirmed by a transbronchial or open lung biopsy. Histopathology is very important for predicting response to treatment (usual interstitial pneumonitis worse than desquamative interstitial pneumonitis). Autoantibodies (e.g. rheumatoid factor) are frequently found on blood tests. Corticosteroids and immunosuppressives are used with the best responses being seen in patients with significant cellular inflammation and less fibrosis. However, benefits are limited and complete commission is rare.

Other conditions causing pulmonary fibrosis are listed in Table 22.

Extrinsic allergic alveolitis

There are many rare examples of conditions causing extrinsic allergic alveolitis: for example, maple bark stripper's lung! You need to be aware of the much more common, but still quite rare, **bird fancier's lung**, from keeping either pigeons or budgerigars. Pathologically, the condition is characterised by the formation of granuloma with subsequent fibrosis. The damage is initiated by a specific precipitating antibody. Lung function shows a restrictive pattern with progressive reduction in lung volumes and transfer factor. Precipitating antibodies to the antigen are positive.

In **pigeon fancier's lung**, exposure is often episodic. Therefore, the picture is an acute illness several hours after exposure to the antigen. Patients have fever, myalgia, cough, breathlessness and, on examination, crackles. In budgerigar fancier's lung, there is often constant exposure, with progressive breathlessness and cough.

The final picture on a chest radiograph or CT is severe *upper lobe* fibrosis with cavitation. In the early stages, diffuse micronodules are seen. Auscultatory findings are a mixture of inspiratory crackles and wheezes. Finger clubbing is *uncommon*. Pulmonary function tests show a restrictive pattern with reduced transfer factor and hypoxaemia at rest or commonly with exercise. The first line of management is to stop the exposure to the antigen. Some patients may be helped by corticosteroids.

Sarcoidosis

Sarcoidosis is important both in its own right and as a major differential diagnosis with respiratory tuberculosis. The aetiology of sarcoidosis is unknown. It usually occurs in young adulthood, with a slight female preponderance. It is more common in temperate zones and in Afro-Caribbeans than Caucasians. Sarcoidosis can affect many different systems, but predominantly affects the hilar lymph nodes and the lungs. Up to half of patients can have systemic features (malaise, arthralgia, fever).

Pathology

There is activation of T cells with granuloma formation in the organ affected. There is no central necrosis, unlike in

Table 22 Causes of pulmonary fibrosis other than cryptogenic fibrosing alveolitis

Type	Examples	Special features
Sarcoidosis		Hilar lymphadenopathy; significant radiograph abnormalities; few symptoms
Drugs	Cytotoxics, e.g. bleomycin, busulfan, methotrexate, etc. Others: amiodarone, nitrofurantoin	First indication is reduction of transfer factor
Autoimmune disease	Rheumatoid arthritis (RF (rheumatoid factor) almost invariably strongly positive)	Three types: (i) diffuse fibrosis (ii) nodular: particularly with pneumoconiosis – Caplan's syndrome (iii) focal fibrosis
	Systemic sclerosis Mixed connective tissue disease Systemic lupus erythematosus (SLE) Ankylosing spondylitis	Pleurisy, vasculitis Upper lobe fibrosis
Occupational	Pneumoconiosis	Spectrum of fine mottling to progressive massive fibrosis; may be nodular (with RA)
	Asbestosis	Basal, pleural calcification Other associations: mesothelioma, bronchial carcinoma
	Silicosis	Eggshell calcification in hilar nodes
Extrinisic allergic alveolitis	Pigeon fancier's lung Budgerigar fancier's lung	Upper lobe, episodic symptoms Insidious; precipitins strongly positive

Two

tuberculosis. In the lungs, broncho-alveolar lavage may contain a large number of T lymphocytes. In the fluid, or in the serum, increased levels of **angiotensin-converting enzyme** (ACE) may be found but is of limited value in diagnosis or monitoring the response to treatment. **Anergy** is found with depressed peripheral T cell immunity (p. 382; delayed hypersensitivity). As the disease progresses, pulmonary fibrosis occurs.

Clinical presentation

The clinical manifestations of sarcoid depend on the organ affected. In the eye, blindness can occur secondary to uveitis. Erythema nodosum, keloid and lupus pernio are skin manifestations. The central nervous system can be involved with neuritis, space-occupying lesions and sterile meningitis. In the heart, the characteristic manifestation is conduction disturbance. Sarcoidosis is one cause of a pyrexia of unknown origin (p. 427).

The most common site of sarcoid is the lung, where sarcoidosis is classified into four stages:

I. hilar lymphadenopathy alone: may have erythema nodosum
II. hilar lymphadenopathy and pulmonary infiltrate
III. pulmonary infiltrate alone.
IV. fibrosis.

Stage I is usually asymptomatic and self-limiting, whereas stage IV implies some irreversible changes.

Investigations

Most patients in stage I are picked up by a routine chest radiograph showing hilar shadowing. In stages II–IV, parenchymal shadowing is apparent in both lung fields. High-resolution CT scanning may be helpful, particularly in differentiating active alveolitis from fibrosis. Serum ACE is more likely to be elevated. Pulmonary function testing shows a reduced transfer factor and a restrictive defect. Hypercalciuria may be present and, occasionally, hypercalcaemia.

Immunologically, there is an increase in cells (predominantly T lymphocytes) in broncho-alveolar lavage fluid and anergy to intradermal tuberculin testing.

Management

Most stage I thoracic cases resolve spontaneously. With progressive disease and deteriorating pulmonary function, corticosteroids should be given. They should also be prescribed for extrathoracic involvement. Other immunosuppressive drugs are also used (e.g. methotrexate, hydroxychloroquine).

Vasculitis

Wegener's granulomatosis

In Wegener's granulomatosis, there is a widespread granulomatous vasculitis affecting the lungs, kidneys and upper respiratory tract. The vasculitis affects the medium and small arteries, arterioles and venules. It commonly presents with haemoptysis, breathlessness, pleuritic pain, general malaise and low-grade pyrexia.

Investigations show bilateral pulmonary nodules that may cavitate. There is *no* hilar lymphadenopathy. ANCA (p. 345) are usually present, consistent with vasculitis. The extent of the renal involvement determines survival. Treatment is with corticosteroids and cyclophosphamide.

Fortunately, with treatment, the prognosis is good, with remission in most patients.

Goodpasture's syndrome

Goodpasture's syndrome is predominantly a disease of young men, presenting with pulmonary haemorrhage and glomerulonephritis (p. 176); either may dominate the clinical picture. The diagnostic hallmark is the presence of **antiglomerular basement membrane antibody** and deposition of immune complex in the basement membrane on renal biopsy. Proven treatments are dialysis, plasma exchange (to remove the antibody) and cytotoxic therapy.

2.6 Miscellaneous respiratory disease

Learning objectives

You should:
- be aware of a range of conditions that may affect the lung
- know the specific features of some of the different conditions.

Case Study

Rosie has brought Fred to the clinic, even though he does not admit that he has a problem apart from his weight. She is 'being driven mad' at night by his snoring, which builds to a peak, then he seems to stop breathing, such that 'I think he is not going to start again.' Fred says that he does not sleep very well and often finds that he is sleepy during the day, which worries him as he drives a delivery van.

Sleep apnoea syndrome

It is helpful to be aware of the definitions used by the Scottish Intercollegiate Guidelines Network (SIGN) and the BTS (http://www.brit-thoracic.org.uk/):

- apnoea — a 10 sec breathing pause
- hypopnoea — a 10 sec event where there is continued breathing but ventilation is reduced by at least 50% from previous baseline during sleep
- obstructive sleep apnoea/hypopnoea syndrome (OSAHS) — the coexistence of excessive daytime sleepiness with irregular breathing at night.
- apnoea/hypopnoea index (AHI) — the frequency of apnoea and hypopnoea hourly (used to assess severity).

In sleep apnoea, the patient experiences a reduction in muscle tone in the upper pharyngeal airways), which causes obstruction. In response, respiratory effort is increased and the patient becomes more wakeful. This is repeated many times during the night so that the patient sleeps poorly and is somnolent during the day.

The presentation is usually with snoring (partner may complain), day-time drowsiness and reduced concentration. Other features include restlessness during the night (again discuss with partner) and irritability. A standard questionnaire (Epworth) is useful in the assessment and patients should be seen by a specialist, particularly if the problem may be affecting driving or working (e.g. machinery). On examination, you must record:

- weight and height (obesity is common)
- neck circumference (shirt size)
- any evidence of nasal or pharyngeal airway obstruction
- blood pressure (often hypertensive).

A specialist centre would perform sleep studies to establish the diagnosis and severity (severe AHI >30/hr). The first line of management is to encourage the patient to lose weight, avoid alcohol or sleeping tablets and sleep on their back. Continuous positive airways pressure (CPAP) is used if the problem is moderate or severe. Some patients benefit from intra-oral devices to increase the patency of the upper airways.

It is very important that the patient is told to inform the driving licensing authorities (DVLA in the UK) and that they must not drive if they feel sleepy.

Acute respiratory distress syndrome

Acute respiratory distress syndrome (ARDS) is the most serious manifestation of acute lung injury. It is associated with prior:

- sepsis (p. 410)
- hypotension/shock (p. 411)
- smoke inhalation
- trauma
- aspiration
- other systemic diseases.

The initial damage is to the pulmonary capillary endothelium, causing an increase in permeability with a leak into the interstitium/alveoli of plasma and red cells. The precise mechanisms are complicated. The management of ARDS is covered in Chapter 10 (p. 412).

2.7 Pleural disease

Learning objectives

You should be able to:
- diagnose patients as having disease of the pleura/pleural space
- outline the investigation and management.

Case Study

The doctors are struggling to diagnose Alice's problem with some fluid round her lung. She says that they are sure that it is not due to her heart, even though she was only in hospital a few weeks ago with a heart attack and a chest infection. Her worry is that they now have said that they need to take a small piece of the lining of the chest to look at under a microscope and they may want to use a 'flexible telescope' to look inside her chest.

The pleural space is bounded by the **parietal** pleura, lining the thoracic cavity and mediastinum. The **visceral** pleura covers the lungs and is rich in blood vessels and lymphatics. Unlike the parietal pleura, it has no pain fibres. The pressure within the space is *negative*, approximately −5 cmH$_2$O.

Pleuritic pain

The major causes of pleuritic pain are infection, pulmonary embolus, malignancy and trauma. The last may be caused by fractured ribs, which may occur during bouts of coughing (**cough fracture**), particularly in elderly people. Your approach to solving the problem must involve combining information from the history, examination and investigations.

Pain should always be relieved, not only because of the distress to the patient but also because of the associated splinting of the ribcage; the poor respiratory effort and cough may lead to hypostatic pneumonia or respiratory failure (in a compromised patient). NSAIDs are useful to relieve bone pain and inflammation. Strong opiates may be needed; if they are used, beware of respiratory depression.

Pleural effusion

The layers of the pleura are usually separated by a thin layer of fluid acting as a lubricant. Clinically, an effusion cannot be detected below 500 ml. Effusions may be loculated (for example, in the transverse fissure) and it may be difficult to determine whether the opacity is caused by fluid or pleural thickening. Ultrasound examination is usually performed to confirm the diagnosis.

There are many different causes of a pleural effusion; your first step in determining the aetiology is to set it in the context of the patient's general history and examination. A diagnostic aspiration is often of value (Table 23). Fluid should always be sent for biochemical analysis (protein and, possibly, LDH, glucose and amylase), microbiology (Gram stain, culture and possible examination/culture for tuberculosis) and cytology (malignancy, including lymphoma and mesothelioma). Often, the aetiology will be clear simply on the clinical findings. In trying to establish the diagnosis from the pleural aspiration results, it is useful to divide the causes into:

- transudates (protein <20 g/l): usually result from cardiac failure; may be caused by hypoalbuminaemia
- exudates (protein >30 g/l): multiple causes; consider infection (including tuberculosis), malignancy, connective tissue disease (rheumatoid disease) or pulmonary infarction.

Although a recent meta-analysis reported that a pleural fluid protein concentration of greater than 30 g/l had a high sensitivity and specificity for diagnosis of an exudate, Light's criteria can also be useful:

- pleural fluid serum protein ratio > 0.5
- pleural fluid serum LDH ratio > 0.6
- pleural fluid LDH > two-thirds of normal serum value.

Further information, particularly in suspected tuberculosis (p. 78) and malignancy (p. 80), can be gained from a pleural biopsy, which can be done under ultrasound or endoscopic guidance (thorascopy). If the patient has been

Two

Table 23 Diagnostic information from pleural fluid

Diagnosis	Appearance	Protein	Sugar	Amylase	Culture	Cytology
Heart failure	Clear	Transudate				
Hypoproteinaemia	Clear	Transudate				
Tuberculosis	Clear	Exudate	Low		Bacilli: low yield	Lymphocytes
Malignancy, including mesothelioma	Blood-stained	Exudate		High: pancreatic		Malignant cells
Pulmonary embolus	Blood-stained	Exudate				Lymphocytes
Rheumatoid disease	Clear	Exudate	Low			
Pneumonia (parapneumonic)	Clear or purulent	Exudate	Normal		Usually negative	Leucocytes
Empyema	Opaque pus (offensive)	Exudate	Low		Bacteria, especially anaerobes	Pus cells
Chylous	White	Exudate			Negative	
Pancreatitis	May have blood	Exudate		High		

Transudate = < 20 g/dl protein; exudate = > 30 g/dl or defined by Light's criteria (see text).

exposed to asbestos, even slightly, you should consider a mesothelioma (p. 99).

Initial management of an effusion is aimed at making an aetiological diagnosis, then treating as appropriate. Small effusions may be aspirated to dryness. A **haemothorax** (trauma) must be aspirated to prevent subsequent organisation and fibrosis. A further reason is that blood is a good culture medium. If the fluid is chyle, this is most likely caused by a malignant block of the thoracic duct, though trauma should be excluded.

Large symptomatic effusions of whatever aetiology require insertion of an intercostal drain. Rapid aspiration is contraindicated; it may distress the patient and, rarely, may precipitate pulmonary oedema. Malignant effusions often reaccumulate; these should be drained, then a sclerosing agent such as talc or tetracycline instilled to achieve adhesion of the pleural layers (pleurodesis) and consequent obliteration of the pleural space.

Infection of the pleural space

There are four major types of infection in the pleural space:

- pleurisy
- parapneumonic effusion
- empyema — grossly purulent pleural effusion
- tuberculous empyema.

Occasionally pleural infection is a marker of subdiaphragmatic disease (i.e. liver abscess) or systemic disease such as endocarditis.

Pleurisy

Pleurisy refers to a sharp chest pain on inspiration, with features of infection. It may be a manifestation of lobar pneumonia or caused by a virus infection (e.g. Coxsackie virus). Management requires a chest radiograph and white cell count. If these are abnormal, then the patient should be managed as if they have pneumonia, with adequate analgesia. If normal, analgesia alone will suffice.

Parapneumonic effusions

Parapneumonic effusions are divided into:

- simple: negative on culture and resolves without loculation or drainage
- complicated: positive culture or Gram stain, loculates and requires drainage.

Parapneumonic effusions follow documented pneumonia in the majority of patients. For example, more than 50% of patients with pneumococcal pneumonia develop pleural effusion. In these cases, the most important action is to determine whether it is a simple parapneumonic effusion or a complicated one. This can best be done by assessing the pH or glucose of the pleural fluid following aspiration; if low (pH < 7.2 or glucose < 2.5 μmol/l), it is likely to be a complicated effusion.

Empyema

Occasionally patients develop anaerobic empyema without a clear-cut preceding chest infection. These patients present with a subacute course over several weeks with weakness, anorexia and weight loss and few signs referable to the chest, and little or no fever. Pleural fluid from these patients is foul-smelling and purulent but a good recovery follows antibiotic and chest tube drainage. The most common organisms include Gram-negative aerobes, such as *Escherichia coli*, and anaerobes.

Management of complicated parapneumonic effusions and empyemas

Early drainage of empyemas and complicated parapneumonic effusions is important to minimise loculation and a subsequent restrictive respiratory defect by reduced lung movement. Occasionally chest tube drainage is unsatisfactory and open surgical drainage is necessary for resolution.

Tuberculous empyema

Pleural effusion is a relatively common manifestation of post-primary tuberculosis. These patients usually present with breathlessness, fever, weight loss and occasionally chest pain. Sometimes the effusions are very large, rendering the patient breathless at rest.

Diagnosis

The characteristics of a tuberculous pleural effusion are shown in Table 22. Drainage of large amounts of fluid may yield rapid temporary relief from breathlessness. Mycobacteria are isolated from pleural fluid in less than 20% of patients and so a pleural biopsy is usually necessary to confirm the diagnosis (95%); the granulomas are seen histologically. Only occasionally do patients have concurrent parenchymal pulmonary tuberculosis. Sputa for smear and culture for tuberculosis are usually negative.

Pneumothorax

You will see young males (occasionally females) with sudden breathlessness and pleuritic chest pain caused by a spontaneous pneumothorax. On examination, you may find reduced breath sounds and increased percussion note, though the diagnosis is more frequently confirmed by the radiograph and not by the examination findings. Management is often by aspiration, as the leak usually closes spontaneously. In patients with asthma or chronic bronchitis and emphysema, even a small pneumothorax may compromise ventilation and requires insertion of an intercostal drain. Pneumothorax secondary to trauma is managed similarly. Insertion of a chest drain is *mandatory* if a patient with a pneumothorax, however small, requires ventilation. You should be aware that many cases of pneumothorax are linked to underlying lung disease such as COPD; those should be managed in consultation with a specialist respiratory unit.

A *tension* pneumothorax, with increasing ventilatory embarrassment, is a medical emergency requiring immediate reduction in the intrathoracic pressure. The patient will have a combination of:

- increasing/severe breathlessness
- cyanosis
- deviated trachea
- absence of breath sounds on one side.

Asbestosis

In patients exposed to asbestos over a period of years, basal pulmonary fibrosis occurs together with pleural plaques and calcification. The cumulative amount and type of fibre inhaled are strongly related to the degree of fibrosis and likelihood of cancer. You must take a careful occupational history including working in the shipyards, with boilers, in demolition or as laggers. The patient is usually clubbed and breathless, and has a cough. A chest radiograph shows predominantly basal changes, including plaques and sheet calcification. Asbestos bodies are usually present in the sputum in severe disease. Frequently those with asbestosis succumb to bronchial carcinoma (fivefold increase in risk); the effect of cigarette smoking is synergistic.

Mesothelioma may occur after only minimal exposure to blue asbestos (**crocidolite**). There are about 1000 new cases per year in the UK. It develops many years after asbestos exposure and presents with chest wall pain, which may be ill-defined and is often intractable. Breathlessness is common. A chest radiograph shows the lung being gradually encased with malignant tissue and fibrosis. An effusion is often present. An ultrasound or a CT scan will help to delineate tumour from fluid. A biopsy will confirm the diagnosis; some patients develop nodules along the course of the biopsy track. The tumour can spread through the diaphragm, though distant metastases are rare. There is no curative treatment. Pain control may require specialist advice.

Two

Self-assessment: questions

Multiple choice questions

Any or all of each set of five statements may be true or false. Choose your answers and see the reasoning behind the correct answer on pages 109–110.

1. Hypoventilation occurs in the following:
   a. Central sleep apnoea syndrome
   b. Severe kyphoscoliosis
   c. Anxiety
   d. Benzodiazepine overdose
   e. Exercise

2. The following shift the oxygen haemoglobin curve to the right:
   a. Increase in temperature
   b. Fall in hydrogen ion concentration
   c. Increase in carbon dioxide concentration
   d. Hypothermia
   e. Hyperventilation

3. Pneumothorax is a recognised complication of:
   a. Rib fracture
   b. A bulla
   c. Kyphoscoliosis
   d. Cryptogenic fibrosing alveolitis
   e. *Pneumocystis jirovecii* (*carinii*) pneumonia

4. The following are features of fibrosing alveolitis:
   a. Cough
   b. Clubbing of the fingers in the majority of cases
   c. Cyanosis in the early stages
   d. Circulating antibodies to alveolar tissues
   e. Haemoptysis

5. Mesotheliomas of the pleura:
   a. Only occur after prolonged heavy exposure to asbestos
   b. Respond to radiotherapy
   c. Pain is often the major symptom
   d. Metastasise early
   e. An ultrasound examination may be useful

6. Radical surgery for carcinoma of the bronchus is contraindicated with the following:
   a. Peripheral neuropathy
   b. Hypertrophic pulmonary osteoarthropathy
   c. Superior vena caval (SVC) obstruction
   d. Obstruction of the bronchus
   e. FEV_1 (forced expired volume in 1 sec) of 0.8 litres

7. A 35-year-old man with atopic asthma is admitted with an acute attack:
   a. High-dose oxygen should be avoided
   b. A normal Pco_2 always indicates a mild attack
   c. The patient should be sedated
   d. Green sputum almost always implies bacterial infection
   e. You should not give nebulised salbutamol if his pulse rate is >100 beats/min

8. In a patient with restrictive lung disease:
   a. The FEV_1 is usually within normal limits
   b. The ratio of FEV_1:FVC (forced vital capacity) is reduced
   c. A raised $Paco_2$ is common in the early stages
   d. Occupation of the patient is important in the differential diagnosis
   e. Clubbing may be found

9. Useful drugs for tuberculosis include:
   a. Piperacillin
   b. Isoniazid
   c. Ciprofloxacin
   d. Ethambutol
   e. Amikacin

10. Causes of life-threatening pneumonia or pneumonitis in adults include:
    a. *Pneumocystis jirovecii (carinii)*
    b. Influenza A virus
    c. Respiratory syncytial virus
    d. *Staphylococcus aureus*
    e. *Legionella pneumophila*

11. Important causes of pneumonia in immunosuppressed patients include:
    a. Cytomegalovirus
    b. *Legionella* spp.
    c. *Mycoplasma pneumoniae*
    d. *Aspergillus fumigatus*
    e. *Streptococcus pneumoniae*

12. Chronic bronchial sepsis:
    a. Is an uncommon feature of cystic fibrosis
    b. Typically is caused by unusual, difficult-to-grow bacteria
    c. May lead to haemoptysis
    d. Can usually be cured with oral antibiotics
    e. May lead to pulmonary fibrosis

13. Pleural aspiration is useful in the following situations:
    a. In diagnosing mesothelioma
    b. Pleural tuberculosis
    c. Viral pleurisy
    d. Empyema
    e. Relieving breathlessness in patients with malignant effusions

Single best answer multiple choice questions

For each numbered questions, only ONE of the options lettered a–e is correct.

1. A 72-year-old man is admitted with an exacerbation of his chronic obstructive pulmonary disease (COPD). He has become increasingly breathless and tired. His peak flow rate is 100 l/min. The patient is conscious and orientated and is able to cooperate with his management. Arterial blood gases on air show:

    pH   7.25
    P_{CO_2} 9 kPa (67 mm Hg)
    P_{O_2} 6.5 kPa (49 mm Hg)

    Which is the most appropriate management?

    a. Non-invasive ventilation
    b. Intubation and ventilation
    c. 100% oxygen via a face mask
    d. Intravenous corticosteroid
    e. Intravenous theophylline

2. A 34-year-old woman has been coughing up blood for about a week and she has had similar episodes over the last few years. She says that when she was a child, she was in hospital for a few weeks with 'a bad chest infection'. Since then, she has always had a productive cough and requires antibiotics a few times a year (but she still smokes). Which is the most likely diagnosis?

    a. Asthma
    b. Chronic bronchitis and empysema
    c. Pulmonary emboli
    d. Bronchial carcinoma
    e. Bronchiectasis

3. A 68-year-old man was treated with intravenous antibiotics for 5 days because of a left lower lobe pneumonia. On review in the outpatient department 8 weeks later, he has improved but still has a troublesome cough with some flecks of blood in the sputum. On examination, there is dullness to percussion at the left base, with some bronchial breathing and coarse crackles. Vocal resonance is increased. What is the most likely diagnosis?

    a. Parapneumonic effusion
    b. Pulmonary infarction
    c. Empyema
    d. Carcinoma of the bronchus
    e. Recurrent chest infection

4. A 34-year-old man presents to the accident and emergency department with an acute attack of asthma. He usually takes regular inhaled corticosteroids and occasionally inhaled salbutamol. Which would best indicate that the attack was severe?

    a. Oxygen saturation 94%
    b. Arterial P_{CO_2} 6.5 kPa (49 mm Hg)
    c. Pulse rate 120/min regular
    d. Marked wheeze all over the chest
    e. Using the accessory muscles of respiration.

5. A 69-year-old man has a dull left-sided chest pain, which has been getting steadily worse over several months. He retired as a pipe-lagger a few years earlier and has been a life-long non-smoker. On examination, he looks unwell, with a stony dull percussion note at the left base, reduced breath sounds and vocal resonance. What is the most likely diagnosis?

    a. Empyema
    b. Bronchial carcinoma
    c. Tuberculosis
    d. Connective tissue disease
    e. Mesothelioma

Extended matched questions

EMQ 1

Theme: Respiratory signs

Options
1. Asthma
2. Bronchial carcinoma with lobar collapse
3. Chronic bronchitis and emphysema (COPD)
4. Cryptogenic fibrosing alveolitis
5. Lobar pneumonia
6. Lymphangitis carcinomatosis
7. Pleural effusion
8. Pneumothorax
9. Pulmonary oedema

Choose the most likely diagnosis for each of the following patients. Each option can be used more than once.

A. A 20-year-old woman is admitted with acute shortness of breath. She smokes 20 cigarettes a day. On examination, you find that she is using her accessory muscles of respiration, and breath sounds are vesicular but reduced. There are widespread wheezes. She has a temperature of 37.5°C.

B. A 62-year-old woman is admitted with marked shortness of breath that has been developing over 2 weeks. She had a mastectomy 3 years prior to this episode. She has smoked 15 cigarettes a day for many years. On examination, she has a temperature of 36.8°C. In her respiratory system, you find a dull percussion note, reduced vesicular breath sounds and vocal fremitus over most of the posterior chest on the left side.

C. A 23-year-old man is admitted with sudden shortness of breath. He smokes about 30 cigarettes a day. On examination, he is distressed and his temperature is 36.9°C. In his respiratory system, breath sounds are absent on the left side, percussion note is resonant and vocal fremitus is reduced.

D. A 47-year-old man is admitted with a 4-day history of shortness of breath. He has smoked 40 cigarettes a day for 20 years. On examination, his temperature is 38.7°C. In his respiratory system the percussion note is dull, vocal resonance is increased at his left base and there is bronchial breathing.

E. A 72-year-old man presents with a 9-month history of increasing shortness of breath. He is a non-smoker. On examination, he is clubbed. His temperature is 36.8°C and in his respiratory system there are showers of late inspiratory fine crackles.

EMQ 2

Theme: Diagnostic tests
Options
1. Blood culture
2. Bronchoscopy
3. CT scan of thorax
4. Lung biopsy
5. PA chest radiograph
6. Pleural biopsy
7. Spirometry
8. Sputum culture
9. Sputum cytology
10. Transfer factor and lung volumes

For patients A–E, select the test that is likely to give the best diagnostic information.

A. A 20-year-old woman presents to casualty with severe shortness of breath. This has come on over a few minutes and is associated with a sharp pain over her left chest. On examination, she is tachypnoeic and centrally cyanosed, with an oxygen saturation of 78%. Breath sounds are absent over the left chest and her heart sounds are very quiet and only heard just to the left of the sternum.

B. A 64-year-old pipe-lagger presents with an 18-month history of worsening breathlessness. He smokes approximately 20 cigarettes per day. On examination, he is not clubbed but has some coarse crackles over both lung bases.

C. A 74-year-old woman has a 3-month history of increasing breathlessness. In the past she has had bouts of palpitations, but these have been controlled by drug treatment for the last 6 months. On examination, there are no abnormal physical signs.

D. A 25-year-old woman has been troubled with bouts of wheezing and cough for about 2 years. These seem to be worse after exercise or if she has a cold.

On examination, she has a few scattered wheezes but nothing else of note.

E. A 16-year-old boy has a 2-week history of cough and some breathlessness. He remembers that it stemmed from when something 'seemed to go down the wrong way' when he was eating peanuts. On examination he has a fixed inspiratory wheeze over his right chest.

EMQ 3

Theme: Breathlessness
Options
1. Aspiration pneumonia
2. Asthma
3. Bronchiectasis
4. Empyema
5. Exacerbation of COPD
6. Fibrosing alveolitis
7. Left ventricular failure
8. Lymphangitis carcinomatosis
9. Pneumothorax
10. Pleural effusion
11. Pulmonary embolism
12. Pulmonary tuberculosis

For each patient with breathlessness, select the most likely diagnosis.

A. A 79-year-old man is admitted with a total anterior cerebral stroke. Two days later, following a choking episode, he becomes breathless, with a temperature of 38°C and coarse crackles at his left base.

B. A 54-year-old man gives a history of a productive cough over many years, which often requires antibiotics. He is seen by his general practitioner because of breathlessness and increased sputum, which has turned green. On examination, he has coarse carckles on the right side posteriorly and he is clubbed.

C. A 64-year-old woman has become increasingly breathless over several weeks with a persistent dry cough. She is very distressed by her dyspnoea, but on examination, apart from the tachypnoea, there are no abnormalities and her chest radiograph appears normal.

D. A 59-year-old woman is admitted with a swinging pyrexia and general malaise. She had been treated by her general practitioner recently for a chest infection and had seemed to improve. On examination, her temperature is 37.8°C and there is stony dullness to percussion at the right base, with decreased breath sounds and vocal resonance.

E. A 72-year-old man has a 1-year history of progressive breathlessness. On examination, he is clubbed and has fine inspiratory crackles.

Objective structured clinical examination (OSCE) stations

OSCE 1

This is a 5-minute station to take a history of a simulated patient with a respiratory problem.

Examiner: This patient has chest pain. Please take a history from her and I will then ask you what you think the problem is.

Student: Hello, my name is Sarah Walsh. Is it alright if I take a history from you?
Patient: Fine.
S: Can you tell me what the problem is?
P: I have had this pain in the left side of my chest for about 2 days.
S: Is it a stabbing pain?
P: Yes.
S: Does breathing make it worse?
P: Yes.
S: I suppose that coughing also affects it?
P: Yes.

Examiner: Can I stop you there. What do you think the problem is?
S: Pleurisy.
E: What else would you want to know to confirm your diagnosis?

OSCE 2

In the year 5 OSCE, you enter a station where there is an elderly man sitting on the edge of the bed and holding on to the sides. His breathing seems laboured.

Examiner: This is Mr Hill, who has a problem with his chest. Please can you examine his respiratory system? At the end, I will ask you to present your findings.

OSCE 3

Examiner: This man has been on anti-TB medication for nearly 4 weeks and is reattending clinic. Ask him how he feels and discuss what action should be taken now.

The patient tells you that he has TB of the spine, with terrible pain over the last 7 months. He has had scans and a needle biopsy. He was started on TB tablets nearly 4 weeks ago. It was difficult to take them all, but he persisted and took everything prescribed (rifater 5 tablets, ethambutol 1000 mg and a vitamin daily). He has been feeling off-colour for about 10 days. He is nauseous, tired and off his food; yesterday he vomited. His daughter thinks he looks ill and maybe slightly yellow. The GP surgery did a blood test last Friday but he hasn't had the results yet. It was a real struggle getting to the clinic today. He has no bleeding or bruising, is taking no other tablets or alcohol, has no tunnel vision and does not use i.v. drugs. No one else is ill at home.

What would you do next?

Case history questions

Case history 1

At an insurance medical examination, a 56-year-old boiler worker is found to have finger clubbing and has recently noticed that he is short of breath on exertion. He is a long-standing smoker and has had a cough for a number of years. His hobbies include keeping and breeding budgerigars. He has never been in hospital.

On examination, the only other findings are bilateral basal crepitations. He is not cyanosed. His chest radiograph shows bilateral basal fine reticular shadowing.

Lung function testing shows:

Vital capacity 2.5 litres (reduced)
FEV_1 1.9 litres (reduced)
FEV_1/FVC 68% (normal)
Total lung capacity (TLC) 4.4 litres (reduced)
CO diffusion 6.5 ml CO/min per mmHg (reduced)
PaO_2 10.3 kPa (77 mmHg)
$PaCO_2$ 5.1 kPa (38 mmHg)

1. Intepret the abnormalities present on his investigations.
2. Give two possible diagnoses.
3. What further investigations may be helpful?
4. What would happen if the patient exercised?

Case history 2

You are a surgical house officer and are called at the weekend to see a 65-year-old patient on the orthopaedic ward who had a left hip replacement 5 days before. Apart from being a smoker and having a regular cough, she was previously well. The nurses report that she has a low-grade fever (38°C), is coughing and seems 'not herself'. She is alert but slightly confused, with a respiratory rate of 28/min and with crackles and bronchial breathing at the left base.

In the following questions, decide whether the options offered are true or false.

1. Your immediate clinical diagnosis(es) is (are):
   a. Left ventricular failure
   b. Diabetic ketoacidosis
   c. Atypical pneumonia
   d. Smoker's cough and chronic airflow limitation
   e. Hospital-acquired pneumonia

2. The following data are *essential* in your immediate management plan:
   a. Whether she keeps birds at home
   b. An old chest X-ray film
   c. The antibiotic prophylaxis she received for her hip operation
   d. The result of a ventilation/perfusion ($\dot{V}/\dot{Q}$) lung scan or pulmonary arteriogram
   e. Arterial blood gas result

3. Appropriate management steps in the first hour after seeing her are:
   a. Arterial blood gases
   b. Chest radiograph
   c. Blood culture
   d. Discussion with the microbiologist on call about antibiotic therapy
   e. Administration of oxygen

4. Subsequent steps over next 8 hours should include:
   a. Rechecking arterial gases while the patient is breathing oxygen
   b. Consideration of full anticoagulation with a more senior physician and orthopaedic team
   c. Repeat chest radiograph after 6–8 hours for signs of improvement
   d. Explanation of condition to anxious relatives
   e. Consideration of transfer to the intensive care unit if her condition deteriorates

Case history 3

A 48-year-old female presents with a 2-week history of haemoptysis. In the recent past, she has had two episodes of left upper lobe pneumonia. On examination, there are no systemic signs of disease, the trachea is slightly deviated to the left, tactile fremitus is reduced at the left apex and wheeze is localised to the left side of chest. A chest radiograph shows loss of volume in the left upper lobe.

1. What is the likely diagnosis?
2. What is the definitive diagnostic test?

Case history 4

The following results are obtained from a pleural aspirate:

Straw-coloured
Protein 35 g/l
Cells: Predominantly lymphocytes
Glucose 0.5 mmol/l
Culture: No growth
Cytology: No malignant cells seen

1. What are your differential diagnoses?
2. What further investigations would you request?

Case history 5

A 40-year-old man is referred to a chest clinic because of increasing shortness of breath of gradual onset. He has a family history of respiratory disease. Pulmonary function tests (predicted values in parentheses) show:

FEV_1 (forced expired volume in 1 sec) 1.2 (3.7) litres
FVC (forced vital capacity) 3.0 (4.2) litres
TLC (total lung capacity) 7.2 (5.3) litres
Transfer factor 12.5 (26)

1. What is the diagnosis?
2. What further investigations should be carried out?

Case history 6

A 44-year-old man presents with a 6-month history of a dry cough and increasing dyspnoea. On examination he is clubbed, has a normal cardiovascular system, is short of breath at rest and has showers of fine crepitations at both bases.
   Blood gases show:

pH 7.4
PO_2 6.4 kPa (48 mmHg)
PCO_2 3.7 kPa (28 mmHg)
HCO_3^- 15 mmol/l

1. What is the likely diagnosis?
2. Explain the blood gas result.

Case history 7

A 60-year-old man presents with a few weeks' history of a severe dry cough and rapidly increasing shortness of breath. He had a resection for carcinoma of the stomach 18 months previously. There is no previous respiratory or cardiac history. On examination, he is markedly tachypnoeic at rest, but his chest is clear on auscultation. There are no other signs. He has the following pulmonary function results (predicted values in parentheses):

FEV_1 1.8 (3.1) litres
FVC 2.0 (4.2) litres
TLC 3.0 (5.0) litres
Transfer factor 12 (22)

1. What do the pulmonary function tests show?
2. What is the likely diagnosis?
3. Give two investigations you would request and explain why.

Case history 8

A 28-year-old female with a known psychiatric history presents with her relatives to the accident and emergency department. She refuses to give a history but has marked hyperventilation and the following blood gases:

pH 7.58
PO_2 15.3 kPa (115 mmHg)
PCO_2 3.5 kPa (26 mmHg)
HCO_3^- 18 mmol/l.

1. What do the gases show?
2. Give three urgent investigations that should be carried out.

Key features questions

1. A 25-year-old man presents to the accident and emergency department with a history of painful bumps on his shins that have been coming and going over a few weeks. He describes them as being red and hard. Just before they started, he felt unwell, with aching joints and a temperature, and thought that he was coming down with a virus. The only thing of note in his past history was that he was in Jamaica visiting his family home a few months ago. On examination, apart from the red, painful nodules over the anterior aspect of his tibia, there are no other abnormalities. In your investigations, blood tests are normal, but his chest radiograph shows bilateral hilar lymphadenopathy.

What is the diagnosis and what supports this? How would you manage him?

2. A 72-year-old woman presents with frequent episodes of coughing up blood over the previous 4 weeks. She has otherwise been well. On examination, there are no abnormal findings. A plain chest radiograph shows a cavitating mass in the left upper zone, which is confirmed on a CT scan together with metastatic spread to the liver. Other investigations show an FEV$_1$ of 0.6 l and an FVC of 2.4 l. Oxygen saturation is 89% on room air.

Why is palliative radiotherapy the best management?

3. You see a 31-year-old man in the accident and emergency department because he has been coughing up blood for the last 4 days. You find out that he has had five similar episodes over the last 18 months. He has been smoking 20 cigarettes a day for the last 15 years and also he thinks that he had whooping cough when he was a little boy. He also tells you that he has frequently visited the doctor for chest infections and sinusitis in which he coughs up foul-tasting sputum.

What is your working diagnosis and why?

4. A 39-year-old man is referred to the outpatient department as an urgent case by his general practitioner, as the patient has become increasing unwell over the last few weeks with weight loss and anorexia. He is complaining of a cough and has coughed up a small amount of blood. Over the last few months, he has noticed increasing nasal stuffiness and his nose has been bleeding. In clinic, he looks unwell and his temperature is 37.8°C. A dipstick of his urine shows microscopic haematuria. You decide to admit him as an urgent case. Blood tests come back showing that his creatinine is 393 µmol/l and he has an ESR of 93 mm/hr. You look at the chest radiograph and it shows several ill-defined opacities (1–2 cm) in the upper zones.

What one blood test would you do to confirm your diagnosis? Why do you suspect this diagnosis?

Data interpretation questions

1. Table 24 is a peak flow chart from a paint factory worker.
   a. What is the diagnosis?
   b. What is the most likely cause in this person?

2. A 49-year-old smoker who has a central abdominal scar presents acutely ill and breathless with these vital signs: temperature, 39.2°C; respiratory rate, 40 breaths/min; pulse, 125 beats/min; blood pressure, 100/70 mmHg. His hands are cold and he is peripherally cyanosed. The pulse oximeter shows an oxygen saturation of 78%. His arterial blood gas results return within a group of five different samples (Table 25).
   a. Which of the five samples is likely to be his and why?
   b. Give a differential diagnosis.

Table 24 Peak flow chart (l/min) for data interpretation 1

	Mon	Tues	Weds	Thurs	Fri	Sat	Sun	Mon	Tues
Work/hols	Work	Work	Work	Work	Work	Hols	Hols	Hols	Hols
Maximum	550	300	250	200	200	200	300	450	500
Minimum	450	480	400	350	300	380	420	520	520

Table 25 Arterial blood gas results for data interpretation 2

	1	2	3	4	5
pH	7.43	7.55	7.22	7.40	7.20
Po$_2$ kPa (mmHg)	11.7 (88)	12.7 (95)	7.5 (56)	11.1 (83)	6.8 (51)
Pco$_2$ kPa (mmHg)	4.5 (34)	3.3 (25)	3.3 (25)	4.0 (30)	6.7 (50)
HCO$_3^-$ mmol/l	18	33	16	19	22

c. What underlying diseases might you reasonably expect?

d. List four key investigations.

e. Suggest an immediate management plan.

Picture questions

1. Look at Figure 24.

   a. Describe the abnormalities and give the diagnosis.

   b. What might be the underlying cause?

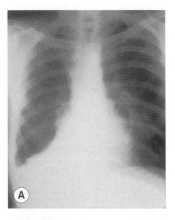

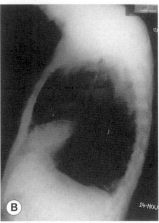

Fig. 24 Two chest radiographs for analysis.

2. Look at Figure 25.

   a. Describe the abnormalities and give the diagnosis.

   b. What might be the underlying cause?

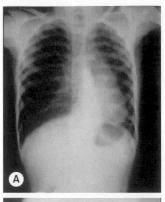

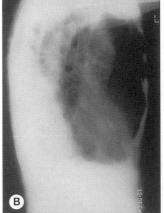

Fig. 25 Two chest radiographs for analysis.

3. Figure 26 is a postero-anterior (PA) chest radiograph from a man with a 6-month history of progressive breathlessness.

   a. Describe the abnormality.

   b. What would be your differential diagnosis?

   c. What would you look for on examination?

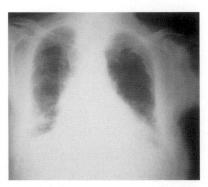

Fig. 26 A PA chest radiograph.

4. This 67-year-old man presented with haemoptysis and weight loss over a few months.

   a. What does the PA radiograph (Fig. 27) show?

   b. What is the likely diagnosis and what other causes would you consider and (possibly) discount?

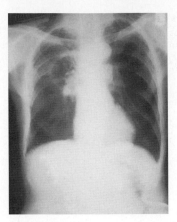

Fig. 27 A PA radiograph.

5. Figure 28 is a PA chest radiograph of a 58-year-old schizophrenic man who sleeps rough in London.
   a. Give three abnormalities you can see.
   b. What investigations would you now do? (Give at least four.)
   c. What would you expect to find and/or grow in his sputum?
   d. Where should he be looked after initially?
   e. What treatment would you prescribe?
   f. Do you foresee any problems with his treatment?

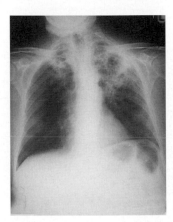

Fig. 28 A PA radiograph.

6. A 25-year-old man was out jogging when he developed chest tightness and shortness of breath. This rapidly progressed and he collapsed on the pavement. An emergency ambulance was called and he was brought to casualty. The radiographer was in accident and emergency and did the antero-posterior (AP) chest film shown in Figure 29.
   a. What does it show?
   b. What signs might the man have?
   c. What would be your immediate management?

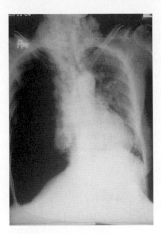

Fig. 29 An AP radiograph.

7. The chest radiograph (Fig. 30) was obtained from a 46-year-old who has been unwell for 3 days with fever, rigors and increasing shortness of breath. Bilateral coarse crepitations and disorientation are clinically obvious. His total white cell count is $2900 \times 10^6/l$, his Po_2 7.6 kPa (57 mm Hg) on air, Pco_2 3.8 kPa (28 mm Hg), pH 7.37, base excess −7.5, urea 9.9 mmol/l, creatinine 128 μmol/l and all other tests normal.

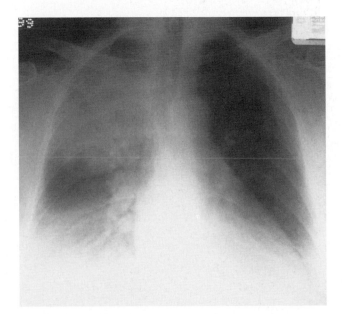

Fig. 30 A chest radiograph.

   a. What does the chest radiograph show?
   b. Assuming he has pneumonia, how would you grade it?
   c. In casualty they gave him cefotaxime 1 g stat. Would you change this or add to it? If so, why?
   d. What will you tell his family about his illness?

Short notes

Write short notes on the following:

1. Ten facts you know about asthma (*without consulting any books*). List three important principles of management of acute asthma and their rationale.

2. The causes of chronic airflow limitation; make a table, giving differences and similarities.

3. Describe how you would instruct a patient in measuring a peak flow rate.

4. Atypical pneumonia.

5. Respiratory infection in the immunocompromised patient.

6. Management of oxygen therapy and analgesia in pneumonia.

7. Indications for physiotherapy in chest disease.

Self-assessment: answers

Multiple choice answers

1. a. **True.** Alveolar hypoventilation is a key feature.

   b. **True.** Severe kyphoscoliosis can produce mechanical ventilation problems because of the changed curvature of the spine.

   c. **False.** Anxiety is associated with hyperventilation.

   d. **True.** Drugs such as benzodiazepines depress the respiratory centre.

   e. **False.** Alveolar ventilation is increased during exercise in normal people.

2. a. **True.** In working muscle, there is an increase in temperature which moves the curve to the *right* which is the *right* thing to do.

   b. **False.** An acidosis not alkalosis shifts the curve to the right.

   c. **True.** CO_2 retention produces an acidosis.

   d. **False.**

   e. **False.** Hyperventilation produces an alkalosis which shifts the curve to the left.

3. a. **True.** Pneumothorax can occur secondary to trauma.

   b. **True.** Any cavitating or cystic/bullous lung lesion can cause a pneumothorax. Bullae can be single or multiple. They are particularly common in emphysema including α_1-antitrypsin deficiency.

   c. **False.**

   d. **False.**

   c. **True.** And lung abscesses (e.g. *Staphylococcus aureus*) can lead to pneumothorax.

4. a. **True.** Patients usually present with cough and breathlessness.

   b. **True.** Clubbing occurs in about 60% of patients but is not essential for the diagnosis.

   c. **False.** Cyanosis is a relatively late sign.

   d. **False.** The aetiology is unknown and circulating antibodies are not found.

   e. **False.** If a patient has haemoptysis you should think of another cause.

5. a. **False.** Exposure may be trivial with a long delay before appearance of the tumour.

   b. **False.** The tumour is resistant to radiotherapy and chemotherapy.

   c. **True.** Pain is often a very troublesome symptom.

   d. **False.** The tumour can spread through the diaphragm; distant metastases are rare.

   e. **True.** It may show the irregular pleural thickening.

6. a. **False.** Peripheral neuropathy is a non-metastatic complication and may respond to curative resection.

   b. **False.** As with 6a, it may respond to surgical resection. There are other non-metastatic manifestations which you should know (Fig. 22).

   c. **True.** SVC obstruction usually denotes extensive mediastinal invasion.

   d. **False.**

   e. **True.** A very low FEV_1 would be a contraindication because of inadequate respiratory reserve following resection.

7. a. **False.** A high concentration of oxygen should be administered to all patients on arrival at hospital.

   b. **False.** Normocarbia is a bad sign signalling failing alveolar ventilation.

   c. **False.** Sedation *must* be avoided.

   d. **False.** Green sputum is normal in some patients.

   e. **False.** A β_2-agonist such as salbutamol should be administered via a nebuliser immediately.

8. a. **False.** FEV_1 is often low.

   b. **False.** The ratio is usually unchanged in restrictive disease.

   c. **False.** The early pattern is type 1 respiratory failure with hypoxia and low $Paco_2$.

   d. **True.** A number of restrictive lung diseases are caused by environmental factors, relating to occupation and hobbies.

   e. **True.**

9. a. **False.** Piperacillin has no activity.

   b. **True.** Isoniazid is a major, first-line agent.

   c. **True.** Ciprofloxacin is a useful agent, less active than rifampicin; it may obscure infection in patients treated before diagnosis considered.

   d. **True.** Ethambutol is another major, but second-line agent.

   e. **True.** Amikacin is a useful i.v. second-line agent.

10. a. **True.** *Pneumocystis carinii* infection is usually seen in AIDS, but also in lymphoma, steroid-treated, transplant and hypogammaglobulinaemic patients.

    b. **True.** Primary influenzal pneumonia or complicated by bacteria, e.g. *Staph. aureus*.

    c. **False.** Respiratory syncytial virus is a problem in immunosuppressed children and bone marrow transplant patients.

    d. **True.** *S. aureus* pneumonia is often rapidly fatal, especially following influenza.

    e. **True.** *L. pneumophila* pneumonia carries a high mortality if not treated appropriately.

11. a. **True.** Cytomegalovirus pneumonia occurs primarily in transplant patients.

b. **True.** *Legionella* infection is associated with solid organ transplant recipients and other steroid-treated patients.

c. **False.** *M. pneumoniae* is very rarely a problem.

d. **True.** *A. fumigatus* is an increasing problem in all immunocompromised groups. May be fatal in 7 days.

e. **True.** *S. pneumoniae* is primarily a problem in chronic chest patients, children and the community. It is not a major problem in immunosuppressed patients except in AIDS, when it is 100 times more common, but with a lower mortality.

12. a. **False.** It is the primary feature of cystic fibrosis.

b. **False.** It is usually caused by common organisms.

c. **True.** Haemoptysis is also seen with dry bronchiectasis, chronic bronchial sepsis and aspergillomas.

d. **False.** It may be ameliorated but not cured. Some patients require i.v. antibiotics for improvement.

e. **True.** It produces a fibrotic reaction.

13. a. **False.** For the diagnosis of mesothelioma, a pleural biopsy/surgery is required.

b. **False.** A pleural aspirate may show lymphocytes but is rarely culture-positive; a pleural biopsy is better.

c. **False.** Viral pleurisy does not cause an effusion, just pain.

d. **True.** An empyema will require tube or surgical drainage for treatment.

e. **True.** Drainage in malignant effusions is often very helpful if litres of fluid are removed or a shunt can be inserted.

Single best answer multiple choice answers

1. **a is correct.** The patient has moderate type 2 respiratory failure with hypoxia, hypercarbia and acidosis. Non-invasive ventilation has been shown to be an effective treatment for short-term support. It is used in conscious patients who are able to cooperate and who have moderate acidosis (pH 7.25–7.35). As well as in COPD (main use), it can also be of benefit in patients with neuromuscular disease.

2. **e is correct.** The productive cough, recurrent chest infections and the childhood admission suggest bronchiectasis, possibly as a consequence of whooping cough. The age of the patient would make a carcinoma unlikely, as would the recurrent haemoptysis over a few years. Pulmonary emboli are a possibility, but there are no other risk factors for thrombo-embolic disease.

3. **d is correct.** The physical signs are consistent with an unresolved left lower lobe consolidation, which should have disappeared by the time of review. There are no features suggestive of a new infection. This points to an obstruction of a major bronchus, probably due to a carcinoma. At this stage, the radiograph (and CT scan) would show (partial) collapse of the lobe.

4. **b is correct.** All of the options occur in an acute asthmatic attack including a tachycardia (which can be due to inhaled β_2-agonists as well as asthma). However, the P_{CO_2} should be low in asthma because of the high respiratory drive. In patients who are tiring (ventilatory failure) or with severe bronchoconstriction, the P_{CO_2} starts to rise and the patient may need ventilation if there is not a rapid response to the immediate management.

5. **e is correct.** The examination findings are of either a pleural effusion or pleural thickening (or both). Bronchial carcinoma is rare in a non-smoker. The history is too long for empyema and you would expect more systemic features. The occupational history of lagging pipes suggests exposure to asbestos and makes the diagnosis of mesothelioma the most probable.

Extended matched answers
EMQ 1

A. **1.** The signs are of airflow obstruction (wheezes). Given the age, it is very unlikely that the cause is chronic bronchitis and emphysema. The mild pyrexia suggests that the asthma attack has been triggered by an infection.

B. **7.** The previous mastectomy suggests malignancy as the underlying cause (as could the smoking). The signs are of a very large pleural effusion. Lymphangitis carcinomatosis presents with intense breathlessness and cough, but there is often very little to find on examination (a few fine crackles at the bases).

C. **8.** In a young man presenting with sudden onset of breathlessness, the main differential diagnoses are asthma (but you might expect a previous history, wheeze and less sudden onset) and pneumothorax. The clinical signs point to the latter but with no evidence of 'tension'.

D. **5.** This patient is pyrexic with a short illness. The signs are of lobar consolidation.

E. **4.** The long time course would be very unusual for lymphangitis carcinomatosis. He is clubbed and the late inspiratory crackles are typical of cryptogenic fibrosing alveolitis.

EMQ 2

A. **5.** The symptoms and signs are of respiratory distress caused by a tension pneumothorax. This is a medical emergency and you need to confirm your diagnosis as quickly as possible. In extreme cases, you should intervene on the clinical evidence alone. A PA chest film will confirm the diagnosis with mediastinal shift.

B. **3.** The history and examination findings point to asbestosis. A PA chest radiograph may support this, but the best diagnostic information is given by a CT scan of the thorax (pleural and lung disease).

C. **10.** Most likely this patient is developing pulmonary fibrosis secondary to amiodarone treatment. A PA chest radiograph will show changes as the disease progresses, but the earliest confirmatory evidence will be from a reduced transfer factor.

D. **7.** The history is typical of asthma and is best confirmed by spirometry.

E. **2.** This patient has probably inhaled a foreign body, which is obstructing a major bronchus. Bronchoscopy will confirm this and will allow removal.

EMQ 3

A. **1.** Swallowing problems are common after a stroke and aspiration pneumonia can occur even in patients who are 'nil by mouth' because of aspiration of saliva.

B. **3.** The history could be due to COPD, but the clubbing implies (in this case) chronic sepsis, which is consistent with bronchiectasis.

C. **8.** The progressive disabling breathlessness over a relatively short period, together with the normal examination findings, should make you suspect lymphangitis and the chest radiograph may be normal. A differential diagnosis would be a pulmonary embolus, but more commonly the breathlessness would vary and the chest radiograph may be abnormal.

D. **4.** The physical signs indicate a pleural effusion, but the history suggests an infection that has been partially treated and has resulted in an empyema.

E. **6.** The clubbing could suggest a bronchial carcinoma, but the long history of progressive symptoms points to pulmonary fibrosis.

Responses to OSCE stations

OSCE 1

In this case, the student has arrived at a diagnosis of pleurisy (which is correct) but would score poorly on the station. Why?

- The opening was good — asking the patient's permission and introducing herself.
- The initial question was open: 'tell me . . .'
- After this, the student asked a series of closed questions.
- The diagnostic thinking was fixed around pleurisy.
- Even though the eventual diagnosis in the station was pleurisy secondary to infection, the history is of

pleuritic chest pain — of which there are other important causes (e.g. this patient could have been a young woman on the oral contraceptive pill and the theme of the station might have been pulmonary embolism and associated risk factors).

Suggestions for further practice

You should practise taking histories from patients with another student observing. You can then receive feedback from him/her about the **communication skills** aspect of the history as well as the information that you have elicited.

OSCE 2

As with all OSCE stations assessing examination skills, it is important to have a system that includes:

- inspection — general and the relevant system
- palpation
- percussion
- auscultation.

These steps should be followed carefully and not just for 'show' for the examiner. In this case, this is the classical position of a patient with COPD who is holding on so that he can use his accessory muscles of respiration, which you must comment on together with his respiratory rate, breathing through pursed lips and any cyanosis. For this patient (apart from the above), consider the following:

- *Hands*. Flap, warm peripheries and bounding pulse point to carbon dioxide retention.
- *Head/mouth*. Central cyanosis
- *Inspection*. Equal movement of both sides, any scars (pneumonectomy), indrawing of intercostal muscles.
- *Palpation*. Tracheal deviation (very difficult sign), tactile vocal resonance (difficult sign) and chest expansion.
- *Percussion*. Compare both sides and comment on any differences.
- *Auscultation*. Listen for the normal vesicular breath sounds or whether there is any bronchial breathing (rare). Comment on added sounds:
  — crackles (crepitations) — generalised, localised; quality (fine, coarse)
  — wheezes (rhonchi) — generalised, localised.
- Examine for vocal resonance and comment on any differences between the two sides.

OSCE 3

After some history has been elucidated, you should ask for the hospital and GP liver function tests (you will want to phone the GP for results).

The hospital baseline LFTs show:

Bilirubin 18 (normal range 1–20 µmol/l)
Albumin 37 (33–49 g/l)
Alkaline phosphatase 88 (25–110 IU/l)
Alanine aminotransferase 32 (5–45 IU/l)
Gamma-glutamyl transferase 40 (<65 IU/l)

Results from the GP show:

Bilirubin 26
Albumin 35
Alkaline phosphatase 145
Alanine aminotransferase 160
Gamma-glutamyl transferase 228

The LFTs have 'gone off', showing a hepatitic picture. The patient is ill. You must stop the anti-TB treatment immediately and arrange careful assessment and follow-up of LFTs.

You will gain marks for:

- eliciting symptoms of nausea, fatigue, anorexia, tinge of yellow
- requesting LFTs
- identifying abnormal LFTs and hepatitic picture
- attributing this tentatively to the anti-TB drugs
- rechecking LFTs and the International Normalised Ratio (urea and glucose) urgently and considering admitting the patient to hospital.

Case history answers

Case history 1

1. He has a moderate restrictive lung defect with hypoxia and impaired transfer factor.

2. Given the history, there are several possibilities:
   a. cryptogenic fibrosing alveolitis (p. 94)
   b. lymphangitis carcinomatosis (p. 84)
   c. asbestosis (p. 99)
   d. extrinsic allergic alveolitis: bird fancier's lung (p. 94)
   e. miscellaneous conditions such as sarcoidosis, rheumatoid disease, systemic lupus erythematosus (SLE; p. 353). No other findings suggestive of these.

3. Avian precipitins, antinuclear factor, rheumatoid factor, bronchoscopy and lavage (asbestosis fibres), and transbronchial biopsy. Pleural plaques may sometimes be visible on CT scanning. It is important

to diagnose occupational disease as he may be eligible for compensation.

4. The patient would become more hypoxic and he would develop hypocarbia. These are caused by ventilation : perfusion mismatching (p. 50). On exercise, this worsens with perfusion of non-ventilated lung areas and a consequent increase in alveolar:arterial oxygen gradient. The increased respiratory drive caused by the hypoxia stimulates excess loss of carbon dioxide.

General discussion
The patient is a smoker but has a short history, with occupational and social exposure to possible hazardous agents. Important points on radiograph shadowing are shown in Table 26.

Case history 2

1. a. **False.** Unlikely for two reasons: bronchial breathing and fever. However, a myocardial infarction during or after surgery is not uncommon and this is a major cause of deteriorating pulmonary function post-operatively.
   b. **False.** Unlikely as no clues in history, but if she were diabetic then an infection with or without surgery could certainly have precipitated this. The patient needs blood sugar measurement.
   c. **False.** Unlikely but possible. Many hospitals have *Legionella* in the water systems and this comes in the differential diagnosis of hospital-acquired pneumonia.
   d. **False.** Too ill for these alone.
   e. **True.** The most common infection post-operatively, especially in the elderly and immobile patient, and more likely in smokers.

2. a. **False.** Desirable but not essential.
   b. **False.** Desirable but not essential.
   c. **True.** Use the British National Formulary. Every surgeon has a different regimen. Your prescription of antibiotics should *not* be the same

Table 26 Comparison of chest radiograph findings and physical signs and symptoms

Possible diagnoses	Radiograph findings	Symptoms and signs
Asbestosis	Linear pleural calcification, lower zone fibrosis	Depend on degree of fibrosis; signs minimal
Lymphangitis carcinomatosis	Minimal abnormalities	Cough, very breathless
Cryptogenic fibrosing alveolitis	Basal shadowing, honeycombing	Late fine inspiratory crepitations, clubbed
Extrinsic allergic alveolitis	Upper lobe mainly	Pigeons – acute symptoms; budgies – chronic symptoms
Sarcoidosis	Severe chest radiograph changes	Moderate symptoms
Aspergilloma	Upper zone, cavitation with marked pleural thickening	Often no symptoms; occasionally haemoptysis
Post-primary tuberculosis	Upper zone, cavitation, bilateral	May have few physical signs

class of antibiotic(s) as used for prophylaxis, as the bacteria causing pneumonia are much more likely to be resistant to it.

d. **False.** Although a pulmonary embolism and/or infarction is possible, you should initially manage her without these data.

e. **True.** Vital for management, to assess oxygenation, carbon dioxide retention and pH. Blood gases are essential in the management of all patients in hospital with pneumonia.

3. a. **True.** See answer to 2e.

b. **True.** For features of pneumonia.

c. **True.** Some patients are bacteraemic with pneumonia, but she may have bacteraemia from another cause and have a separate pulmonary problem.

d. **True.** Unless you recently discussed a very similar case, microbiological advice about appropriate antibiotics is usually invaluable.

e. **True.** The best level depends on the arterial blood gases.

4. a. **True.** This is vital. If you started the oxygen because the patient was hypoxic, the gases should be rechecked.

b. **True.** Post-operative patients such as this are usually on subcutaneous heparin anyway. The risk of bleeding into the operative site is high and so a senior medical opinion is appropriate.

c. **False.** No use at all. Radiographic resolution follows clinical improvement and in the case of *Legionella* pneumonia can take 4–6 weeks to clear.

d. **True.** This needs to be done judiciously as this patient is not under you but under the orthopaedic team, and you do not yet know how the patient will respond. But as a 'medical expert' for the surgeons, your broad outline of the problem as you observe it, with cautious optimism about outcome, would be appropriate.

e. **True.** This is the key reason for *you* to reassess the patient, including blood gases.

Case history 3

1. Common things being commonest, the most likely diagnosis is a bronchial carcinoma. The patient is in the right age group, she has had two episodes of *upper* lobe pneumonia (rare, mostly lower lobe) and has haemoptysis. You are not told whether she is a smoker and when the episodes of pneumonia occurred. The examination findings are consistent with a partial collapse of the left upper lobe and the wheeze implies local obstruction. An alternative, but much rarer, diagnosis would be a bronchial adenoma. A further possibility is that the lobe was damaged by tuberculosis at some time in the past and the recent problems result from complications of this (e.g. bronchiectasis, pneumonia, aspergilloma). You should always consider active tuberculosis

(treatable) and that adenocarcinomas occur at the site of lung scarring.

2. The definitive diagnostic test is a bronchoscopy (p. 82). Other tests would be sputum for acid-fast bacilli, culture for *Mycobacterium tuberculosis* and cytology (malignant cells).

Case history 4

1. Note the lymphocytes and the low sugar. This pattern is consistent with either tuberculosis (common; Ch. 2) or rheumatoid disease (relatively rare; Ch. 8). Further information from the history may help, though an effusion may be the first manifestation of rheumatoid disease.

2. Rheumatoid factor can be measured. Culture for acid-fast bacilli should be undertaken and Mantoux testing requested. A pleural biopsy will be more likely to give a positive result for tubercle than simply culture of the fluid. Caseating granulomas may be seen on histology. A thoracoscopy may be carried out in a specialist unit; this allows biopsy of the pleura under direct vision and gives the highest diagnostic yield.

Case history 5

1. The pulmonary function tests should be analysed and put into the context of the description of the patient. The patient has marked airflow limitation with reduced transfer factor and increased total lung capacity. The family history in a relatively young man points to α_1-antitrypsin deficiency (p. 85).

2. A chest radiograph may show marked lower lobe changes with bullae. The serum level of α_1-antitrypsin can be measured.

Case history 6

1. The history of progressive breathlessness, clubbing and showers of fine crepitations is consistent with a diagnosis of cryptogenic fibrosing alveolitis.

2. Analysis of the blood gases shows hypoxia with a compensated respiratory alkalosis.

Case history 7

1. The patient has a restrictive pattern and a reduced transfer factor with a previous history of carcinoma of the stomach. The present problem is one of rapidly worsening respiratory symptoms but, apart from the tachypnoea, there are no abnormal physical signs.

2. The overall picture is lymphangitis carcinomatosis.

3. Blood gases may show hypoxia with a respiratory alkalosis. A chest radiograph may show fine basal shadowing with honeycombing. A transbronchial biopsy may give a definitive tissue diagnosis.

Case history 8

1. You will see similar patients in casualty. The blood gases show a primary respiratory alkalosis

(pH 7.58) and a metabolic acidosis. The history of a psychiatric illness is supportive of a diagnosis of salicylate overdose. In the early stages this stimulates the respiratory centre, giving hypocarbia. Later a metabolic acidosis (falling pH) supervenes and finally the respiratory centre is depressed, giving a combined respiratory and metabolic acidosis.

2. Confirm the diagnosis with a blood salicylate level. A level above 500 mg/l indicates severe poisoning. The aim of treatment is to make the patient fluid-replete (with hyperventilation, sweating and possible vomiting, it is likely that she is hypovolaemic) and then alkalinise the urine. The latter is because salicylate is a weak acid and can exist in its ionised or its unionised form within the range of pH found in the body. If the pH is high (alkaline) in the urine, salicylate is ionised and cannot diffuse back across the tubule once it has been filtered at the glomerulus. Apart from checking the salicylate levels and the blood gases, check the blood glucose (may see either hypo- or hyperglycaemia), urea and electrolytes (hypo-/hypernatraemia, hypokalaemia), prothrombin time/bleeding time (may be prolonged) and a chest radiograph (non-cardiogenic pulmonary oedema in late stages). You could also request lactate levels and take blood for a subsequent toxicology screen. If in any doubt over a deliberate or accidental poisoning, you should contact one of the National Poison Units urgently for advice.

Key features answers

1. The most likely diagnosis is sarcoidosis. Key features are the probable ethnic background, systemic upset, painful nodules on lower limbs (erythema nodosum) and the bilateral hilar lymphadenopathy. The overall picture is stage I disease (hilar lymphadenopathy with erythema nodosum); most patients will not progress from this and will recover, so no action is necessary, apart from regular follow-up.

2. The clinical picture is one of a bronchial carcinoma and there are a number of treatment options possible. Prior to this, you would want to confirm the diagnosis, if possible by biopsy. Curative surgery would be the aim in a patient with non-small cell carcinoma, but the metastatic spread to the liver excludes this option. In addition, the pulmonary function tests and the hypoxia suggest underlying COPD, which would rule out a pneumonectomy or a lobectomy. Radical radiotherapy is similarly used to achieve a long-lasting remission in a patient with limited disease. Chemotherapy is an option, but would be for palliation and the patient's main symptom is haemoptysis. This is best managed by local treatment (e.g. palliative radiotherapy) in the same way that a solitary bone metastasis is managed.

3. The most probable diagnosis is bronchiectasis. However, there is a list of differential diagnoses and you need to be able to sift the information to decide which is the most likely. You should consider a bronchial carcinoma in view of the smoking history, even with the patient's relatively young age. However, the recurrent nature of the episodes over a period of 18 months makes this unlikely. A bronchial adenoma can present with recurrent haemoptysis, but this is rare and the patient has also had recurrent chest infections, though these can occur due to bronchial obstruction. A plain chest radiograph would be a mandatory investigation. Recurrent pulmonary emboli can present with haemoptysis, but there are no risk factors in the history; the patient is male, so the question of risk with the oral contraceptive pill does not come into play. The diagnosis of bronchiectasis is supported by the patient's age, history of whooping cough and recurrent infections. On examination, you may find that the patient has finger clubbing and has localised coarse crackles in a lung field. A plain chest radiograph may show ring shadows and localised streaky fibrosis, but a CT scan will be more useful in delineating the extent of the problem

4. You should request a serum antineutrophil cytoplasmic antibody (ANCA) as a matter of urgency and contact a renal physician by phone. The patient mostly likely has Wegener's granulomatosis (p. 95) on the basis of respiratory and kidney involvement (and has renal failure — which will be progressive). The respiratory tract can be involved from the nasopharynx downwards (nasal stuffiness) and typically there is nodular shadowing in both lung fields. ANCA can be divided into cytoplasmic (C) and perinuclear (P). In patients with active Wegener's granulomatosis, almost all the patients will be positive to ANCA (mostly C).

Data interpretation answers

1. a. The peak flow values indicate occupational asthma with worsening pulmonary function during the working week and improvement when not at work.

   b. In a paint factory, the most likely trigger is toluene diisocyanate.

2. a. Blood gas sample 3. Hypoxia with metabolic acidosis caused by sepsis syndrome. You already know that he is hypoxic because of the low oxygen saturation on the pulse oximeter. He is shocked (low blood pressure and cold, cyanosed peripheries) and likely to have a metabolic acidosis.

   b. Septic shock: probably Gram-positive but could be Gram-negative (p. 410). Possibly meningococcaemia.

   c. A previous splenectomy (pneumococcal sepsis), AIDS (*Pneumocystis* pneumonia) (unlikely as septic shock is infrequent) or alcoholism (pneumococcal sepsis).

d. Blood cultures, chest radiograph, differential white cell count, bronchoscopy (if oxygen corrects the hypoxia), ultrasound of abdomen to look for a spleen, urea and electrolytes (as renal failure likely) and blood sugar (as he has a metabolic acidosis).

e. High-flow oxygen (as he has a low CO_2 and is severely hypoxic do not be too concerned about a rising CO_2 — it is more important to correct hypoxia rapidly); i.v. broad-spectrum antibiotics, such as cefotaxime and a single dose of gentamicin (acute renal failure is likely, so beware aminoglycoside toxicity); i.v. fluids; refer to intensive care unit (see septic shock, p. 410).

Picture answers

1. a. The postero-anterior (PA) film (Fig. 23A) shows a wedge-shaped opacity adjacent to the right heart border that is indistinct. The lateral film (Fig. 23B) confirms that this is caused by right middle lobe consolidation with the abnormality visible in the anterior mediastinum between the horizontal and oblique fissures.

   b. The most likely cause is a pneumonia, but disease triggered by a carcinoma should also be considered. Rarely it can be caused by a bronchial adenoma in a young person, giving rise to secondary infection behind an obstruction.

2. a. These radiographs are harder to interpret. The PA film shows a shift of the lower mediastinum (heart) to the left. There is a narrow triangular opacity behind the heart adjacent to the spinal column. The lateral film shows this to be in the posterior part of the chest. The appearances are classical of a left lower lobe collapse. Remember the location of the lower lobe posteriorly.

   b. The most likely cause is a carcinoma, but it could be the result of mucus plugging in, for example, asthma (perhaps complicated by bronchopulmonary aspergillosis).

3. a. He has hazy opacification of the lower (predominantly) lung fields bilaterally.

   b. Given the history, the most likely diagnosis is fibrosing alveolitis. Lymphangitis carcinomatosis could give a similar picture, but the length of the history is too long. Occupational lung disease (for example, asbestosis) should be considered, though there are no calcified plaques. Autoimmune disease should also be considered, e.g. systemic lupus erythematosus (SLE) or rheumatoid disease. Check the relevant autoantibodies; remember there is a high prevalence of false positives, but these are not usually of a high titre. Extrinsic allergic alveolitis predominantly affects the upper zones.

   c. On examination, the patient may be tachypnoeic at rest or after minimal exertion (getting on to the examination couch). In the late stages, cyanosis may be evident. Look for clubbing (most likely in *cryptogenic* fibrosing alveolitis). On auscultation, there will be the typical showers of late inspiratory crepitations.

4. a. The patient has a cavitating lesion adjacent to the upper mediastinum with increased density of the hila (lymphadenopathy). There are increased lung markings in the right upper zone, suggesting a partial collapse.

   b. The most likely cause, given the history, is a cavitating bronchial carcinoma. However, there are other possibilities. The walls of the cavity are too dense for a simple bulla and the hilar abnormality goes against this. Sometimes, a bulla becomes infected with an aspergilloma, which can cause haemoptysis and may be expectorated. Again the hilar lymphadenopathy goes against this. In a lung abscess, the history would be much shorter, with severe constitutional disturbance.

5. a. Cavitary disease at both apices and an elevated left diaphragm consistent with substantial left upper lobe contraction.

   b. (i) Three sputa for tuberculosis smear and culture; (ii) sputum for routine microbiology; (iii) full blood count and erythrocyte sedimentation rate (ESR); and (iv) biochemistry, including liver function tests and albumin. Tuberculin skin tests are probably unnecessary. Most other tests can await the outcome of the acid-fast bacilli smear.

   c. Positive smear for acid-fast bacilli. In gross cavitary disease, the smear is usually strongly positive. If the smear is negative, he should undergo bronchoscopy as soon as possible.

   d. In a single room with negative pressure ventilation in hospital.

   e. Rifampicin, isoniazid, pyrazinamide, ethambutol and pyridoxine. It is imperative to prescribe pyridoxine in a malnourished patient; otherwise the isoniazid may induce pellagra.

   f. As he is unlikely to be compliant, he will need directly supervised treatment on discharge.

6. a. The chest radiograph shows a right pneumothorax, with mediastinal shift to the left (demonstrated by tracheal deviation and displacement of the heart) and compression of the left lung. He has a tension pneumothorax.

   b. The signs would be: (i) respiratory embarrassment (cyanosis, tachypnoea, tachycardia); (ii) signs of the pneumothorax (reduced breath sounds, increased percussion note on the right); and (iii) signs of 'tension' (pulsus paradoxus, tracheal deviation, displaced apex beat).

   c. Your management would be: (i) high concentration of oxygen ('100%' — not really achievable) and (ii) *immediate* insertion of intercostal drain (or any means of releasing the 'tension').

7. a. This is a poor-quality chest radiograph (as is common in severely ill patients) showing bilateral lower lobe consolidation, consistent with bilateral pneumonia.

b. Severe.

c. The issues and questions in your mind are (or should be): cefotaxime covers *Streptococcus pneumoniae* well, including penicillin-resistant isolates (unless they are causing meningitis, in which case vancomycin and rifampicin are required). (Does he have meningitis? Is his disorientation simply sepsis or has he disseminated? You need to check if he has neck stiffness.) Could he have an atypical pneumonia? (Legionnaire's disease and *Mycoplasma* may casue severe illness, but he has no hyponatraemia (more common in legionnaire's disease.) As he is very ill, you might add ciprofloxacin (excellent for legionnaire's disease) or a new macrolide, i.e. clarithromycin. Does he have a very unusual case of pneumonia, i.e. *Pseudomonas aeruginosa, Acinetobacter* spp., etc? (Ask microbiology; you could add ciprofloxacin/gentamicin.)

d. He is very ill and may not survive (in fact, his overall chance of survival is ~60% with excellent supportive care). So the message is '50/50 chance of survival, take each day as it comes; doing everything we can; excellent supportive care key to survival.'

Short notes answers

1. Refer to text (p. 89).

2. Refer to text (Table 13).

3. You should be able to give clear instructions in the steps for using a peak flow meter (p. 72). Similarly, you should be able to explain to a patient how to use a metered-dose inhaler (MDI).

4. See the sections on *Mycoplasma, C. psittaci,* Q fever, *Legionella, C. pneumoniae* and viral pneumonias.

5. Major pathogens include:
   - Ordinary bacteria and Gram-negative bacteria, *Pneumocystis jirovecii (carinii)* (p. 388).
   - Cytomegalovirus is a major problem in bone marrow, and heart and lung transplant patients and is life-threatening. Infection with cytomegalovirus presents with cough and breathlessness, usually with fever and a pneumonitis; it is diagnosed by bronchoscopy and treated with ganciclovir and hyperimmune globulin i.v. Infection has a high mortality, especially if diagnosed late.

   - *Aspergillus.* Invasive aspergillosis is the invasion of tissue by *Aspergillus* spp. Therefore, it develops in previously normal lung or sinuses. It is common (5–25%) in leukaemia, bone marrow, liver, heart and lung transplant recipients and sometimes advanced AIDS. Symptoms are usually minor; cough, mild fever and chest pain are typical. CT scans are more sensitive than plain chest radiographs in diagnosis. It may spread to the brain. It is fatal if untreated. Voriconazole is the drug of choice.

6. *Oxygen.* All patients with pneumonia in hospital require supplemental oxygen. The percentage required depends on their needs and whether they retain carbon dioxide. *The greatest danger is in leaving a patient with a low oxygen.* Patients with chronic respiratory disease, exhausted patients or those with major neuromuscular problems require monitoring of blood gases to ensure that there is not a significant rise in carbon dioxide. This may require you to make small changes in oxygen concentration and repeat arterial gases an hour later. Previously well patients should be given high oxygen concentrations (e.g. ≥60% oxygen) and can be monitored simply with pulse oximetry.
   Analgesia. In pneumonia this is only required for patients with pleurisy. Be careful that your choice will not suppress the respiratory drive and allow carbon dioxide to accumulate.

7. Physiotherapy is indicated as a treatment in:
   - wet bronchiectasis
   - cystic fibrosis
   - productive lobar pneumonia and bronchopneumonia
   - aspiration pneumonia
   - ventilator pneumonia
   - infective exacerbations of COPD
   - palliative care for carcinoma of bronchus
   - pneumothorax with drain in situ.

   It is also used to help in investigation:

   - induced sputum in AIDS for *Pneumocystis* and tuberculosis
   - sputum production for assessment of infection.

   Physiotherapists should also be involved in patient education:

   - in management of acute asthma (e.g. postural advice, breathing pattern, inhaler technique)
   - in cystic fibrosis and bronchiectasis (postural drainage).

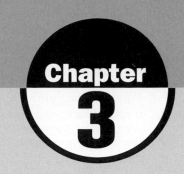
Gastrointestinal, hepatobiliary and pancreatic disease

3.1 Clinical aspects

Learning objectives

You should be able to:
- link the common symptoms and signs in gastrointestinal (GI) disease with disease processes
- construct a logical investigation plan based on the symptoms and signs
- utilise appropriately the range of investigations for the GI tract, particularly endoscopy and imaging
- describe principles of management of the common problems and diseases.

Case Study

Edith is an 84-year-old woman who is brought to the elderly care outpatient clinic by Fred, her husband, who is her main carer. You find it difficult to get a history from Edith because she has a dysphasia as well as a right hemiparesis from a stroke over a year ago. Fred tells you that over several months, it seems that she has been having difficulty in swallowing her food. This seems to be getting worse and he now has her on a 'sloppy' diet. She does not seem to have any difficulty with her cups of tea. Apart from aspirin, she is on omeprazole long-term because of recurrent heartburn.

Common symptoms

Dysphagia

You must take swallowing difficulties seriously. The first step is a careful history. Patients will often localise the difficulty to high (i.e. throat/pharynx) or lower (oesophageal) obstruction. Dysphagia is a common accompaniment of neurological disease (p. 216), but usually there will be other symptoms and signs. A very important discriminating feature is difficulty with different consistencies of food:

- in neurological disease — liquids
- in local disease — solid food.

In a patient with longstanding heartburn (see below), with dysphagia over several months, a benign **stricture** may have occurred. However, you must exclude oesophageal carcinoma. Rarer causes of dysphagia include **achalasia** and **systemic sclerosis** (p. 355). Always be very wary of making the diagnosis of a psychological cause for swallowing difficulties (globus hystericus). It is very rare and there should be other evidence of psychiatric illness.

Heartburn

Heartburn is a common symptom and is caused by reflux oesophagitis. It increases with age and is often severe in pregnancy because of relaxation of the oesophageal sphincter. Patients complain of an ill-defined burning sensation behind the sternum. It may be worsened by stooping or lying flat, which increases the reflux. Less commonly, heartburn may be caused by oesophageal **candidiasis**. Recent-onset heartburn in a patient with associated symptoms (e.g. weight loss) should be investigated.

Indigestion/dyspepsia

Most patients do not give a 'classical' description of dyspepsia, but rather one of many variations. The typical description of ulcer pain is epigastric discomfort that is relieved by eating and occurs a few hours after meals or during the night. A valuable question is whether they take regular antacids. There is no reliable way of differentiating between gastritis, gastric ulcer or duodenal ulcer at the bedside. If the patient is aged over 55 years or if they have associated symptoms (e.g. weight loss, iron deficiency anaemia, vomiting or dysphagia), an urgent endoscopy should be arranged.

Abdominal pain

The following framework is useful in abdominal pain.

Is the pain of recent onset?

If acute and severe, it suggests an acute problem such as perforation or acute pancreatitis; if longstanding, it might suggest a peptic ulcer (periodicity) or chronic pancreatitis.

Where is the pain?

If epigastric, it suggests a peptic ulcer; if right hypochondrial, biliary disease; if periumbilical, peritoneal irritation. Lower abdominal pain is linked to colonic or bladder disease.

Where does it radiate to?

Shoulder tip pain suggests diaphragmatic irritation; pain going through into the back is linked to pancreatic disease though duodenal ulceration or biliary disease can also cause back pain.

What helps/worsens the pain?

Local heat (hot water bottle) may help chronic pancreatic pain. Diaphragmatic irritation may be worsened by deep breathing/coughing.

What is the character of the pain?

Intestinal obstruction may cause typical colic pain. Biliary colic is not typically 'colicky' as it comes in waves lasting about 30 minutes. Chronic pancreatitis causes a severe unremitting pain described as 'boring' through into the back.

Are there any associated features?

Intestinal obstruction may be accompanied by vomiting and abdominal distension. Weight loss is always worrying, but it may be associated with malabsorption.

Abdominal distension

Many people complain of abdominal distension, but it is usually a subjective feeling. It is associated with functional bowel disease/irritable bowel syndrome and sometimes the distension can be seen. Rarely, you will see patients with distension caused by ascites or intestinal obstruction.

Vomiting

The vomiting centre is in the medulla close to the **chemoreceptor trigger zone**. It is stimulated through the zone by the vestibular apparatus, by central connections (e.g. olfactory) or by vagal afferents from the GI tract.

Vomiting has three phases:

1. nausea and excess autonomic activity with sweating, salivation and pallor

2. retching with closure of the glottis, cessation of respiration and contraction of the diaphragm and abdominal muscles

3. expulsion of the gastric contents with relaxation of the lower oesophageal sphincter and cardia, and contractions of the abdominal muscles.

In a patient with nausea and vomiting, you should consider:

- GI disease, including food poisoning (common)
- drugs (common in hospitals)
- systemic disease, including neurological problems.

You have to consider whether the patient is compromised by the loss of fluid and electrolytes as well as by reduced intake. The principles of management are:

- replace the fluid and electrolytes lost
- treat the underlying cause; sometimes this is not possible
- symptomatic relief.

You should know the mechanisms of action of the common antiemetics (Table 27).

Haematemesis

Haematemesis is common. First, you should make sure that the patient is not shocked due to a reduced blood volume (systolic BP > 100 mmHg, pulse < 100 beats/min). Tachycardia is a worrying sign. Occasionally, patients can have a (relative) bradycardia because of β-blockers or as a result of vagal stimulation.

After this, take a history. It can be difficult to estimate the volume of blood lost as it is a frightening symptom. The history may suggest peptic ulceration and you should enquire about the use of non-steroidal anti-inflammatory drugs (non-selective NSAIDs, and COX-2 inhibitors) and antiplatelet drugs (aspirin and clopidogrel). Occasionally, a **Mallory–Weiss tear** is indicated by violent retching followed by vomiting fresh blood.

The patient may be known to have liver disease/portal hypertension (varices) or a history of chronic heavy alcohol ingestion may be given. A bleeding diathesis is possible and the appropriate investigations (clotting, fibrin degradation products, platelets) should be carried out. Sometimes, the most difficult story to unravel is vomiting 'coffee grounds', but it is better to be cautious and assume upper GI bleeding.

Table 27 Mechanism of action of common antiemetics

Drug	Action	Comments
Metoclopramide	Dopamine antagonism	Crosses blood–brain barrier; side-effect – parkinsonism
Domperidone	Dopamine antagonism	Acts on peripheral receptors
Prochlorperazine	Dopamine and cholinergic antagonism	Side-effects – parkinsonism, constipation
Ondansetron	5-Hydroxytryptamine (5-HT$_3$) antagonism	Useful in cancer chemotherapy

Diarrhoea

People use different terms to describe their bowel habit. With any possibly abnormal bowel habit, you need to find out its time course, variability and associated symptoms. To some people, diarrhoea means a single explosive bowel movement; to others it means increased frequency of passing stools.

Passing large volumes of watery faeces is indicative of organic bowel disease. Bloody diarrhoea points to a colonic problem. *Steatorrhoea* means a motion with high fat content and is usually described as being bulky, offensive and difficult to flush away. Appearance of oil/fat globules in stools suggests pancreatic malabsorption. Patients with chronic diarrhoea (more than 4 weeks and stool weight > 200 g/day) need further assessment and investigation. Routine blood tests (full blood count, liver function tests, calcium, B$_{12}$, folate, thyroid function tests) stool cultures (for infectious causes) and serology (coeliac disease) are needed as well as imaging, depending on the possible aetiology of the diarrhoea (e.g. small or large bowel, pancreas).

Constipation

Many people complain of constipation using passing a motion once per day as their yardstick. In reality, the range of normality is much greater. As with diarrhoea, it is a recent change in bowel habit that is worrying. You need to have a clear idea of the person's diet (roughage) and medication; many drugs cause constipation, including narcotic analgesics (e.g. codeine) and tricyclic antidepressants (anticholinergic effect).

Melaena

The passage of a black, offensive tarry motion indicates high GI tract bleeding. The major diagnostic pitfall is concurrent treatment with iron preparations (which also can cause either diarrhoea or constipation).

Faecal incontinence

Faecal incontinence is very distressing. It may be associated with urgency and a clear history of an acute bowel problem. More commonly it occurs in elderly, often disabled, people. There are two chronic types:

- neurogenic faecal incontinence
- overflow.

In neurogenic incontinence, the patient passes formed motions with no adequate warning. It is often linked to eating (**gastro-colic reflex**). The underlying process is usually cerebrovascular or degenerative neurological disease. Management is either by the carers anticipating the bowel habit or by promoting constipation (e.g. using codeine), together with regular enemas.

In overflow incontinence, the patient is constipated. Examination confirms that the rectum is full of faeces and there is leakage of faeculent material. The management is regular enemas, removal of any predisposing factors and prescription of a laxative. If the faeces are soft, then a stimulant such as senna should be used. If the faeces are hard, then a high-roughage diet should be advised, with the addition of bulking agents (ispaghula husk) or osmotic laxatives such as lactulose.

Rectal bleeding

Patients with haemorrhoids or anal fissures (often painful) may complain of the passage of bright red blood. However, you should be cautious about assigning bleeding to a minor problem and failing to consider serious disease such as inflammatory bowel disease or malignancy, especially as they are treatable.

Jaundice

Jaundice becomes clinically detectable at around double the upper limit of the bilirubin concentration in the blood (30–40 µmol/l). You should consider an infective cause and ask about potential recent risk factors, such as blood transfusion or travel abroad. In obstructive jaundice, the patient may volunteer that the urine has been dark and that the motions are pale. On examination, you should carefully palpate for an enlarged gall bladder (**Courvoisier's sign — pancreatic or bile duct carcinoma**). Remember that, in an older person, gall stone obstruction is at least as common as malignant blockage as a cause of jaundice.

Jaundice may signify decompensated chronic liver disease and you should examine accordingly. In long-standing problems such as **primary biliary cirrhosis**, the pigmentation may be deep with evidence of pruritus — excoriation of the skin (irritation due to deposition of bile salts).

Weight loss/anorexia

Weight loss is a common presenting problem, either in association with other features or alone. The first task is to try to quantify the loss. You should always weigh the patient as a baseline. A framework for diagnosis is:

- inadequate intake, e.g. depression
- malabsorption, e.g. coeliac disease
- disturbed metabolism; thyrotoxicosis
- malignancy, e.g. GI or in another system
- systemic disease, e.g. tuberculosis.

Investigations

Plain radiographs

There is limited usefulness for plain radiographs in GI disease. Only a small proportion of gall stones are calcified. Chronic pancreatitis is associated with calcification. In a suspected perforated viscus, an erect film may show gas under the diaphragm. Gas is also seen in patients who have had recent surgery and it may outline the biliary tree. In the absence of a surgical explanation, the sign may point to a cholangitis.

You should order erect and supine films in a patient with possible bowel obstruction and look for fluid levels as clues to the level of the obstruction (small or large bowel obstruction).

Barium studies

Barium swallow

If a patient has severe heartburn or if food is 'sticking', a barium swallow may be useful to show a stricture (benign or malignant), a hiatus hernia, oesophagitis (but better to request endoscopy) or filling defects caused by varices.

Videofluoroscopy

Videofluoroscopy is useful in non-obstructive dysphagia. It will show any abnormalities within the three phases of swallowing (oral, pharyngeal and oesophageal) and aspiration.

Barium meal

Although endoscopy has become the investigation of choice for suspected gastroduodenal disease, a good-quality barium meal interpreted by an experienced radiologist can give structural and motility information, complementary to biopsy/culture.

Barium follow-through/small bowel enema

Visualisation of the small bowel can be achieved in one of two ways. Either the barium is taken orally and followed as it moves through the small intestine, or a catheter is placed in the upper jejunum and barium is administered direct. The latter approach will give better imaging but is more invasive.

Barium enema

The main indications for a barium enema are:

- a recent change in bowel habit
- to delineate the extent of suspected inflammatory bowel disease
- unexplained iron deficiency anaemia
- rectal bleeding.

A significant proportion of barium enemas fail to exclude pathology because of poor bowel preparation. This requires strong laxatives and some patients find it unpleasant. Many old people are unable to retain the enema. The alternative investigation is colonoscopy (see below), but this has similar drawbacks.

Computed tomography (CT) and magnetic resonance imaging (MRI)

The use of CT and MRI in GI disease continues to grow and it is now the preferred investigation in a number of conditions. However, in most centres ultrasound remains the first test for hepatobiliary or pancreatic disease, including guided biopsy. CT can be useful in:

- small bowel obstruction, where it can show the site and also the cause (including ischaemia)
- staging for colonic cancers, including distant metastases and recurrence
- primary detection of colo-rectal tumours in older patients unable to undergo colonoscopy or barium enema
- seeking morphological evidence of cirrhosis, spenomegaly and the presence of ascites
- evaluation of acute pancreatitis (using contrast) and its complications
- differentiating chronic pancreatitis from pancreatic carcinoma
- staging pancreatic carcinoma.

MRI is also being evaluated in GI disease and can be used when giving contrast is contraindicated (allergy or renal insuffiency). Magnetic resonance cholangiopancreatography (MRCP) is a newer, non-invasive technique (biliary tree fluid is hyperintense on T_2-weighted images) that can be used to diagnose stones, strictures or bile duct dilatations but, unlike ERCP, it cannot be used as a treatment.

Endoscopy

Detailed discussion of the different types of endoscopy is given with the relevant GI problems.

Laparoscopy

In place of the laparotomy, which is a major surgical procedure, suspected GI pathology is increasingly investigated using a laparoscope. Insufflation of the peritoneal cavity with carbon dioxide is required. This means that, as with instrumentation of the biliary tree or laparotomy, gas may be seen subsequently on plain radiographs for a short period of time.

Ultrasound

Ultrasound scanning is key investigation of GI (intra-abdominal) disease. Like CT imaging, it is particularly useful in hepatobiliary or pancreatic disease, but there is also interest in its role in bowel disease. Ultrasonography is dependent on the experience of the operator and the clinical information given to them. The latter allows the operator to direct the examination to the appropriate area and to give a more definite report as to the likelihood of disease being present.

Biopsy

A key investigation may be histological examination or culture. For example, in gastric disease, testing for *Helicobacter pylori* is important, particularly in those with relapsing peptic ulceration. *H. pylori* infection is usually detected by urease activity on a mucosal biopsy obtained at endoscopy. It can also be detected using a urea breath test, serology ('near-patient' testing) or a stool antigen test. Histological examination is also required in gastric ulcers to exclude an adenocarcinoma. In other parts of the bowel, biopsy is essential: for example, in coeliac or inflammatory bowel disease. A biopsy is often taken using ultrasound or CT guidance. Alternatively, direct endoscopic visualisation may be preferable.

3.2 The oesophagus

Learning objectives

You should be able to:

- link oesophageal pathophysiology with the three common symptoms
- construct a differential diagnosis
- plan investigation and management.

Case Study

Rhajib is a middle-aged man who has been assessed by the cardiologists and then referred to the GI clinic. He has had four bouts of central chest pain, which he describes as being 'a tightness' in the centre of his chest, with no radiation. These have woken him up from sleep and he has been admitted each time. He does not have any risk factors apart from his age and ethnicity. The cardiologists are asking whether the underlying problem might be gastrointestinal.

The major symptoms of oesophageal disease are:

- dysphagia
- heartburn
- painful swallowing (odynophagia); this is unusual and is linked to infections such as candidiasis or herpes simplex.

Disorders of motility

Normal motility

The function of the oesophagus is to convey food from the pharynx to the stomach. There are two muscular layers, circular and longitudinal, with a gradual transition from striated to smooth muscle. Normally, there is a resting tone in the lower pharyngeal constrictor muscles producing an upper oesophageal sphincter; similarly, there is a lower oesophageal sphincter preventing reflux of stomach contents. When swallowing is initiated, a **primary peristaltic wave** causes relaxation of the upper sphincter and a coordinated wave of contraction moving the bolus of food down to the lower sphincter, which relaxes and allows passage into the stomach. Secondary peristaltic waves strip the oesophagus of any residual foodstuffs.

Achalasia

Rarely, the ganglionic cells controlling the coordinated peristalsis and the relaxation of the lower oesophagus degenerate, causing achalasia. The person presents with progressive dysphagia with regurgitation of undigested food several hours after eating. Recurrent aspiration pneumonias occur. Plain chest radiography may show a fluid level behind the heart. On a barium swallow, there is oesophageal dilatation with a smooth outline tapering down to the lower oesophageal sphincter.

Other disorders of motility

In older people, spasm of the oesophagus causes chest pain that may mimic angina or even a myocardial infarction. A barium swallow may show a *corkscrew* oesophagus and manometric recordings demonstrate the disordered motility. The difficulty is that these features may be present without symptoms, and in symptomatic patients the relationship may not be causal. Treatment is with nitrates and calcium antagonists, which relax smooth muscle.

In systemic sclerosis (p. 355), there is commonly gross disturbance of oesophageal motility, which may produce dysphagia and heartburn. Occasionally, an autonomic neuropathy (diabetes mellitus) may affect the oesophagus.

Hiatus hernia and oesophagitis

Clinical presentation

A sliding hiatus hernia is increasingly common with age. Much more rare is the rolling hiatus hernia in which the stomach rolls up into the chest cavity alongside the oesophagus. In a sliding hiatus hernia, reflux causes the problems. The person may be obese and the symptoms may be worsened by substances that relax the lower oesophageal sphincter, such as alcohol. Similarly, the hormonal changes of pregnancy may precipitate severe heartburn. If the symptoms are longstanding, then it is reasonable to assume that they are caused by reflux oesophagitis, but recent onset of swallowing problems in a middle-aged or older person should lead to suspicion of cancer.

Occasionally, reflux oesophagitis presents with a haematemesis or anaemia. Again, be wary of assuming that the cause of an iron deficiency anaemia is a mild oesophagitis, thereby missing a large bowel carcinoma.

Investigations

Often no investigation is required, providing the probability of other causes is low. A full blood count will show any anaemia. A barium swallow will demonstrate a hiatus hernia, but this does not prove causation. Some mucosal irregularity may help to confirm the presence of oesophagitis. The investigation of choice is endoscopy, which allows direct visualisation of the oesophagus and biopsy of any suspicious area.

Management

There are three steps in management:

- symptomatic relief
- reducing acid to promote healing
- increasing lower oesophageal sphincter tone and gastric emptying.

For many people, a simple antacid will suffice, together with advice about weight loss and avoiding tight clothing or excessive bending. Coupled with this, in more severe cases, you should advise patients to sleep with the head of the bed elevated.

In patients with marked oesophagitis with severe symptoms, acid secretion should be reduced. A histamine receptor (H_2) blocker such as ranitidine will produce healing in about 50% of people. A proton pump inhibitor, such as omeprazole, will cause almost immediate relief in virtually all patients, together with quick healing and these drugs are often used as the first-line therapy.

In the long term, if the simple measures described above do not suffice, prokinetic agents such as domperidone (a peripheral dopamine antagonist) will help to prevent recurrence. It is rare that patients with reflux require surgery.

Complications

There are two long-term complications of reflux that you should be aware of.

Strictures The years of inflammation from reflux can produce scarring and constriction at the lower end of the oesophagus. Patients present with increasing dysphagia, poor nutrition and aspiration pneumonia. Endoscopy is mandatory to exclude malignancy and is therapeutic as dilatation produces dramatic relief. The stricture tends to recur but can be redilated. Proton pump inhibitors may reduce the recurrence rate.

Metaplasia The other consequence of long-term inflammation is metaplasia of the epithelium. Normally, the oesophagus is lined with stratified squamous epithelium,

Three

but this may change into columnar epithelium in the lower part over a variable length (**Barrett's oesophagus**). It is visible on endoscopy above the oesophageal–gastric junction and should be confirmed on biopsy. It is premalignant and repeated surveillance endoscopy may be required (every 2 years) with intense acid suppression.

Oesophageal carcinoma

Most oesophageal carcinomas occur in the middle and lower third of the oesophagus and are squamous cell carcinomas with varying degrees of differentiation. The majority occur in the sixth and seventh decades of life. The incidence shows considerable worldwide variation. In the UK, the main associations are with smoking and heavy alcohol intake. Barrett's oesophagus (see above) is premalignant for adenocarcinoma and there has been an increase in this cancer in the lower third of the oesophagus or gastro–oesophageal junction.

Clinical presentation

Any middle-aged or elderly person with progressive dysphagia may have carcinoma of the oesophagus. Sometimes, people develop retrosternal pain as a result of local infiltration and may have haematemesis or anaemia. You must enquire about general well-being and any 'alarm' symptoms (e.g. weight loss, vomiting and anaemia). Eventually, aphagia occurs for both solids and liquids, with a high probability of aspiration pneumonia. On examination, you may find some enlargement of the cervical lymph nodes and hepatomegaly.

Investigations

Basic investigations may show an iron deficiency anaemia, a high alkaline phosphatase indicative of hepatic metastases and, on a chest radiograph, involvement of the hilar nodes. In a severely malnourished and water-depleted patient, hypoproteinaemia, high urea and hypernatraemia may occur.

A barium swallow will show the level of the lesion and, characteristically, the stricture is irregular in outline. Sometimes the carcinoma is ulcerated or polypoid. Urgent endoscopy is the investigation of choice, allowing direct visualisation with biopsy. An ultrasound scan of the liver will demonstrate hepatic metastases. If curative surgery is being contemplated, spiral CT or MRI will show the extent of any spread.

Management

Initially, management is directed towards adequate hydration and improving the patient's nutritional state. Overall, the long-term prognosis is poor with only 10–15% of people surviving 5 years. In the lower part of the oesophagus, curative surgery is sometimes possible (20% of cases). In the upper part, radiotherapy is used. Survival may be improved by combining radiotherapy and chemotherapy, sometimes to reduce tumour bulk as a prelude to surgery.

Often, the only approach is palliation, in which the major aim is to preserve swallowing. Laser therapy can be used for debulking, and radiotherapy may be useful.

Stents may be inserted endoscopically to protect the lumen. Alternatively, if the lumen cannot be opened or if the patient is finding it difficult to sustain eating and drinking,

a percutaneous endoscopic gastrostomy (PEG) tube may be inserted.

3.3 The stomach and duodenum

Case Study

You are called to the accident and emergency department on an urgent bleep because of a middle-aged patient who has been brought by ambulance in shock. Nobody knows his name, but he was found by some passers-by on the pavement where he was vomiting blood and asking for help. Since then, things have deteriorated; he has brought up copious amounts of blood in the resuscitation area and the nurses have been unable to record a blood pressure. The patient is in some distress and is not responding to questions.

Normal structure and function

The stomach has three functions:

- acting as a reservoir, mixing the food and passing it into the duodenum in small volumes
- secreting acid and pepsinogen to aid digestion
- secreting intrinsic factor for vitamin B_{12} absorption.

Food is passed down into the 'C'-shaped duodenum, in the second part of which there is the **ampulla of Vater** with opening of the pancreatic and common bile ducts.

The stomach consists of three parts: the fundus, the body and the antrum, which extends into the pylorus. There are waves of muscular contraction that aid in mixing food and moving it down towards the pylorus. The pylorus (hypertrophy of the circular muscle layer) acts as a sphincter governing passage of food into the duodenum.

The upper two-thirds of the stomach contains parietal cells, which secrete acid, and chief cells, secreting pepsinogen. The antrum contains mucus-secreting cells and G cells producing gastrin. Acid secretion is under neural (vagal) and hormonal (gastrin — stimulatory; vasoactive intestinal peptide (VIP) somatostatin — inhibitory) control. Common to both is the release of histamine, which stimulates hydrogen ion production and secretion. The sites of action of inhibitory drugs are shown in Figure 31.

Gastritis

Gastritis can be divided into acute and chronic forms.

The presentations of acute gastritis are:

- dyspepsia
- bleeding from acute mucosal ulceration (occasionally)
- as an incidental finding at endoscopy.

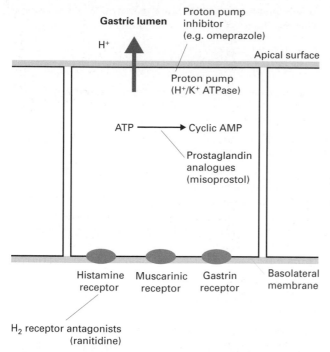

Fig. 31 The sites of action of drugs that inhibit hydrogen ion secretion by a gastric parietal cell. AMP/ATP, adenosine mono-/triphosphate.

Acute gastritis is associated with NSAID ingestion (including aspirin) and heavy alcohol (binge) drinking. Very sick patients in intensive care can develop acute ulceration with bleeding, which relates to disturbance in gastric blood flow.

Chronic gastritis is seen in association with *Helicobacter pylori* infection (see below), chemical irritation (for example, bile reflux) or as an autoimmune response. In the last cause, antibodies are directed against gastric parietal cells and intrinsic factor, which may produce pernicious anaemia. There are different histopathological stages that may culminate in atrophic gastritis. If this occurs, premalignant changes may be found, with an increased risk of gastric carcinoma.

Most cases of acute gastritis respond to simple antacids and removal of the cause. Sometimes, in both acute and chronic gastritis, proton pump inhibitors or H_2 receptor antagonists can alleviate dyspepsia.

Peptic ulcer

Peptic ulceration is a common disease, affecting approximately 1 in 6 people in the UK at some time, with increasing incidence with age. It shows considerable worldwide variation. It is more common in men. Associated factors are smoking, ingestion of NSAIDs, hyperparathyroidism, blood group O and, importantly, *H. pylori* infection.

Pathogenesis

The mechanisms leading to a peptic ulcer include:

* factors acting against the mucosal barrier — acid secretion

* factors weakening the mucosal barrier — composition of the mucus, impaired production of prostaglandins, *H. pylori* infection and reduced blood flow (acute).

You should not simply consider excess acid secretion as a cause of ulceration; most people with a gastric ulcer have normal or low acid secretion. In duodenal ulceration, many people are hypersecretors, but other factors play a role (e.g. *H. pylori* infection). Rarely ulcers are associated with the **Zollinger–Ellison syndrome**, which is due to a pancreatic tumour producing large quantities of gastrin and hence acid.

Clinical presentation

Patients may present with 'indigestion'. You should always explore what is meant by this, rather than simply translating it into dyspepsia. The pain is usually in the epigastrium and can be described as a gnawing or a hunger pain. It may come on several hours after eating or wake the person during the night. Eating may relieve the pain. You must enquire about *periodicity*; that is, the pain will be present (not continously) over a few months/weeks and then subsides, before returning after an interval. You should always ask about smoking/ alcohol and NSAID ingestion as well as any previous diagnosis of peptic ulcer, its complications or surgery.

Frequently, the ulcer will present with a complication, particularly in older people when the resulting mortality may be high. Complications are:

* Perforation causing peritonitis and shock; corticosteroid therapy may mask these signs.
* GI haemorrhage, causing either a haematemesis or melaena (see below)
* Anaemia: either symptomatic or diagnosed on a full blood count.
* Outflow tract obstruction resulting from severe scarring of the pylorus. Rarely seen now, the history is of repeated vomiting over several months, weight loss and severe electrolyte and fluid disturbance.

Investigations

You should always request a full blood count and, if this is abnormal, measure iron status. In all emergency patients with upper abdominal pain, you should request serum amylase estimation. An electrocardiograph (ECG) may be needed if there is a possibility of a myocardial infarction. If the patient has been compromised by severe vomiting, you should check urea and electrolytes.

Your aim is to confirm the suspected diagnosis. Endoscopy is required in any patient with active bleeding as it can visualise the source of bleeding and enable specimens to be taken for culture of *H. pylori*. In severe haemorrhage, the bleeding artery may be injected with adrenaline (epinephrine; up to 95% haemostasis) or coagulated using a heat probe. A repeat endoscopy (or barium meal) may be needed to assess response to therapy, diagnose relapse or confirm healing — particularly in gastric ulcers, which sometimes prove to be malignant.

Management

Patients should be advised on smoking and alcohol ingestion. The necessity of continuing with NSAID therapy should be carefully considered. If necessary, these can be continued with either misoprostol or a proton pump inhibitor (see below). Many patients can be switched to simple analgesics. Some people will need a course of iron supplements; others may need antimicrobials for *H. pylori* (see below).

The need for surgery has dropped dramatically since the introduction of the H₂ antagonists and the subsequent development of the proton pump inhibitors. The main indication for surgery is management of complications, particularly perforation and, rarely, outflow tract obstruction. Occasionally, surgery is required in patients who continue to have severe haemorrhage.

Specific drug therapy

Antacids

Antacids are often used by people with intermittent mild dyspepsia. It is often worth enquiring about use of 'white medicines', as this may give you a clearer idea of a longer-term problem. Antacids give symptomatic relief but have little role in healing or prophylaxis.

Proton pump inhibitors

There are several proton pump inhibitors (PPIs) available, e.g. lansoprazole, omeprazole, rabeprazole and pantoprazole. These have proven to be effective in a number of overlapping conditions:

- Proven peptic ulceration combined with testing and treating for *H. pylori* infection.
- Proven NSAID-induced ulcer when patients must continue with these (e.g. in rheumatoid arthritis).
- Severe gastro-oesophageal reflux disorder (GORD) including oesophageal ulceration or Barrett's oesophagus. In mild disease antacids or H₂ receptor antagonists are alternative therapies.
- Non-ulcer dyspepsia (endoscopy), but PPIs should only be used if the symptoms appear to be acid-related.
- Mild dyspepsia in general practice. Treatment is on either a 'step-up' (antacids not effective) or a 'step-down' (healing followed by maintenance dose) basis. Where possible, a definite diagnosis should be made.
- Acute upper GI bleeding. Use intravenous therapy.

In all patients, the optimum dose to achieve healing should be used, followed by the lowest dose that provides on-going symptom relief. The least expensive drug should be prescribed. All the PPIs have a low incidence of side-effects (<2.5%) but these include headache and diarrhoea. As the PPIs are metabolised through the cytochrome P450 system (see below), drug interactions are possible but are usually not clinically relevant.

The H₂ receptor antagonists

An alternative to a PPI is an antagonist that acts at the histamine H₂ receptor, e.g. ranitidine. These drugs can be given in divided doses, though a single dose at night may be preferable for suppressing nocturnal acid secretion. They can be used in:

- *healing proven peptic ulcers:* very effective in duodenal ulcers, less so with gastric ulcers
- *chronic therapy to prevent relapse:* moderately effective
- *chronic non-ulcer dyspepsia:* moderately effective
- *severe oesophagitis:* heal about half of cases (PPI more effective)
- prevention of ulceration in patients who need NSAIDs: a limited role.

Unlike the PPIs, the H₂ receptor antagonists have no impact on acute bleeding.

All of the H₂ receptor antagonists are well tolerated, with no proven long-term problems. You should be aware of some of the side-effects and potential drug interactions specific to cimetidine. It is an enzyme inhibitor at the cytochrome P450 system, which is a heterogeneous group of enzymes involved in the metabolism of many drugs. Cimetidine significantly inhibits the metabolism of *phenytoin, warfarin* and *theophylline*.

Prostaglandin analogues

Misoprostol is an analogue of prostaglandin E₂; it acts by reducing gastrin and acid secretion as well as by promoting the mucosal barrier. The main side-effect is diarrhoea. It is relatively little used, but can be prescribed as prophylaxis against gastric damage by NSAIDs (a PPI or H₂ antagonist is the usual preferred option), but the first consideration is to stop NSAIDs if possible.

Drugs acting on the mucosal barrier

Sulcralfate is occasionally used as it helps to preserve the mucosal barrier. It is a complex of aluminium hydroxide and sucrose. The main side-effect is constipation.

Bismuth also promotes the mucosal barrier and is bactericidal with antibiotics for *H. pylori* infection. It is best taken as a tablet as the liquid form has an unpleasant taste. Side-effects include constipation and black stools.

Helicobacter pylori

The link between *H. pylori* and gastroduodenal disease is important not simply because of understanding the basic mechanisms, but also for choice of therapy.

Many people are infected with *H. pylori* and more than half the population over the age of 50 have evidence of gastritis. The general need to eradicate the organism has been contentious, though many clinicians do so.

However, antimicrobial therapy is an important element in the treatment of peptic ulceration, with 70–80% of patients with duodenal ulcer testing positive. It is now routine to check for infection in patients with a peptic ulcer by urease assay, histology, serology or a breath test. The management is a combination of a specific antiulcer drug together with one or more antimicrobials. One of the most effective regimens is a PPI combined with amoxicillin and clarithromycin. Such triple therapy can result in healing in 85–90% of cases. There is a recurrence rate of 10–20%.

In addition to the proven association with peptic ulcer disease, there may be links between *H. pylori* infection and development of gastric carcinoma and lymphoma.

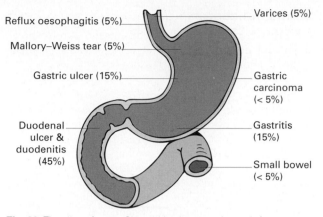

Reflux oesophagitis (5%)

Mallory–Weiss tear (5%)

Gastric ulcer (15%)

Duodenal ulcer & duodenitis (45%)

Varices (5%)

Gastric carcinoma (< 5%)

Gastritis (15%)

Small bowel (< 5%)

Fig. 32 The sites of upper GI tract bleeding, together with frequencies.

Acute gastrointestinal bleeding

Acute GI bleeding can present with haematemesis, coffee ground vomiting or melaena. The causes of an acute bleed are shown in Figure 32. Most cases result from peptic ulceration or duodenitis/gastritis, but other possible causes may be suggested by the history or examination, e.g. a *Mallory–Weiss tear* or *varices* (p. 149).

The emergency management of severe haematemesis is shown in the box. Mortality from acute GI haemorrhage increases with:

- age (>65 years)
- hypotension
- pre-existing comorbidity.

Clinical Box: Emergency treatment: management of severe haematemesis

Put on latex gloves (as the patient may have hepatitis B or C or HIV)

1. Assess for hypovolaemia: blood pressure, heart rate, peripheral perfusion
2. Establish venous access, preferably into a large central vein with large-bore cannula
3. Take blood for urgent cross-match (8 units whole blood)
4. Give a plasma expander such as gelofusine rapidly
5. Ask for senior help urgently
6. Give high-concentration inspired oxygen
7. Gather information (from patient, carer, ambulance personnel, etc.) for cause
8. Examine patient: cause and other problems (e.g. ascites)
9. If delay in cross-match, consider transfusing O-negative blood (universal donor)
10. Take blood for:
    - Haemoglobin (possibly pre-existent anaemia)
    - Clotting (bleeding diathesis)
    - Urea and electrolytes (renal function)
    - Blood gases in severely shocked patients.

You should tell the surgical team on call when a patient is admitted with severe acute bleeding. This allows time for assessment and intervention before the patient becomes moribund.

Most patients should have an endoscopy on the next available list, preferably the day following admission. It may need to be done sooner, but the rule is resuscitate first. Patients should be started on high-dose PPIs intravenously. Therapeutic options at endoscopy include:

- adrenaline (epinephrine) injections for bleeding ulcers
- heat coagulation
- banding or sclerotherapy for varices.

If the haemoglobin is <100 g/l, a transfusion should be started. One unit of blood will raise the haemoglobin by approximately 10 g/l. If the patient is not anaemic, the haemoglobin should be repeated as haemodilution takes place over the 48 hours following a significant bleed. Renal function should be monitored. All patients with haematemesis should receive iron therapy to replenish the iron stores.

The ongoing management is dependent on the cause and is discussed in the relevant sections. Investigation and management of chronic iron deficiency anaemia is discussed on page 268.

Gastric tumours

Most gastric tumours are malignant. Occasionally, smooth muscle benign tumours are found (leiomyoma). A small proportion of malignant tumours are lymphomas (<5%) and these carry a better prognosis. Most gastric tumours are adenocarcinomas.

Adenocarcinoma

The incidence of gastric adenocarcinomas is falling but is still high in the UK. It is more common in men. The tumours are associated with chronic atrophic gastritis and pernicious anaemia.

Clinical presentation

Most tumours present late, commonly with epigastric pain, anorexia and weight loss. The diagnosis should be suspected in any patient with onset of dyspepsia over the age of 50 years, particularly with any other 'alarm' symptoms. The pain from a tumour can be indistinguishable from that of a peptic ulcer. Tumours often bleed, leading to an iron deficiency anaemia and, occasionally, a brisk haematemesis. Sometimes, the presentation is with metastatic disease: enlarged lymph node on the left side of the neck (Virchow's node), ascites, hepatomegaly, and bone or brain metastases. Non-metastatic manifestations (paraneoplastic syndromes) are seen (e.g. thrombophlebitis migrans or thromboembolic disease). The cachexia may be striking. Lymphadenopathy may be present and, in the abdomen, an epigastric mass is common. Other findings may be irregular hepatomegaly and ascites.

Investigations

Adenocarcinomas commonly arise in the antrum and may cause outlet obstruction. They often take the form of an ulcer with raised edges, but sometimes they are polypoid and occasionally may be diffusely infiltrative, producing **linitis plastica**.

Endoscopy is the diagnostic investigation of choice, allowing direct visualisation and biopsy. Sometimes the biopsies may be negative and may have to be repeated. A barium meal can give high diagnostic probability but cannot provide histopathological confirmation. It is the better investigation in diffuse infiltrating carcinoma as it will demonstrate the shrunken non-relaxing stomach.

Basic tests include a full blood count (anaemia) and liver function tests (metastatic disease); a chest radiograph may show pulmonary metastases or lymph node spread. Ultrasound can show liver metastases or abdominal lymph node involvement. If a curative resection is being considered, a staging assessment (using the TNM — tumour, nodes, metastases — system) is carried out using spiral CT of the thorax and abdomen.

Management

Because of the late presentation, curative resection is not possible for most tumours. Of all patients with gastric carcinoma, around 20% will survive 5 years. Early diagnosis and resection of mucosa and submucosal tumours can be curative with around 75% 5-year survival, but few in the UK are identified early. Palliative chemotherapy can increase quality of life and survival in locally advanced or metastatic disease. A palliative resection with bypass may be feasible.

3.4 The small intestine

Learning objectives

You should be able to:
- discuss the interrelationship between the structure and the function of the small intestine, which is the key to the common symptoms
- describe the common disease processes affecting the small intestine and how these affect the normal structure and function.

Case Study

Sue has come back to the GI clinic for review. She is a 32-year-old woman who has not been feeling well for several months and has lost some weight. Investigations show that her haemoglobin is 101 g/l and her mean cell volume is 86 fl, but a blood film has been reported as showing a 'dimorphic' picture. Her total protein is 58 g/l and albumin is 29 g/l. Sue is keen to have an explanation for the results and to know what can be done for her.

Small intestinal disease should be considered in any person with one or more of:

- weight loss
- nutritional deficiencies
- abdominal pain
- diarrhoea including steatorrhoea.

Normal function

The prime functions of the small intestine are to break down and absorb nutrients. It also provides a barrier against noxious agents.

Motility

Peristaltic action (controlled by the innervation of the bowel and gut hormones) continues the mixing of food started by the stomach and moves the contents through the small bowel, allowing absorption along its length.

Disruption of peristalsis can lead to stasis (permitting bacterial overgrowth), ileus (e.g. postoperative) or colicky pain (e.g. obstruction). The prime innervation of the gut is through the parasympathetic system, and gut motility is affected by commonly used drugs. For example, tricyclic antidepressant drugs have an anticholinergic effect and cause troublesome constipation. You should ask about drugs in any patient with a disturbed bowel habit.

Secretion and breakdown

Coordinated with the movement of food through the small intestine is the secretion of bile, and of fluids from the pancreas and intestinal mucosa. The secreted fluids:

- Manipulate the pH through high bicarbonate concentration. Excess loss of small intestinal fluid (e.g. fistula) may cause a metabolic acidosis.
- Produce a semi-liquid to facilitate the digestive process. This means that a total of 8 litres has to be (re)absorbed by the small intestine every day; interference with this results in watery diarrhoea.
- Break down and absorb fat, by the action of lipase (pancreas) and by the formation of micelles (bile). Lipase deficiency may result in steatorrhoea.
- Digest protein through the action of proteolytic enzymes. Pancreatic disease may cause protein malnutrition.
- Break down carbohydrates through a combination of pancreatic amylase and oligo/disaccharidases.

Absorption

The small intestine has a very large surface area in contact with the bowel contents, which facilitates transport. The mucosa is folded and there are projections of villi, each of which is covered by microvilli. Within the core of the villi are capillaries and lymphatic channels. The absorptive columnar epithelial cells are formed at the base of the crypts and migrate to the top before being shed. The turn-over time is 3–4 days and this accounts for the sensitivity of the gut mucosa to antimitotic drugs or radiotherapy.

Absorption takes place through three mechanisms:

- passive diffusion, dependent on concentration gradients
- active transport, requiring a carrier protein and energy
- facilitated transport, requiring a specific mechanism but with no energy requirements.

Glucose absorption is linked to sodium transport into the intestinal lumen. There are specific transport systems for different classes of amino acid. Fat is more complicated, with breakdown into monoglycerides and fatty acids and incorporation with bile salts into micelles. The fat products are absorbed across the cell and, after re-esterification, triglycerides, cholesterol and phospholipids are incorporated into chylomicrons for transport in the lymph.

Other than the major nutrients, the small intestine absorbs water, fat-soluble vitamins, essential metals and trace elements. Calcium, iron and folic acid are absorbed in the duodenum and upper jejunum, while vitamin B_{12} and bile salts are absorbed in the terminal ileum. All other nutrients are absorbed throughout the length of the small intestine. Damage to the mucosa (e.g. coeliac disease) or reduction in length of the small intestine (e.g. surgical resection) may grossly impair the absorptive capacity of the gut and lead to global malnutrition or to particular deficiencies.

Defence

The intestinal mucosa forms a barrier to potential harm from a large range of different antigens. Lymphoid tissue is present throughout the small intestine (GALT: gut-associated lymphoid tissue) and is either scattered or aggregated (**Peyer's patches**). There are mechanisms whereby antigens can be recognised and lymphocytes either sensitised or activated. Secretory IgA is an important element in defence (p. 380).

Malabsorption

Coeliac disease

Coeliac disease is also known as gluten-sensitive enteropathy (a better description) and non-tropical sprue.

Aetiology and epidemiology

Coeliac disease is caused by sensitivity to the protein gluten, which is contained in wheat. Gluten is split into a number of peptides, of which α-gliadin is the main antigenic component.

Geographically, there is a wide variation in prevalence. An association with antigens HLA-B8 and DRW3 is seen. A bimodal age-related incidence exists, with peaks in young children and in the third and fourth decades of life, but people present at any age and coeliac disease should be considered in anyone with malabsorption, including elderly people. There is under-diagnosis of coeliac disease, so you should have a low threshold for serological screening.

Pathological features

The dominant problem is villous atropy. Alongside this, there is a thickening of the mucosa and a chronic inflammatory cell infiltrate with a predominance of T lymphocytes. The disease tends to be most severe in the proximal small bowel, less so in the terminal ileum.

Clinical presentation

The dominant features are simply those of malabsorption rather than any specific pointers to coeliac disease. You may find evidence of bowel problems (abdominal distension, diarrhoea) or nutritional deficiencies (weight loss, oedema, vitamin K and/or vitamin D deficiency). Most patients will have a general lassitude. There is an associa-

tion with a rare condition called **dermatitis herpetiformis**, which is an intensely pruritic, vesicular skin eruption. Treatment is with dapsone and a gluten-free diet.

Investigations

Nutritional status You should estimate the nutritional status of the patient through the **body mass index** (weight (kg)/height^2 (m^2)). The normal range is 18.5–25.

Immunology Patients suspected of having coeliac disease can be screened using measurement of endomysial antigliadin antibodies. These are highly sensitive markers (90% of untreated patients).

Haematology Most patients will have anaemia. Both folate and iron deficiency occur so the picture may be dimorphic, meaning that some red blood cells are microcytic and some are macrocytic. Vitamin B_{12} deficiency is less common, as the terminal ileum tends to be relatively spared.

Biochemistry The patient may have marked hypoproteinaemia and hypoalbuminaemia, as well as hypocalcaemia (vitamin D).

Tests of malabsorption Although many tests of malabsorption are described, they are difficult to perform with an acceptable degree of diagnostic accuracy and are not of great help in most patients with possible malabsorption.

Intestinal biopsy If coeliac disease is suspected, an intestinal biopsy should be arranged. Usually this is a distal duodenal biopsy obtained at gastroscopy (previously a jejunal biopsy was used). The characteristic features of villous atrophy will be seen, and, when the patient is put on a gluten-free diet, the changes will resolve.

Management

The main treatment is a gluten-free (wheat, rye and barley) diet. The dietitian will advise the patient on this, but you need to support the patient as the changes in lifestyle enforced by a strict diet may cause difficulties (Gluten is found in bread, biscuits, cakes, cereals, pasta, beer and many soups and sauces.) Gluten-free products can be obtained on prescription from a general practitioner. Around 70% of patients will respond to gluten exclusion. Often, young people will be reasonably well on a low-gluten rather than a gluten-free diet, but this increases the risk of lymphoma. Dietary supplements may be required in the initial stages of treatment to replenish stores. The disease activity should be monitored by general wellbeing, weight, basic haematology and biochemistry. The endomysial antibody test will usually become negative in a patient adhering to an exclusion diet.

There is a small risk of lymphoma, which is diminished by adherence to a gluten-free diet. The lymphoma can be difficult diagnose and treat.

Blind loop/bacterial overgrowth

Malabsorption caused by bacterial overgrowth occurs by an entirely different mechanism to coeliac disease. Normally, the upper small intestine is relatively sterile because of its high acidity. Bacterial counts increase through its length, with a faecal pattern in the terminal ileum. If structural integrity is disturbed or motility is impaired, bacteria can multiply. This occurs in:

- surgery: 'blind loops'
- multiple small bowel diverticula
- disturbed motility: autonomic neuropathy (diabetes), systemic sclerosis
- achlorhydria: colonisation of the upper small intestine
- small bowel fistulas.

The bacteria may cause some mucosal damage, but the main effects are in cleaving conjugated bile salts (interfering with fat absorption) and metabolising vitamin B_{12} and impairing its binding to intrinsic factor. Folate may be produced, so blood levels are usually normal.

From the above, you can predict that the main clinical features are:

- distension, flatulence
- steatorrhoea
- diarrhoea
- vitamin B_{12} deficiency (usually mild, no neurological features).

You should consider bacterial overgrowth in any patient with the above symptoms/signs who has a history suggestive of a predisposing factor.

Investigations

[^{14}C]-Glycocholate breath test [^{14}C]-labelled bile salts are given orally. Deconjugation by the bacteria releases [^{14}C]-glycine, which is measured through its breakdown into [^{14}C]-carbon dioxide in the small intestine. In healthy people, this occurs in the large intestine much later, so the important feature is the *timing* of the [^{14}C]-carbon dioxide peak (specificity 70% but lower sensitivity).

Hydrogen breath test Oral lactulose is degraded by the bacteria, releasing hydrogen. As with the [^{14}C]-bile salt test, breakdown occurs in healthy people, but in the large intestine. An early rise of hydrogen in the breath indicates production in the jejunum (specificity 80% but lower sensitivity).

Management

The first aim in management is to restore normal bowel function and motility. This may be very difficult to achieve and the mainstay of treatment is the use of antimicrobials such as metronidazole and tetracycline. Repeated courses may be needed.

Short bowel syndrome

Short bowel syndrome is simply a descriptive term implying that a considerable length of the small bowel has been lost and that the remainder is insufficient for digestion and absorption. The most common causes are surgical resection, e.g. in Crohn's disease, and bowel infarction. If the terminal ileum is resected, absorption of vitamin B_{12} is impaired together with the enterohepatic circulation of bile salts. Otherwise, the major problem is global malabsorption. Depending on the length of bowel lost, the person may manage with dietary adjustment and supplementation; otherwise parenteral nutrition is required, supervised by a specialist unit.

Tumours

Resected appendixes may contain small carcinoid tumours, which are derived from neuroendocrine cells. Much more rare is the **carcinoid syndrome**, which occurs with extensive liver metastases from an ileal carcinoid tumour. Large amounts of 5-HT are produced, together with other active substances. Common symptoms are flushing of the upper body, secretory diarrhoea, weight loss, wheezing (bronchospasm), tachycardia and fluctuating blood pressure. Fibrosis of the tricuspid and pulmonary valves may occur. Levels of urinary 5-hydroxyindole acetic acid (a breakdown product of 5-HT) are markedly raised. Imaging (CT, ultrasound) is important for assessing the extent of the disease. Some patients can have surgical resection; for many the treatment is palliative (e.g. 5-HT antagonists). Carcinoid tumours are part of a group of gastroenteropancreatic tumours which may have a genetic element (multiple endocrine neoplasia type 1 or 2). A careful family history is important, possibly with genetic testing.

Inflammatory bowel disease

Crohn's disease is discussed on page 131.

3.5 The large intestine

Case Study

Lawrence has had ulcerative colitis for about 10 years, since he was 31 years old. He has had a couple of bouts that have been severe and has been admitted for one of these. However, he has never felt 'his old self'. Over the last few weeks, things have been getting worse and he has been passing loose motions several times a day, mixed with blood and mucus. His general practitioner has sent him to the medical admissions unit for assessment and treatment.

Normal structure and function

The large bowel starts at the caecum and consists of ascending, transverse, descending and sigmoid sections leading into the rectum. There is an inner circular layer and an incomplete longitudinal layer of smooth muscle. The mucosa is flat, lacking crypts, and has a large number of goblet cells.

The blood supply is important when considering sites of ischaemia and possible resection. The superior mesenteric artery supplies the colon to the splenic flexure, and the inferior mesenteric artery supplies the descending colon and sigmoid section. The splenic flexure and the sigmoid are more vulnerable to ischaemic colitis (see below).

The prime action of the colon is to reduce the water content of the faeces from approximately 2 litres per day to 150 ml.

Normally the rectum is empty; passage of faeces into it produces the desire to defaecate. The internal sphincter and the puborectalis muscle relax, and the acute angle between the rectum and the anus decreases. Defaecation is produced by voluntary relaxation of the external sphincter and contraction of the abdominal muscles.

Diverticular disease

Diverticula are outpouchings of the colon through the muscle layer, usually at the point of entry of small arteries through the submucosa. The term **diverticulosis** implies no inflammation/infection, whereas **diverticulitis** implies their presence. It is probably better to talk about **diverticular disease**, unless there is definite evidence of an acute problem.

The diverticula are thought to be produced by the high intraluminal pressures forcing the mucosa through weaknesses in the bowel wall. They are more common in countries with a low-fibre diet.

The prevalence of diverticular disease increases with age, with most patients over the age of 70 years having diverticula on barium examination. The most common site is the sigmoid colon, but they occur throughout the large bowel.

In most people, diverticular disease is asymptomatic. Some patients experience bouts of constipation and diarrhoea, with left-sided abdominal pain. The differential diagnosis is with colonic carcinoma, which must be excluded.

Occasionally, patients present with an infected inflamed diverticulum (abscess). The patient is ill, with left iliac fossa pain and tenderness, together with fever and leucocytosis. The diverticulum may perforate, causing faeculent peritonitis, which has a high mortality. Sometimes a fistula is formed with the bladder or vagina.

In acute diverticulitis, blood cultures and an abdominal radiograph (for perforation) should be performed. The management is:

- Give i.v. broad-spectrum antibiotics. These should cover coliforms (e.g. cefotaxime) and *Bacteroides* spp. (metronidazole).
- Give i.v. fluids and pain relief.
- Inform the surgical team.

Sometimes, diverticular disease presents with rectal bleeding, which rarely leads to hypovolaemic shock. Mostly, the bleeding stops spontaneously and does not require surgical intervention.

The main management of uncomplicated diverticular disease is reassurance as to the absence of more serious disease and advice on a high-fibre diet.

Irritable bowel syndrome

Functional bowel disorders, including non-ulcer dyspepsia and irritable bowel syndrome (IBS), are very common. IBS is more common in women and occurs in around 10% of the population. There is no clear evidence as to the cause. In IBS, abnormal gut motility and sensitivity to distension may be present. Many patients also have considerable psychological morbidity.

Clinical presentation

In most patients, the history extends over many years. A significant number report recurrent abdominal pain in childhood. Enquire carefully about stresses and psychological disturbances. Many patients with IBS do not consult their doctor but those that do report more severe symptoms associated with psychological distress (anxiety, depression, sleep disturbance). Patients with IBS often have the somatic symptoms. The story is often one of being relatively symptom-free for long periods interspersed with bouts of symptoms. The abdominal pain varies in site, with the commonest site being in the left iliac fossa, but it can be periumbilical or in the right hypochondrium. Alternating constipation and diarrhoea are common, with tenesmus and feelings of incomplete emptying. Patients often complain of abdominal distension and bloating. The stools are often described as ribbon-like or pellet. Mucus may be passed. There are no abnormal findings on examination other than some tenderness.

Investigations

You should resist ordering a series of investigations in patients whom you strongly suspect of having a functional bowel disorder. There is no consistent evidence of disturbed gut motility. Investigate those patients where there are other important features, such as recent foreign travel or:

- onset of symptoms over the age of 40 years
- recent change in symptoms
- other symptoms not usually associated with IBS, such as rectal bleeding or weight loss.

Management

Management of IBS is difficult, with symptoms persisting over many years. The approach should be with a positive diagnosis, an explanation of the symptoms and reassurance about the prognosis. You should remember that many patients will respond to a placebo. You should be aware of psychological problems and treat depression. The mainstay of therapy has been a high-fibre diet, but many patients are made worse with the addition of wheat bran, whilst only a minority improve. The use of antispasmodics such as mebeverine or peppermint oil may help, as can antidepressants.

Tumours

Benign tumours (polyps)

Polyps are very common in developed countries. There are different types.

- *Metaplastic polyps* are small and associated with regeneration; they have no malignant potential.
- *Hamartomatous polyps* are developmental abnormalities. They are seen in the rare **Peutz–Jeghers syndrome** (autosomal dominant inheritance). There is oral mucocutaneous pigmentation and extensive hamartomas in the small and, to some extent, the large bowel. No malignant potential.
- *Adenoma* has malignant potential developing over several years.

The malignant potential of adenomas rises with increasing size (about 10% chance of containing cancer if >1.5 cm), and it is likely that most colonic carcinomas originate in polyps. Adenomas come in different forms: tubular or villous. The latter occasionally are associated with diarrhoea and loss of potassium. Rarely, multiple adenomas are seen, in familial **polyposis coli** (autosomal dominant) and genetic studies may show mutations in the *adenomatosis polyposis coli* (APC) gene.

Most polyps are asymptomatic and only come to light because of a barium enema, sigmoidoscopy or colonoscopy carried out for a different reason. Some large polyps may bleed and can cause a chronic iron deficiency anaemia.

Management

Once identified, all polyps should be removed and sent for histological analysis. Removal can usually be achieved by snaring or diathermy via a colonoscope. Further polyp development is common and repeated surveillance is necessary (usually at 3-year intervals). The management of polyposis coli is pancolectomy with ileoanal anastomosis.

Malignant tumours

Aetiology and epidemiology

Adenocarcinoma of the rectum/colon is the second commonest cause of cancer death in the UK. It is associated with inflammatory bowel disease, adenomas and polyposis coli (rare). It is thought to be linked to a diet high in animal fat, together with low vegetable fibre.

There is a genetic predisposition. The *p53* gene is considered to be central to the development of many tumours. Its role is to prevent *entry* into the S phase of cell replication (DNA replication) until the genetic material has been checked and repaired. If this is abnormal, then the *p53* gene permits the duplication of cells with abnormal genotypes. Very rare syndromes, such as Li–Fraumeni, lead to early development of a wide range of cancers. Much more common is somatic mutation, which is similarly associated with a range of tumours, including colonic carcinoma. Screening programmes for affected families are now in operation, including the *APC* tumour suppressor gene. Mutations of p53 protein and allelic loss of chromosome 18q are both associated with a poor prognosis.

Pathology and staging

Most tumours are adenocarcinomas and can be annular (apple core), ulcerative or polypoid (cauliflower) in appearance. The majority are located in the rectum or sigmoid colon. Histological staging according to the **Duke's classification** is important for predicting survival.

- Stage A: involves mucosa or submucosa only; 95% 5-year survival
- Stage B: tumour has penetrated muscle; >70% 5-year survival
- Stage C: lymph node involvement; <60% 5-year survival
- Stage D: distant metastases (including liver); few 5-year survivors.

Clinical presentation

You should consider colonic carcinoma in any person presenting over the age of 40 years with recent onset of symptoms referable to the large bowel. Change in bowel habit is a common symptom, or rectal bleeding with left-sided tumours. Caecal carcinomas are often asymptomatic until late in the disease and may present with an iron deficiency anaemia. Occasionally, patients with colonic carcinoma present with a constant pain resulting from anal or sacral invasion; some have colicky pain because of bowel obstruction. If the tumour erodes into the vagina or bladder, then faecal material or gas may be passed per urethra or vagina. In advanced disease, the presentation may be cachexia, hepatomegaly or ascites.

In any patient suspected of having large bowel pathology, you must at least perform a rectal examination and arrange a sigmoidoscopy (preferably flexible). A colonoscopy with adequate bowel preparation will also probably be required.

Investigations

On routine blood tests, patients may have an iron deficiency anaemia and, in those with hepatic metastases, alkaline phosphatase may be elevated. Your main aims of investigation are to image the large bowel adequately and, where necessary, obtain a tissue diagnosis. Other than an examination of the rectosigmoid bowel as indicated above, the first investigation is usually a colonoscopy to visualise and biopsy lesions and to remove polyps. An alternative is a double-contrast barium enema with careful bowel preparation, but this does not allow for tissue diagnosis. In frail elderly patients, a CT scan can exclude a colonic carcinoma with reasonable certainty. CT scanning is also used in staging prior to surgery to detect lymph node, liver and more distant (e.g. lung) metastases. It is also used in follow-up of patients following surgery and chemotherapy.

Management

The principal management is surgical resection, with preservation of the anus if possible. Sometimes, this is not feasible and a permanent colostomy is fashioned. Survival is related to Duke's staging. Where resection is not possible, a defunctioning colostomy may be indicated. Laser therapy can help in debulking large tumours and preventing/relieving obstruction. Preoperative radiotherapy is now used in the management of rectal carcinoma.

Adjuvant or palliative combination chemotherapy (including 5-fluorouracil) prolongs survival and improves quality of life.

Inflammatory bowel disease

Chronic inflammatory bowel disease can be divided into:

- Crohn's disease, which affects the GI tract anywhere from mouth to anus
- ulcerative colitis, which is confined to the large bowel.

Both are much more common in developed countries and have a peak incidence in young adult life (10–40 years), but they can occur at any age (15% >60 years).

There are many theories about the causation of both conditions, but nothing has been proven. Environmental factors appear important and disease may be an unusual (immune) response to an infectious agent or some other trigger. Smoking increases the risk of Crohn's disease, but decreases that of ulcerative colitis. Genetic factors contribute but there is no single Mendelian inheritance.

Pathology

The two diseases are contrasted in Table 28. Crohn's disease characteristically 'skips' lengths of bowel and is patchy. It may be defined by pattern (e.g. stricture) or location (e.g. ileal, colonic). It has a particular tendency to involve the terminal ileum. Ulcerative colitis affects the rectum (distal colitis), spreading up the colon (pancolitis).

Crohn's disease affects all the layers of the bowel, producing thickening and matting. There are deep fissures and ulcers in the mucosa: 'cobblestone' appearance. Aphthous ulceration is an early feature. An increase in inflammatory cells and lymphoid hyperplasia are usual and most patients have non-caseating granulomas.

Ulcerative colitis remains confined to the mucosa and submucosa, which is reddened and bleeds readily. There is widespread ulceration with preservation of adjacent mucosa, which has the appearance of polyps (pseudopolyps). In the lamina propria, an inflammatory cell infiltrate is found. Crypt abscesses and goblet cell depletion are usual.

Clinical presentation

The main symptoms are gastrointestinal. Non-GI manifestations are given in Table 29.

Crohn's disease

The main symptoms of Crohn's disease are heterogeneous but include:

- diarrhoea
- abdominal pain
- constitutional disturbance: weight loss.

The symptoms depend on the parts of the bowel affected. Some patients present with acute disease and others with a chronic problem. For example, anal disease may be the problem, with swelling, skin tags, fistulae or perianal abscesses.

Table 28 Histopathological comparison between ulcerative colitis and Crohn's disease

Histological feature	Ulcerative colitis	Crohn's disease
Inflammatory process	Superficial, continuous	Transmural, skip lesions/patchy
Granulomas	Infrequent	Majority
Crypt abscesses	Frequent	Some
Goblet cells	Depleted	Preserved

Table 29 Non-GI complications of inflammatory bowel disease, together with their relative frequency and response to bowel therapy

System	Complication	Crohn's disease	Ulcerative colitis	Response to bowel therapy
Eyes	Uveitis	+	+	Yes
	Episcleritis	+	+	Yes
	Conjunctivitis	+	+	Yes
Skin	Erythema nodosum	++	+	Yes
	Pyoderma gangrenosum	+	+	Yes
Liver	Fatty infiltration	++	++	No
	Pericholangitis	++	++	No
	Sclerosing cholangitis	+	+++	No
	Cirrhosis	+	++	No
Locomotor	Sacroiliitis	+	+	No
	Ankylosing spondylitis	+	+	No
	Peripheral arthropathy	+	+	Yes

Significant active disease is indicated by:

- weight loss
- general malaise
- loss of appetite
- low-grade fever.

The abdominal pain is variable but is often colicky. Most patients have diarrhoea and, in colonic disease, this may contain blood. A significant proportion of patients simply have constitutional upset. Others may present with acute right iliac fossa pain, suggestive of appendicitis.

On examination, apart from extra-GI complications (see below) and low weight (always have patients weighed), very few signs may be present. In the mouth, aphthous ulcers may be seen. There may be some discomfort on abdominal palpation and, occasionally, there is a right iliac fossa mass or fistulae. You must always examine the anal region.

Ulcerative colitis

In almost all patients, the dominant symptom is diarrhoea mixed with blood and mucus. In acute, severe disease, there is usually constitutional upset. In some patients, the disease is limited to a proctitis with diarrhoea, urgency and tenesmus. The frequency of defaecation, both night and day, can be very debilitating and socially very difficult.

The severity of an acute attack can be assessed by:

- constitutional upset
- stool frequency
- fever and tachycardia
- hypoalbuminaemia, anaemia and high erythrocyte sedimentation rate (ESR).

A severe attack requires admission to hospital, particularly if it has not responded to oral and topical therapy, given the potential development of toxic dilatation of the colon.

There are few signs in ulcerative colitis. Patients may have some abdominal distension or be tender to palpation. Rectal examination will show blood and mucus. Table 29 lists non-GI complications.

Investigations

The diseases can be distinguished clinically and radiologically to some extent, but histological differences seen on biopsy are important. In some cases, the conditions cannot be separated.

Blood tests

Using simple blood indices, a measure of disease activity and response to therapy can be achieved. In acute exacerbations, the ESR, plasma viscosity, C-reactive protein (CRP) and other acute-phase reactants (e.g. ferritin) are raised.

Patients may have a normochromic normocytic anaemia, though iron and folate deficiencies should be identified and treated. Although Crohn's disease commonly affects the terminal ileum and vitamin B_{12} levels are low, a megaloblastic anaemia is unusual.

Hypoalbuminaemia is common in severe disease. Abnormalities of liver enzymes should alert you to the presence of hepatobiliary involvement.

Imaging

Your aims are to:

- diagnose inflammatory bowel disease
- distinguish Crohn's from ulcerative colitis
- estimate the extent of the bowel involvement.

A plain abdominal radiograph may show fluid levels suggestive of bowel obstruction or a right iliac fossa mass in Crohn's disease or colonic dilatation (toxic) in ulcerative colitis. A small bowel enema is useful in Crohn's disease, demonstrating strictures, proximal bowel dilatation, 'rose-thorn' ulcers and fistulae. The extent of colonic disease is assessed by a colonoscopy or possibly barium enema (less useful). In Crohn's disease, it will again show deep ulcers and skip areas. In ulcerative colitis, there are loss of haustrations, dilatation and superficial ulceration. The disease is contiguous from the anus. In longstanding disease, the colon is narrow and shortened ('pipestem'). Contrast media can be used to delineate the tract fistulae (Crohn's disease). Ultrasound, CT or MR scanning may be helpful in showing matted bowel, thickened wall, abscesses, hepatobiliary disease or perineal involvement.

Endoscopy (including colonoscopy) allows visualisation and biopsy of the abnormal bowel, particularly of any possibly malignant areas.

Other investigations

Stool cultures and microscopy should always be performed if the patient has diarrhoea. The major differential diagnoses of ulcerative colitis are amoebic and bacillary dysentery. Administration of steroids can be disastrous in these patients. Breath tests can be useful in those patients in whom bacterial overgrowth is suspected because of the damaged small bowel. In patients with possible liver disease, endoscopic retrograde cholangiopancreatography (ERCP) and liver biopsy may be helpful. Magnetic resonance cholangiopancreatography (MRCP) is now available.

Management

You need to know about the drugs used in inflammatory bowel disease and have a grasp of the general approach to management, including the use of surgery. It is very important to spend time explaining the disease to patients so that they can participate in decisions about treatment. Some patients derive benefit from contact with support groups such as the National Association for Colitis and Crohn's Disease. (You should also remember this type of resource when dealing with other illnesses, e.g. Parkinson's Disease Society or Coeliac Society.) Optimum care for patients with inflammatory bowel disease is achieved by teams of doctors, specialist nurses and other key people such as nutritionists.

5-Aminosalicylic acid drugs

The various preparations of 5-aminosalicylic acid are effective in inducing remission in inflammatory bowel disease and in preventing relapse in ulcerative colitis (but not Crohn's disease). Commonly, this was prescribed as sulfasalazine, which was broken down into sulfapyridine and 5-aminosalicylic acid in the large intestine through cleavage of the azo bond. Newer preparations, which are equally effective as sulfasalazine but better tolerated, include:

- mesalazine: enteric-coated tablets with a resin coating that is pH-dependent and releases 5-aminosalicylic acid in the ileum and colon
- slow-release mesalazine (Pentasa): releases 5-aminosalicylic acid more proximally in the gut; useful in small bowel disease
- olsalazine: two molecules of 5-aminosalicylic acid bound by an azo bond that is cleaved by intestinal bacteria
- balsalazide: colonic release preparation that has an azo bond; probably more effective and better tolerated than mesalazine.

The main side-effects are headache, nausea, diarrhoea or blood dyscrasias (particularly agranulocytosis). Interstitial nephritis rarely occurs, so renal function should be monitored. Overall, about 10% of patients cannot tolerate 5-aminosalicylic acid preparations.

Corticosteroids

Corticosteroids are of major benefit in inflammatory bowel disease but have long-term side-effects, such as osteoporosis, skin atrophy and cataracts. Corticosteroids can be used orally, or as enemas when the disease is localised to the rectum and sigmoid colon. Budesonide is a steroid with high topical potency. It causes less adrenocortical suppression and other steroid-induced side-effects than prednisolone because of poor absorption and rapid first-pass metabolism. It is used orally for ileo-caecal Crohn's disease or as an enema for either Crohn's disease or ulcerative colitis. The main role of corticosteroids is in moderate to severe relapse in both Crohn's disease and ulcerative colitis. Steroids do not have a role in maintenance therapy.

Immunosuppression

For patients refractory to, or dependent on, corticosteroids, azathioprine is useful but requires regular monitoring for bone marrow suppression. Its role is in both active disease and maintenance of remission. Ciclosporin is useful in inducing remission in severe ulcerative colitis. Methotrexate has some effect in Crohn's disease but not ulcerative colitis.

Other drugs

Metronidazole Some patients with Crohn's disease are helped by metronidazole either on its own or in combination with ciprofloxacin.

Infliximab This is a mouse:human chimeric antibody against tumour necrosis factor. Given by infusion, it can be used to induce remission in refractory cases of Crohn's disease. It can also be useful in patients with fistulae.

Surgery

Surgery has an important role in the management of inflammatory bowel disease. Most patients with Crohn's disease will require bowel resection at some stage. For ulcerative colitis, a panproctocolectomy with an ileostomy is curative.

For Crohn's disease, the main indications for surgery are:

- failure of medical therapy, with severe ill-health
- persistent bowel obstruction or enteric fistulae
- acute perforation/appendicitis
- chronic perirectal infection
- failure to grow in adolescence
- development of malignancy

Given the high probability of recurrence in Crohn's disease, the surgery undertaken should always be the minimum required.

For ulcerative colitis, surgery should be considered in:

- severe colitis that is not controlled by intensive medical therapy
- acute megacolon, perforation or life-threatening bleeding
- unacceptable side-effects from therapy
- those with high risk for the development of carcinoma; longstanding (>10 years) extensive disease with dysplasia.

Approach to the management of Crohn's disease

You should have some understanding as to how to use the different therapies in Crohn's disease. In acute ileitis, steroids will usually induce a remission. For colitis, these are combined with a 5-aminosalicylic acid preparation. There are *no* proven therapies for maintaining remission.

The bowel complications of Crohn's disease may need specific treatment. Metronidazole may help with fistulae or perianal disease, but some require surgical intervention. Broad-spectrum antibiotics are used in proven bacterial overgrowth.

After bowel resection, or in severe ileitis, the diarrhoea caused by colonic irritation by bile salts can be helped by colestyramine. Extensive bowel resection may require nutritional supplements, including medium-chain triglycerides and parenteral vitamins (fat-soluble: A, D, E, K and B_{12}). Ultimately, a short bowel syndrome may result, necessitating total parenteral nutrition.

Approach to the management of ulcerative colitis

In an acute attack, fluid balance must be maintained and the nutritional state monitored; steroids are prescribed. High-dose oral (i.v. in severe attacks) prednisolone and rectal steroids are used. Mild attacks may be helped by a 5-aminosalicylic acid preparation. You should be alert to the incipient development of perforation or toxic dilatation, which will require surgical intervention.

Maintenance therapy is with a 5-aminosalicylic acid preparation. Steroids are not used.

Prognosis

Crohn's disease

Most patients with Crohn's disease will run a relapsing and remitting course and will require surgery at some stage.

Ulcerative colitis

In patients with localised sigmoproctitis, the prognosis is good, with most going on to long-term remission. In fulminant pancolitis, there is a significant mortality and aggressive therapy is required. A minority of patients will require a colectomy.

In ulcerative colitis, extensive disease over several years (>10 years) is a risk factor for the development of malignancy. Furthermore, there is a higher risk of malignancy with Crohn's colitis than indicated by previous estimates. Regular screening by colonoscopy for malignancy in *longstanding inflammatory colitis* should be advised.

Other inflammatory bowel disease

Non-specific colitis

In some patients, a local sigmoproctitis develops with troublesome diarrhoea. Sigmoidoscopic appearance is non-specific, as is biopsy. An infective cause should always be excluded. Treatment is by steroid enemas.

Ischaemic colitis

In elderly people, colonic ischaemia can occur, particularly around the splenic flexure and the descending colon. The main features are bloody diarrhoea and abdominal pain. A barium enema classically will show 'thumb printing' — indentations of the bowel wall. However, radiological appearances are often non-specific. The preferred investigation is CT scanning. In most patients, the symptoms may resolve spontaneously though they can progress to perforation or a subsequent stricture formation. Management usually consists of maintaining fluid balance and prescribing analgesics.

Radiation colitis

Radiation damage can occur secondarily to therapy directed towards a pelvic tumour. In the acute phase, the patient experiences bloody diarrhoea, tenesmus and abdominal pain. The proctitis can be treated with local steroids. In the late phase, the proctitis may remain troublesome, with bleeding, ulceration and stricture formation.

Bleeding from the lower GI tract

Bleeding from the lower GI tract can be divided into:

- occult: major causes are caecal carcinoma and angiodysplasia (arteriovenous malformations which can be visualised on colonoscopy; this is a relatively common cause of iron deficiency anaemia in elderly people)
- blood mixed with stool: left-sided colonic tumour, inflammatory bowel disease, diverticular disease, infective colitis and angiodysplasia
- fresh blood in small amounts: haemorrhoids, anal fissure, Crohn's disease of the anus, carcinoma of the rectum or anus
- severe bleeding (rare): diverticular disease and ischaemic colitis.

You can usually narrow the possible diagnoses by a careful history and examination. For example, carcinoma of the colon is extremely rare under the age of 40 years.

The management of chronic iron deficiency anaemia is considered on page 268. Faecal occult blood testing is of very limited benefit in reaching a diagnosis.

3.6 Food poisoning and intestinal infection

Learning objectives

You should be able to:
- distinguish clinically between predominantly vomiting and predominantly diarrhoeal illnesses and state the significance of the distinction
- discuss the many causes of vomiting other than food poisoning
- construct an aetiological differential diagnosis for diarrhoea so as to be able to manage the patient appropriately
- describe rehydration management.

Case Study

Nausea, abdominal cramping and vomiting (× 2) preceded diarrhoea in this 29-year-old school teacher. She describes an onset overnight, without fever but 'feeling terrible'. Episodes of watery diarrhoea, without blood, occurred six times today, but this has tailed off towards evening. She reports no foreign travel.

Food poisoning is defined as any disease of an infectious or toxic nature proven or likely to be caused by consumption of food or water. Food poisoning is extremely common, with over 75 000 cases notified annually in the UK. About 10% are acquired abroad. Poor food handling is the reason for most cases. Outbreaks (two or more people) are common.

The clinical presentation can be divided into two groups: predominantly vomiting and predominantly diarrhoea. There is some overlap between the two.

Fever, nausea and vomiting may be the initial features, even though the illness transforms into diarrhoea over the next day or two. Consequently, you need to follow the course of the illness over about 24 hours before deciding that the predominant symptom is vomiting. It is exceptionally rare for vomiting to be the predominant symptom of an intestinal infection for more than 48 hours.

Vomiting illnesses

There are many causes of vomiting (p. 118). However, food poisoning is the most common in previously well people, the major causes of which are (with little or no diarrhoea):

- small round structured viruses (SRSVs) including calicivirus, rotavirus and noroviruses (Norwalk viruses)
- *Bacillus cereus* toxin
- *Staphylococcus aureus* toxin.

The toxins are produced in food and it is these, rather than the bacteria, that cause vomiting. In most diarrhoeal diseases, the causative bacteria reproduce in the GI tract, but in *B. cereus* and *Staph. aureus* food poisoning, bacterial reproduction in the gut is irrelevant.

Clinical presentation

The patient is often doubled over the toilet repeatedly vomiting or lying prostrate in bed. Upper abdominal cramping is severe. Fever is usually absent or low-grade. The abdomen is soft and, apart from a sinus tachycardia, there are usually no abnormal signs. Occasionally, patients will have one or two loose stools, especially if infection is caused by an SRSV.

Investigations

The most useful investigation is to send the implicated food (if not all consumed), along with some vomitus and diarrhoea, to the laboratory for toxin and viral analyses. Stool cultures should also be done.

Management

You should admit the patient to hospital for i.v. fluids if the vomiting is severe, diagnosis is unclear (possible surgical abdomen, etc.) or the patient is diabetic. Otherwise, the patient should be encouraged to drink small volumes of fluids frequently, such as oral rehydration fluid, thin soups and water. You should review the patient again after 12–24 hours if the episode has not resolved.

Diarrhoeal illnesses

There are many causes of infectious and non-infectious diarrhoea. The challenge is to distinguish one from another, for three primary reasons:

- correct management of the patient
- protection of other patients or family
- public health reasons.

Aetiology

Some diarrhoeal diseases are clinically distinguishable, such as haemorrhagic colitis and cholera. Others are sometimes characteristic, such as giardiasis, amoebic dysentery and *Campylobacter* enteritis. The travel or antibiotic history may be the clue to the diagnosis. PPIs and H_2 receptor antagonists increase the risk of intestinal infections.

Toxins

Both *B. cereus* and *Clostridium perfringens* produce toxins that cause self-limited diarrhoea for up to 24 hours. The former is often found in cooked, stored rice and the latter in contaminated meat.

Salmonella *spp.*

Infection is usually community-acquired, about 10% of cases are contracted abroad and some institutional outbreaks have been reported. Salmonellosis has a short incubation period (12–48 hours). Clinically it is not easily distinguishable from *Shigella* or *Campylobacter* infections. It is invasive and often fatal in elderly people and patients with acquired immunodeficiency syndrome (AIDS). It is difficult to eradicate carriage in some people. Carriers are occasionally a source of infection in the community.

Shigella *spp.*

S. sonnei infection is common in the UK. The other three species (*S. dysenteriae*, *S. flexneri* and *S. boydii*) are usually imported. The organism can survive on door and toilet flush handles and is commonly transmitted by children in school or by flies. Excretion in stools is shortened by antibiotic therapy.

Campylobacter *spp.*

Infection is common and is often associated with poultry and milk products; infection with *Campylobacter* has a long incubation period (2–5 days). It causes more abdominal pain than other causes of intestinal infection. It is invasive in hypogammaglobulinaemic and AIDS patients.

Traveller's diarrhoea

Often referred to colloquially as 'Delhi belly' or 'Montezuma's revenge', traveller's diarrhoea is common in visitors to the developing world. It is often attributable to enteropathogenic and other *Escherichia coli* isolates. Patients usually have watery, non-bloody diarrhoea without fever; if they have either bloody diarrhoea or fever, an invasive infection (such as *Salmonella*) is more probable. Usually traveller's diarrhoea is self-limiting over 1–5 days. Careful selection of food and drink substantially reduces the risk.

Haemorrhagic colitis

Haemorrhagic colitis is caused by the same toxin-producing *E. coli* as is haemolytic uraemic syndrome (*E. coli* O157). It is characterised by sudden onset and extremely bloody diarrhoea, without fever. Person-to-person spread is well documented. Mortality rates are high in elderly people (40%).

Clostridium difficile

Cl. difficile causes a severe form of antibiotic-associated diarrhoea. At its worst, a necrotic membrane overlies the colonic mucosa (pseudomembranous colitis). *Clostridium* spores are acquired from other patients. During or after antibiotic therapy, spores germinate in the gut, producing *Cl. difficile* toxin. The toxin causes a non-bloody, watery diarrhoea in which millions of spore-forming bacteria are found. Patients may be mildly ill or extremely ill and toxic. Ileus and toxic dilatation of the colon are occasionally seen. Isolation of patients, together with restriction of antibiotic prescribing, are the keys to controlling an outbreak.

Cholera

Caused by *Vibrio cholerae*, cholera is a rare imported cause of severe watery diarrhoea that can lead to hypovolaemic shock in 12 hours. Fluid requirement in the first 24 hours is typically 30–40 litres. Special cultures are required in the laboratory for identification.

Viral diarrhoea

Rotavirus infection occasionally affects adults. Stools do not contain blood or white cells. The viruses are spread by fomites (e.g. inanimate objects such as toys or door handles). Other viruses are sometimes implicated.

Entamoeba histolytica

E. histolytica causes several infectious syndromes including asymptomatic cyst passage, acute amoebic dysentery, chronic non-dysenteric colitis, amoeboma and amoebic liver abscess (p. 141). The first two are most common. In amoebic dysentery, blood, mucus and white cells are passed in the stool by a patient who is otherwise not particularly ill. As it may be relatively chronic, it can be mistaken for ulcerative colitis, with serious consequences if corticosteroids are given. There is an antibody test for amoebiasis. Treatment with metronidazole followed by diloxanide furoate is curative.

Giardia lamblia

G. lamblia is a protozoan that is usually acquired abroad, occasionally in the UK. The typical patient complains of 3–5 bulky stools a day, pale in colour with much griping abdominal pain and wind. They may lose weight. Symptoms fluctuate. The cysts appear in the stool intermittently, making diagnosis difficult; empirical therapy with metronidazole is warranted. There is a 10% relapse rate.

Other protozoa

Several other protozoa cause diarrhoea, which is usually acute in onset but may become chronic. Almost all patients have a travel history, except those with *Cryptosporidium* diarrhoea, which is often acquired in the UK. Treatment differs depending on the protozoan.

Clinical presentation

The spectrum of illness in infectious diarrhoea ranges from the trivial 'upset stomach' with a few loose stools over 1–3 days to the life-threatening. You must distinguish the illest patients from the rest, which can be difficult, particularly in elderly people, who have a higher mortality. You may need to see and examine the patient repeatedly to decide the best course of action.

History

You will find it helpful to consider the following features to arrive at an early presumptive diagnosis (Table 30).

1. Has the patient been abroad? If so, consider traveller's diarrhoea, amoebic and *Shigella* dysentery and other protozoal causes (e.g. *Giardia, Cyclospora*, etc.).
2. Has the patient been in hospital or a nursing home recently? If so, consider *Cl. difficile* or *Salmonella*.
3. Is the patient receiving antibiotics or have they just finished a course? If so, consider *Cl. difficile*.
4. Is the diarrhoea frankly bloody? If so, consider haemorrhagic colitis, *Shigella* or amoebic dysentery, or ulcerative colitis.
5. Is there some blood in the stool? If so, consider *Salmonella, Campylobacter* and *Shigella* infection and inflammatory bowel disease.
6. Is there any blood in the stool? If not, consider traveller's diarrhoea, cholera, *Cl. difficile*, and viral and protozoal causes.
7. Has the diarrhoeal episode been continuing for more than a week? If so, consider non-infectious causes, giardiasis and other protozoa, *Salmonella* infection and immunodeficiency (e.g. AIDS).

Some infectious diarrhoeal illnesses are related to specific exposures. For example, *Crytosporidium* diarrhoea is more frequently associated with visits to farms, haemorrhagic colitis with beef products, especially beefburgers,

and *Campylobacter* infection with poultry. However, only in the context of an outbreak is it usually possible to ascertain the food or other source reliably.

Pain

Abdominal pain and tenesmus are particularly related to large bowel involvement and are found in *Campylobacter, Salmonella* and *Shigella* infections. Grumbling mild abdominal pain and chronic diarrhoea is typical of giardiasis.

Physical signs

Signs of sodium and water depletion are described on page 194. Common physical signs in acute infectious diarrhoea vary with the organism and the patient:

- Fever is typical of *Salmonella, Shigella, Campylobacter* and *Cl. difficile* infection (Table 30)
- Dehydration (sodium and water depletion) is common if the diarrhoea is severe (e.g. >10 stools daily) and particularly if associated with vomiting; elderly people are especially prone.
- Abdominal distension may be mild but if marked could indicate dilatation of the colon. This is seen particularly in *Salmonella, Campylobacter* and *Cl. difficile* infections.

Occasionally, patients are extremely unwell with features of sepsis (e.g. fever, tachycardia, renal impairment) and diarrhoea. They usually have invasive *Salmonella* infections caused by the more virulent species, such as *S. cholerasuis* or *S. dublin*. Such patients often develop acute renal failure and shock, and may die within 3 or 4 days of first symptoms.

Investigations

Stools should be sent to the laboratory in all cases for (standard) culture, which will yield evidence of infection with *Salmonella, Shigella* or *Campylobacter* spp.

- If the stool is bloody, culture for *E. coli* O157.
- If *Cl. difficile* is a possible diagnosis, request *Cl. difficile* toxin estimation.
- If a viral diarrhoea is possible (no blood, other members of family affected), request virology.
- If the stool is not bloody, request ova, cysts and parasites, particularly if the patient has been abroad.
- If the stool is bloody and the patient has been abroad, then request a 'hot stool', meaning direct observation of the stool for amoebae, together with standard and *E. coli* cultures.

The white cell count may be elevated in bacterial diarrhoea. Urea, creatinine and electrolytes should be measured in all patients admitted to hospital, to guide intravenous therapy. Stool white cells are helpful in presumptive diagnosis (Table 30). A blood culture is essential in all patients admitted to hospital with diarrhoea, even if afebrile. Abdominal radiographs are not useful unless the abdomen is distended and an alternative (surgical) diagnosis or constipation with overflow is likely.

If stool cultures are negative and diarrhoea continues, sigmoidoscopy and rectal biopsy are indicated to diagnose inflammatory bowel disease (p. 132).

Table 30 Distinguishing characteristics of the causes of acute intestinal infection

	Salmonella	*Shigella*	*Campylobacter*	Traveller's diarrhoea	Haemorrhagic colitis	*Clostridium difficile*	Viral infection including rotavirus	*Entamoeba histolytica*	Other protozoa*
Blood in stools	-/+	-/++	-/+	-	+++	-	-	++	-
Abdominal pain	++	+	+++	+	+	+	-	+	+/++
Tenesmus	++	++	++/+++	-	++	+	-	++	-
Fever	++	++	+++	-/+	-	++	-/++	+	-/+
Vomiting	++	++	++	+	+	++	+++	+	+
Acquired in UK	++	++	++	+	++	++	++	-	+/++
White cells in stool	++	+++	++	+	+	+++	-	-/+	-
Incubation periods	12–48-hr	12–48 hr	2–5 days		3–9 days	N/A		5–14 days	
Requires antibiotic treatment	S	S	S	N	N	Y	N	Y	S

Y, yes; N, no; S, sometimes, depending on condition of patient and/or infecting species; N/A, not applicable.
* *Giardia lamblia, Cryptosporidium parvum, Cyclospora* spp, *Isospora belli* and *Blastocystis hominis.*

Three

Management

All patients admitted to hospital with diarrhoea must be placed in a single room. The local infectious disease unit should be involved, especially for very ill patients and those from abroad, as the diagnostic capabilities of their laboratories are often better tailored to tropical problems and they have much clinical expertise in this area.

Fluid replacement

Dehydrated patients require sodium and water replacement (usually 3–4 litres daily) with either oral or i.v. rehydration solution. Potassium depletion is common and requires replacement. In the acute phase, patients should avoid milk products because of temporary lactase deficiency.

Antidiarrhoeal remedies

These are relatively ineffective and sometimes dangerous. Loperamide is the best but should be used *only* in patients with traveller's diarrhoea who have no systemic features of illness (e.g. no fever or vomiting) and only for 1–2 days. Loperamide should *not* be prescribed for children, elderly people, or anyone with either bloody diarrhoea, or a possible alternative diagnosis or moderate to severe diarrhoea (e.g. >six stools daily), as it may lead to toxic dilatation of the colon.

Antimicrobial therapy

Antibiotics are necessary for certain patients only. Table 31 indicates which are the preferred agents for which pathogen. Until the pathogen is known, the following groups require empiric antimicrobial therapy, usually with oral or intravenous quinolones (e.g. ciprofloxacin):

- immunocompromised patients
- very ill patients (high fever, frequent stools (e.g. >10–20 per day), severe dehydration, renal impairment, etc.)
- patients over 60 years of age.

Overall, quinolones shorten diarrhoea by 24 hours. However, in patients with *Salmonella* infection, their use may not prevent longer-term carriage.

Prevention

At home, thorough cooking of all meat and eggs, handwashing after defaecation and before food preparation, and separation (in the refrigerator) of cooked and uncooked meats are all preventative. Anti-ulcer medications increase risk. In hospital, minimisation of antibiotic usage both in number and duration, is important. Abroad (tropical environments), the points listed above plus avoidance of all uncooked or unpeeled food, mayonnaise and ice, with fastidious attention to sterilised or filtered water, are helpful.

Notification

All patients with food poisoning and/or infectious diarrhoea must be notified to the public health authorities even if the cause of the episode is not identified.

3.7 The liver

Table 31 Antimicrobial treatment for intestinal infection

Organism/syndrome	Patients that should be treated	Preferred antibiotic
Salmonella or *Campylobacter* spp.	Immunocompromised, extremes of age	Ciprofloxacin
Shigella spp.	All symptomatic	Ciprofloxacin, co-trimoxazole
Escherichia coli O157	None, increased morbidity and mortality	–
Traveller's diarrhoea	If desired and therapy available	Ciprofloxacin, loperamide
Clostridium difficile	All symptomatic	Metronidazole (p.o./i.v.), vancomycin (p.o.)
Cholera	All	Tetracycline, ciprofloxacin
Entamoeba histolytica	All	Metronidazole then diloxanide furoate
Giardia lamblia	All	Metronidazole, tinidazole
Cryptosporidium parvum	AIDS patients	Experimental

Case Study

An unkempt 27-year-old is referred for hepatitis C treatment. His antibody test is positive, as is his anti-HBc. His HIV antibody test is negative, as is his HBsAg. He is living with his girlfriend and they are not using contraception.

Normal anatomy and function

The liver lies immediately underneath the right diaphragm, with the left lobe of the liver lying under-neath the heart and left diaphragm.

The liver has a dual blood supply: the hepatic artery, which is a branch of the coeliac axis, and the portal vein, which is formed from the mesenteric vein and the splenic vein. The portal vein drains most of the blood from the GI tract. The venous drainage of the liver passes via a number of hepatic veins into the vena cava.

The liver has six distinct functions:

- It contains the components of the major excretory pathway for many large molecules, producing bilirubin, urea and others.
- It synthesises a number of important specialised proteins, including albumin and all clotting factors.
- It maintains stable levels of amino acids and glucose in the blood.
- It supplies bile salts and bicarbonate to assist in digestion.
- It detoxifies many potential toxins and drugs.
- It is an important immunological organ, processing antigens from the gut and phagocytosis (Kupffer cells).

Major hepatic dysfunction leads to metabolic derangement and bleeding.

Clinical features

Symptoms

Most symptoms of liver disease are indirect and do not immediately focus your attention on the liver. Typical symptoms are:

- anorexia
- fatigue.

Acute liver disease leads to:

- nausea and vomiting
- jaundice
- bleeding
- encephalopathy (if severe, e.g. liver failure).

Chronic liver disease has a multitude of clinical manifestations, which are described in the relevant sections.

Signs

Few signs in *acute* liver disease are specific to the liver. Important signs include:

- jaundice
- hepatomegaly or reduced liver size (as in hyperacute hepatic failure)
- right hypochondrial tenderness
- fever (sometimes).

There are usually no signs associated with mild chronic hepatitis. In contrast, there are a plethora of signs associated with severe chronic liver disease and cirrhosis.

Investigations

Blood tests

Specific tests for liver disease fall essentially into two groups:

- measuring synthetic function (albumin, clotting times, urea and glucose)
- measuring direct liver damage or excretory function (bilirubin, transaminases and other hepatic enzymes).

You should consider abnormal liver function tests in two broad categories:

- cholestatic (raised alkaline phosphatase and bilirubin)
- hepatocellular (raised transaminases: alanine aminotransferase (ALT) and aspartate aminotransferase (AST)). A raised gamma-glutamyl transferase (GGT or gamma-GT) is a sensitive (but not a highly specific) indicator of excess alcohol intake.

A cholestatic pattern suggests obstructive jaundice or cholangitis (such as sclerosing cholangitis). A hepatocellular pattern suggests direct liver cell damage, as in viral hepatitis, hepatotoxicity from drugs, alcohol or ischaemia.

Abnormal liver function tests are extremely common in very sick patients. They are probably multifactorial in origin. Mostly, the abnormalities are mild and no action is required. There are five differential diagnoses that you should consider in very ill patients:

- cholestasis caused by sepsis
- ischaemic hepatitis
- acute hepatitis C or cytomegalovirus infection
- total parenteral nutrition hepatitis
- drug-induced hepatitis.

Sometimes, the abnormalities may be part of multiorgan failure, contributing to the patient's death or prolonged recovery.

A number of specific tests are used to diagnose particular liver diseases (see below).

Imaging

Ultrasound

Ultrasound is extremely useful for:

- identifying gall stones and the diameter of the common bile duct
- assessing the approximate size of the liver and spleen
- detecting liver or splenic abscesses/masses
- detecting subpleural fluid
- targeting liver biopsy.

Ultrasound is quick, inexpensive and non-invasive. The sensitivity for gall stones or abscesses exceeds 90% but is not 100%.

Computed tomography

A CT scan is excellent for visualising liver texture and identifying small abscesses or collections of fluid and pus.

Biopsy

Often the only way to establish the diagnosis of liver disease is to do a biopsy and examine the tissue histologically (p. 147). The main indication is investigation of chronic hepatitis, but it is also used for staging lymphomas and diagnosing tumours.

Acute liver disease

Paracetamol poisoning

Most cases of paracetamol poisoning are intentional and constitute a suicide attempt. Normally, paracetamol is easily detoxified by the liver. Excessive doses overwhelm the normal hepatic detoxification system and so a highly reactive metabolite accumulates. This causes liver damage or failure, and occasionally renal failure.

Few symptoms accompany paracetamol poisoning itself. The history may not be forthcoming from the patient.

Investigations

Measurement of serum paracetamol (and aspirin levels) should be made as soon as possible. In addition, baseline biochemistry (liver function tests, prothrombin time, electrolytes, creatinine and glucose) is important. Consider whether any other drugs have been taken and, if appropriate, consult 'Toxbase' or contact the National Poisons Information Service.

Management

If the patient presents to hospital within 4 hours of ingestion and has taken at least 15 tablets (7.5 g), then you should consider a gastric washout.

Three key pieces of information are needed to manage a patient with paracetamol overdose:

- the interval between taking the overdose and presentation
- the plasma concentration of paracetamol
- whether the patient is an alcoholic or is taking P450 enzyme inducers (e.g. carbamazepine, phenytoin, rifampicin), as these all increase the amount of reactive metabolite produced.

The administration of i.v. acetylcysteine will reduce liver damage by increasing the amount of glutathione available to counteract the effects of the highly reactive metabolite. The decision to treat is based on the plasma concentration of paracetamol (Fig. 33). Treatment should be started as soon as possible. In patients who present 16 hours or more after poisoning, the serum concentration is not a useful guide to the need for treatment. When the timing of the overdose is uncertain, if the overdose is staggered or when presentation to hospital is >16 hours after the overdose, the antidote must be given. The assessment of liver damage can be made by:

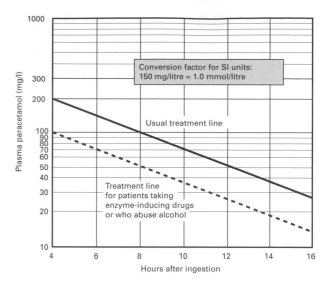

Fig. 33 Treatment graph for paracetamol overdose.

Table 32 Types of toxic reaction occurring in the liver

Reaction	Example
Direct toxicity	Paracetamol, carbon tetrachloride, mushrooms
Idiosyncratic	Isoniazid, propylthiouracil
Allergic hepatitis	Phenytoin, co-amoxiclav, sulphonamides
Cholestatic reaction	Pregnancy, chlorpromazine, captopril, estradiol
Chronic hepatitis	Isoniazid, trazodone
Fibrosis or cirrhosis alone	Methotrexate, vitamin A
Veno-occlusive disease	Cyclophosphamide, other chemotherapy agents, herbal teas
Ischaemic damage	Cocaine, sustained-release nicotinic acid, amphetamines

- serial International Normalised Ratio (INR)
- liver enzymes: aspartate transaminase.

INR is a standardised value for the prothrombin time. In severe liver dysfunction, lower levels of clotting proteins are produced and the INR is prolonged. Such patients should be discussed with a liver specialist and patients who develop hepatic failure (p. 145) should be considered for transplantation.

Hepatotoxicity of other drugs

There are numerous drugs which, rarely, cause liver disease (Table 32). For example, the antituberculous agents isoniazid and rifampicin may cause severe (fatal) liver damage weeks or months after starting treatment.

Early warning signs of liver toxicity include feeling tired, anorexia and abdominal tenderness (right upper quadrant). Jaundice is a late feature. Any of these features should prompt you to do liver function tests immediately. Drug-induced hepatotoxicity may be cholestatic or hepatocellular. Hepatocellular derangements are usually more life-threatening. If the liver function tests are significantly abnormal, the implicated drugs should be stopped immediately.

Gilbert's syndrome

Gilbert's syndrome is a benign inherited disorder that causes jaundice with no other abnormality of liver function tests. The patient has a partial inability to conjugate bilirubin and so unconjugated hyperbilirubinaemia results, especially when the load is increased during infections, operations, following fasting, etc. The major differential diagnosis is haemolytic jaundice (p. 270).

Alcoholic hepatitis

In contrast to hepatic cirrhosis, alcoholic hepatitis is an acute illness associated with acute or chronic alcohol abuse. Patients present with:

- deep jaundice
- right upper quadrant abdominal pain
- tender hepatomegaly
- fever
- raised white cell count
- elevated INR.

Sometimes the patients have spider naevi and palmar erythema, suggesting chronic liver disease. Liver function is somewhat deranged. You can make the diagnosis with a combination of history, physical findings and liver function test abnormalities. The differential diagnoses are:

- extrahepatic obstructive jaundice (e.g. gall stones or pancreatic tumour)
- liver abscess, cholangitis or other infection.

Investigations

Liver function tests, urea and electrolyte measurement, coagulation tests and full blood count are mandatory. Ultrasound will help to exclude other differential diagnoses.

Management

Management is supportive (fluids, nutrition, etc.). Abstinence from alcohol, assuming the patient recovers, is key to long-term survival. Laparotomy and other invasive procedures may lead to early death. The mortality in severe alcoholic hepatitis is 30–60%.

Pyogenic liver infection

The broad differential diagnosis of patients with fever and jaundice or substantially abnormal liver function tests (Table 33), other than in the intensive care unit (p. 139), is:

- cholecystitis (p. 151)
- bacterial liver abscess
- cholangitis (p. 152)
- amoebic liver abscess (p. 142).

Table 33 Clues to the diagnosis of acute infections of the liver

	History	Signs	Investigations
Hepatitis A, B and E	Epidemiology (see text)	Absence of fever when jaundiced; enlarged, diffusely tender liver	Very high AST/ALT and high bilirubin; normal (or low) white cell count and ESR
Leptospirosis (Weil's disease) (p. 420)	Water exposure (well, etc.); sewer worker	Cough; fever; bleeding tendency	Renal impairment; proteinuria; raised white cell count; moderately elevated liver function tests
Glandular fever (p. 419)	Typical age group (teenage, early 20s)	Non-tender lymphadenopathy; sore throat; fever	Atypical lymphocytes on blood film; positive Monospot and Paul–Bunnell test
Bacterial liver abscess	Older age group; underlying pathology; subacute presentation	Fever (usually); right-sided chest signs	Raised white cell count and ESR; mildly abnormal liver function tests; low albumin; abscess on scan
Amoebic liver abscess (p. 429)	Travel abroad in preceding 3–18 months	Fever; hepatic point tenderness; right-sided chest signs	Raised white cell count and ESR; moderately abnormal liver function tests; large abscess(es) on scan
Hydatid cyst of liver	Residence in endemic area, e.g. Wales, developing world	Usually none, sometimes hepatomegaly	Normal liver function tests; normal white cell count; cyst on scan with septae and/or calcified rim; no useful serology

AST, aspartate aminotransferase; ALT, alanine aminotransferase; ESR, erythrocyte sedimentation rate.

Bacterial liver abscess

Bacterial liver abscesses in the developed world are more common than amoebic liver abscesses, whereas the opposite is true in the developing world. They are more common in elderly people and the presentation may be subtle. The aetiology is:

- associated with infection of the biliary tree and portal drainage area and local spread from, for example, a subphrenic abscess
- haematogenous spread from other sites, e.g. lungs
- trauma
- cryptogenic (20–30%).

Predisposing factors include diabetes, alcoholism, corticosteroid therapy, malignancy and immune deficiency.

Clinical presentation The presentation is usually insidious over several weeks. There is usually low-grade fever, raised white cell count and ESR and, sometimes, tender hepatomegaly. Other common features include:

- right-sided pleural effusion and/or crackles
- ascites
- splenomegaly
- mental confusion.

Jaundice and significant abnormalities of liver function are uncommon unless the disease is associated with another source of infection in the biliary tree.

Management The number of organisms that cause liver abscesses is large, including anaerobes, *Streptococcus milleri* and several Gram-negative bacilli. Abscesses are usually polymicrobial. Blood cultures are positive in about 50% of patients but may be so for only one of the organisms involved in the abscess. For this reason, percutaneous aspiration is appropriate to optimise antimicrobial therapy. As much pus as possible should be removed. If the abscess is small, no further action is required other than antibiotic therapy. If the abscess is large, percutaneous drainage may be appropriate. Empirical antibiotics should include:

- pencillin or ampicillin
- metronidazole
- an antibiotic active against Gram-negative bacteria.

Overall mortality is around 10–15%.

Viral hepatitis

There are many causes of hepatitis, most of which cause jaundice but not all. Some are common (e.g. hepatitis A), others less so, but all are important for management reasons. Clues to the clinical diagnoses are shown in Tables 33 and 34.

Hepatitis A

Hepatitis A causes acute self-limiting hepatitis and is extremely common in all parts of the world except Northern Europe, North America and Australasia. In developing countries, it typically presents in children. Most adults born in the UK have not been infected and are at risk.

Clinical presentation Hepatitis A presents with non-specific symptoms, such as malaise and weakness, followed by anorexia, which is usually profound, sometimes nausea and vomiting, and a vague dull right upper quadrant pain. During this phase, there may be fever although typically there is not. The early symptoms last between 3 and 10 days prior to the onset of jaundice, which is associated with dark-coloured urine. The patient starts to feel better shortly after they become jaundiced, which usually lasts between 2 and 3 weeks, although sometimes less in mild cases. Most patients remain tired for some weeks.

Investigations Liver function tests are extremely helpful as patients usually have marked elevations of aminotransferases and bilirubin, with slight increase in alkaline phosphatase and lactate dehydrogenase (LDH) (Fig. 34). The white cell count is normal or low and the plasma vicosity or ESR is not elevated. Renal function is normal unless the patient goes into acute liver failure. The INR is typically prolonged, but usually only slightly. Monitoring of aminotransferases and INR is the most helpful guide to progress. The diagnosis is confirmed by a positive hepatitis A IgM test.

Management Management consists of rest and maintenance of nutrition, if possible. Patients who exercise early after initial recovery are more likely to suffer a relapse of hepatitis. Patients with INR values greater than 2 should be admitted to hospital. Deteriorating hepatic function, which occurs in about 1 in 2000 patients, is an indication for transfer to a liver transplant unit.

Once the liver function tests have returned to normal, alcohol may be consumed again. Banning alcohol is only

Table 34 Hepatitis viruses

	A	B	C	E
Transmission	F/O	I/V, vert, horiz, B/T, sexual	I/V, B/T, sexual	F/O
Incubation period (weeks)	3–6	5–26	2–3	4–20
Chronic carriage	N	Y	Y	N
Causes chronic hepatitis	N	Y	Y	N
Causes hepatocellular carcinoma	N	Y	Y	N(?)
Treatment with interferon beneficial	N	Y	Y	N

F/O, faecal/oral; I/V, intravenous drug abuse; vert, mother to child; horiz, sibling to sibling; B/T, blood transfusion; Y, yes; N, no.

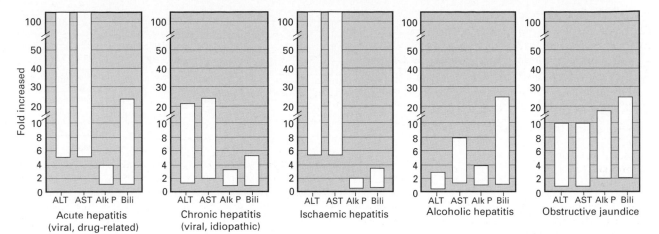

Fig. 34 Elevation of key serum enzymes and proteins in several liver diseases. ALT, alanine aminotransferase; AST, aspartate aminotransferase; Alk P, alkaline phosphatase; Bili, bilirubin.

Table 35 Hepatitis B tests

Test	Interpretation of tests	
	If positive	If negative
Surface antigen tests		
Antigen itself (HBsAg)	Acute hepatitis B or carrier	Non-infectious, not acute hepatitis B
Antibody to surface antigen (anti-HBs)	Prior hepatitis B or prior immunisation	Not protected (if immunised)
Core tests		
IgM test (anti-HBc IgM)	Recent acute hepatitis B	No evidence of recent hepatitis B infection
IgG test (anti-HBc IgG)	Hepatitis B infection in past	Never had hepatitis B
Tests for e antigen		
e antigen itself (HBeAg)	Acute hepatitis B or highly infectious carrier	Not highly infectious
Antibody to e antigen (anti-HBe)	Prior hepatitis B but not highly infectious	Not useful (see text)

appropriate in alcoholic hepatitis or where alcohol withdrawal would carry other general health benefits for the patient.

Hepatitis B

Compared with hepatitis A (Table 34), the incubation period of hepatitis B is much longer. Homosexual patients and those sharing needles are most at risk but most infections are acquired via heterosexual sex. Institutions for the mentally handicapped and medical procedures are occasional sources of infection.

Clinical presentation The presentation is similar to that of hepatitis A, though less acute. There is a slightly greater likelihood of arthritis or rash (a form of serum sickness-like syndrome). The other major distinction between hepatitis A and B is the possibility of carriage and chronic liver disease in patients with hepatitis B (see below).

Investigations You should do the same investigations as you would do for hepatitis A, along with hepatitis B tests (Table 35). If there is doubt about the diagnosis, a liver ultrasound is helpful to exclude other problems.

Hepatitis B surface antigen (HBsAg) is nearly always positive during the acute phase of hepatitis B (Table 35). The problem can be confirmed as an acute episode of hepatitis B (rather than another form of hepatitis on top of chronic hepatitis B carriage) using the hepatitis B core IgM test (anti-HBc IgM). This test is only useful in patients who are acutely ill with jaundice or have just recovered. The anti-HBc IgG test is used to find out if a patient has ever had hepatitis B.

Management The management of acute hepatitis B is very similar to that of hepatitis A. Patients with hepatitis B may develop fulminant liver failure as in hepatitis A.

Chronic infection There are over 200 million people with chronic hepatitis B infection worldwide, particularly in South-east Asia. In Europe and the USA, about 1 in 1000 of the population are carriers. Patients with hepatitis B need to be followed up to establish whether they are or have become chronic carriers (see Fig. 35). The likelihood of a patient who develops jaundice becoming a chronic carrier is substantially less than for patients who have 'silent' (anicteric) hepatitis B, which is quite common. If patients remain HBeAg-positive, they are termed 'supercarriers' because

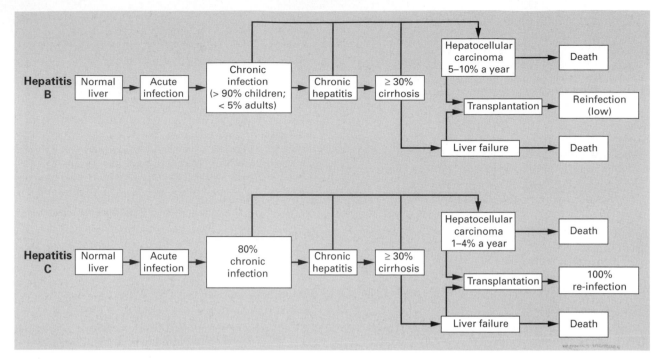

Fig. 35 Natural history of hepatitis B and C infection.

they are so infectious. Mutant viruses that are deficient in e antigen (and do not elicit an e antibody response) may cause even more aggressive hepatitis.

Hepatitis C

The presentation of hepatitis C is milder than that of A and B and is rarely seen clinically. It essentially always follows a blood transfusion or sharing of needles. Sexual transmission is uncommon but does occur. Transmission of hepatitis C vertically to neonates is also uncommon (10%).

Clinical presentation Symptoms and signs are similar to those of hepatitis A and B. Patients are frequently not jaundiced with acute hepatitis C.

Investigations Raised transaminases with or without an elevated bilirubin are typical. Hepatitis C antibodies are positive late during the acute phase and persist for a long time. Persistent infection is confirmed by detecting viral RNA in blood.

Management Patients with acute hepatitis C must be followed up to establish whether they become chronic carriers or not (Fig. 35). This requires measurement of liver function and hepatitis C RNA in the blood. Patients with circulating hepatitis C RNA may develop chronic liver disease and are potentially infectious. Patients who are hepatitis C RNA-positive or who have hepatitis C antibodies and abnormal liver function tests should be managed as if they have chronic hepatitis (see below). There are estimated to be over 150 million people with chronic hepatitis C infection worldwide.

Acute liver failure

Acute liver failure has three facets:

- encephalopathy
- jaundice

- markers of extreme hepatic malfunction (e.g. prolonged INR).

The causes of acute liver failure in patients referred to a liver unit in the UK are:

- paracetamol overdose (55%)
- hepatitis A (5%)
- hepatitis B (10%)
- non-A, non-B hepatitis (20%)
- other causes (10%).

Clinical presentation

There are few physical signs of acute liver failure other than jaundice and encephalopathy. The liver may be so small that there is no overlying dullness to percussion.

Encephalopathy Encephalopathy may be mild or profound. Conscious level varies from drowsy to unresponsive to pain. There are some distinctive features of hepatic encephalopathy:

- specific cognitive abnormalities
- liver flap
- hepatic foetor (sweet-smelling breath).

If the patient is not unconscious, test for liver flap and specific cognitive abnormalities. Spatial awareness is grossly impaired. Common tests include drawing a five-pointed star and putting the numbers and hands on a clockface. Patients tend to put all the numbers in one or two quadrants.

Investigations

Your investigation should include:

- liver function tests (showing high transaminases and bilirubin)

- arterial blood gases (respiratory alkalosis caused by hyperventilation or metabolic acidosis associated with poisoning)
- INR (very prolonged)
- blood glucose (usually low)
- serum creatinine (usually elevated)
- blood cultures (Gram-negative sepsis, including cholangitis, is an important differential diagnosis).

Management

Cerebral oedema Cerebral oedema results from loss of cell membrane integrity and alteration in the permeability of the blood–brain barrier. The very high intracerebral pressures produced lead to a reduction in cerebral perfusion, diffuse cerebral ischaemia and sometimes herniation of the brainstem. Rises in intracranial pressure are often sudden and unpredictable. The clinical features of cerebral oedema include systemic hypertension, bradycardia, increased muscle tone progressing to decerebrate posturing and abnormal pupillary reflexes. Unfortunately, these signs occur late and intervention based on their appearance rarely improves outcome. Intracerebral monitoring of intracranial pressure with a probe may be used to guide treatment. Patients should be kept supine. If cerebral oedema is documented clinically or with a probe, mannitol (20%) should be infused rapidly. Other cerebral oedema-reducing measures such as dexamethasone are not effective in liver failure.

Coagulopathy Coagulopathy (as measured by a prolonged INR) results from the reduced synthesis of several clotting factors, though there are more complex events that contribute to bleeding, including reduced platelet function. Fresh frozen plasma should be given if there is bleeding. Vitamin K is of limited value.

Oliguric renal failure Approximately 50% of patients develop oliguric renal failure, and this worsens the prognosis. This is sometimes called the hepatorenal syndrome. Renal failure may be directly caused by paracetamol overdose, poisoning by other toxins or by leptospirosis.

Hypoxaemia Hypoxaemia is common and may necessitate ventilation. High inspired oxygen concentrations should be given. Epoprostenol (prostacyclin) improves peripheral oxygen delivery.

Hypoglycaemia Hypoglycaemia is common and is related to defective gluconeogenesis as well as high circulating insulin levels resulting from inadequate hepatic uptake. Blood glucose levels should be monitored frequently and 50% glucose administered via a central line as appropriate. Hypokalaemia can occur as a result of this and sometimes large amounts of potassium are required to maintain normokalaemia.

Infection Bacterial and candidal infections are common. Patients have faulty neutrophil function and impaired cell-mediated immunity. Frequent blood and other cultures, with appropriate antibiotic or antifungal therapy, are commonly required.

Outcome of liver failure and transplantation

Liver failure can be divided into three broad categories depending on the interval between the appearance of jaundice and encephalopathy (Table 36). The outcome depends on which group the patient falls into.

Transplantation (p. 391) is particularly indicated for those with acute and subacute liver failure as the prognosis is especially poor.

Chronic hepatitis

Chronic hepatitis is essentially a histopathological diagnosis. Previously it was classified into chronic persistent and chronic active (or chronic aggressive) hepatitis, but these classes have been abandoned. Chronic hepatitis is graded histologically into minimal, mild, moderate and severe inflammatory activity, together with mild, moderate or severe fibrosis. Mild disease remains restricted to the portal tracts. The severity increases to include disease damaging the border between lobules (limiting plate) including bile duct proliferation, extensive inflammatory cell infiltrate and fibrosis. In cirrhosis there is loss of lobular architecture with identifiable central veins and peripheral portal tracts and replacement of these with regenerating nodules.

Certain forms of chronic hepatitis have characteristic features that allow a specific aetiological diagnosis. Examples include alcoholism (fatty infiltration, Mallory's hyaline bodies and a central zonal type of liver damage), α_1-antitrypsin deficiency (intracellular periodic acid–Schiff base (PAS)-positive material) and granulomatous hepatitis.

Clinical presentation

Chronic hepatitis presents in three ways:

- abnormal liver function tests
- hepatomegaly
- markers of active hepatitis B or hepatitis C infection.

Chronic hepatitis is often discovered accidentally when liver function test abnormalities are found. Some patients present with fatigue. Patients who are particularly ill may have a fever and other manifestations of disease, as in autoimmune chronic hepatitis and granulomatous hepatitis. Some patients with chronic hepatitis C, granulomatous

Table 36 Subgroups and outcome of acute liver failure

	Interval between jaundice and encephalopathy (days)	Outcome without transplantation (% survival)
Hyperacute liver failure	0–7	35
Acute liver failure	8–28	7
Subacute liver failure	More than 28	15

hepatitis or haemochromatosis have normal liver function tests but have hepatomegaly.

Causes of chronic hepatitis

Deficiency of α₁-antitrypsin

Deficiency of α_1-antitrypsin is an uncommon inherited problem in which the enzyme produced by the patient is abnormal and unable to be exported out of the liver, where it is made. This leads to accumulation and chronic liver disease (usually in childhood). The systemic deficiency causes emphysema (p. 85). Variations in the degree of deficiency lead to differing levels of severity of disease. Because α_1-antitrypsin is an acute-phase protein, tests for deficiency can only be done successfully when the patient does not have any degree of acute inflammation Phenotyping confirms the deficiency. There is no treatment, although smoking should be avoided.

Haemochromatosis

Haemochromatosis is an autosomal recessive condition leading to increased iron absorption from the gut and deposition in the body. The carrier frequency is 10% and the disorder affects approximately 1 in 300 of the northern European population. The specific gene for haemochromatosis (HFE) is tightly linked to the human leucocyte antigen (HLA) — A region on the short arm of chromosome 6. A genetic test (polymerase chain reaction) to detect the point mutation (C282Y) in the gene HFE is now available and a second missense mutation (H63D) has been identified. Between them, the mutations account for approximately 95% of all cases. There is variable penetrance, but the clinical manifestations are:

- diabetes mellitus
- bronzed appearance
- symmetrical arthritis (knees, metacarpophalangeal (MCP) joints)
- gynaecomastia
- hypogonadism
- hepatomegaly, hepatic cirrhosis and hepatocellular carcinoma.

Liver function may be normal but hepatomegaly is present. Serum iron and/or ferritin is usually very high. Liver biopsy shows large liver stores of iron. It is best prevented by screening and venesection.

Wilson's disease

Wilson's disease is a very rare disorder of copper metabolism inherited as an autosomal recessive trait, with the gene regulating copper transport in the liver located on chromosome 13. Heterozygotes have no clinical features. The biochemical stages in homozygotes are:

1. defect in copper excretion from hepatic lysosymes to bile
2. increased copper in liver
3. reduced caeruloplasmin levels in blood (carries copper)
4. increased free copper in blood
5. increased urinary copper excretion
6. deposition of copper in tissues (brain, kidney, etc.).

In Wilson's disease, many of the above indices overlap into the normal range. Chronic liver disease is often the first manifestation in childhood/young adulthood. In some, an acute hepatitis/fulminant hepatic failure may be the first presentation. As the copper starts to spill out of the liver, the patient may develop acute haemolysis, renal tubular acidosis and/or neurological features (extrapyramidal system). In the early stages, response to D-penicillamine is good, with increased urinary copper excretion.

Autoimmune hepatitis

Autoimmune hepatitis occurs mostly in females. It is subdivided into types 1 and 2, both associated with other autoimmune diseases such as ulcerative colitis, pericarditis, thyroiditis, migratory arthritis and fibrosing alveolitis. The diagnosis is suggested by abnormal liver function tests, positive autoantibody tests and raised gamma globulins. The onset is often insidious and may lead to cirrhosis relatively rapidly. Immunosuppressive therapy is usually successful in type 1 disease.

Type 1
- Autoantibodies: ANA, smooth muscle, ANCA, anti-actin
- Age: any
- Severity: variable
- Treatment failure: infrequent

Type 2
- Autoantibodies: liver, kidney microsomes
- Age: childhood, adolescence
- Severity: usually severe
- Treatment failure: frequent

Primary biliary cirrhosis

Primary biliary cirrhosis is a chronic obstructive cholangitis usually seen in middle-aged women. Presymptomatic cases are now commonly found as a result of liver function tests requested for other reasons. Progression of the disease is relatively slow. Patients present with marked fatigue, pruritus, because of retention of bile salts, and abnormal liver function tests typical of cholestasis. The dominant pathological feature is destruction of small to medium-sized bile ducts mediated by CD4 and CD8 lymphocytes. On examination, the patient is often hyperpigmented (bile salt deposition) with hepatosplenomegaly. Ultrasound is used to exclude obstruction. The antimitochondrial antibodies are detectable in high titre in almost all patients. The patients also have a raised serum IgM. Ursodeoxycholic acid (UDCA) is used to slow progression of the disease and colestyramine (sequesters bile salts) can help the pruritus. Liver transplantation can be used.

Granulomatous hepatitis

Granulomatous hepatitis is a hotch-potch of around 30 diseases caused by both infectious and non-infectious agents. Around 10% of normal people have hepatic granulomas on biopsy. Therefore, granulomatous hepatitis implies hepatic dysfunction or generalised illness and the presence of granulomas. Causes include:

- classical causes of granulomas such as tuberculosis and sarcoidosis
- tropical parasitic diseases such as schistosomiasis

- Q fever
- chronic fungal disease (e.g. histoplasmosis).

Sometimes granulomatous hepatitis is the cause of pyrexia of unknown origin (PUO, p. 427). Treatment is directed towards the underlying cause, although sometimes none is required.

Investigations

The management of chronic hepatitis requires knowledge of the underlying cause and assessment of the extent of inflammation and fibrosis. Therefore, serological tests to identify the cause and a liver biopsy are essential.

Serological tests

Useful tests for the diagnosis of chronic hepatitis are shown in Table 37.

Liver biopsy

A liver biopsy is one of the most invasive 'medical' investigations and warrants detailed discussion with the patient. The primary risk is bleeding, which occurs to a minor degree following almost all liver biopsies. Occasionally, it is severe, unrelenting and ultimately fatal. The overall risk of death is 1 in 2000 liver biopsies, but there are some factors that make some biopsies more risky than others:

- abnormal clotting times
- cirrhosis
- abnormal platelet function
- ascites.

If you are involved in organising a liver biopsy you need to:

- seek written consent
- ask about any recent drug ingestion, including aspirin, NSAIDs
- make a clinical assessment with regard to the likelihood of cirrhosis, e.g. spider naevi, evidence of oesophageal varices, radiological reports suggesting cirrhosis, etc.
- measure clotting times and platelet count
- group and save serum for cross-match.

Although liver biopsy may be done on a day case basis, the patient must be in a bed and spend a minimum of 4 hours resting after the biopsy. This is partly for observation for possible bleeding problems. Many patients complain of pain in the right lower chest or the right shoulder following liver biopsy. If the pain and pulse rate are increasing and the patient looks unwell, you should summon senior colleagues immediately and arrange for cross-matching of at least 4 units of whole blood.

The information gained from a liver biopsy is often vital to the diagnosis and management of patients with chronic hepatitis, as the liver function tests only give part of the picture. For patients on treatment, it may be necessary to repeat the liver biopsy at intervals of 6 or 12 months to ascertain whether there has been any response to treatment and whether it should be continued.

Management

Management is guided by the cause and extent of disease.

Chronic hepatitis B is currently treated with interferon-alpha or lamivudine, and hepatitis C with interferon-alpha (or pegylated interferon-alpha) and the antiviral agent ribavirin (pregnancy must be avoided). Response rates are ~50%.

Immunosuppressive therapy is required for patients with autoimmune chronic hepatitis, as is copper chelation for Wilson's disease, abstention from alcohol for alcoholic liver disease and specific treatment for the underlying cause of granulomatous hepatitis. Progressive deterioration in younger patients may be an indication for transplantation.

Table 37 Investigations for chronic hepatitis

Cause	Abnormal liver function tests	Blood test useful for establishing aetiology
Hepatitis B	Yes	HBsAg
Hepatitis C (HCV)	Yes or no	Anti-HCV, PCR for HCV
Haemochromatosis	Yes or no	Serum iron and iron-binding capacity, ferritin, *HFE* gene PCR
Deficiency of α_1-antitrypsin (AAT)	Yes	Serum levels and phenotype of AAT if normal C-reactive protein
Wilson's disease	Yes	Copper and caeruloplasmin levels
Chronic hepatitis of unknown aetiology	Yes	None
Primary biliary cirrhosis	Yes	Antimitochondrial antibodies
Autoimmune chronic hepatitis	Yes	ANA, smooth muscle and anti-LKM antibodies
Alcoholic liver disease	Yes	Blood alcohol (sometimes)
Granulomatous hepatitis	Yes or no	Sometimes, e.g. Q fever, schistosomiasis, gammaglobulins

HBsAg, hepatitis B surface antigen; PCR, polymerase chain reaction; ANA, antinuclear antibody; LKM, liver–kidney microsomal antibody.

Cirrhosis of the liver

Case Study

After 40 years of sustained alcohol abuse, it is not surprising that the man in your surgery is plethoric with a protuberant abdomen and palmar erythema. He also has a pyrexia and is complaining of new abdominal pain. He has generalised moderate peritonism on examination.

Hepatic cirrhosis is the end-stage of many chronic inflammatory processes of the liver. It is characterised histologically by fibrosis and regenerating nodules. The most common cause is excess alcohol consumption; others include all the causes of chronic hepatitis. There is a parallel between the development of fibrosis in the liver and the clinical manifestations. Progressive fibrosis leading to cirrhosis can sometimes be arrested or slowed by correction of the underlying cause.

Clinical presentation

The clinical manifestations of cirrhosis include:

- palmar erythema
- more than five spider naevi on the face or upper trunk
- evidence of portal hypertension
- evidence of deranged hepatic synthetic function.

Numerous other associated clinical features may be present (Table 38). Some are not very specific. These include ankle oedema, which has multiple causes, and haemorrhoids, which are common in the normal population. However, when several of these features are present, the possibility of cirrhosis should rise in your mind.

Recognising alcohol abuse

There are some clues to the diagnosis of alcohol abuse:

- raised mean red cell volume
- hypertension
- raised gamma-GT

Table 38 Clinical findings in patients with cirrhosis

Cause	Clinical features
Cirrhosis itself	Spider naevi
	Gynaecomastia
	Testicular atrophy
	Palmar erythema (also rheumatoid arthritis, pregnancy, etc.)
	Dupuytren's contracture
	Low-grade PUO
Portal hypertension	Splenomegaly
	Ascites
	Oesophageal varices and/or GI haemorrhage
	Haemorrhoids
Hypoalbuminaemia	White nails (leuconychia)
	Ankle oedema
	Sacral oedema
Poor nutritional status	
Lack of adequate intake	Proximal muscle wasting and myopathy
Lack of adequate caloric intake and utilisation	Weight loss
Folate, iron, riboflavin, pyrodoxine deficiency	Glossitis/angular cheilitis
Chronic thiamine deficiency	Ankle oedema and ascites, global cardiac dysfunction, Korsakoff's psychosis
Acute thiamine and other nutritional deficiencies	Wernicke's encephalopathy and retinal haemorrhage
Prolonged bleeding time	Bruising, GI haemorrhage
Prolonged INR, reduced platelet function, vitamin C deficiency	
Reduced immune function	Subacute bacterial peritonitis
	Pneumococcal pneumonia
	Bacteraemia
	Pulmonary tuberculosis
	Skin sepsis
Cerebral problems	Dementia
Directly caused by alcohol or chronic subdural haematomas	Korsakoff's psychosis, Wernicke's encephalopathy

PUO, pyrexia of unknown origin; INR, International Normalised Ratio for prothrombin time.

- raised uric acid
- asymptomatic rib fractures found on chest radiograph.

Direct questions about alcohol intake sometimes are helpful (> 3–4 units/day in men, 2–3 in women). The CAGE questionnaire may be useful; a yes answer to three or four questions indicates problematic drinking. The questions are:

1. Have you ever felt you should cut (C) down your drinking?
2. Have you ever been annoyed (A) by criticism of your drinking?
3. Have you ever felt guilty (G) about your drinking?
4. Do you drink in the morning (eye (E) opener)?

These should be supplemented by questions on maximum daily and total weekly consumption. Other screening questionnaires are also in use (e.g. AUDIT, FAST).

Alcoholism is extremely destructive (Box 6) and the rate of cirrhosis in the UK has increased rapidly.

Portal hypertension

Portal hypertension is caused by increased resistance to flow of the blood draining the GI system and spleen, leading to venous engorgement. As the resistance to flow increases so venous connections between the portal and systemic circulation open up:

- around the lower oesophagus: oesophageal and stomach varices
- around the rectum: haemorrhoids
- around the umbilicus: rare caput medusae and other dilated veins over the anterior abdominal wall
- dilated splenic vein: splenomegaly.

Oesophageal varices

Bleeding of oesophageal varices is common and partially preventable by propranolol or variceal band obliteration. Bleeding varices can be very difficult to control. Transjugular intrahepatic portosystemic shunt (TIPS) is useful when all other treatments have failed. Approximately 50% of patients with oesophageal varices bleed from another site within the GI tract, usually a gastric or duodenal ulcer. The varices may be in the stomach and difficult to access, and clotting and platelet abnormalities may aggravate the bleeding tendency.

The presence of large amounts of blood in the GI tract produces additional absorption of toxic compounds, such as ammonia and bilirubin, which the diseased liver cannot metabolise, and this leads to encephalopathy.

In varices, reduction of portal pressure can be achieved by infusion of somatostatin (octreotide) or vasopressin. Emergency sclerotherapy is of proven value. Only rarely is it necessary to use balloon tamponade (Sengstaken–Blakemore tube).

Ascites

The other major effect of portal hypertension is the development of ascites, which only occurs with sinusoidal obstruction *within* the liver, not in obstruction of the portal vein. The reason is that cirrhosis is associated with alterations in sodium and water handling by the kidney because of increased activity of the renin–aldosterone system. Figure 36 shows the mechanisms leading to ascites. Without understanding these, it is difficult to treat appropriately.

Management

A graded approach is required, depending on the severity of the ascites and the patient's compliance with diet and therapy. Excessive diuretic use will lead to hypovolaemia, electrolyte disturbance, significant prerenal impairment and sometimes renal failure. All treatment should be introduced gradually with careful observation in hospital, monitoring weight and salt and water balance. The steps in therapy are as follows:

1. sodium-restricted diet only: 10% response
2. sodium restriction plus spironolactone 100–200 mg daily: extra 50% response
3. sodium restriction plus spironolactone 200 mg daily plus furosemide 40 mg daily: extra 25% response.

During the time that these are introduced, renal function and urine output should be measured. Drug doses should be gradually increased.

Patients with ascites refractory to other measures may be candidates for liver transplantation.

Box 6: The effects of chronic excess alcohol consumption

Physical effects
- Hepatic: fatty inflammation, alcoholic hepatitis, cirrhosis
- Pancreatitis
- Gastritis
- Peripheral neuropathy
- Korsakoff's encephalopathy
- Wernicke's encephalopathy
- Chronic subdural haematomas
- Cardiomyopathy

Psychological effects
- Suicide
- Withdrawal
- Depression
- Anxiety states
- Morbid jealousy
- Dementia

Social effects
- Financial problems
- Employment problems
- Marital breakdown
- Violence
- Sexual dysfunction: lack of libido, impotence
- Legal problems: drunk driving, manslaughter, theft

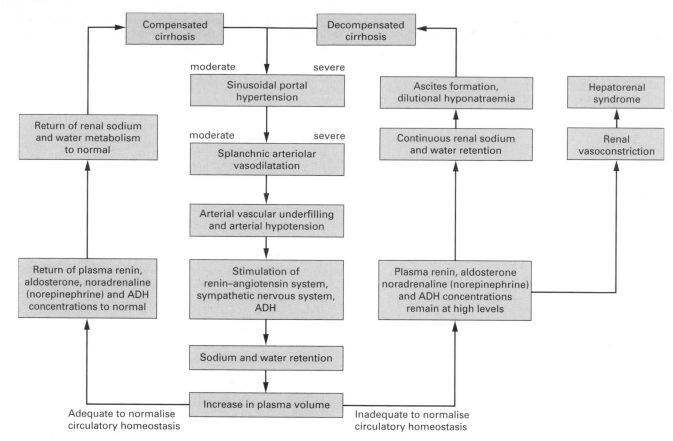

Fig. 36 The mechanisms leading to ascites. ADH, antidiuretic hormone.

Spontaneous bacterial peritonitis

Occasionally, ascites becomes infected from passage of gut bacteria into the intestinal lymph vessels and ascitic fluid. It occurs in about 10% of patients with ascites. It is almost always caused by Gram-negative bacteria such as *E. coli*. Risk factors include:

- GI haemorrhage
- raised serum bilirubin
- low ascitic fluid protein (low complement and immunoglobulin content)
- prior spontaneous bacterial peritonitis.

Patients present with abdominal pain and usually fever but sometimes only with general deterioration. On examination there is marked ascites with a very tender abdomen, often with rebound tenderness.

In suspected bacterial peritonitis, ascitic fluid should be taken for a white cell count and differential, protein, glucose, amylase, Gram stain and culture.

Treatment is with a broad-spectrum antibiotic such as cefotaxime. Mortality is 20–40%. Recurrences can be prevented with ciprofloxacin.

Tumours

Benign tumours

Adenomas are very rare. They are associated with use of the oral contraceptive pill and anabolic steroids. They can present with shock caused by intraperitoneal rupture and haemorrhage. Haemangiomas are being found fairly com-

monly with all the screening that is done for other reasons. They are usually small and clinically irrelevant.

Malignant tumours

Primary tumours

Compared with metastatic disease, you will see very few primary hepatocellular carcinomas. They are associated with cirrhosis from any aetiology. In other parts of the world, the vast majority of patients with a hepatocellular carcinoma are hepatitis B antigen-positive.

The presentation is usually non-specific with general deterioration in a patient with known cirrhosis. Some will complain of abdominal pain; others will have abdominal swelling caused by ascites. The possibility should be considered in any unwell patient with known chronic liver disease.

Liver function tests are usually unhelpful. *Serum α-feto-protein* is often markedly increased and is then diagnostic. Ultrasound or CT scan imaging will show the tumour, which is usually solitary. A biopsy should not be done if any attempt is to be made at resection because the tumour can seed along the needle track.

The outlook is bleak with only a few patients surviving beyond 3 months. If the tumour is confined to one lobe, it can be resected, but this is rare. Early detection may be possible in patients with cirrhosis by screening for α-feto-protein and by liver ultrasound every 6 months. Some patients gain temporary remission with chemotherapy (fluorouracil, cisplatin, doxorubicin) either systemically or direct into the hepatic artery, possibly combined with particle embolisation (normal liver can be supplied by the portal vein).

Secondary tumours

By far the most common liver tumour you will see is a metastasis, particularly from the GI tract, bronchus and breast. Often, it is the first presentation of the primary tumour. Patients may complain of general malaise, weight loss and non-specific abdominal pain. Patients may have hepatomegaly (irregular edge), but not all.

A raised alkaline phosphatase is consistent with the diagnosis but is common and non-specific so imaging with ultrasound or CT is necessary. As with primary tumours, a biopsy may be carried out, but again may be contraindicated if resection is being considered for isolated or small number of metastases (e.g. from carcinoma of the colon). Often, there is little active therapy that can be offered for multiple metastases, though patients with (for example) breast disease may respond.

3.8 The biliary system

Learning objectives

You should be able to:
- describe the different clinical patterns of biliary disease and how these affect management.

Case Study

The consultant is quizzing you about Joan Smithson, one of your patients on the ward. She is 82 years old and has been admitted because of a urinary tract infection. As part of the series of investigations that you ordered, an ultrasound examination of her abdomen has shown that Ms Smithson's gall bladder contains multiple gall stones and your consultant is asking you whether Ms Smithson can go home or whether anything else needs to be done.

Anatomy and physiology

The role of the biliary system is to collect the bile salts and bilirubin secreted by the hepatocytes and deliver these to the small intestine. The function of bile salts is to form micelles so that key lipid-soluble substances such as cholesterol triglycerides (largest amount) and phospholipids can be absorbed.

Bile canaliculi transfer bile salts from the hepatocytes to interlobular bile ductules in the portal tracts. These converge into the right and left hepatic duct, and then into the common hepatic duct. Outside the liver, the cystic duct joins the gall bladder where about 50 ml of bile can be stored. The common bile duct starts at the junction of the cystic duct with the common hepatic duct and runs to enter the second part of the duodenum with the pancreatic duct at the **ampulla of Vater**. The **sphincter of Oddi** prevents passage of bile into the small intestine in the absence of food.

Bile acids are synthesised from cholesterol in the hepatocytes. Conjugation (with taurine or glycine) increases the solubility. The bile acids are secreted in the bile, metabolised to some extent by bacteria in the small intestine and then almost all reabsorbed in the terminal ileum. Subsequently, they are resecreted by the liver. This recirculation takes place several times per day.

Failure of bile salt absorption (for example, in Crohn's disease or after ileal resection) can cause colonic irritation and diarrhoea, which can be relieved by using colestyramine to bind the bile salts. The ability of the drug to deplete the bile acid pool can help to alleviate the skin irritation and pruritus in prolonged obstructive jaundice.

The prime action of bile acids is to act as detergents. They aggregate into micelles so that there is a water-soluble envelope surrounding a hydrophobic (lipophilic) core, which allows the transport of cholesterol triglycerides and phospholipids (particularly lethicin). Imbalance leads to aggregation and formation of gall stones.

Gall stones and cholecystitis

Gall stones are more common in women and become increasingly prevalent with age. The major factors leading to stones are:

- supersaturation of bile with cholesterol
- impaired gall bladder motility
- bile stasis.

Pigment stones are mostly seen when there is prolonged increased red cell turnover: for example, in hereditary spherocytosis.

Clinical presentation

There are three presentations.

Asymptomatic

Most gall stones are asymptomatic and remain so. Often they are identified incidentally during ultrasound scanning.

Symptomatic

There is intermittent pain in the right upper quadrant, classically occurring after food and lasting several hours (biliary colic). The pain may be severe and require narcotic analgesics for relief. Once symptoms have occurred, they tend to recur and worsen, with increased risk of cholecystitis and pancreatitis.

Complicated

The most common complications are cholecystitis and duct obstruction together with cholangitis or pancreatitis. Acute cholecystitis with cystic duct obstruction can lead to abscess formation, gall bladder perforation or mucocoele. Finally, chronic cholecystitis causes a scarred, shrunken, non-functioning gall bladder. Carcinoma is an uncommon long-term problem.

Investigations

Pointers to gall stones may be the typical history described above, raised serum bilirubin and alkaline phosphatase. If you suspect gall stones, you should request an ultrasound examination, which has a sensitivity and specificity of over 90% for identification of stones. The gall bladder may be small and thick-walled. The width of the common bile duct is important (<8 mm) as dilatation indicates extrahepatic biliary obstruction.

Acute cholecystitis is usually diagnosed on the history, physical examination and ultrasound findings.

Management

Management of gall stones can be either medical or surgical. The first decision is whether to do anything at all. Where stones are diagnosed by chance and the patient is asymptomatic, it is reasonable to do nothing.

Non-surgical treatment

This includes gall stone dissolution, extracorporeal shock wave lithotripsy and mechanical litholysis. However, these are suitable for few patients and have a higher gall stone recurrence rate.

Surgery

The principal therapy is cholecystectomy; the aims are to remove the stones and avoid the risk of future recurrence. The operation can be done 'open' or using a laparoscope. The latter is associated with reduced pain, scarring, length of stay and convalescence.

Common bile duct stones

Stones in the common bile duct may either be passed spontaneously or have to be removed. They present with right hypochondrial pain, jaundice and fever (caused by ascending cholangitis). Surgical exploration may be necessary, but many stones can be removed using ERCP.

Ascending cholangitis

Infection of the biliary tree has high morbidity and significant mortality. It is usually associated with stones and can present with an unexplained pyrexia, or it may cause Gram-negative septicaemia with shock. A plain abdominal radiograph may show stones (10% radio-opaque) or gas in the biliary tree.

Treatment is with i.v. fluids, high-flow oxygen and antimicrobials. A reasonable choice is a combination of cefotaxime (a broad spectrum of activity against Gram-negative organisms) and metronidazole (anaerobes).

At some stage, subsequent to an ultrasound scan, ERCP is often performed, looking for stones in the common bile duct or a stricture.

Tumours

Cholangiocarcinoma is a relatively rare tumour that is usually associated with gall stones in elderly people. There is also an association with primary sclerosing cholangitis with or without ulcerative colitis. The tumour is much more common in South-East Asia (liver flukes). It presents with obstructive jaundice, which may be painless. Ultrasound is the first-line investigation. MR scanning, MRCP and ERCP can determine the extent of the disease. Most tumours are inoperable and the management is symptomatic, with the relief of biliary obstruction using a stent inserted via an ERCP.

The most common cause of obstructive jaundice in elderly people is gall stones. When the obstruction results from malignant disease this is usually a carcinoma at the head of the pancreas or metastatic disease in the lymph nodes at the porta hepatis.

3.9 The pancreas

Learning objectives

You need to be able to:
- discuss the normal structure and function of the pancreas and how derangement leads to the common presentations of pancreatic disease
- construct a plan of investigation and subsequent management of a patient with suspected pancreatic disease.

Case Study

You are called to see Alex, who was admitted yesterday with severe epigastric pain and a high amylase. Since then, he seems to have got worse and the nurses are worried about him as he is still in severe pain and his blood pressure is 84/52 mmHg. The nurses are asking you to review his management and whether he should be on a high-dependency unit.

Normal structure and function

The pancreas is situated retroperitoneally with the second part of the duodenum wrapping around the head. The tail of the pancreas lies over the spleen. The exocrine secretion is drained by a branching system of ducts, draining into the main pancreatic duct. This usually enters the second part of the duodenum together with the common bile duct at the ampulla of Vater. There is considerable anatomical variation.

The vast majority of the pancreatic cells are concerned with its exocrine function. Release of **secretin** from acid stimulation of the duodenum causes production of water, electrolytes and bicarbonate from the pancreas. **Cholecystokinin** is released when fat and amino acids enter the duodenum. As well as stimulating gall bladder contraction and relaxation of the sphincter of Oddi, it promotes pancreatic enzyme secretion and is trophic to the pancreas.

The main pancreatic enzymes and their substrates are:

- fat: lipase, phospholipase
- starch: amylase
- protein: chymotrypsin and trypsin. Importantly, these proteolytic enzymes are secreted in an inactive form and activation within the gland is seen with acute pancreatitis.

The endocrine function of the pancreas is served by the **islets of Langerhans**. Within these, most cells are beta-cells, secreting insulin. Others are alpha-cells, releasing glucagon, D-cells producing somatostatin and PP-cells secreting pancreatic polypeptide. Rarely, specific tumours of these cells produce symptoms through excess hormone production.

Pancreatitis

Inflammation of the pancreas can be acute or chronic; both of these can be relapsing.

Acute pancreatitis

You should always consider acute pancreatitis as a possible diagnosis in a patient with an acute abdomen and a cause can be found in at least 80% of cases of pancreatitis. Most cases are associated with either gall stones or high alcohol intake. There are other much rarer associations, such as with hyperlipidaemia, hyperparathyroidism, hypothermia, AIDS and drugs (e.g. corticosteroids). The trigger for the attack may be an alcoholic binge or passing of a gall stone causing a temporary increase in the intraductal pressure. Activation of phospholipase and proteases sets up an ongoing inflammatory response.

Clinical presentation

Abdominal pain is the dominant symptom, which is usually central/epigastric and may radiate through to the back. It is severe and the patient is often in great distress with pallor and sweating. Shock may develop with hypotension, poor peripheral perfusion and tachypnoea. Ask about possible triggers, as outlined above. On examination, other than the signs of shock, the patient will have tenderness, rigidity and guarding. Occasionally with severe haemorrhagic pancreatitis, there may be bruising in the flanks (**Grey–Turner's sign**) or around the umbilicus (**Cullen's sign**).

Investigations

The main differential diagnoses are:

- perforated peptic ulcer
- acute cholecystitis
- myocardial infarction.

Your investigations should exclude these and establish the diagnosis of acute pancreatitis as well as looking for evidence of complications. A rise in serum amylase more than fivefold above the upper limit of normal is highly specific for the diagnosis. An alternative is lipase (which is only produced by the pancreas). Lower rises occur with the other conditions and results should be considered in conjunction with the clinical features.

Other biochemical features indicating severe disease are hypoalbuminaemia, hypocalcaemia (corrected) and a rise in urea and creatinine (which may progress to overt acute renal failure). The blood sugar may be elevated and sometimes needs control with insulin. Prolongation of the prothrombin time, elevated fibrin degradation products (FDPs) and thrombocytopenia indicate disseminated intravascular coagulation (DIC). Hypoxia resulting from ventilation/perfusion mismatching and a metabolic acidosis are commonly found on blood gas analysis.

An ultrasound scan will help to exclude acute cholecystitis and identify gall stones. Ultrasound is relatively poor at identifying pancreatic disease, especially in the body or tail of the pancreas. A CT scan is better than ultrasound for visualising the pancreas and para-aortic nodes and is the imaging modality of choice. The pancreas may be oedematous with evidence of necrosis. Ascites may be present or there may be collections of fluid around the pancreas. A plain abdominal radiograph helps to exclude a perforated viscus and may show the *sentinel* sign of a distended loop of small bowel surrounding the pancreas.

Management

There is no specific treatment of pancreatitis other than supportive management:

- pain relief with opiates: avoid morphine as it causes spasm in the sphincter of Oddi
- nil by mouth, i.v. fluids, and antibiotics (probably reduces mortality)
- regular aspiration through a nasogastric tube: nausea and vomiting are common
- high-flow oxygen
- urgent ERCP in those with gall stones (particularly with obstruction or cholangitis).

The pain usually subsides after a couple of days. In severe cases, the patient may need to be admitted to the intensive care unit. In those patients with organ failure that persists for more than 48 hours, the mortality rate is over 50%, but it is very low for other patients. It is important to be aware of factors that predict a high mortality (Box 7).

Complications

Early complications These are shock, DIC, renal failure, hypoxia, ileus and hypo-/hyperglycaemia.

Late complications These include pseudocyst, ascites, pleural effusions (high amylase concentrations), abscess formation and candidaemia (p. 415).

Box 7: Indicators of poor prognosis in acute pancreatitis

Clinical features
- Age > 60 years
- Obesity
- Associated with gall stones
- Hypotension
- Grey–Turner sign*: flank bruising
- Cullen's sign*: periumbilical bruising
- Ascites (particularly if haemorrhagic)

Investigation results
- High C-reactive protein
- Low albumin
- Low corrected calcium (N.B. Hypercalcaemia is associated with pancreatitis)
- Low haemoglobin, high white cell count
- Increased blood glucose
- Increased serum urea
- Low arterial oxygen partial pressure (Po_2)

*Indicates haemorrhagic pancreatitis.

A pseudocyst may be suspected because of continuing ileus, pain and a smooth epigastric swelling. It is diagnosed using ultrasound and may require drainage, though most resolve spontaneously.

Abscesses have a high morbidity and mortality. The responsible organism is often *E. coli* and apart from broad-spectrum antibiotics (cefotaxime, metronidazole), drainage is required.

In patients with persistent symptoms and >30% pancreatic necrosis, aspiration, antibiotics, surgical debridement and necrosecting may be used.

Chronic pancreatitis

Chronic pancreatitis is strongly associated with heavy, continuing alcohol intake. It is also seen in patients with cystic fibrosis. In some patients the case is unknown. It is thought that protein plugs block the small ducts, leading to damage to the exocrine and endocrine cells. A large fibrotic response takes place, the ducts dilate and calcification occurs in the gland. The condition is non-reversible, but will stabilise if the person stops drinking.

Clinical presentation

The dominant symptom is chronic pain. It is usually centred around the upper abdomen but may radiate through to the back. Some patients find relief by sitting forward. The condition may run a relapsing and remitting course, with episodes of severe pain and features of acute pancreatitis.

You can predict the other symptoms from the functions of the pancreas. Malabsorption causes weight loss. Reduction in lipase secretion causes steatorrhoea. The patient complains of bulky offensive faeces that are difficult to flush away. Damage to the endocrine function leads to diabetes mellitus, which may be non-insulin-dependent or insulin-dependent, according to the degree of beta-cell damage.

Investigations

The main differential diagnosis is pancreatic carcinoma.

A plain radiograph may show intra-gland calcification. Ultrasound will demonstrate the small, shrunken fibrotic gland with ductal dilatation. Cysts may be present. An ERCP can show the disruption of the normal pancreatic anatomy, and MRCP is being increasingly used. A CT scan is usually abnormal in late disease but a normal scan is possible in early to moderate disease and so does not rule out the condition. The amylase levels are not usually raised except where the condition runs a relapsing course. Biochemical and haematological investigations may show evidence of malabsorption. Faecal fat collections will show the large increase in fat excretion.

Management

The course of the condition is long. The main therapeutic aims are to stop alcohol intake and to treat the symptoms.

The pain from chronic pancreatitis is often severe and may lead to depression. It commonly requires narcotic analgesics and patients may need the expertise of a pain clinic.

Malabsorption may be helped by pancreatic enzyme supplements. A histamine H_2 antagonist is used to prevent very low pH values occurring in the duodenum and limiting residual enzyme activity. Medium-chain triglycerides (MCT) are given, as these do not require breakdown before absorption. Supplementation with fat-soluble vitamins (A, D, E, K) may be needed.

Tumours

Benign (endocrine activity) tumours

The pancreas can give rise to a number of rare tumours that are hormonally active, e.g. VIPoma, glucagonoma, insulinoma.

Malignant tumours

Adenocarcinoma of the pancreas is rising in incidence. It is more common in males and with increasing age. The tumour is associated with smoking, but there are no other proven strong aetiological links. There are some cases in association with a familial/genetic predisposition. Most tumours are in the head of the pancreas.

Clinical presentation

Most patients present late in the course of the disease. Pain, similar to that of chronic pancreatitis, is common, as is painless obstructive jaundice. Many people simply present with lethargy and weight loss. On examination, the patient may be jaundiced, and often has hepatomegaly and/or an abdominal mass resulting from lymph node involvement. You may find ascites. A known association is thrombophlebitis, which may be superficial and migratory.

Investigations

Serum biochemistry may show a high alkaline phosphatase and bilirubin, but these are non-specific features. Ultrasound can usually demonstrate the tumour or metastatic spread. It can also guide a biopsy for histopathological confirmation. Sometimes CT, MRI, MRCP or ERCP may be useful.

Management

Operative resection is usually not feasible and, where resection is undertaken, the perioperative mortality is high and the results are poor. There are very few survivors at 5 years.

Surgery may help by creating biliary or intestinal bypass to alleviate the symptoms. ERCP can also be used to relieve jaundice by the insertion of stents. There is some evidence for palliation with gemcitabine as a single agent. Early and regular use of appropriate narcotic analgesics should be practised to prevent pain occurring rather than taking it away. There is also benefit from coeliac plexus block and advice from a pain specialist is useful.

Self-assessment: questions

Any or all of each set of five statements may be true or false. Choose your answers and see the reasoning behind the correct answer on pages 164–165.

Multiple choice questions

1. In the small intestine:
   a. If there is bile salt deficiency, micellar formation is reduced
   b. Long-chain triglycerides are transported from the gut in the lymph as chylomicrons
   c. There is no lymphatic tissue
   d. The entire mucosa is turned over every 2–3 weeks
   e. Is the site of most nutrient absorption

2. Histological features more consistent with ulcerative colitis than Crohn's disease are:
   a. Depleted goblet cells
   b. Crypt abscesses
   c. Granulomas
   d. Diffuse lymphocytic infiltrate
   e. Mucosal involvement only

3. Colorectal cancer:
   a. May arise from a metaplastic polyp
   b. Most often occurs in the rectum and sigmoid
   c. Entails further polyps in most cases
   d. Involving local lymph nodes does not affect prognosis
   e. With obstruction is more common in right-compared with left-sided lesions

4. Angiodysplasia of the colon:
   a. Is more common in the caecum and ascending colon
   b. Is associated with a macrocytic anaemia
   c. Is best shown by barium enema
   d. Usually requires surgery
   e. Is a congenital lesion

5. Causes of acute pancreatitis include:
   a. Alcohol
   b. Hypocalcaemia
   c. Hyperlipidaemia
   d. Self-poisoning with diazepam
   e. Endoscopic retrograde cholangiopancreatography (ERCP)

6. Recognised side-effects of sulfasalazine include:
   a. Irreversible oligospermia
   b. Haemolysis
   c. Folate deficiency
   d. Teratogenicity
   e. Acute pancreatitis

7. In coeliac disease:
   a. The patient will almost always have had symptoms since childhood
   b. Diagnosis is best on colonic biopsy
   c. There is an association with HLA-B8
   d. The diagnosis is incorrect if a patient fails to respond to a gluten-free diet
   e. There is a requirement for a diet free from wheat, barley and rye

8. Features of non-ulcer dyspepsia include:
   a. Epigastric pain
   b. Abdominal fullness after meals
   c. Response to proton pump inhibitors
   d. Being more common in men than women
   e. A clear clinical separation from peptic ulcer

9. Pseudomembranous colitis:
   a. Can only be diagnosed by sigmoidoscopy
   b. Is usually a relatively mild self-limited disease
   c. Can only be acquired in hospital
   d. Usually responds to treatment with oral metronidazole
   e. Has a >10% relapse rate after therapy

10. In a large ward where two of the nurses have had much vomiting and some diarrhoea over a 48-hour period, you should:
    a. Send the patients home
    b. Culture stools (and vomitus) for viruses
    c. Treat everyone with metronidazole
    d. Exclude visitors from the ward
    e. Prevent the patients (affected or not) leaving the ward for investigations, physiotherapy, etc.

11. The differential diagnosis of acute bloody diarrhoea includes:
    a. Amoebic dysentery
    b. *Campylobacter* enteritis
    c. Haemorrhagic colitis caused by *E. coli*
    d. Traveller's diarrhoea
    e. Cholera

12. The following episodes of illness should be reported to the local consultant in communicable disease control (CCDC):
    a. Rotavirus infection of a family
    b. A couple who both have acute diarrhoea and vomiting 3 days after an Indian meal
    c. A nursery nurse with *Salmonella* group D enteritis
    d. Three people admitted over 24 hours with acute vomiting who had attended a wedding reception 36 hours before

e. A teenager admitted with acute bronchospasm and laryngeal oedema after eating a Chinese spring roll containing prawns

13. The following are correct:
    a. Hepatitis B can be acquired from serous fluid from a wound
    b. Hepatitis C is not a cause of hepatocellular carcinoma
    c. Hepatitis A is a cause of chronic liver disease
    d. Hepatitis E can be acquired by sharing needles
    e. A person with only a hepatitis B core IgG test positive is infectious for hepatitis B

14. Direct complications of acute viral hepatitis include:
    a. Aplastic anaemia
    b. Fulminant hepatic failure
    c. Chronic hepatitis
    d. Renal failure
    e. Fetal death during pregnancy

15. The following are causes of chronic hepatitis:
    a. Hepatitis C
    b. Deficiency of α_1-antitrypsin
    c. Gilbert's syndrome
    d. Sarcoidosis
    e. Rifampicin therapy

16. A 'fatty liver' may represent:
    a. An obese person
    b. Alcoholism
    c. Hepatitis C infection
    d. Acute vitamin A poisoning
    e. An ultrasound artefact

17. With regard to cirrhosis of the liver:
    a. Oesophageal varices are almost always present
    b. There is a >60% likelihood of GI bleeding
    c. It may be caused by schistosomiasis
    d. If itching is a prominent symptom, the diagnosis is likely to be primary biliary cirrhosis
    e. It may cause low-grade fever, without apparent infection

18. Complications of acute liver failure include:
    a. Cerebral oedema
    b. Bleeding
    c. Drug hypersensitivity
    d. Candidaemia
    e. Hypoglycaemia

Single best answer multiple choice questions

For each numbered option, only ONE of the options lettered a–e is correct.

1. You are asked to see a 31-year-old woman who is 36 weeks pregnant. She is complaining of passing fresh blood per rectum when she goes to the toilet. There has also been a lot of itching and pain. What is the most likely diagnosis?
   a. Rectal prolapse
   b. Crohn's disease
   c. Fissure in ano
   d. Diverticular disease
   e. Haemorrhoids

2. A 65-year-old woman presents to the accident and emergency department with a 4-hour history of severe periumbilical pain. On examination, her pulse is 130 beats/min irregularly irregular, blood pressure is 84/52 mmHg and she has marked tenderness on central abdominal palpation. What is the most likely diagnosis?
   a. Cholecystitis
   b. Arterial embolism
   c. Perforated peptic ulcer
   d. Acute pancreatitis
   e. Ruptured aortic aneurysm

3. A 41-year-old woman presents to the accident and emergency department with history of increasing abdominal pain since the previous day. She is known to the gastroenterologists as she has a 15-year history of ulcerative colitis. On examination, her pulse is 120 beats/min regular, blood pressure 92/64 mmHg and temperature 37.9°C. There is marked abdominal distension, particularly in the flanks, with some rebound tenderness and a reduction in bowel sounds. What is the most likely diagnosis?
   a. Pseudomembranous colitis
   b. Sigmoid volvulus
   c. Toxic megacolon
   d. Intussusception of the large bowel
   e. Diverticular abscess

4. A 22-year-old woman is seen by her general practitioner because of a 4-month history of episodes of lower abdominal pain and loose motions. She has lost about 3 kg in weight during this time. In the past, she has had a perianal abscess. What is the most likely diagnosis?
   a. Ulcerative colitis
   b. Endometriosis
   c. Irritable bowel disease
   d. Crohn's disease
   e. Pelvic inflammatory disease

5. An 85-year-old woman is admitted with jaundice. She has also not been well for a few days with some right hypochondrial pain and 'shivers and shakes'. On examination, her temperature is 38.5°C and she is tender in the right hypochondrium, but there are no masses. Result of investigations are:

Haemoglobin 129 g/l
White cell count 16.4 (predominantly neutrophils)
Alanine amino transferase 83 IU/l
Alkaline phosphatase 867 IU/l
Bilirubin 89 μmol/l

What would be the best initial investigation to establish the diagnosis?

a. Ultrasound
b. ERCP
c. MRCP
d. CT scan
e. Plain abdominal radiograph

Extended matched questions

EMQ 1

Theme: Diagnostic tests
Options
1. Barium swallow
2. Colonoscopy
3. CT scan of abdomen
4. Endoscopic retrograde cholangiopancreatography (ERCP)
5. Erect chest radiograph
6. Flexible sigmoidoscopy
7. Gastroscopy
8. Jejunal biopsy
9. Liver biopsy
10. Ultrasound of the abdomen

For patients A–E select the test that is most likely to establish the diagnosis.

A. A 76-year old man has had altered bowel habit for about 3 months. On examination, there is nothing abnormal in the abdomen, but on rectal examination, you can feel something firm at the tip of your finger and there is blood on the glove. The prostate feels normal.

B. A 53-year-old man with severe inflammatory arthritis presents with sudden onset of severe upper abdominal pain. On examination, he is shocked, his abdomen is rigid with marked guarding and rebound tenderness in the epigastrium.

C. A 47-year-old woman with a known heavy alcohol intake presents with a severe haematemesis. On examination, her pulse is 110 beats/min regular and blood pressure is 94/62 mmHg. There are no abnormalities on abdominal examination apart from mild splenomegaly.

D. An otherwise fit 85-year-old woman has had an unexplained iron deficiency anaemia for several months. On examination, there are no abnormalities. A recent gastroscopy was normal.

E. A 57-year-old man presents with severe upper abdominal pain and weight loss over the previous 3 months. The pain radiates through to his back. There is no previous history and he is a non-drinker. On examination, there are no abnormalities.

EMQ 2

Theme: Next step in treatment
Options
1. Azathioprine
2. Bendroflumethiazide
3. Captopril
4. Cefotaxime
5. Corticosteroid enemas
6. Ispaghula husk (Fybogel)
7. Furosemide
8. Lactulose
9. Mannitol
10. Metronidazole
11. Nystatin suspension
12. Octreotide
13. Omeprazole
14. Propranolol
15. Ranitidine
16. Senna
17. Spironolactone

For patients A–E with alcoholism, suggest the next step in treatment.

A. A 33-year-old woman with constipation over several weeks. On examination, you find that her colon is loaded with faeces and she has soft faeces filling the rectum.

B. A 68-year-old man presents in a malnourished state. He is complaining of pain on swallowing. On examination, you find that his pharynx is red. Oesophagoscopy shows diffuse oesophagitis with white patches.

C. A 63-year-old man presents with increasing swelling of his abdomen. On examination, you demonstrate shifting dullness and a fluid thrill. He is otherwise well and is apyrexial.

D. A 25-year-old man presents with severe haematemesis. On examination, he is continuing to bleed and his condition is deteriorating despite resuscitation.

E. A 53-year-old man has developed a burning retrosternal pain, which is worse when he lies flat. On examination, there is nothing to find. A gastroscopy shows a severe oesophagitis with some ulceration just above the sphincter. Biopsies show no evidence of a carcinoma.

EMQ 3

Theme: Liver enlargement

Options

1. Acute infective hepatitis
2. Acute poisoning
3. Alcoholic cirrhosis
4. Hepatoma
5. Haemochromatosis
6. Heart failure
7. Metabolic syndrome (syndrome X)
8. Metastatic liver disease
9. Polycythaemia rubra vera
10. Primary hepatocellular carcinoma
11. Primary biliary cirrhosis

For each case, choose the most likely cause of the hepatic enlargement.

A. A 60-year-old woman is seen in the outpatient department because of itching, which she had developed over the previous 3 months. She has also been very tired. On examination, she has excoriation of the skin and is pigmented. There are also xanthelasma.

B. A 70-year-old man with a body mass index of 30 kg/m² is seen because of possible angina. In his investigations, his random blood sugar is 17.2 mmol/l.

C. A 78-year-old woman is readmitted to hospital because of severe breathlessness, leg oedema and some right hypochondrial pain. She was only discharged 3 weeks ago following admission with an acute myocardial infarction. On examination, she has tender hepatomegaly.

D. An 82-year-old woman is seen in the outpatient clinic because of a transient ischaemic attack (TIA) 1 week earlier. On examination, she has hepatosplenomegaly. She also tells you that she tends to itch when she is having a bath, which has been puzzling her.

E. A 59-year-old man with longstanding cirrhosis is seen in clinic. On examination, you find that he has an enlarged irregular liver.

Objective structured clinical examination (OSCE) stations

OSCE 1

This is a station for abdominal examination.

Examiner: I would like you to examine this patient's abdomen. You do not have to examine the groin/pubis area. Please talk me through what you are doing and any abnormalities you find.

During the examination, the following dialogue takes place.

Student: There seems to be a mass in both the right and left hypochondrium.

Examiner: So what do you think they are?

Student: Probably hepatosplenomegaly.

Examiner: So why do you think that?

Student: Well, in the right hypochondrium, I can feel a smooth edge moving with respiration approximately 4 cm below the costal margin. There is also a similar area of dullness to percussion, which is continuous with the area of liver dullness over the chest. In the left hypochondrium, there is a mass that moves with respiration and is extending down about 6 cm towards the right iliac fossa. I cannot get above it.

Examiner: If you were not sure whether it was a spleen, are there any manoeuvres that would help in the examination?

Student: I can ask the patient to roll on to their left side with their knees drawn up.

Examiner: How would that help?

Student: The spleen falls away from the costal margin and is easy to feel — particularly if it is just 'tippable'.

Examiner: Why is it not a kidney?

Student: Well, it is not ballotable and over the kidney there is sometimes an area of resonance because of the overlying bowel.

Examiner: Carry on with the examination.

OSCE 2

Station 1

Examiner: Please take a history from this 46-year-old woman who has been brought to her general practitioner because her husband thinks that she is drinking excessively.

History (observed by examiner): When you introduce yourself, you notice that she appears a bit anxious and withdrawn.

She tells you that she usually drinks about half to one bottle of wine in the evening 'with my meal' and finishes the bottle when she is watching television. She does say that this has increased a bit over the last few months and she looks forward to opening the bottle in the evening, but she finds that it does not relax her as much as it used to. After a row with her husband over her drinking, she did agree to stop, but had to start again after a few days as she felt too shaky. Sometimes this happens in the morning (and she has had a drink to 'calm her nerves'). Because of the row, she often hides a bottle away in the kitchen so that she can drink when she is cooking. There have also been quite a few rows about money, but then she drinks to forget these.

She and her husband used to have a good social life, but after a few quite drunken evenings, their friends have not been in contact and seem to be avoiding them. Anyway, she does not feel like going out of the house much these days except for things like appointments (though she forgot the dentist's recently).

On direct questioning, she does agree that she feels 'a bit low' and has not been sleeping too well.

Station 2
Examiner:
  a. What is your differential diagnosis?
  b. What particular features suggests alcohol dependence?
  c. If she has depression, how would you manage it?
  d. How would you manage her alcohol withdrawal (if she agrees)?

OSCE 3

This is a combined abdominal examination and results station.

Examiner: Please examine this (male) patient's hands and comment as you do so.
Student: The patient has bilateral palmar erythema and Dupuytren's contracture of the fourth finger on the right hand.
Examiner: Please comment on his nails.
Student: The nails are well looked after without obvious disease, damager or pitting, but they may be a little pale.
Examiner: Now look at these results and comment (she hands the student a set of results):

Bilirubin	19 (1–20 µmol)
Albumin	22 (33–49 g/l)
Globulin	45 (21–38 g/l)
Alkaline phosphatase	145 (25–110 IU/l)
Alanine amino transferase	62 (5–45 IU/l)
Creatinine	98 (60–120 µmol/l)
Urea	4.3 (2.7–7.5 mmol/l)

Student: He has a very low albumin and slightly elevated alkaline phosphatase and ALT.
Examiner: If you were to examine this patient's abdomen what might you find?
Student: A swollen abdomen with ascites and an enlarged and tender liver. No splenomegaly. No jaundice.
Examiner: What do you think the unifying diagnosis is for the hands and biochemistry abnormalities?
Student: Probably cirrhosis of the liver, caused by alcohol.

Case history questions

Case history 1

You see a 79-year-old woman in the general medicine outpatient clinic because of poor mobility. It transpires that this is because of marked osteoarthrosis of both knees. A full blood count shows a haemoglobin of 108 g/l and a mean cell volume (MCV) of 70 µl.

1. What would you do now?

A few days later, you are on call and she presents to the accident and emergency department with brisk rectal bleeding.

2. What should you do?

Subsequently, a barium enema does not show any abnormalities other than severe diverticular disease. She is keen to go home and when you review her 4 weeks later, she still has a significant iron-deficient anaemia.

3. Outline a management plan.

Case history 2

You are a house officer on call for medicine. A 69-year-old woman presents with severe, constant, low central chest pain of several hours' duration. The only medical history of note is that she is awaiting a cholecystectomy for gall stones. She also admits to drinking 'a couple of bottles of sherry a week'.

1. What are you going to do now?
2. A diagnosis of acute pancreatitis is made; how would you treat this?

She is making a reasonable recovery, but when you examine her at 7 days, she has a smooth swelling in her epigastrium.

3. What do you think this is and what actions should you take?

Case history 3

A 27-year-old i.v. drug abuser is admitted with cellulitis of his left groin. You treat him with cefuroxime and metronidazole and his skin improves. However, his liver function tests remain abnormal as follows (normal range in parentheses):

Bilirubin 16 (1–20 IU/l)
Albumin 32 (35–50 IU/l)
Alkaline phosphatase 101 (30–130 IU/l)
Aspartate aminotransferase 123 (11–55 IU/l)
Gamma-glutamyl transpeptidase 63 (10–43 IU/l)

1. What is your initial differential diagnosis?
2. What other tests would you request?
3. What would you advise with respect to sexual practice?

Case history 4

You admit a verbose marketing executive, 39 years old, to hospital one evening because of a possible head injury. He weighs 95 kg and vital signs are temperature 36.8°C, pulse 95 beats/min regular, blood pressure 130/95 mmHg, respiratory rate 14/min. He has a 2 cm laceration on his left temple and his clothes are filthy, as he fell in the rain on his way home from work. He has no other signs of injury or abnormalities on neurological or general examination.

His plain skull radiographs are normal and so you arrange 2-hourly neurological observations and an overnight stay.

You are telephoned at 6.30 a.m. by the night sister because your patient tried to get up and leave but fell over and bruised his left thigh. He is being argumentative. He looks pale and sweaty and appears anxious and jittery. You try to examine him neurologically, but he is uncooperative. His pulse is 130 beats/min and weak and his respiratory rate 24/min. His thigh has a large bruise on it. He insists on going home, although he does not appear rational.

1. What are your diagnostic considerations?
2. What should you do?

An hour later he is calmer and willing to undergo further tests.

3. What additional history would you like?
4. How might you obtain a more complete history?
5. What further tests and assessments would you want to do?

Case history 5

You admit a 44-year-old Pakistani woman from accident and emergency with a low-grade fever and bloody diarrhoea. She arrived from Lahore 2 days previously. The stool is offensive and contains blood and mucus. She has moderate left lower quadrant pain on deep palpation.

1. What are the three most likely pathogens?
2. What are three useful tests you can do that evening?

You admit her to hospital and treat her initially with i.v. fluids and oral rehydration solution (e.g. Dioralyte). The next morning she is more unwell and still has bloody diarrhoea.

3. What specific tests can the laboratory do on her stool to help you make a therapeutic decision?

Case history 6

You are called to a ward you are covering on a Sunday because two patients have developed diarrhoea. One is 76 years old and came in 3 days ago from a nursing home where she had not responded to oral cefalexin for a cough. She has been treated with intravenous and oral ampicillin since admission. The other patient is a 'long-stay' case who is bed- and chair-bound following a stroke 10 weeks ago. She has an indwelling urinary catheter.

The nurse in charge tells you that the diarrhoea is voluminous in both but not bloody. The fluid intake in both patients is suboptimal. She has started fluid charts on both.

1. What should you do now with respect to the management of each patient?
2. If you decide to treat one or other patient, what should you use?
3. What action should the nurse in charge take with respect to the patients?

Case history 7

You see a 57-year-old man in the outpatient clinic who is complaining of a feeling of incomplete emptying when he goes to pass a motion. He has had some constipation over the last 4 months and has been taking regular senna. In the past, he has had some heartburn and investigations showed a mild iron deficiency anaemia. He has been on regular iron therapy for 6 months. On examination, you find that his descending colon is full of faeces, but his rectum is empty on per rectum examination.

1. What would be your initial management plan?
2. Figure 37 is one of the films from his barium enema:
   a. What are the abnormalities?
   b. What is the likely diagnosis?

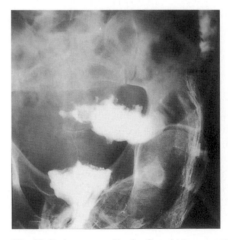

Fig. 37 Barium enema film for Case history question 7.

Key features questions

1. A 19-year-old drunken female student comes to the accident and emergency department late on a Friday night with a history of vomiting that started with food; she is now vomiting fresh blood. Her boyfriend says that she has been drinking a lot since coming to university a couple of years previously. On examination, her pulse is 90 beats/min and her blood pressure is 120/72 mmHg, falling to 116/70 when sitting up.

List three features that are crucial to assessing blood loss. What is the most likely diagnosis and why?

2. A 43-year-old man is seen at his general practitioner with abdominal pain that has been present on and off for about 2 months. He describes it as a gnawing pain that does not radiate and seems to come on a couple of hours after eating. His weight has been steady, though he has vomited with the pain quite regularly over the last few weeks. The GP notices that the patient did consult with one of her partners a few years ago and he admits to taking Gaviscon from time to time. He is a smoker and drinks a couple of pints on Friday and Saturday nights. On examination, there is minimal epigastric tenderness but no masses, and the liver does not appear enlarged. The GP takes blood for a full blood count and this shows:

Haemoglobin 131 g/l
Mean cell volume 88 fl
Platelets 340
White cell count 8.7×10^9/l

Give three features that the GP uses in deciding whether to refer this man for an urgent endoscopy.

3. You are the house officer (foundation trainee) on call for medicine and are asked to see a 56-year-old woman who has come to the accident and emergency department with severe abdominal pain that is radiating through to her back. The pain has been present constantly for about 24 hours and is getting worse. In the previous medical history, she was diagnosed with gall stones a couple of years ago on a scan for abdominal pain (which she says is totally different to the pain she is now getting). She is a lifelong non-smoker and teetotaller. She is not on any drugs. On examination, she is obese and in pain. Her temperature is 36.8°C, pulse 120 beats/min regular and blood pressure 98/60 mmHg. In her abdomen, there is marked epigastric tenderness, but no guarding or rebound. Her investigations show:

Oxygen saturation (air) 91%
pH 7.29
$PaCO_2$ 4.5 kPa (33 mm Hg)
PaO_2 10.8 kPa (81 mm Hg)
Haemoglobin 109 g/l
White cell count 17×10^9/l (predominantly neutrophils)

Blood glucose (random) 11.4 mmol/l
Amylase 1500 IU/l
Corrected calcium 2.5 mmol/l
Bilirubin 10 µmol/l
Aspartate aminotransferase 40 IU/l
Alkaline phosphatase 90 IU/l
Urea 5.4 mmol/l
Na 137 mmol/l
K 4.5 mmol/l

What key features would you use to assess her prognosis?

4. The following histopathological report is received on a patient with a 3-month history of bloody diarrhoea:
   The specimens consist of several samples of large bowel mucosa. All show abnormalities of the glandular architecture. Crypt abscesses are present with inflammation and evidence of ulceration. There is a diffuse inflammatory infiltrate in the lamina propria, but this does not extend into the submucosa. There is depletion of the goblet cells. No granulomata are seen.

What four key features would you use in making the histopathological diagnosis?

Data interpretation questions

Table 39 gives the liver function test results for nine patients whose presenting complaints are shown below. Suggest a diagnosis for each patient.

1. Vomiting patient 22 years of age, referred by GP
2. A 47-year-old with fever and abdominal pain
3. A 19-year-old college student with sore throat
4. A 44-year-old hill walker admitted with fever
5. A 52-year-old retailing executive investigated for ankle swelling
6. An intensive care unit patient (third week) with acute respiratory distress syndrome and renal impairment just started on haemofiltration

Table 39 Liver function test results for nine patients (normal range in parentheses) for data interpretation

Patient	1	2	3	4	5	6	7	8	9
Bilirubin (1–20 µmol/l)	123	145	45	48	16	22	75	11	9
Albumin (35–50 g/l)	34	31	38	29	21	23	19	39	43
Alkaline phosphatase (30–130 IU/l)	165	470	135	210	95	220	350	75	92
Aspartate aminotransferase (11–55 IU/l)	2365	227	550	350	65	195	750	110	27
Creatinine (blood 60–120 µmol/l)	92	75	80	225	125	370	225	75	95
International normalised ratio (≤1.0)	1.2	1.1	1.1	1.9	2.5	1.5	4.8	1.0	1.1
White cell count (4–11×10⁹/l)	4.3	17.1	9.3	15.3	7.4	13.4	12.5	8.5	6.3

7. A 21-year-old evasive unemployed woman 72 hours after acute admission with vague abdominal pain and unwell

8. A 'routine' blood test preoperation on a 49-year-old woman who had a major car accident 12 years ago

9. A 44-year-old male ex-prisoner, now a car mechanic with 2 cm hepatomegaly

Picture questions

1. Figure 38 is a CT scan of the liver in a 69-year-old woman with a pyrexia of unknown origin (PUO) of 2 weeks' duration. She has mildly deranged liver function tests, a total white cell count of $12.8 \times 10^9/l$ with 80% neutrophils, mild normochromic normocytic anaemia, an erythrocyte sedimentation rate (ESR) of 68 mm/hr and a serum albumin of 29 g/l. She has no abnormal physical findings.

   a. Describe the abnormality.
   b. What is the likely diagnosis?
   c. What investigations are now appropriate (give two)?
   d. How should she be managed?

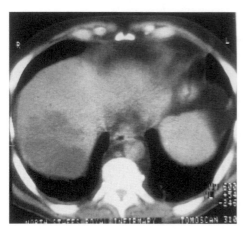

Fig. 38 A CT scan of the liver for Picture question 1.

2. Figure 39 is a chest radiograph taken preoperatively of a 78-year-old man, who is having peripheral vascular surgery.

   a. Give three abnormalities.
   b. What action should be taken?

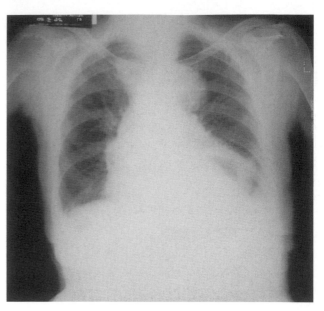

Fig. 39 A chest radiograph for Picture question 2.

3. Figure 40 is a barium enema in a 25-year-old woman with a 6-month history of general malaise, weight loss and bloody diarrhoea with mucus.

   a. Describe the abnormalities.
   b. What is the diagnosis?
   c. What would be your initial management?

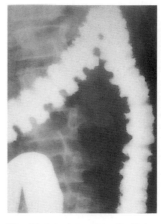

Fig. 40 A barium enema for Picture question 3.

Short notes

Write short notes on the following:

1. A patient is admitted from outpatients who is said to be malnourished and malabsorption is suspected. Outline your approach, including the investigations that you would initially request.

2. A 64-year-old man in the outpatient clinic was diagnosed as having a peptic ulcer 8 weeks previously at endoscopy. Unfortunately, he is still

complaining of the same symptoms of upper abdominal pain. What should be done?

3. What is your management plan for a patient with jaundice and severe pain caused by a carcinoma of the pancreas which is inoperable?

4. You see a man of 48 years in clinic who is complaining of difficulty in swallowing. Discuss the key features that you will want to explore with him.

5. You have requested an ultrasound scan on a 75-year-old woman with a suspected aortic aneurysm. The report comes back 'Aorta clearly seen, no aneurysm. Multiple stones seen in the gall bladder'. What are you going to do?

6. Discuss the different therapies used in inflammatory bowel disease. What would you use to maintain remission in a patient with ulcerative colitis? What side-effects would you discuss with the patient?

Self-assessment: answers

Multiple choice answers

1. a. **True.** Bile salts are essential for micelle formation.
    b. **False.** Fat is broken down to monoglycerides and fatty acids in the gut, absorbed across the cell and then re-esterified to short-chain triglycerides for transport as chylomicrons.
    c. **False.** Lymphatic tissue is prominent in the gut, e.g. Peyer's patches.
    d. **False.** The gut turns over its mucosa every 2–3 days.
    e. **True.** The small intestine is the main area for the breakdown and absorption of nutrients.

2. a. **True.** Goblet cells are depleted in ulcerative colitis.
    b. **True.** Ulcerative colitis is a mucosal disease associated with crypt abscesses.
    c. **False.** Granulomas are uncommon.
    d. **False.** A polymorph infiltration occurs.
    e. **True.** Ulcerative colitis is a superficial inflammation which is continuous from the rectum.

3. a. **False.** Metaplastic polyps have no malignant potential.
    b. **True.**
    c. **False.** Additional polyps do occur but only in about one-third of patients.
    d. **False.** Prognosis is assessed by Duke's staging; lymph node involvement is stage 3 with <60% 5-year survival.
    e. **False.** Rectal bleeding and obstruction are more common with left-sided lesions.

4. a. **True.** It usually occurs in the right side of the colon.
    b. **False.** It causes iron deficiency anaemia.
    c. **False.** It is visualised on colonoscopy.
    d. **False.** There is no effective specific treatment but diathermy can be used.
    e. **False.** It is an acquired abnormality of the vascular system.

5. a. **True.** Most cases are associated with gall stones or high alcohol intake.
    b. **False.** Hypocalcaemia can occur during acute attacks, but *hypercalcaemia* is a cause of acute pancreatitis.
    c. **True.** There is an association with hyperlipidaemia, but it is an uncommon cause.
    d. **False.**
    e. **True.** ERCP is used in the diagnosis of pancreatic and biliary disease but can precipitate an acute attack.

6. a. **False.** Causes reversible oligospermia.
    b. **True.** In a small number of patients.
    c. **True.**
    d. **False.** It is safe in pregnancy.
    e. **True.**

7. a. **False.** Peaks of incidence occur in young children and in adults aged 20–40 years.
    b. **False.** A duodenal or jejunal biopsy is needed.
    c. **True.** It is associated with HLA-B8 and HLA-DRW3 antigens.
    d. **False.** Failure to respond to diet usually means poor compliance, but secondary lactose intolerance, associated infection and nutritional deficiencies should also be considered.
    e. **True.** All contain gluten.

8. a. **True.** Both ulcers and non-ulcer dyspepsia give epigastric pain.
    b. **True.**
    c. **True.** Patients do respond to proton pump inhibitors and this cannot be used as a diagnostic test to separate non-ulcer dyspepsia from that caused by a peptic ulcer.
    d. **False.** Women are more often affected.
    e. **False.** There is no way of differentiating clinically.

9. a. **True.** It is a visual/pathological diagnosis. However, *Clostridium difficile*-related diarrhoea can be diagnosed by detecting cytotoxin in stool, and pseudomembranous colitis inferred.
    b. **False.** It is often fatal in the elderly debilitated patient; it requires treatment.
    c. **False.** However, most infections are acquired in hospital.
    d. **True.** Over 90% response rate (but not 100%).
    e. **True.** However, these patients usually respond to retreatment with oral metronidazole or vancomycin.

10. a. **False.** Impracticable and would further spread the likely cause.
    b. **False.** The likely cause is norovirus (Norwalk virus) or another of the 'small round structured viruses' (SRSVs), which are diagnosed by electron microscopy, polymerase chain reaction or enzyme-linked immunosorbent assay and are not cultured.
    c. **False.** *Cl. difficile* diarrhoea is the most important differential diagnosis but vomiting is less common with this and it rarely affects the staff, so a viral aetiology is more likely. You would send stools for detection of *Cl. difficile* toxin, though.
    d. **True.** To prevent further spread, unless necessary for, say, a dying patient.

e. **True.** Unless the investigation was absolutely vital.

11. a. **True.** This has much mucus and tenesmus.

   b. **True.** The amount of blood is usually small.

   c. **True.** The classic cause, with mostly blood and little stool and no fever.

   d. **False.** This is a watery diarrhoea caused by *E. coli*.

   e. **False.** Cholera has very watery diarrhoea in large volumes (rice-water stool).

12. a. **True.** Although rotaviruses can be transmitted via many routes, only one of which is food and water.

   b. **True.** This is likely to be *Campylobacter* because of the incubation period; the CCDCs will instruct environmental health officers to inspect the restaurant. There may also be other cases you do not know about.

   c. **True.** *Salmonella* infection is notifiable, and given her work with small babies who are at risk of *Salmonella* meningitis, etc., she should not be allowed back to work until her stools are negative.

   d. **True.** Notify by telephone as it may be a large outbreak with affected people spread all over the country. The caterers will need to be inspected. The investigation by the CCDCs may form the basis of a prosecution by the bride's family (also consider alcoholic gastritis!).

   e. **False.** Clearly the patient is allergic to something in the spring roll, possibly prawns. He needs to be referred to an allergist/immunologist for detailed advice on what foods to avoid, etc.

13. a. **True.** This is the likely mode of horizontal transmission among siblings in developing countries.

   b. **False.** Hepatitis C can lead to chronic liver disease and its sequelae (see Fig. 32).

   c. **False.** Hepatitis A causes an acute self-limiting disease.

   d. **False.** It is a waterborne disease.

   e. **False.** Only those who are HBsAg-positive are infectious.

14. a. **True.** Generally rare but life-threatening and more common in Asia.

   b. **True.** It only occurs in about 1 in 2000 jaundiced patients with hepatitis A.

   c. **True.** If hepatitis B and C viruses are involved.

   d. **False.** Unless the patient first has fulminant hepatic failure. If renal impairment or failure is present, consider leptospirosis, haemolytic uraemic syndrome or acute poisoning, e.g. paracetamol.

   e. **True.** But only in hepatitis E, which is often severe and life-threatening in pregnancy.

15. a. **True.** About 20% of hepatitis C infections lead to cirrhosis.

   b. **True.** This is rare and untreatable.

   c. **False.** Gilbert's syndrome involves a rise in unconjugated bilirubin only.

   d. **True.** Granulomatous hepatitis, usually evidence of disease in other organs.

   e. **False.** A cause of acute hepatitis. It is vital to stop rifampicin (and isoniazid) or seek immediate expert help if abnormal liver function tests are found in patients taking these.

16. a. **True.** Increasingly common (non-alcoholic fatty liver — NAFL — or non-alcoholic steatohepatitis — NASH). It is part of the metabolic syndrome (syndrome X) which links obesity, type 2 diabetes and cardiovascular disease, possibly due to insulin resistance.

   b. **True.** A common 'early' abnormality.

   c. **True.**

   d. **False.** Vitamin A poisoning is caused by eating fish or polar bear liver and causes severe headache, cerebral oedema, flushing of the face and skin, peeling of the nose and, in severe cases, death. Chronic vitamin A ingestion may lead to cirrhosis.

   e. **False.** But is often found on ultrasound.

17. a. **True.** As a result of portal hypertension.

   b. **False.** About one-third of patients develop bleeding varices. Sometimes they have gastric ulcers or other causes of bleeding.

   c. **True.** In Asia and Africa: *Schistosoma japonicum* and *S. mansoni*.

   d. **True.**

   e. **True.** But beware subacute bacterial peritonitis, tuberculosis and other occult infections.

18. a. **True.** The most likely cause of death.

   b. **True.** Especially nose bleeds and/or GI bleeding.

   c. **False.** Although drug toxicity is a problem because of failure to metabolise many drugs.

   d. **True.** However, it usually follows serious bacterial infection.

   e. **True.** Blood glucose requires constant monitoring and treatment.

Single best answer multiple choice answers

1. **e is correct.** Rectal prolapse and diverticular disease are both problems that occur at an older age. There is no other history that might suggest Crohn's disease (even though perianal problems are a feature). Pain is the dominant feature in a fissure. Haemorrhoids are common in pregnancy, and pruritus, as well as bleeding and pain, is common.

2. **b is correct.** The main clue is the irregular pulse, signifying atrial fibrillation. Patients have a risk of

arterial embolisation leading to bowel infarction and shock as the bowel dies. It is a surgical emergency and requires bowel resection. If she survives and the major part of her small intestine has been removed, then she may have a short bowel syndrome requiring nutritional support.

3. **c is correct.** This is a descriptive term for dilatation of the colon in association with an acute toxic colitis. The principle features are a non-obstructive dilatation of the colon accompanied by systemic toxicity (e.g. fever, tachycardia and hypotension). It can complicate conditions causing colitis. In elderly patients, a common cause is pseudomembranous colitis (*Clostridium difficile*), but in this patient there is no history of recent antibiotic use. One precipitating factor in patients with ulcerative colitis is discontinuation of maintenance treatment (e.g. sulfasalazine or 5-aminosalicylic acid).

4. **d is correct.** The history is consistent with inflammatory bowel disease, particularly with the weight loss (though you should check that this has not been intentional). Both endometriosis and pelvic inflammatory disease cause lower abdominal pain and occasionally can be associated with altered bowel habit. The pointer to Crohn's disease is the previous history of a perianal abscess.

5. **a is correct.** The patient history and examination suggest biliary sepsis and the liver function tests are consistent with biliary obstruction. The most likely cause is gall stones (although a carcinoma of the head of the pancreas could present with an ascending cholangitis).

Extended matched answers

EMQ 1

A. **6.** In a patient with altered bowel habit, the first examination is often a barium enema or a colonoscopy. However, there is an abnormality on rectal examination in this patient that should be easily visible on flexible sigmoidoscopy and can be biopsied.

B. **5.** The history is of an acute abdomen with pointers towards the upper GI tract. The arthritis suggests treatment with non-steroidal anti-inflammatory drugs (NSAIDs), which would predispose to a perforated peptic ulcer. The presence of free gas under the diaphragm would confirm the perforated viscus.

C. **7.** The alcohol intake and splenomegaly are strongly suggestive of varices. Although a liver biopsy might confirm cirrhosis, this is not the immediate concern. A barium swallow would show oesophageal varices but would not allow direct treatment.

D. **2.** In this patient, the most important diagnostic task is to examine the colon thoroughly. Caecal carcinomas often do not cause obstructive symptoms but present with an unexplained anaemia. Similarly,

colonic angiodysplasia is best diagnosed by direct visualisation after good bowel preparation.

E. **10.** The history might suggest gastric pathology, but pain radiating through to the back is typical of pancreatic disease (particularly carcinoma). Chronic pancreatitis may present with severe unremitting pain, but there is no previous history and he does not drink.

EMQ 2

A. **16.** In this patient, there is no evidence of any serious cause of constipation. The motion is soft, so a stimulant laxative would be the first treatment (as well as stopping any drugs causing constipation — if this is possible).

B. **11.** The history, examination and endoscopy findings all point to *Candida* infection.

C. **17.** There are no clues suggestive of bacterial peritonitis. Ascites should initially be treated with bed rest, salt restriction and spironolactone.

D. **12.** In this situation, it is reasonable to assume that the cause of his bleeding is varices (while organising a gastroscopy). In a deteriorating situation, you need to reduce his portal venous pressure quickly — terlipressin (glypressin) or octreotide can be used (as well as contacting the intensive care team).

E. **13.** The severity of his oesophagitis warrants treatment with a proton pump inhibitor.

EMQ 3

A. **11.** Tiredness is a dominant feature with pruritus developing due to the bile salt deposition in the skin. About 25% of patients will have an enlarged liver (also splenomegaly due to portal hypertension).

B. **7.** There is increasing recognition of the link between obesity (particular central distribution — waist size), heart disease, type 2 diabetes and fatty infiltration of the liver. This is also known as non-alcoholic fatty liver disease (NAFLD) and is linked to insulin resistance.

C. **6.** Only the liver capsule has pain fibres and acute stretching of these due to liver congestion (e.g. heart failure) or hepatic necrosis (viral, poisoning or alcoholic binge) can cause severe pain with tenderness.

D. **9.** Patients with PRV can present with thrombotic events such as strokes or TIAs. On examination, splenomegaly may be detected (hepatomegaly less common). Itching when hot is a particular feature.

E. **10.** Alcoholic liver disease is a possibility, but a patient with longstanding cirrhosis would be expected to have a shrunken, non-palpable liver. An irregular liver edge points towards a tumour and fits best with a hepatocellular carcinoma developing in a cirrhotic liver rather than metastatic disease or a benign hepatoma.

Responses to OSCE stations

OSCE 1

Clearly, this student is doing very well!

Hepatosplenomegaly is often a stable physical sign, so patients can be brought up for examinations and reasonable consistency can be achieved for each student in the degree of difficulty of the patient he/she is asked to examine.

The key steps in examining the abdomen are:

- inspection: general, hands, head and neck, abdomen
- position of patient
- palpation
  - general
  - liver
  - spleen
  - kidneys
- percussion
  - shifting dullness
  - liver
  - bladder
- auscultation
- hernia orifices
- genitalia
- rectal examination.

Suggestions for further practice Apart from gastrointestinal and liver clinics, other specialties in which you will encounter patients with abdominal signs include:

- Haematology clinics: you will find many patients with hepatosplenomegaly, and the clinics are the best places to convince yourself of what an enlarged spleen feels like.
- Renal units: easily palpable kidneys are rare in general medicine; in an examination, the most likely cause of enlarged kidneys would be polycystic disease.
- Oncology units: patients may have gastrointestinal tumours and hepatic metastases.

OSCE 2

These linked stations are common in OSCEs with an observed history-taking, followed by questions about the information that you have elicited. In the former, your communication skills will be important (open versus closed questions, summarising, reflecting any emotion back to the patient and acknowledging this (e.g. 'you appear to be quite anxious'). You should also consider the use of ICE:

- I — ideas (patients)
- C — concerns
- E — expectations.

The key aspects that you need to elicit in station 1 then come back in your discussion at station 2.

a. The differential diagnosis is a primary alcohol dependence syndrome, depression or possible an anxiety disorder.

b. Alcohol dependence
  - craving — could not do without it for a few days and looking forward to her drink
  - increased tolerance — finding that the effects are not as strong and also drinking more
  - withdrawals — shaking.

  There have also been major social consequences of her drinking, with social isolation and interference with day-to-day life (e.g. missing appointments).

c. You would indicate that you would do a formal mental state examination in this patient and this would include screening for depression or anxiety. The initial management of any low mood (or anxiety) is for the patient to abstain from alcohol (with reassurance that this is likely to bring about an improvement in mood) and then re-evaluate. Depression and alcohol dependence are inter-related, with one often leading to the other, so the patient may have an underlying depression, which should be treated.

d. Her alcohol withdrawal should be managed by a tapering regimen of benzodiazepines with vitamin supplementation (B_1 thiamine). Chlordiazepoxide is often used over 1 week. If she has had fits before (which could be alcohol-related) or if she is frail with other physical comorbidities, then she should be admitted to hospital.

  Remember that it is very important to support her as much as possible in coming off alcohol. Most patients relapse within a year and referral to the alcohol dependence team would be beneficial (providing she is motivated to attend). Underlying factors (e.g. depression) should be treated.

OSCE 3

The student does well on the hands, missing the white nails (leuconychia) initially but recovering well. The student understands the results offered. Correctly the student suggests ascites, but incorrectly guesses the liver to be enlarged, whereas it is likely to be shrunken. The student might have mentioned distended veins over the abdomen consistent with oesophageal varices (even a 'caput medusae') or spider naevi (usually on the chest, neck or face). Correctly the student clinically diagnoses hepatic cirrhosis. As Dupuytren's contracture is more common in alcoholics and alcohol is the most common cause of cirrhosis, this was either a good point or a shrewd clinical diagnosis!

Case history answers

Case history 1

1. She has a mild, microcytic anaemia. You should look carefully at the blood count report to see what other information is given. There may be a low mean corpuscular haemoglobin concentration (MCHC) and an increased red cell distribution width. The reticulocyte count may be increased and, if the patient is actively bleeding, there may be a raised platelet count. A blood film would confirm the

presence of small red cells together with hypochromia. At this stage, you should confirm the iron deficiency anaemia with serum ferritin, or serum iron and total iron-binding capacity. You should also consider why she is anaemic. The temptation is to treat simply with iron supplements on the basis that the anaemia is only mild.

In an elderly person, there may be an element of poor nutrition, but more likely she has organic disease. You should enquire carefully about upper GI symptoms and also whether she is, or has recently been, taking NSAIDs because of her arthritis. The other main concern is that she has an occult large bowel carcinoma.

2. You should establish i.v. access; if she is hypovolaemic, you should use a plasma expander such as Gelofusine whilst waiting for cross-matched blood and the haemoglobin. Renal function should be measured. In significant GI bleeding, you should inform the on-call surgical team so that, if intervention is needed, it does not come too late.

Assuming that the bleeding stops and that a transfusion has been given, the next step is to decide on investigations to determine the cause. Occasionally, anal disease can haemorrhage, but the most likely problem is a large bowel carcinoma, diverticular disease or angiodysplasia. It is reasonable to request a barium enema, but in this case no cause for the bleeding is found.

3. You need to consider whether the patient has been complying with therapy; iron supplements can produce GI upset. You need to consider the value of the barium enema. Was the examination a complete one or was there considerable faecal loading? You need to decide whether to accept that the probable cause was diverticular disease, whether a carcinoma was missed or whether you should look for angiodysplasia. If you wish to pursue one of these, you need to request a colonoscopy. Sometimes angiography can be used to diagnose angiodysplasia. Occasionally, despite intensive and repeated investigation, no cause for GI bleeding is found, in which case management is by iron supplements and transfusion.

Case history 2

1. The differential diagnoses are myocardial ischaemia, aortic dissection (but no history of pain through to the back or arterial insufficiency) and an intra-abdominal catastrophe (biliary colic, perforated peptic ulcer or acute pancreatitis). Your next step would be a focused examination looking for supportive evidence of one of the possibilities. There may also be signs which help to exclude a diagnosis. For example, absence of abdominal tenderness would be strongly against the diagnosis of a perforated peptic ulcer. In addition, you should look for signs of shock, such as hypotension and tachypnoea.

Investigations are again targeted towards your differential diagnosis. In all patients with chest pain, you should request an urgent ECG and chest radiograph. Serum levels of cardiac creatine kinase (CK) can be measured. If the pain has been present for more than 12 hours, estimation of troponin T can be used to exclude myocardial infarction. A serum amylase should also be checked. It may be mildly elevated in the other conditions, but gross elevation is diagnostic of acute pancreatitis. In any patients who are shocked, you should also perform blood gas analysis, check urea and electrolytes and measure urine output. If you suspect a perforated peptic ulcer, then a plain upright chest radiograph is indicated.

2. You are told that the patient has acute pancreatitis. Clues to this in the history are the heavy alcohol intake (you should also consider why — this may be associated with depression) and gall stones. Management is supportive (p. 154). Remember fluids, oxygen, antibiotics and pain relief.

3. She almost certainly has a pancreatic pseudocyst. Ascites can also occur in severe cases, but this would cause generalised swelling. You should request an ultrasound scan to confirm the diagnosis. Many small collections of fluid resolve spontaneously, but some need drainage. Remember the other complications of pancreatitis (p. 154).

Case history 3

1. The initial differential diagnosis is:
   * chronic hepatitis: hepatitis B or C, drug-induced hepatotoxicity or alcohol abuse
   * granulomatous hepatitis
   * cirrhosis of liver (low albumin is more consistent with acute illness but can also be a feature of cirrhosis).

2. Tests that should be requested are:
   * hepatitis B surface antigen and anti-HBc IgG
   * hepatitis C antibody
   * HIV (if he gives consent)
   * ultrasound of the liver
   * smooth muscle and antimitochondrial antibodies
   * clotting screen
   * serum ferritin.

3. If hepatitis B surface antigen or hepatitis C RNA is positive, then advise safe sex and undertake immunisation of any partners for hepatitis B if they are not already positive.

Consider liver biopsy and treatment, but compliance can be the limiting factor.

Case history 4

1. Delirium tremens (alcohol withdrawal) is by far the most likely diagnosis, although it is usually manifest 24–36 hours after admission. However,

hypoglycaemia, serious sepsis and intracranial bleeding must be excluded. Disorientation may also be caused by concussion.

2. Steps that should be undertaken are:
   - blood monitoring (BM) stix immediately
   - blood culture and white cell count
   - sedation with chlordiazepoxide and frequent neurological observations
   - re-examine him carefully when he is quieter, seeking neurological signs and signs of hepatic cirrhosis
   - CT scan of brain (when sedated)
   - if febrile or with features of pneumonia or sepsis, investigate as you would any pneumonia (chest radiograph, blood gases, etc.) and treat empirically with antibiotics, e.g. cefotaxime.

3. Additional history:
   - Is he a drinker? (Use CAGE questionnaire, p. 149.)
   - Has he travelled anywhere? (Malaria, typhoid)
   - Does he have any past medical history of note?
   - Has his behaviour changed lately? (? Manic/depressive, hyperthyroidism, intracranial pathology, such as encephalitis, meningioma)

4. Speak to a close relative or work colleague in confidence later that day.

5. Further tests:
   - Assess his liver function status (? cirrhosis): albumin, clotting, ? endoscopy for oesophageal varices.
   - Assess him neurologically: CT scan, lumbar puncture.
   - Assess his endocrine status, especially thyroid function.
   - Refer him for psychiatric assessment.

Case history 5

1. *Shigella, Entamoeba histolytica, Salmonella* infections.

2. Useful tests:
   - stool culture
   - urea and electrolytes
   - blood culture
   - full blood count and differential.

3. Stool microscopy on a 'hot stool' for amoebae, red and white cells and parasites. (The bedpan (or a generous portion of stool without urine) should be taken directly to the laboratory.)

Case history 6

1. Examine each patient with respect to fluid state and any intra-abdominal pathology. It is easy to assume that they have the same problem, but it may be coincidental. Measure urea and electrolytes and send stool for culture and *Clostridium difficile* toxin. Use i.v. fluids if oral rehydration solution is not adequate.

2. If *Cl. difficile* is implicated, use oral metronidazole; for *Salmonella* or other bacterial diarrhoea, use ciprofloxacin. If diarrhoea is severe, it is appropriate to start therapy before test results are available.

3. Put each patient in a separate cubicle. Inform the infection control sister as soon as possible. Have the area around each patient's present bed cleaned to reduce dispersal of clostridial spores.

Case history 7

1. The patient is complaining of a change in bowel habit, which must be taken seriously. Iron therapy can cause constipation, but you should not assume that this is the cause. The empty rectum with a full descending colon suggests an obstructive lesion. A common error is for an iron deficiency anaemia to be ascribed to 'reflux oesophagitis'; many of these patients have lower bowel disease and, unless a barium meal or gastroscopy shows a definite cause, a barium enema or colonoscopy should be carried out.

   You need to repeat the blood count and check the iron status. As the patient may have a large bowel carcinoma, you should request liver function tests and ultrasound. A high alkaline phosphatase would suggest liver metastases. You need to examine the lower bowel; a flexible or rigid sigmoidoscope will enable you to visualise the rectum and lower sigmoid colon. If a barium enema is inconclusive, colonoscopy would be indicated.

2. a. With barium studies, always try to orientate yourself. This film shows the rectum and lower sigmoid colon. The hip, pelvis and sacroiliac joint are visible. There is a gross filling defect, with a thin line of barium in communication with the sigmoid colon. Even if you cannot see the thin column, you can deduce that obstruction is not total by the filling of the sigmoid colon. The appearances are described as an 'apple core'.

   b. A rectal carcinoma. The tumour must have been just beyond the tip of the finger on rectal examination.

Key features answers

1. The most important features are concerned with assessing circulating blood volume (rather than assessing the volume from the patient's history). The key factors are that **her blood pressure** is normal, with **minimal drop** on sitting up (though this will underestimate the postural drop on standing). She does not have **a tachycardia**.

   The most likely diagnosis is a Mallory–Weiss tear, based on the history of vomiting blood after a sustained bout of vomiting (probably brought on by alcohol). Although she appears to drink heavily, this has probably only been for a few years, so cirrhosis and varices are unlikely (at this stage).

2. The patient describes dyspepsia, which could be due to a peptic ulcer. The GP will probably refer him for

an endoscopy to establish a diagnosis prior to treatment. She could also take blood for *Helicobacter pylori* serology (or request a stool antigen) and treat with triple therapy. The main question is whether she is missing a gastric carcinoma. The previous history and taking Gaviscon all point to benign disease, but the patient could have a malignant gastric ulcer. The key features are:

- weight — steady
- full blood count — normal
- vomiting — frequently for last few weeks.

   The presence of vomiting (which is unusual in uncomplicated peptic ulcer disease) would indicate that an urgent endoscopy is justified.

3. This patient has acute pancreatitis. You should consider a perforated viscus (but there is no evidence of significant peritonism — a chest radiograph would be useful to exclude gas under the diaphragm) and also acute cholecystitis or cholangitis (but her liver function tests are normal and the pain is not typical).

   It is very important to assess the severity of the pancreatitis as this guides the management. The associated factors for a poor prognosis are given in the text (Box 7). For this patient these are:

- obesity
- gall stones (she will need an urgent ultrasound and possibly ERCP)
- hypotension
- low oxygen saturation (she also has a metabolic acidosis, indicating impending shock)
- elevated glucose
- low haemoglobin and elevated white cell count.

   She has a normal urea and corrected calcium (at this stage). However, resuscitation and discussion with senior colleagues are required, with transfer to the high-dependency unit.

4. The diagnosis is ulcerative colitis. The key features are:
- no granuloma
- inflammatory process confined to mucosa (superficial)
- goblet cells depleted
- crypt abscesses.

Data interpretation answers

1. Typical hepatocellular liver function test abnormalities, with normal white cell count and typical clinical presentation: acute hepatitis, probably A but could be B, C or E or possibly Epstein–Barr virus (EBV).

2. Typical cholestatic liver function test abnormalities, with fever and a raised white cell count: cholecystitis, cholangitis, liver abscess.

3. Consistent with viral hepatitis but not very high aspartate aminotransferase (AST). Must account for

the sore throat: glandular fever, could be hepatitis A (but why sore throat?) or primary HIV.

4. Mixed cholestatic/hepatitic picture with fever and impaired renal function. Leptospirosis (p. 420), haemorrhagic fever with renal syndrome (Hantaan virus), severe sepsis including liver abscess or cholangitis, alcoholic hepatitis.

5. Note the low albumin and raised INR, typical of acute or chronic liver failure: alcoholic cirrhosis (consider heart failure, thiamine deficiency). Impaired renal function may occur with severe cirrhosis because of poor renal perfusion and diuretic therapy.

6. Note the typically low albumin of patients in the intensive care unit (ICU) (non-specific). Raised white cell count alerts you to infection: sepsis including candidaemia, total parenteral nutrition (TPN)-induced hepatitis (mild), drug-induced hepatitis.

7. Typical biochemical features of acute liver failure with renal impairment: for example, caused by paracetamol poisoning, hepatitis A, B or C, drugs. Look for liver flap and encephalopathy.

8. Isolated raised AST typical of chronic hepatitis, most likely C but consider B and autoimmune disease. Consider primary sclerosing cholangitis (but alkaline phosphatase normal).

9. Hepatitis C (or B), haemochromatosis, alcoholic liver disease, emphysema (caused by downward displacement of the liver without enlargement).

Picture answers

1. a. Low attenuation irregular area posteriorly in the right lobe of the liver.

   b. Bacterial liver abscess. Usually amoebic abscesses are more clearly circumscribed and found in younger people; metastases or liver tumours are virtually always more clearly outlined and often of higher attenuation.

   c. (i) Direct aspiration of abscess contents for Gram stain and aerobic and anaerobic culture, (ii) amoebic serology and/or (iii) blood culture.

   d. Intravenous antibiotics to cover the likely organisms and to penetrate into a large abscess cavity, e.g. ampicillin (*Streptococcus milleri*), third-generation cephalosporin (Gram-negatives) and metronidazole (anaerobes).

2. a. He has cardiomegaly (cardiothoracic ratio >0.5), an unfolded aorta (prominent aortic knuckle) and a hiatus hernia (gas bubble behind the left heart border).

   b. You would probably do nothing. The anaesthetist may want to assess his cardiovascular function in more depth. You may want to question him about any symptoms of reflux oesophagitis. Patients with 'rolling' (portion of stomach rolling alongside the oesophagus) rather than the very common 'sliding' hiatus hernia are more at risk of complications such as gastric volvulus. However, if the patient is asymptomatic, you would do nothing.

3. a. The barium enema visualises the transverse and descending colon. There are fine spiculating superficial ulcers throughout, giving a fuzzy contour. There are also examples of 'collarstud' ulcers and 'pseudopolyps' — luminal filling defects that are inflamed mucosal islands between ulcer craters. The colon in the lower left of the picture has lost its haustration pattern and is featureless ('hosepipe').

    b. The history points to inflammatory bowel disease and the barium enema confirms ulcerative colitis.

    c. Given the severity of the disease, the patient needs admission. Initial management would be oral and rectal corticosteroids.

Short notes answers

1. There is very little information about the patient (which is often the case for a house officer; patients will 'turn up' on the ward). An initial step would be to recap the history and examination findings. There are two interdependent problems. The first is whether the patient is malnourished. Find out about the length of the history and try to quantify any weight loss. Arrange for the patient to be weighed and *you* should record this in the patient's notes. Ideally, the height of the patient should be measured to calculate the **body mass index** (weight (kg)/height^2 (m^2)). Are there any are other pointers towards nutritional deficiency? Is there marked oedema, or possible ascites, indicating protein malnutrition? Is there evidence of folate or vitamin B$_{12}$ deficiency, e.g. a peripheral neuropathy (p. 243)?

    Having decided that the patient is malnourished, the second question is then why? Is it because of a poor diet? This can be difficult to assess and a dietary assessment by a nutritionist might help. Is there a previous history of bowel problems? The patient may have had a gastrectomy years ago, extensive gut resection or surgery that has created a blind loop. The patient may have a disease such as systemic sclerosis, which, because of the interference with gut motility, has permitted bacterial overgrowth. Are there pointers from the history, or examination findings suggestive of inflammatory bowel disease?

    It may then be decided that the patient is malnourished and that GI disease is suspected. The investigations take the same logical approach:

    *   Document the degree of malnourishment: iron, total iron-binding capacity, vitamin B$_{12}$, folate, calcium, alkaline phosphatase and plasma albumin should all be measured.

    *   What is the underlying disease? In coeliac disease, a distal duodenal or jejunal biopsy may be requested; for bacterial overgrowth, a hydrogen breath test may be required.

2. The first task is to look back at the records from 8 weeks ago and check the details. Was the ulcer in the stomach? If a gastric ulcer, then were biopsies taken and are the results in the notes? Even if the biopsies were negative, the patient needs a repeat endoscopy to assess healing, as there can be false-negative biopsies with gastric carcinoma.

    Assuming that he has a proven duodenal ulcer, why have the symptoms persisted? Is the ulcer a coincidental finding with another cause for his symptoms, e.g. myocardial ischaemia? If the dyspepsia is caused by a duodenal ulcer, what therapy was he prescribed (if any!) and has he been complying with it? Was he tested initially for *H. pylori* infection and prescribed triple therapy (two antibiotics plus a proton pump inhibitor)? If he was given a proton pump inhibitor, almost all ulcers should have healed by 8 weeks. If an H$_2$ antagonist was prescribed, the healing rate is slower. It may be worth continuing with the therapy, changing to a proton pump inhibitor or repeating an endoscopy. This last option should include urease measurement or other tests for *H. pylori* (p. 124).

3. In dealing with a patient who has a terminal carcinoma, it is important not to focus on physical symptoms to the detriment of the psychological care. Involvement of the MacMillan nurses or a palliative care team should be strongly considered. There is also a high probability of a reactive depression. In this patient there are two goals: relief of jaundice and pain control.

    The jaundice may be managed by insertion of a stent using ERCP. Alternatively, surgical bypass may be used. If the jaundice cannot be relieved, the pruritus may be helped by antihistamines and/or colestyramine to bind the bile salts. Pancreatic insufficiency may also be a problem, with steatorrhoea (p. 119).

    Pain relief should start with simple analgesics such as paracetamol, stepping up through codeine and dihydrocodeine to morphine. Bone pain may be helped by the use of NSAIDs or radiotherapy, though adenocarcinomas tend not to be very radiosensitive. If morphine is used, it should be rationally prescribed. Initially, the patient is placed on regular oral morphine (4-hourly), with supplementation for breakthrough pain. A pain chart will indicate the degree of control obtained. The dose of morphine is adjusted according to the amount of PRN dosing being used. Finally, the 4-hourly dosing is converted to sustained release morphine. Always prescribe a PRN dose for ready access to pain relief. A prophylactic laxative should be prescribed whenever using narcotic analgesics. Consulting a pain specialist will be useful; they may be able to perform a nerve block as well as advising on drug treatment.

4. You must allow the patient to describe his difficulty. Is it dysphagia, nasal regurgitation or aspiration (violent coughing on eating)? The main differential diagnoses are neurological or oesophageal disease. What is the context of the symptoms? Does the patient have a history suggestive of neurological disease or does he give a story of longstanding heartburn? Is the problem more with liquids (neurological) or solids (obstructive)? If we assume that the pointer is towards GI disease, then the main differential diagnoses are a benign stricture and carcinoma. Even with a long history of reflux and heartburn, it cannot be assumed that the problem is benign. A barium swallow may help, but oesophagoscopy will allow direct visualisation (after an oesophageal toilet to clear out the debris) and biopsy.

5. Given that the patient has gall stones, you need to know whether these are asymptomatic. If so, then the correct course of action would be to do nothing. If she gives a history of recurrent right upper quadrant pain and the gall bladder is shrunken and scarred on ultrasound scan, you may discuss the possible need for surgery and say that you would like to send her for a surgical opinion. Remember that abdominal pain may have other causes and do not assume that it is necessarily caused by the gall stones.

6. The question is 'open', asking you to state your knowledge of drug therapy in inflammatory bowel disease. It then closes down to maintenance and potential side-effects (p. 133).

Chapter 4

Renal disease, and fluid–electrolyte and acid–base balance

4.1 Background

Learning objectives

You should:

- feel confident about diagnosing renal failure on the basis of abnormal biochemistry
- understand those aspects of renal physiology which explain renal failure and its treatment
- understand how the kidneys, heart and circulation form a functional unit in the regulation of fluid and electrolyte balance
- understand how abnormalities of renal perfusion can affect renal function
- understand how renal function is affected by urinary outflow.

Case Study

The case of an elderly patient admitted seriously ill with renal failure illustrates how the physiological functions of the kidney can go wrong in disease. She is in left ventricular failure and hypertensive due to salt and water overload. She is life-threateningly hyperkalaemic, acidotic, and twitching and confused due to uraemia. It is thought she has acute rather than chronic renal failure because she is not anaemic.

You may regard renal disease as very difficult to understand, and feel that your training has given you little experience of it. However, about one patient in three on any acute medical ward has abnormal renal function. The dif-

ficulty arises because many renal diseases are asymptomatic in their early stages, most of the symptoms and signs of renal disease are non-specific, and the diagnosis is usually based on abnormal 'Us and Es' (urea and electrolytes) or proteinuria. You may feel uncomfortable about making such an important diagnosis as renal failure from a mere laboratory report.

Another problem arises because many practising clinicians are shaky on the assessment of fluid/electrolyte balance. Many a patient with heart failure is wrongly given saline because they 'look dry'. A reader who comes to the end of this chapter able to distinguish a volume-depleted patient from one who is volume-overloaded and able to look with interest and understanding at biochemistry results has the basic skills to recognise and manage renal disease.

This chapter will show that renal function and fluid/electrolyte homeostasis are inextricably linked and that the kidneys form a functional unit with the heart and circulation. The emphasis is more on phy-siological concepts than structural pathology, which is covered in pathology and reference textbooks. However, the traditional anatomical framework makes it easier to remember the causes of renal disease (Box 8).

Renal anatomy

The kidneys are 8–13 cm in length and situated retroperitoneally at the level of T12–L3, the right one being 1–2 cm lower than the left. Each has one or more main renal arteries entering at the hilum, dividing into interlobular arteries, which run radially out to the cortico-medullary junction and then into the arcuate arteries and ultimately through the afferent arterioles to the glomerular capillaries. The functional unit is the nephron (Fig. 41).

The glomerulus, the anatomy of which is shown in Figure 42, can be thought of as an epithelial pouch invaginated by a tuft of capillaries running from the afferent to the efferent arteriole. The endothelial and epithelial cell junctions and basement membrane constitute a semipermeable filter. The other cellular element of the glomerulus is the mesangium. The mesangial cells are contractile and can alter blood flow and the glomerular filtration rate (GFR). They are commonly involved in glomerular disease.

Box 8: Causes of renal disease

Prerenal factors

- Something wrong with the circulation
  - Volume depletion/shock, e.g. blood loss, excess gastrointestinal (GI) losses, burns
  - Fall in peripheral vascular resistance, e.g. caused by sepsis
  - Heart failure
  - Hypertension

- Something wrong with the renal vasculature
  - Renal arterial disease
  - Renal venous disease
  - Drug-induced shutdown of renal perfusion, e.g. therapy with angiotensin-converting enzyme (ACE) inhibitors or non-steroidal anti-inflammatory drugs (NSAIDs)

- Something wrong with the blood
  - Hypoxia
  - Infection
  - Toxin

Renal factors

- Glomerular disease
- Tubular disease
- Parenchymal/interstitial disease

Postrenal factors

- Diseases of the renal papillae, renal pelvis, ureters, bladder or urethra

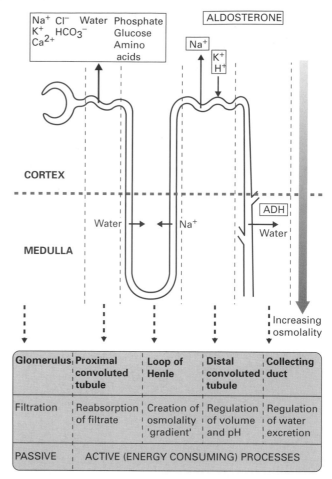

Fig. 41 The anatomy and physiology of the nephron. The site of action of the two principal hormones controlling water and electrolyte levels is shown. ADH, antidiuretic hormone. (Adpated from: Textbook of Medicine, ed. Souhami and Moxham, Churchill Livingstone, Edinburgh, 1997.)

The juxtaglomerular apparatus is formed by the afferent arteriole and distal tubule of the same nephron.

Renal physiology

Filtration and flow

The kidneys receive 25% of cardiac output (about 1200 ml/min). About 20% of the blood volume which enters the glomeruli passes through the glomerular filter, which is permeable to every component of blood except cells and large protein molecules, to form the glomerular filtrate. The glomerular basement membrane is negatively charged and this charge barrier retains anionic proteins such as albumin which are small enough to pass through the pores. Damage to the glomerular basement membrane disrupts the charge barrier before it disrupts pore size, making albumin an exquisitely sensitive marker of glomerular damage.

Filtration is a **passive** process determined by the pressure balance across the capillary wall. Haemostatic pressure in the glomerular capillaries causes filtration. It is opposed by the hydrostatic pressure in the urinary space and the oncotic pressure exerted by proteins in glomerular capillary blood. Figure 43 illustrates these opposing pressures diagrammatically.

In order to understand renal disease, a crucial concept is the distinction between **filtration** and **flow**. Nitrogenous waste can only reach the urine by filtration since it is not actively secreted into the tubule. Maintenance of filtration is, therefore, crucial to homeostasis. It is maintained by

renal autoregulation over a wide range of systolic pressures (80–200 mmHg). Filtration only fails if there are insufficient functioning nephrons or the perfusion pressure falls below the lower limit of autoregulation. The latter can be caused by one of the prerenal processes listed in the anatomical classification in Box 8 or if there is increased pressure in the tubule, as in ureteric obstruction.

Within the physiological range of perfusion pressures, rate of urine flow can be vastly different — for example, after celebrating your examination results compared with when you play squash on a hot summer afternoon. In both situations, a glomerular filtrate amounting to 180 litres/24 hours is needed to clear nitrogenous waste, and about 90% of the fluid is obligatorily reabsorbed to prevent circulatory collapse. It is in the handling of the remaining 10% of filtrate that the controlling mechanisms operate; they can alter flow between a minimum of 0.5 and a maximum of over 20 litres/24 hours. There are two controlling mechanisms.

Sodium reabsorption

This is the main factor which determines extracellular fluid **volume**; it is controlled primarily by the rennin–

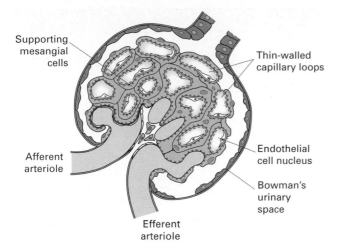

A

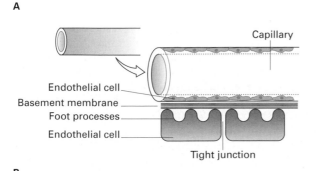

B

Fig. 42 The glomerulus. **A** Anatomy of a whole glomerulus. **B** Detail of the filtration surface comprising endothelial cells, basement membrane and foot processes of epithelial cells.

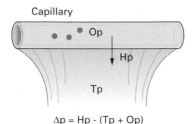

$$\Delta p = Hp - (Tp + Op)$$

Where
Δp = net pressure acting across glomerular capillary
Hp = Capillary hydrostatic pressure
Tp = Tubular pressure
Op = Oncotic pressure

Fig. 43 Pressure gradients across the capillary wall.

angiotensin–aldosterone system and the natriuretic peptides.

Water reabsorption

This determines extracellular fluid **osmolality**; it is controlled by **antidiuretic hormone** (ADH, arginine vasopressin; p. 296).

Filtration should be regarded as the 'waste disposal' function and urine flow the regulator of volume and osmolality.

Tubular 'processing' of the glomerular filtrate

Urine reaches the proximal convoluted tubule as a cell-free ultrafiltrate of plasma. Two-thirds is reabsorbed in this segment as a consequence of active sodium reabsorption. Water in the renal tubule diffuses passively down the concentration gradient created by sodium reabsorption and there is little change in urine osmolality from one end of the pro-ximal tubule to the other. Chloride, potassium, calcium, phosphate, glucose and amino acids are also reabsorbed in this segment.

Another tubular function is acidification of the urine. Water and carbon dioxide combine in the tubular cells to form carbonic acid, catalysed by the enzyme carbonic anhydrase. Dissociation into hydrogen and bicarbonate ions yields free hydrogen ions, which are pumped into tubular fluid in exchange for sodium. The hydrogen ions are buffered by recombination with bicarbonate to yield water and diffusible carbon dioxide, and by combination with phosphate buffers and ammonia. The net effect is absorption of bicarbonate and increase in the acidity of urine.

The loop of Henle progressively increases the osmolality of the renal interstitium from cortex to medulla by 'countercurrent multiplication' (summarised in any physiology textbook) and removes a further 15% of filtrate, primarily by reabsorption of water. It is in the distal convoluted tubule and collecting duct that the mechanisms which control the non-obligatory handling of sodium and water operate. **Aldosterone** increases sodium reabsorption in exchange for potassium. About 15% of glomerular filtrate flows from the distal tubule to the collecting ducts where it passes through an increasingly hyperosmolar interstitium. ADH, secreted primarily in response to changes in plasma osmolality, regulates the permeability of the collecting ducts to water and, together with aldosterone, controls urine flow.

Endocrine function

The endocrine functions of the kidney can be summarised as:

- secretion of renin by the juxtaglomerular apparatus; this controls angiotensin and aldosterone secretion in response to volume depletion and hyponatraemia
- erythropoietin synthesis in response to anaemia and hypoxia
- 1α-hydroxylation of vitamin D, controlled by parathyroid hormone.

Urea and creatinine as markers of renal disease

The renal handling of urea and creatinine deserves special mention, not just because these are important nitrogenous waste products but also because they are measured in every patient and are a key to understanding fluid and electrolyte biochemistry.

Creatinine

In health, there is a steady rate of creatinine synthesis from the turnover of muscle protein. Creatinine is freely filtered and a small proportion is actively secreted by the proximal tubule; very little is reabsorbed. Plasma creatinine concentration is thus primarily determined by GFR. Unless there is accelerated muscle catabolism, an increase in plasma creatinine signifies a fall in GFR.

Urea

General protein catabolism produces urea, synthesis of which is dependent on intact liver function. Urea production is, therefore, more labile than creatinine production, rising in catabolic states (and after eating a large protein meal) and falling in liver failure. More important still, between 10 and 70% of urea within the filtrate is reabsorbed, depending on the rate of urine flow. Thus plasma urea concentration can be increased by both reduced **filtration** and reduced **flow**. The relationship between plasma urea and creatinine concentrations can be used to distinguish between these two very different physiological conditions. If urea alone is raised, the cause is reduced flow (e.g. caused by reduced renal perfusion within the range that can be compensated for by autoregulation). If both are raised, there is hypofiltration ('renal failure'). Remember that a small increase in urea may result from protein catabolism after large protein meals or GI bleeding.

Summary of renal physiology

When considering renal disease and its management, it is useful to have the following simple framework of renal function in your mind:

- clearance of nitrogenous waste
- regulation of sodium, potassium and water balance
- retention of essential proteins
- regulation of blood pressure
- regulation of acid–base homeostasis
- endocrine function: erythropoietin synthesis and 1α-hydroxylation of vitamin D.

Renal pathology

Glomerular disease

The nephrons are vulnerable to abnormal oxygenation, to abnormal perfusion and to toxins in the incoming blood. The glomeruli can also be damaged by immunological processes, notably autoantibodies to glomerular structures (e.g. antiglomerular basement membrane in Goodpasture's syndrome) and circulating immune complexes. Glomerulonephritis may also follow infection or complicate connective disease or malignancy. Some metabolic processes, of which diabetes mellitus is the most common example, also cause diffuse glomerular damage. The effects of glomerular disease are proteinuria, haematuria, hypertension and hypofiltration (renal failure).

Tubular disease

Tubular disease may be congenital (e.g. Fanconi syndrome) or acquired (e.g. multiple myeloma). It causes abnormal water/electrolyte handling and acidosis, as discussed on page 186.

> **Box 9:** Other causes of polyuria and polydipsia
>
> **Common causes**
> - Anxiety or habit
> - Diabetes mellitus
>
> **Uncommon causes**
> - Diabetes insipidus
>   - Nephrogenic
>   - Cranial
> - Hypokalaemia
> - Hypercalcaemia

Postrenal disease

Obstruction to the urinary tract is an important cause of renal dysfunction; remember, however, that there is so much reserve capacity in the two kidneys that both must be obstructed for there to be significant renal failure. Infection and stones often present with their own symptoms long before they cause renal failure.

Symptoms and signs

The symptoms and signs can be separated into those of any underlying disease and those of renal disease itself.

The symptoms of renal disease can be elusive. Urinary frequency and dysuria suggest lower urinary tract disease. Polyuria and nocturia, the earliest symptoms of chronic renal failure, are caused by failure of renal tubular sodium reabsorption and/or collecting duct disease. Renal failure is only one cause of polyuria and polydipsia. Others are listed in Box 9.

Table 40 lists the symptoms and signs of renal disease. You should remember that the symptoms and signs of **uraemia** (failure to excrete nitrogenous waste) do not occur until the GFR is severely impaired (<20 ml/min).

No assessment of a patient with renal disease is complete without an assessment of blood volume (as described on p. 192). This is because:

- volume depletion (shock, 'dehydration') impairs renal perfusion and can cause or worsen renal failure
- renal failure impairs salt and water excretion and can cause volume overload
- heart failure impairs renal perfusion and can ultimately cause renal failure
- the kidneys are intimately related to the control of blood pressure.

These points emphasise a crucial concept: the heart and kidneys are a functioning unit in terms of fluid balance. At the bedside, the haemodynamic effects of 'heart failure' (p. 22) and 'renal failure' can be indistinguishable. Another important relationship is between renal disease and hypertension. Both fluid retention and renin oversecretion exacerbate, and can be caused by, renal disease and both cause hypertension. You must measure blood pressure carefully and assess your patient carefully for the complications of hypertension (p. 43).

Table 40 Symptoms and signs of renal failure

	Symptoms	Signs
Failure to excrete nitrogenous waste	Pruritus	Uraemic foetor
	Nausea, anorexia, vomiting, dyspepsia	Pale, sallow skin
	Lethargy	Scratch marks
	Chest pain	Pericardial or pleural rub
	Mental dullness/confusion	Cognitive impairment, twitching, fits and/or coma
	Paraesthesiae	
	Hiccoughs	Sensori-motor neuropathy (rare)
Protein loss and failure to regulate fluid/ electrolyte balance and blood pressure	Thirst	Oedema
	Polyuria	Signs of left ± right heart failure
	Nocturia	Hypertension or hypotension
	Oliguria or anuria	Hypertension retinopathy
	Weakness (hypo- or hyperkalaemia)	
	Breathlessness	
Acidosis	Breathlessness	Kussmaul respiration
	Confusion	Cognitive impairment
Failure of endocrine function		
Anaemia	Lethargy	Pallor
	Dyspnoea	
Impaired hydroxylation of vitamin D	Bone pain	Signs of osteomalacia or rickets (proximal myopathy, tender pelvis, etc.)
Underlying disease		
Urinary tract disease	Haematuria	Loin tenderness
	Loin pain	Palpable bladder
	Dysuria	
Inherited renal disorders	Deafness: for example, in Alport's syndrome	Palpable kidneys: for example, in polycystic disease
Systemic disease	For example, symptoms of diabetes and its complications	For example, vasculitic rash in systemic vasculitis

4.2 Investigation of renal disease

Learning objectives

You should:
- know the range of investigations for renal disease and understand their use in different clinical situations
- appreciate that proteinuria and haematuria are easy to detect with a dipstick, usually indicative of renal/urinary tract disease and all too often overlooked at an early stage when referral, investigation and treatment could preserve renal function.

Case Study

A healthy man in his thirties is shocked to be refused life insurance because he has dipstick-positive proteinuria at a medical. Urine microscopy shows no cells or casts. Estimated GFR, blood count, immunological assessment and renal ultrasound scan are normal. An early-morning albumin:creatinine ratio is normal. The diagnosis is benign orthostatic proteinuria and he gets insurance after all.

Urine analysis

Stick testing

Dipsticks can accurately measure pH and detect the presence of blood, protein and white cells. Urine testing for albumin is an essential adjunct to physical examination since healthy people do not have 'dipstick-positive' proteinuria except during intercurrent illness or menstruation and, in some cases, in the upright posture ('benign orthostatic proteinuria'). Proteinuria needs further investigation. Its causes (with the most common in bold) are:

- general
  — fever
- benign orthostatic proteinuria
- abnormal plasma protein
  — myeloma (p. 279; but note that free immunoglobulin light chains, Bence Jones protein, are not detected by standard dipsticks)
- glomerular disease
  — hypertension
  — **diabetes**
  — **acute or chronic glomerulonephritis**
  — pre-eclampsia

- tubular disease
  — acute tubular necrosis
- other renal diseases
  — renal tumours or cysts
  — **chronic pyelonephritis**
  — renal tuberculosis
  — interstitial nephropathy
- lower urinary tract disease
  — **urinary tract infection**
  — tumour.

Microscopy and culture

Both microscopy and culture can give valuable information. The presence of red and/or white cells signifies infection or structural pathology at any level from the glomerulus to the bladder. The presence of casts must be taken seriously. Red cell casts are pathognomonic of glomerular disease. Hyaline or granular casts may be caused by disease of the glomeruli or tubules.

Culture should be performed on a fresh, midstream urine sample. Infection is distinguished from contamination by the presence of white cells and growth of pathogenic rather than commensal organisms.

Urine biochemistry

Unlike plasma biochemistry, there are no clearly defined normal ranges for any urinary solute except protein (less than 150 mg/24 hr). When proteinuria is detected, it can be quantitated either as the ratio of protein or albumin to creatinine in an early morning urine sample, or as a total amount of protein excreted in a 24-hour urine collection. Low-grade proteinuria (an increased albumin : creatinine ratio) is termed 'microalbuminuria'. Dipstick-positive proteinuria is termed 'persistent proteinuria'. The heaviest proteinuria is termed 'nephrotic range proteinuria'.

In health, the urinary excretion of sodium and potassium reflects intake and is determined by food preferences rather than physiology. In disease, measurement of urinary sodium or potassium can tell you whether or not depletion or overload of these solutes is caused by abnormal renal handling. Similarly, creatinine excretion varies widely between individuals of different muscle bulk, but measurement of its clearance in a 24-hour urine sample (excretion in relation to plasma concentration) gives an estimate of GFR. Timed urine collections are notoriously incomplete and GFR can better be estimated from serum creatinine alone. In acute renal failure, measurement of the ratio of urine to plasma urea concentration can help you decide whether the problem is impaired renal perfusion with intact glomerular function (ratio >8) or whether the capacity to concentrate urea is lost (ratio <8).

Plasma biochemistry

Plasma creatinine concentration is a useful proxy for GFR, provided you remember that the steady-state serum creatinine concentration is also determined by muscle bulk. Therefore, a wasted elderly patient may have significant renal failure at a creatinine concentration that is normal for a muscular rugby player. This is reflected in the wide 'normal' range for serum creatinine. Changes in serum creatinine within an individual can be a sensitive guide to changes in renal function, although serum creatinine rises in a near-exponential relationship to GFR. Therefore, a rise in creatinine from 130 to 140 µmol/l may signify the same proportional loss of renal function as a rise from 400 to 600 µmol/l. Plasma creatinine does not rise above normal until over 50% of glomerular filtration is lost. Plasma urea is usually measured together with creatinine for the reasons discussed on page 175.

Measurement of potassium is important because renal failure impairs its excretion, sometimes further exacerbated by drugs (p. 197). Hyperkalaemia is a potentially fatal complication of renal disease. Renal failure may also cause acidosis through failure of the tubular processes described on page 176.

Measurement of glomerular filtration rate

GFR can be measured isotopically ($[^{51}Cr]$-labelled ethylenediaminetetraacetic acid (EDTA)) or chemically (inulin clearance); these measurements are usually confined to specialist nephrological practice. More practically, it can be estimated ('eGFR') by the Cockcroft and Gault formula:

$$\frac{140 - age\,(years) \times weight\,(kg)}{creatinine\,\mu\,mol/l} \times k$$

where k is 1.23 in females and 1.05 in males, or by the modification of diet in renal disease (MDRD) formula, which is being adopted for routine reporting by biochemistry laboratories across the UK.

Autoimmune profile

The glomerulus is a target for some autoantibodies and can be damaged by circulating immune complex, so immunological assessment is an important part of the investigation of renal disease. Relevant antibodies include antineutrophil cytoplasmic antibodies, glomerular basement membrane antibodies, antinuclear factor and antibodies to double-stranded DNA. Measurement of complement is another way of detecting autoimmune activity.

Imaging

Plain radiography and intravenous urography (IVU)

A plain radiograph can show calculi and the renal outlines but provides little other useful information. IVU gives good definition of the kidneys and indicates whether they are functional, but opacification is poor in renal failure. Moreover, even modern 'non-ionic' contrast media present a considerable osmotic load, which can cause heart failure and precipitate acute renal failure, particularly in patients with myeloma or diabetes. You must ensure that such patients are not volume-depleted at the time of contrast radiology or the risk is increased further still.

Ultrasound

In the hands of a skilled radiologist, ultrasound gives detailed information about the structure of the kidneys and urinary tract. It cannot, however, assess function. Because ultrasound is non-invasive and very informative, it is usually the first and often the only form of imaging in both acute and chronic renal disease.

Computed tomography

Computed tomography (CT) gives detailed information about abnormalities within the renal parenchyma and the relationship of organs of the urinary tract to surrounding structures.

Magnetic resonance imaging

Magnetic resonance imaging (MRI) is a non-invasive technique and may be more informative than CT for certain intra-abdominal/pelvic conditions (e.g. prostate/bladder disease). MR angiography is the most useful screening test for renovascular disease.

Antegrade and retrograde pyelography

The renal pelvis and ureters can be cannulated endoscopically and imaged following contrast injection. These techniques are used in obstructive uropathy, in which cannulation may relieve obstruction as well as demonstrating its anatomical level and cause.

Cystography

Cystography is used primarily in paediatric practice. It is performed by instilling contrast into the bladder to demonstrate ureteric reflux during micturition ('micturating cystogramy').

Angiography

Digital angiography allows detailed non-invasive imaging of the renal arterial circulation but has been largely superseded by MR and CT angiography in the investigation of renovascular disease. Renal venography is used to investigate suspected renal vein thrombosis, although this can also be detected non-invasively by duplex/Doppler ultrasound.

Isotope renography

Isotope studies are used not just to image the kidneys but also to measure renal function. For example, asymmetrical uptake between the two kidneys supports a diagnosis of unilateral renal artery stenosis. Delayed clearance of isotope suggests obstruction. Scans using dimercaptosuccinic acid (DMSA) are routinely used in paediatric practice to detect renal scars in reflux nephropathy.

Biopsy

Biopsy is performed by placing a biopsy needle into the kidney substance through a posterior loin approach under ultrasound guidance in a conscious patient. Cooperation is needed because the kidneys move several centimetres with respiration and the patient must stop breathing when the biopsy is taken. Serious complications are rare (<0.5%), the most serious being haemorrhage. Renal biopsy is indicated for the investigation of acute or chronic renal failure of unknown cause, or unexplained persistent proteinuria,

particularly in the nephrotic range, and haematuria. It is primarily indicated to diagnose diffuse disease of the glomeruli, tubules and interstitium. The biopsy sample is analysed by light microscopy, electron microscopy, immunofluorescence and immunohistochemistry.

4.3 Clinical presentations of renal disease

Learning objectives

You should:
* understand the common presentations of renal disease
* understand the causes and management of the common diseases.

Case Study

A diabetic bank manager, able to continue working despite stage 4 chronic kidney disease, is being considered for a 'preemptive' renal transplant before he even starts dialysis. He is receiving an ACE inhibitor, erythropoeitin and a calcium-free phosphate-binding agent to minimise his long-term morbidity.

Table 41 shows a 'matrix' correlating pathologies with clinical presentations. This section first discusses the clinical presentations and then gives details about specific pathologies. There has been recent change in the classification of chronic kidney disease, as shown in Table 42. Where the term 'renal failure' is used in the text that follows, it refers to stages 3–5 chronic kidney disease.

Renal failure

Renal failure may be acute, chronic or 'acute-on-chronic'. There are three potentially **reversible** factors which can cause or exacerbate renal failure:

* impaired perfusion
* urinary obstruction
* infection.

Impaired perfusion not only causes renal failure but can be made worse by it since uraemic anorexia and vomiting cause volume depletion. You should approach a patient with renal failure with the following questions in mind:

* What is the patient's blood volume?
* Have obstruction and infection been excluded?

In addition, the size of the kidneys (easily measured by ultrasound; p. 178) gives you important information about the chronicity of the problem.

Acute renal failure

Epidemiology

Acute renal failure requiring dialysis has an annual incidence of approximately 70 cases per million. Of these:

* 60% are caused by prerenal disease leading to acute tubular necrosis (includes, for example,

Table 41 Clinical presentation of renal/urological disease

Pathology	Clinical presentation							
	Acute nephritis	Acute renal failure	Chronic renal failure	Nephrotic syndrome	Tubular disease	Haematuria	Pain	Symptomless mass
Glomerulonephritis	+	+	+	+		+		
Renovascular disease		+	+					
Renal involvement in systemic disease	+	+	+	+	+	+	+	
Congenital/inherited diseases			+	+	+			+*
Renal tumours						+	+	+
Stone			+			+	+	
Infection			±	+			+	+

*Polycystic kidneys.

Table 42 Classification of chronic kidney disease

Stage	eGFR (ml/min)	Description
1	>90	Normal or low-normal GFR but classified as abnormal because of urinary
2	60–90	abnormality (e.g. proteinuria) or structural abnormality (e.g. cysts in polycystic kidney disease)
3	30–59	Moderate chronic kidney disease; now recognised that 4% of adult Western population falls into this category
4	15–29	Severe kidney disease – 'uraemia'
5	<15	End-stage renal disease

rhabdomyolysis in which free myoglobin damages the tubules)
- 10% are caused by urinary obstruction
- 10–15% result from vasculitides and rapidly progressive glomerulonephritis
- 10% are caused by drugs (e.g. ACE inhibitors, gentamicin) and interstitial nephropathies
- 10% are due to structural abnormalities of renal vasculature:
  — large vessel occlusion (renovascular disease)
  — small vessel occlusion: accelerated hypertension, disseminated intravascular coagulation (DIC) (p. 285), haemolytic–uraemic syndrome, thrombotic thrombocytopenic purpura, systemic sclerosis, pre-eclampsia
  — acute cortical necrosis.

Pathology

The diseases that cause acute renal failure are rapid in their onset and usually prerenal. Bladder outflow obstruction can cause acute renal failure but post-renal disease proximal to the bladder rarely causes truly acute (as opposed to acute-on-chronic) renal failure because both ureters would have to be occluded simultaneously unless there is a congenital absence of, or pre-existing disease in, one kidney. Likewise, there are few renal parenchymal diseases that cause simultaneous acute failure of 1.3 million nephrons; glomerular vasculitides and rapidly progressive glomerulonephritis due to Goodpasture's syndrome, lupus nephritis or renal vasculitis are striking exceptions.

Since each kidney has a separate arterial supply, the same logic might apply to vascular causes, except that aortic disease may involve both renal arteries simultaneously. Prerenal factors leading to renal ischaemia are the most common cause of acute renal failure and are most often seen in the context of severe illness *exogenous* to the kidneys.

The most important concept in the understanding of acute renal failure is that *failure of renal perfusion can progress from a functional abnormality (reversible if perfusion is restored) to established renal damage (acute tubular or, much less commonly, cortical necrosis).*

Clinical presentation

As often as not, renal failure is diagnosed in an already 'ill' patient. The diagnosis may be made biochemically or from the development of oliguria or anuria. Oliguria is defined as a urine flow less than the obligatory minimum for nitrogen excretion (0.51/24 hours). Complete anuria usually signifies urinary obstruction. Oliguria/anuria are not *necessary* conditions for the diagnosis of acute renal failure, since flow may be maintained despite hypofiltration. Progression from oliguria/anuria to polyuria is common during recovery from acute tubular necrosis. Patients with polyuric acute renal failure have an impaired ability to control *flow* (they have, effectively nephrogenic diabetes insipidus) and are extremely vulnerable to volume depletion, which can secondarily exacerbate their renal failure. Other symptoms of renal failure are as shown in Table 40. The symptoms in any individual patient depend on the severity and duration of their disease but do not usually include the effects of renal endocrine failure since these take time to develop.

The clinical assessment of patients with acute renal failure should concentrate on:

- duration: is the disease truly acute, or is there evidence of a previous abnormality of renal function ('acute-on-chronic')?
- symptoms and signs of causative diseases, either specifically renal or multisystem
- assessment of blood volume (p. 192)
- assessment of cardiac function
- exclusion of obstruction: rectal and vaginal examinations are essential in all patients
- assessment for the other features listed in Table 40.

Investigations

Biochemistry You should measure plasma sodium, potassium, urea and creatinine and venous bicarbonate. Arterial blood gas sampling is not necessary for diagnosing metabolic acidosis but may be indicated for assessing pulmonary gas exchange. Measurement of urea and sodium in a 'spot' urine sample helps to distinguish between failure of perfusion and 'established' renal failure; in the former, urinary sodium is low (<20 mmol/l) and the ratio of urinary to plasma urea >8 due to a homeostatic effect of the rennin–angiotensin–aldosterone system.

Urinalysis Culture and microscopy of fresh urine for cells and casts is essential in all cases.

Imaging *Immediate* ultrasound is indicated to assess renal size and exclude bladder outflow obstruction, hydronephrosis and other lower urinary tract disease. One possible problem is that hydronephrosis may not be seen in obstructive uropathy if the patient is also severely volume-depleted. A chest radiograph is needed to assess heart size and look for signs of pulmonary oedema.

Haematology Normochromic anaemia is suggestive of **chronic** renal failure. Other haematological changes such as thrombocytopenia, fragmentation of red cells, etc. may give clues to underlying microvascular disease (e.g. DIC or haemolytic–uraemic syndrome).

Electrocardiograph (ECG) This may show ischaemic heart disease but the most immediate reason for obtaining one is to detect bradycardia and broadening of the QRS complex which is premonitory of cardiac asystole in severe hyperkalaemia.

Renal biopsy The procedure and indications are described on page 179.

Other investigations These are indicated by your suspected cause of renal failure and should include the immunological tests listed above.

Management

Fluid therapy Just as assessment of blood volume is crucial to the diagnosis of acute renal failure, fluid therapy is central to its management. In many cases, the need for fluid can be determined by clinical signs (Fig. 48, below). In a high-dependency or intensive care unit, a pulmonary arterial flow catheter should be used. Management is guided not just by the initial assessment but by frequent bedside reassessment of blood volume and close observation of fluid balance and weight. A urinary catheter can introduce infection and is best avoided in any patient who is able to cooperate, but most patients are very ill so it is needed for accurate hour-to-hour monitoring of output. It is mandatory to weigh the patient daily to assess net gains and losses. The aim of fluid therapy is to achieve adequate but not excessive volume replacement. The choice of fluid depends on the context. Blood loss is treated by blood transfusion. Patients with a reduced colloid osmotic pressure may need 'colloid' infusions. In other cases, saline is the fluid of choice because volume-depleted patients need volume expansion with **salt** and **water**, sometimes with dextrose to correct imbalances in the plasma sodium concentration.

Management of fluid overload A loop diuretic (furosemide or bumetanide) should be given i.v. in high dose and repeated as necessary. A diuretic may also be given as a therapeutic trial to re-establish urine flow in a volume-depleted patient who has been adequately treated with i. v. saline. The signs of fluid overload are indistinguishable from heart failure and impaired cardiac function may be a contributing factor. Any dysrhythmia should be treated and the patient may need inotropic support. Low-dose dopamine specifically improves glomerular perfusion and may be given conjointly with dobutamine for maximum inotropic effect. Logical as their use may seem, neither loop diuretics or dopamine alter the renal functional outcome of people with acute renal failure. Fluid overload that does not respond to these measures is an indication for dialysis (see below).

Obstruction If present, obstruction must be relieved. In the case of bladder outflow obstruction, a urethral or suprapubic catheter should be passed. In ureteric obstruction, a drainage catheter can be positioned in one or both renal pelvices percutaneously (nephrostomy).

Hyperkalaemia Failure of tubular potassium excretion is potentially the most serious metabolic complication of acute renal failure since it can cause fatal ventricular fibrillation or asystole. A serum potassium concentration >7 mmol/l is a medical emergency and should be managed as described on page 197.

Diet and fluid intake The fluid and sodium intake should be adjusted to maintain a normal blood volume, allowing for insensible loss (500 mg/24 hours, higher if pyrexial). Patients who are volume-overloaded should be salt and water-restricted; those who are volume-depleted should drink freely and may need salt supplements. Potassium intake should be restricted. Nutrition is a very important part of the management of acute renal failure. Carbohydrate must be the predominant source of calories and patients should take as high a calorie intake as is commensurate with their fluid and potassium allowances. A protein intake of 0.9–1.0 g/kg body weight is often recommended. If oral feeding is impracticable, enteral or parenteral nutrition should be started without delay.

Dialysis for acute renal failure Dialysis is indicated for:

- nitrogen retention (uraemic symptoms or 'high' blood urea: threshold individualised to the patient)
- pericarditis or neurological complications of uraemia
- intractable fluid retention, even if primarily caused by cardiac failure
- severe hyperkalaemia (potassium >6.5 mmol/l or less if ECG changed)
- acidosis (pH <7.1) or other electrolyte disturbance.

Haemodialysis is used in preference to peritoneal dialysis for acute renal failure. In the intensive care or high-dependency unit, continuous renal replacement therapy is preferred because it removes fluid more slowly and is better tolerated by patients with cardiovascular instability.

Prognosis

Partly because it often develops in the context of multiorgan failure and partly because it causes severe catabolism and widespread tissue damage, acute renal failure has an overall mortality of around 50% in those who reach the stage of needing dialysis. If the patient survives, most of the prerenal causes of acute renal failure have an excellent renal prognosis.

Chronic renal failure

Epidemiology

The overall annual incidence of end-stage renal failure in the UK is approximately 100 cases per million; the incidence increases with age. The causes are:

- diabetic nephropathy: 25% (highest incidence in Asians and Afro-Caribbeans)
- chronic glomerulonephritis: 20%
- chronic reflux nephropathy: 15%
- hypertension and renovascular disease: 15%
- polycystic kidney disease: 10%
- obstructive uropathy: 10%
- other: 5%.

Pathology

Figure 44 shows causes of chronic renal failure. An important point to understand is that it can become self-

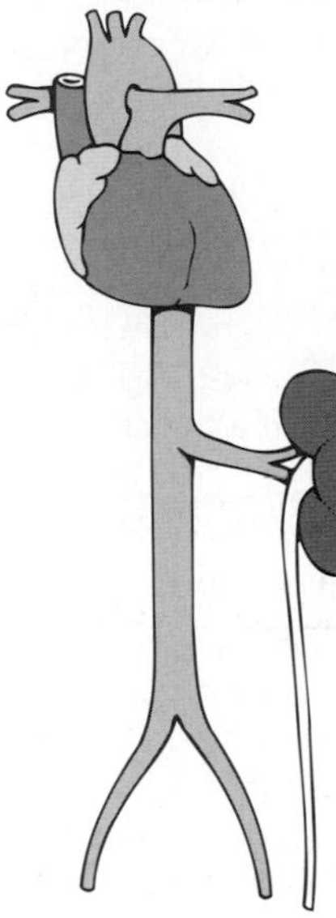

Prerenal:
- Cardiogenic
  Severe cardiac failure
- Vascular
  Renal artery stenosis;
  Intrarenal atherosclerosis
  Hypertension

Renal:
- Immunological /vasculitis
  Glomerulonephritis – primary or
  secondar to systemic disease
- Other microvascular disease
  Diabetes
- Neoplastic
  Multiple myeloma
- Toxic
  Ciclosporin, NSAIDs
- Tubulo-interstitial nephropathy
- Infection and/or reflux
  Chronic pyelonephritis
  Renal tuberculosis
- Cystic diseases
  Polycystic kidneys

Postrenal:
- Disease of the renal pelvis
  Stone
  Pelvi-ureteric obstruction
- Bilateral ureteric obstruction
  Retroperitoneal tumour or fibrosis
  Pelvic or bladder tumour or fibrosis
- Obstruction of solitary kidney
- Bladder outflow obstruction
  Urethral stenosis
  Prostate hypotrophy

Fig. 44 Causes of chronic renal failure.

perpetuating because loss of functioning nephrons causes glomerular hypertension, which leads to further nephron loss. For this reason, treatment rarely reverses established chronic renal failure (though it slows its progression). Renal function may deteriorate progressively despite correction of an underlying disease.

Clinical presentation
The presentation varies from a chance biochemical finding to the most florid and fully developed uraemia. A typical presentation is with non-specific lethargy and anaemia with or without urinary symptoms. Unlike in acute renal failure, the symptoms of bone disease may be prominent. Clinical assessment follows exactly the same steps as described under acute renal failure (p. 181), including exclusion of reversible factors.

Investigations
Investigation follows the same principles as in acute renal failure except that there are some investigations — for example, micturating cystography — which are specific to diseases causing chronic renal failure. Renal biopsy is indicated if no diagnosis has been made, the renal anatomy is normal and renal failure is not too far advanced.

Management
Management consists of:

- treating underlying causes
- optimising fluid/clectrolyte balance and nutrition
- retarding the progression of chronic renal failure
- treating complications
- renal replacement for end-stage renal failure.

Fluid/electrolyte management Patients with chronic failure may be fluid-overloaded or fluid-depleted. Their fluid and salt intake should be adjusted to achieve euvolaemia. Dietary potassium restriction is usually necessary. When diuretics are needed, care must be taken not to cause volume depletion and prerenal uraemia. Potassium-conserving diuretics are relatively contraindicated.

Acid–base management In some cases, chronic treatment with oral bicarbonate is needed to correct acidosis.

Diet Restriction of dietary protein below 1 g/kg body weight daily can improve hydrostatic pressures within the glomeruli and attenuate the self-perpetuating renal deterioration. Vigorous protein restriction was previously recommended to delay the need for dialysis, but that delay was achieved at the expense of malnutrition and increased mortality. Now it is only used in some patients deemed unsuitable for dialysis. Dietary phosphate restriction helps reduce the severity of renal bone disease.

Antihypertensive therapy There is strong evidence that, for at least some causes of chronic renal failure, antihypertensive therapy can halt or attenuate renal deterioration. ACE inhibitors/angiotensin 2 receptor blockers are particularly beneficial but can be harmful if the patient has renal artery stenosis or is volume-depleted. Close monitoring of renal function after starting ACE inhibitors/angiotensin 2 receptor blockers is essential and 'arteriopaths' may need renography or angiography to exclude renal artery stenosis before starting them.

Hyperlipidaemia Most patients with chronic renal failure have moderate combined hyperlipidaemia, a factor contributing to the formidably high cardiovascular morbidity and mortality. Fasting lipids should be checked periodically and treated (as described on p. 313). That is not without difficulty, because fat restriction is yet another imposition on the renal patient's diet, so early use of a statin is commonplace.

Anaemia When the eGFR is below 30 ml/min normochromic normocytic anaemia is common. Treatment with iron (given intravenously because it is poorly absorbed by mouth) and subcutaneous erythropoietin can improve quality of life, cardiovascular mortality and overall survival.

Renal replacement Renal replacement therapy is indicated for patients with advanced renal failure whose general state of health, psychosocial wellbeing and support are such that it is likely to improve the quality as well as the quantity of life. Renal replacement should be planned and discussed with patients well in advance of end-stage renal failure. It is started when uraemia seriously affects their wellbeing (GFR often ≤10 ml/min) or complications develop. Transplantation, where possible, achieves a higher level of rehabilitation than maintenance (home or hospital) haemodialysis or continuous ambulatory peritoneal dialysis.

Prescribing in renal disease
At its simplest, this can be covered in five words: 'refer to *British National Formulary*'. This should be carried in every

Table 43 Important drug effects in renal failure

	Drug	Effect	Action
Accumulation	Digoxin	Potential toxicity	Reduce dose, monitor drug level
	Aminoglycosides	Ototoxicity	Use prescribing nomogram, monitor levels
	Sulphonylureas	Hypoglycaemia	Use non-renally excreted drugs, e.g. gliclazide
Nephrotoxicity	Aminoglycosides	Tubular toxicity in acute renal failure	Use prescribing nomogram, monitor levels
	Radiographic contrast media	Acute-on-chronic renal failure	Ensure patients are adequately hydrated before radiographic procedures
May have side-effects	NSAIDs	Fluid retention Worsened GFR	Use with caution Monitor serum creatinine
	ACE inhibitors/angiotensin receptor antagonists	Worsened renal function in renal artery stenosis	Avoid in severe renal artery stenosis, monitor creatinine
		Hyperkalaemia	Monitor serum K^+ and creatinine
Less effective in renal failure	Diuretics		Increase effectiveness by using loop diuretics, giving i.v., using high dose
Contraindicated or to be used cautiously*	Potassium-sparing diuretics	Hyperkalaemia	
	Nitrofurantoin	Renal tubular necrosis, peripheral neuropathy	
	Tetracycline	Worsened uraemia	
	Metformin	Lactic acidosis	

ACE, angiotensin-converting enzyme; GFR, glomerular filtration rate; NSAID, non-steroidal anti-inflammatory drug.
*Avoid in stages 4–5 chronic kidney disease; monitor renal function and serum potassium.

doctor's pocket or briefcase and gives detailed information about drugs that affect or are affected by renal disease. The ways in which renal disease affects the action of drugs and how drugs can damage the kidneys are summarised in Table 43.

Renal bone disease

Pathophysiology

The pathogenetic mechanisms, summarised in Figure 45, are relatively specific to chronic renal failure. Renal tubular phosphate retention and failure to 1α-hydroxylate vitamin D lead to osteomalacia and secondary hyperparathyroidism, with failure of mineralisation and increased osteoclastic bone resorption. There may also be osteosclerosis, which causes the 'rugger jersey spine' appearance on plain radiographs.

Clinical presentation and biochemical features

There may be weakness, bone pain, deformity and fractures. Plasma calcium is usually normal or low. Plasma phosphate is high. Alkaline phosphatase is high if there is significant bone disease. Serum parathyroid hormone is raised.

Management

Phosphate-binding agents should be given to all patients with established chronic renal failure. Calcium carbonate has previously been the mainstay of treatment because it is cheap and provides supplemental calcium as well. However, there is increasing concern about vascular calcification, to which renal patients are very prone, as a risk factor for arterial events. For that reason, non-calcium-containing phosphate binders (e.g. sevelamer, a polymer) are taking its place. 1,25-Dihydroxycholecalciferol or an analogue is used to treat hypocalcaemia and suppress secondary hyperparathyroidism. Tertiary hyperparathyroidism is diagnosed when the patient becomes hyperalcaemic and treated by parathyroidectomy.

Acute-on-chronic renal failure

Patients with chronic renal failure are vulnerable to the prerenal and postrenal diseases summarised on page 174 and the effects of intercurrent illness and urinary infection, all of which can acutely exacerbate chronic renal failure. The clinical features, investigation and management are as for acute renal failure. The search for exacerbating factors, volume depletion in particular, is paramount. With prompt and effective treatment, it is usually possible to reverse the functional deterioration.

Nephrotic syndrome

Nephrotic syndrome is a chronic condition defined by the triad of:

- proteinuria (>3 g/24 hours)
- hypoproteinaemia (serum albumin <25 g/l)
- oedema.

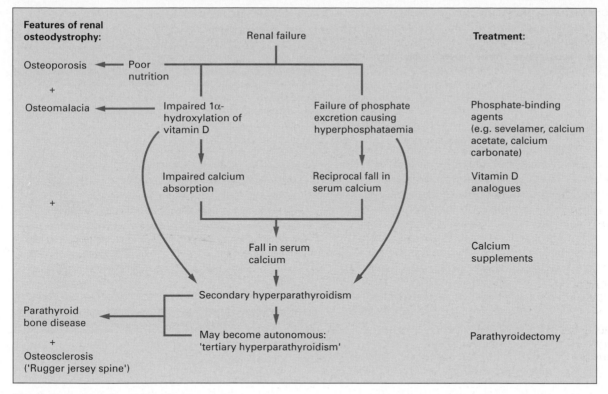

Fig. 45 Mechanisms of renal bone disease.

It is to be distinguished from nephritic syndrome, although both syndromes may be caused by glomerulonephritis. Proteinuria is the primary abnormality; hypoproteinaemia ensues and this lowers plasma oncotic pressure so that salt and water leak from capillaries into the interstitial space, often causing gross oedema. Plasma volume is reduced and there is compensatory hyperaldosteronism, which increases total body sodium content. Nephrotic syndrome signifies increased permeability of the glomerular filter caused by glomerular disease.

Causes

The most classical cause of nephrotic syndrome is **minimal change nephropathy** in children. A more complete list is given in Box 10.

The most common causes are glomerulonephritis, diabetes and drugs.

Complications and management

Apart from salt retention (oedema, pleural and pericardial effusions, ascites), patients may suffer from malnutrition and increased susceptibility to infection as an effect of protein loss. Hypercholesterolaemia and hypercoagulability predispose to coronary artery disease. Nephrotic syndrome predisposes to one quite specific complication, renal vein thrombosis, which should be suspected in any nephrotic patient whose proteinuria or renal function worsens abruptly. It is diagnosed by renal venography or Doppler ultrasound and treated with anticoagulants both to preserve renal function and prevent pulmonary embolism.

Box 10: Causes of nephrotic syndrome

Glomerulonephritis
- Primary
  - Minimal change disease
  - Other glomerulonephritides
- Secondary
  - Autoimmune disease such as systemic lupus erythematosus (SLE)
  - Neoplasia: carcinoma, lymphoma, leukaemia
  - Infection: subacute bacterial endocarditis, malaria, hepatitis B
  - Drugs/toxins: gold, other heavy metals, penicillamine, i.v. drug abuse

Other immunological disease
- Amyloid

Metabolic
- Diabetes mellitus

Myeloma
- 'Myeloma kidney'

Vascular
- Renal vein thrombosis

Diuretics are prescribed for oedema but their use is problematic because they may further contract an already reduced plasma volume and worsen renal perfusion. If plasma volume contraction prevents effective diuretic therapy, colloid may be infused to increase plasma colloid oncotic pressure and provide a temporary 'bridge' between the interstitial fluid and glomeruli. Minimal change disease responds well to corticosteroids or other immunosuppressives; some causes of nephrotic syndrome are unremitting even with treatment. In that situation, ACE inhibitors or angiotensin receptor blockers can be used to reduce proteinuria.

Acute nephritic syndrome

At its most florid, the acute nephritic syndrome consists of oliguria and oedema of the face, hands and legs. The urine is 'smoky' because of glomerular haematuria, proteinuria and urinary casts. Historically, the most common cause was streptococcal infection, but poststreptococcal nephritis is now rare in the developed world. The acute nephritic syndrome is more commonly caused by rapidly progressive glomerulonephritis, often associated with systemic vasculitis or connective tissue disorders. It may also follow a range of non-streptococcal infections. It may be benign and self-limiting or lead to acute renal failure. Management is as described for other causes of acute renal failure, with specific treatment aimed at any underlying cause.

Renal tubular acidosis

Renal tubular acidosis (RTA) is a name to strike terror into the heart of all but the nephrologist or the physician who has recently passed MRCP. In fact, the principles are simple and follow exactly from the description of tubular function (p. 175).

- There is failure of bicarbonate reabsorption (type 2, proximal tubular) or hydrogen ion secretion (type 1, distal tubular), leading to reduced serum bicarbonate and metabolic acidosis.
- The urine is inappropriately alkaline.
- There is a compensatory rise in serum chloride to maintain electrical neutrality, a 'hyperchloraemic acidosis'.
- There may be other tubular dysfunctions, such as increased leakage of sodium, potassium, glucose, calcium, amino acids and phosphate (type 2 RTA).
- The disease may be congenital or acquired.
- There may be calcification of the kidneys, particularly at the cortico-medullary junction, nephrocalcinosis (type 1 RTA).
- The tubular phosphate leak may cause a vitamin D-resistant form of rickets (renal rickets).

The best-recognised form of renal tubular acidosis is **Fanconi syndrome**. This inherited disorder is caused by proximal tubular dysfunction and comprises glycosuria, aminoaciduria, 'renal rickets' and renal tubular acidosis. Acquired renal tubular disease may result from multiple myeloma, connective tissue disease, heavy metal poisoning, acquired aldosterone deficiency and chronic parenchymal kidney disease. Treatment is with alkali, phosphate, sodium and potassium. The synthetic analogue of aldosterone, fludrocortisone, can be used to treat renal sodium loss and hypovolaemia.

4.4 Specific renal and urinary tract diseases

Learning objectives

You should:
- understand the features and investigation of parenchymal and vascular renal diseases
- be able to identify the possible underlying causes and how to treat the disease and its secondary effects
- be able to distinguish acute cystitis from the urethral syndrome in young women
- be able to distinguish upper tract infection (pyelonephritis) from lower tract infection (cystitis)
- be conversant with the concept of a complicated urinary tract infection and how it is distinguished from a simple urinary infection
- be able to interpret a urine microscopy and culture report.

Case Study

After a night of severe chills and teeth chattering, a woman in the 34th week of pregnancy presents in primary care. Her temperature in 38.3°C, her BP is 90/60 mmHg and she looks unwell. She has protein ++ on urine dipstick but no ankle oedema. She is told that a urinary infection does not pose a serious threat to her pregnancy.

The clinical presentations described so far are core knowledge. Many individual renal diseases, including the glomerulonephritides, are 'non-core'. A description of them can be found in a reference textbook.

The ways in which individual **systemic diseases** affect the kidneys are best learned when studying the diseases themselves.

Parenchymal and vascular diseases

Interstitial nephropathy

Glomerulopathy is one renal response to injury; another is interstitial or 'tubulo-interstitial' nephropathy, where the tubules and interstitium bear the brunt of disease. The classical stereotype is analgesic nephropathy, but this is now uncommon. Important causes include:

- vesico-ureteric reflux leading to reflux nephropathy (the major cause of chronic pyleonephritis)
- chronic urinary obstruction
- idiopathic
- drugs (e.g. lithium, NSAIDs).

Less common causes include:

- connective tissue disease
- neoplasia
- metabolic causes: hypercalcaemia, hypokalaemia, gout
- sarcoidosis.

Interstitial nephropathy presents with moderate proteinuria, acute or chronic renal failure or renal tubular dysfunction. Diagnosis rests on clinical suspicion and, where appropriate, renal biopsy. Treatment is by correction of underlying causes; in some patients, steroids are effective. The disease may progress to end-stage renal failure.

Renal papillary necrosis

Renal papillary necrosis is caused by ischaemic necrosis and sloughing of renal papillae. It is characterised by:

- loin pain (sometimes of a colicky nature)
- haematuria
- variable degrees of renal impairment.

It is an acute and uncommon variant of interstitial nephropathy, most commonly caused by drugs/toxins and acute infections, particularly in diabetes mellitus.

Renovascular disease

Narrowing of the renal artery or its tributaries proximal to the glomeruli reduces glomerular pressure and increases renin secretion, irrespective of systemic pressure. This may result from a single narrowing of a main renal artery or diffuse intrarenal arterial disease. Renal artery stenosis may cause hypertension and, if bilateral, renal failure. Renal arterial disease is suggested by otherwise unexplained renal failure or hypertension in a patient with peripheral vascular and/or generalised arterial disease; arterial (femoral, epigastric, etc.) bruits are the chief clinical sign. Renovascular disease should also be suspected in a patient whose renal function worsens when given an ACE inhibitor, because these drugs adversely affect the compensatory haemodynamic response to renal arterial disease. Because of this risk, renal function should be measured frequently after initiation of ACE inhibitor therapy in arteriopaths or elderly patients.

Ultrasound may show a small kidney on the side of unilateral renal artery stenosis; angiography is the definitive investigation. Renal artery stenosis can be treated by:

- angioplasty
- stenting
- surgery.

Renal vein thrombosis has been mentioned under nephrotic syndrome.

Cystic disease

There are three main forms of cystic disease:

- solitary benign cysts
- cysts associated with renal cell carcinoma
- polycystic disease.

A solitary cyst may be found by chance on abdominal examination or ultrasound or in the investigation of loin pain and/or haematuria. Most solitary cysts are benign. If in doubt, cyst fluid may be aspirated percutaneously for cytological examination.

Autosomal dorminant polycystic disease is an important diagnosis because it accounts for about 10% of cases of end-stage renal failure, typically presenting between 40 and 50 years of age. Patients may also present with:

- loin pain
- haematuria
- symptoms and signs related to the sometimes massively enlarged kidneys.

In established disease, the appearances on ultrasound or CT are pathognomonic and the diagnosis can even be made by abdominal examination (large, irregular masses in both loins). The disease follows an autosomal dominant pattern of inheritance and progresses slowly but inexorably towards end-stage renal failure. Treatment is with:

- good control of blood pressure
- general management of chronic renal failure
- dialysis when the end stage is reached.

There are liver cysts in 70% of patients and 25% have berry aneurysms, which may lead to subarachnoid haemorrhage. Chromosomal markers have been identified and genetic counselling must be offered in all cases.

Neoplasia

Neoplasia can be classified into:

- urothelial tumours
- renal cell carcinoma
- exogenous or secondary tumours directly or indirectly affecting the urinary tract, the renal parenchyma, the renal circulation, the glomeruli and/ or the tubules.

Haematuria and pain are the main symptoms; the exact distribution and nature of the pain depend on the site, size and invasiveness of the tumour. Renal adenocarcinoma is a tumour notorious for its systemic effects. In addition to its local effects, it may present with:

- pyrexia of unknown origin
- weight loss and systemic malaise
- bony or pulmonary metastases
- hypercalcaemia
- polycythaemia.

Relevant investigations are urinalysis, ultrasound, CT, intravenous pyelography and cystoscopy. Table 44 summarises key facts about tumours of the kidneys and urinary tract.

Urinary stones

Stones may present with:

- pain and/or haematuria
- symptoms of infection
- renal failure in patients with a solitary kidney or chronic disease.

They may be a chance radiographic finding. Most stones are radio-opaque. Those that are not can be detected with IVU or ultrasound. The management is with analgesics, a high fluid intake and, occasionally, lithotripsy or surgery for large stones or acute obstruction.

The 'medical' approach to stones is to measure urinary calcium excretion and consider underlying causes which predispose to stone formation. These are:

Four

Table 44 Tumours of kidney and urinary tract

Type	Demography	Clinical features	Management
Renal adenocarcinoma	Male > female, adults	Pyrexia of unknown origin, malaise, loin pain, haematuria, mass effects of local invasion, metastases, hypercalcaemia, polycythaemia	Surgery, embolisation (chemotherapy, radiotherapy)
Nephroblastoma (Wilms' tumour)	Infants or children	Mass, haematuria, pain	Surgery, chemotherapy, radiotherapy
Transitional cell carcinoma			
Kidney and ureters	Adults	Haematuria, mass, hydronephrosis	Surgery
Bladder	Adults	Haematuria, urinary symptoms (including obstruction)	Superficial: regular cystoscopic surveillance, diathermy, intravesical chemotherapy Invasive: cystectomy, radiotherapy, chemotherapy

- chronic infection
- hypercalcaemia
- hyperuricaemia
- cystinuria.

A small minority of patients with stones will have one of these diseases. The majority have hypercalciuria or hyperoxaluria, for which the management is a high fluid intake and avoidance of foods with high calcium or urate contents. Hypercalciuria can be treated with thiazide diuretics. The treatment of hypercalcaemia is discussed on page 360. Hyperuricaemia is treated with allopurinol. Cystinuria is managed by alkalinisation of the urine and with penicillamine.

Urinary tract infections

Clinical syndromes

Several different bacterial diseases of adults come under the heading of 'urinary tract infection'. They can be grouped as follows:

- cystitis and acute urethral syndrome in young women
- acute uncomplicated pyelonephritis in women
- urinary tract infection in young men
- catheter-associated urinary tract infection
- asymptomatic bacteriuria in elderly people
- complicated urinary tract infection.

Infection can also be caused by *Mycobacterium tuberculosis*, fungi and parasites. Many viruses are excreted in the urine but only adenoviruses and BK virus cause infection.

Diagnosing urinary tract infection

Diagnosis rests on microscopy and culture of an appropriately collected specimen (Table 45). Rapid tests include the detection of nitrates, dehydrogenase activity and proteinuria, and are often automated.

Occasionally, pyuria occurs without a positive culture ('sterile pyuria'). This may occur in elderly people and is rarely significant unless symptoms are also present. Causes are:

- a partially treated urinary tract infection
- fastidious bacteria, e.g. *Lactobacilli*, *Corynebacteria*, streptococci
- urinary tract tuberculosis
- papillary necrosis.

In symptomatic patients with sterile pyuria, it is important to culture urine for *M. tuberculosis* and fastidious organisms.

Cystitis

Cystitis in young women

Cystitis is common, affecting about 1 million women annually in the UK. Typically, they present acutely ill with frequency, urgency and dysuria. Physical signs are few and fever is usually absent. There are several risk factors, including:

- sexual intercourse
- the use of a contraceptive diaphragm and spermicide
- not micturating after intercourse
- a history of prior cystitis.

Over 85% of cases are caused by *Escherichia coli* and *Staphylococcus saprophyticus*, the remainder being caused by other Gram-negative rods. A midstream urine specimen will usually contain more than 10^5 organisms/ml and >10 white cell/mm^3 (>10 × 10^6 cells/l).

Treatment regimens include single doses or short courses of amoxicillin, trimethoprim, co-trimoxazole or a quinolone, depending on the local prevalence of resistance. Women should be advised to drink plenty of fluids and to urinate immediately after intercourse.

Table 45 Laboratory diagnosis of urinary infection in various clinical settings

Urinary findings	Cystitis	Acute urethral syndrome	Pyelonephritis	Catheterised patient[a]	Complicated UTI	Elderly nursing home patient[a]
White cell count	+++	−/+	+/++	−/++	−/+++	+/++
Significant bacterial count	$>10^5$/ml	?	$>10^4$/ml	$>10^4$/ml	Variable	$>10^4$/ml
Common pathogens	Escherichia coli, Staphylococcus saprophyticus	Negative[b]	E. coli	Any	Proteus spp., Mycobacterium tuberculosis, Candida spp., Pseudomonas spp.	E. coli

UTI, urinary tract infection.
[a] Clinical assessment essential as asymptomatic bacteriuria common and does not require therapy.
[b] Special cultures required (see text).

Recurrent cystitis

A significant number of women suffer from recurrent cystitis. Risk factors include:

- the Lewis blood group secretor phenotype
- increased vaginal colonisation with E. coli or other Gram-negative rods, sometimes related to diaphragm use
- urinary tract abnormalities, present in <5% and easily excluded by renal ultrasound.

Antibiotic prophylaxis may be administered either continuously, after intercourse or on first symptoms.

Recurrent infection in older women

Older, particularly multiparous, women may have a cystocele preventing complete bladder emptying during micturition. Postmenopausal loss of urethral elasticity and increased E. coli colonisation of the vagina may also contribute. Oestrogen pessaries often substantially reduce the frequency of urinary infection in postmenopausal women.

Acute urethral syndrome

Acute urethral syndrome refers to a clinical syndrome in young women akin to cystitis but with negative urine culture and microscopy. Symptoms are generally milder but more chronic than in cystitis. Like cystitis, this problem is common. Sexually transmitted infections such as those caused by Chlamydia spp. need to be excluded (p. 423). A large percentage of these women, particularly if the infection is chronic, appear to have bacterial infection and inflammation of the periurethral tissues of the distal ureter. The causative organisms are frequently unusual and missed in routine urine cultures. A urethral swab and/or the first portion of urine during micturition from such patients is usually positive. Antibiotic management should be directed at the pathogen isolated and continued for longer than the standard urinary tract infection course (e.g. 10–14 days).

Acute pyelonephritis in women

The spectrum of illness is wide. Clinical features include:

- fever (common)
- back or loin pain (common)
- chills and rigors (common)
- nausea and vomiting
- hypotension and features of the sepsis syndrome (p. 410) (occasional).

Severe pain and radiation of the pain into the groin are rare but, if present, suggest a renal calculus. Pyelonephritis is proportionally more common in pregnancy, partly because of dilatation of the ureters and decreased ureteral peristalsis, and may lead to premature labour. Asymptomatic pyelonephritis sometimes accompanies cystitis.

Diagnosis

Over 80% of acute pyelonephritis in young women is caused by invasive E. coli strains that have specific virulence mechanisms. Blood cultures are often positive, especially in the more severely ill patients. The urine usually shows pyuria and is culture-positive. The 10^5/ml cut-off for bacteriuria used for cystitis does not apply to pyelonephritis, as at least 20% of patients with acute pyelonephritis have less than this number of bacteria in their urine.

Acute pyelonephritis in older patients or with other organisms is most likely to represent a complicated urinary tract infection, even though the presentation is very similar (see below).

Investigations

Investigations for abnormalities of the urinary tract (e.g. reflux, scarring, stones, diverticulae) are unrevealing in most young women with pyelonephritis. Indications for investigation include:

- slow resolution of infection
- more than one episode
- prior urinary infection in childhood

Four

- unusual features, e.g. haematuria, impaired renal function, colicky pain, etc.

Management

The vast majority of patients with pyelonephritis require admission to hospital. Intravenous antibiotics are appropriate for all but the mildest cases. Aminoglycosides, quinolones or third-generation cephalosporins are most appropriate. Patients should have a repeat urine culture and renal ultrasound to seek a perinephric abscess if they have not responded after 3 days. Second- or third-generation cephalosporins are the preferred agents in pregnancy.

Urinary tract infections in men

Urinary tract infections are rare in men up to the age of 60. The same uropathogenic *E. coli* strains that cause pyelonephritis in young women cause cystitis and occasionally pyelonephritis in men. Risk factors include anal intercourse, no circumcision and a female sexual partner with vaginal colonisation by uropathogenic *E. coli*. Occasionally urinary infections are complicated by epididymitis and/or prostatitis. Oral antibiotics are usually appropriate. Investigations for a structural urological abnormality are usually negative but should be undertaken if the organism isolated is unusual or the patient has more than one episode. Likewise, chronic prostatitis should be excluded.

Epididymitis

Epididymitis is a common infection that varies in aetiology depending on the age of the patient. Over 35 years of age it is usually caused by Gram-negative rods, sometimes Gram-positive cocci. Under the age of 35 years, *Neisseria gonorrhoeae* and *Chlamydia trachomatis* are the most common causes. Patients present with painful swelling of the scrotum over 1–2 days. It is often asymmetrical and appears to involve the testis. Fever, dysuria and frequency of micturition are common. In younger patients, urethritis is common and should be sought clinically. A gratifying response to antibiotics is usual.

Catheter-associated urinary tract infection

Urinary catheters may be placed for short- or long-term use. Ascending infection from the use of short-term catheters in hospital is the most common cause of Gram-negative bacteraemia, sometimes with fatal consequences. Therefore, early removal of a catheter is appropriate, if possible. However, in the incontinent patient, catheterisation may prevent skin breakdown and bed sores so, as in all aspects of medicine, a reasonable judgement between two opposing risks is necessary. Careful, aseptic changing and draining of catheter bags and the use of a closed collecting system reduce infection rates.

Diagnosis and management

Bacteriuria of only 10^2/ml drained through a catheter is significant when the patient is symptomatic. Asymptomatic pyuria and bacteriuria are common and do not require therapy. The organisms causing catheter-associated urinary tract infection are much more varied, often multiple, and more likely to be resistant to antibiotics than those causing cystitis in healthy women. Therefore,

broader-spectrum antibiotics, such as quinolones, may be appropriate for treatment. As the infecting bacteria often produce biofilms on catheters, treatment failure or relapse is common and a catheter change or removal is important for eradication.

With respect to long-term catheterisation, intermittent self-catheterisation (as, for example, in paraplegic patients after spinal injury) is far less likely to lead to infective problems than continuous long-term indwelling urinary catheters. Long-term indwelling silastic catheters should be changed every 3 months.

Asymptomatic bacteriuria in elderly people

Bacteriuria is relatively common (up to 40%) in immobile elderly patients, especially in nursing homes, and may or may not reflect disease. Surprisingly, symptomatic infections, including pyelonephritis and/or sepsis, are uncommon. Therefore, screening and treatment of those found to be positive are unjustified. Furthermore, routine cultures of urine in elderly people on admission to hospital are wasteful as asymptomatic bacteriuria and pyuria are more common than urinary infections. Elderly patients with a new confusional state and/or symptoms suggestive of a urinary infection (e.g. frequency, nocturia, etc.) should, however, be treated promptly after cultures have been obtained. Pyuria may be present but is a less useful guide to symptomatic infection in elderly people.

Complicated urinary tract infection

A complicated urinary tract infection is defined as an infection that occurs in patients with a functionally or anatomically abnormal urinary tract, or is caused by pathogens resistant to standard antibiotics (e.g. *M. tuberculosis, Pseudomonas* spp., etc.) or both.

However, these factors are not necessarily discernible when the patient first presents. There is a wide spectrum of presentation, from mild cystitis to life-threatening sepsis syndrome. Clues to the diagnosis of a complicated urinary tract infection include:

- history of renal tract disease, such as stones, surgery, haematuria, etc.
- prior urinary tract infection or bacteriuria
- prior antibiotic therapy (possibly for other problems)
- prior hospitalisation, especially if catheterised
- abnormal renal function on presentation.

All patients with complicated urinary tract infections need referral to a specialist physician and/or a urologist as surgery may be necessary. Unusual antibiotic regimens are also usually necessary and so obtaining a culture before antibiotic treatment is fundamental to good management.

Fungal urinary tract infection

Candida is found in the urine of 5–10% of hospitalised patients. In the intensive care unit it is often synonymous with life-threatening candidaemia and rapid consideration is given to treatment for disseminated candidiasis (p. 423). In other patients, it carries little significance unless accompanied by symptoms or white cells. *C. albicans* is the most common species. *C. glabrata* is also common. Fluconazole is the initial treatment of choice.

Tuberculosis of the urinary tract

Urinary tract disease is a relatively unusual manifestation of tuberculosis. Patients complain of frequency and urgency, with little dysuria. Tuberculosis is a classic cause of sterile pyuria and should be suspected in symptomatic patients in whom straightforward bacterial infection has been excluded and when the patient is from the Indian subcontinent. Tuberculin skin tests are usually strongly positive in these patients.

Early morning urine samples for *M. tuberculosis* culture are frequently requested for 'generally ill patients in whom tuberculosis is a possibility'. Their utility is, however, very poor as they have a low yield and the results take 4–8 weeks to come back. If the diagnosis of urinary tract tuberculosis is a serious possibility, cystoscopy and biopsy of the bladder wall is a quicker way to reach the diagnosis.

Treatment is as for pulmonary tuberculosis (p. 79), for at least 6 months.

Antibiotic management of urinary tract infections

Useful antibiotics for uncomplicated urinary tract infection include trimethoprim (about 80% of infecting organisms are sensitive) and quinolones (about 90%). The duration of therapy for cystitis should not exceed 5 days and 1–3 days is often sufficient. Longer treatment (e.g. 10 days) is required for the acute urethral syndrome.

For ill patients with pyelonephritis, cephalosporins such as cefuroxime or cefotaxime, or quinolones are appropriate. Aminoglycosides are also very useful and effective. For patients with complicated urinary tract infections, empirical therapy with the above is appropriate but coverage for *Pseudomonas* spp. with ciprofloxacin or gentamicin is superior.

4.5 Fluid and electrolyte balance

Learning objectives

You should:
- understand the concept of fluid 'compartments'
- know the 'barriers' that divide the compartments
- understand the mechanisms that control vascular volume and electrolyte homeostasis
- be able to assess vascular volume reliably at the bedside
- be able to interpret abnormalities of plasma sodium, potassium, urea, creatinine, bicarbonate and albumin concentrations and know how to use physical signs to help to interpret them
- understand how to manage common fluid/electrolyte disorders.

Case Study

An epileptic patient, recently started on carbamazepine, is admitted in status epilepticus. Her serum sodium concentration is 112 mmol/l. Carbamazepine is thought to have precipitated her status by causing the syndrome of inappropriate antidiuresis.

For the tissues to function effectively, they have to be perfused with oxygenated blood of the correct electrolyte composition. Perfusion depends upon:

- cardiac pumping
- vascular tone
- maintenance of vascular volume.

This section primarily concerns vascular volume and the electrolyte composition of plasma. Cardiac pumping and vascular tone are discussed in Chapter 1 (p. 8). Remember, however, that renal function, fluid/electrolyte homeostasis and cardiovascular function are intimately related physiologically, biochemically and in their symptoms and signs.

The underpinning physiology may be a distant memory but the moment you collect an on-call bleep for the first time you assume responsibility for interpreting the physical signs and biochemistry of fluid–electrolyte and acid–base balance and maintaining the volume and composition of your patients' fluid compartments. This section will 'lock together' simple physiological concepts with the everyday measurements made by clinicians and show how they relate to disease states. The approach is deliberately simplistic because it is through failing to apply simple physiological concepts that clinical errors are made.

Physiology of fluid and electrolyte balance

Compartments

A 70 kg man has a total fluid content of approximately 42 litres. Figure 46 shows how this divides between a large intracellular and a smaller extracellular compartment. The cell membrane acts as a barrier which maintains the different electrolyte composition of the two compartments by active electrolyte transport. The predominant intracellular cation is potassium and the predominant anions are proteins and phosphate. Sodium and chloride are the predominant extracellular anion and cation, respectively. The extracellular fluid is subdivided into a larger interstitial and smaller vascular compartment. The barrier between them is the capillary wall, which acts as a semi-permeable membrane. The vascular and interstitial fluids have the same electrolyte composition but protein cannot pass across the capillary wall.

Osmolality and filtration

Osmotically active substances, predominantly electrolytes, attract water. The degree of dilution of these solutes is regulated by antidiuretic hormone (ADH; also known as arginine vasopressin) and measured as osmolality. Water diffuses freely between the intracellular and extracellular compartments and their osmolality is, therefore, identical. In the ECF, sodium is the most abundant low molecular weight solute and, therefore (as discussed on p. 174), the sodium content of the extracellular fluid determines its volume. Plasma is protein-rich compared with the

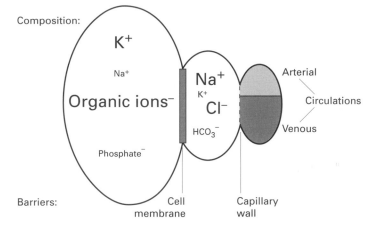

Compartments:	Intracellular fluid (ICF)	Extracellular fluid (ECF)	
		Interstitial	Vascular
Volumes in a 70 kg man (litres)	28	10	5.5

Fig. 46 Fluid compartments.

interstitial fluid. Plasma proteins exert an osmotic force termed the **colloid osmotic pressure**, which maintains **vascular** volume.

The capillaries have a higher hydrostatic pressure than the interstitial compartment, with a gradient between the arterial (high-pressure) and venous (low-pressure) ends. Capillary pressure forces an ultrafiltrate into the interstitial fluid. This process of filtration leaves an increasingly protein-rich fluid in the capillary, which, at its low-pressure venous end, osmotically draws sodium and water back into the vascular compartment. Excessive accumulation of interstitial fluid (oedema) occurs if the colloid osmotic pressure is low (hypoproteinaemia), the capillary wall leaks protein (as in sepsis ('capillary leak syndrome')) or there is increased venous pressure, which opposes the colloid osmotic 'draw' of fluid back into the capillary (as occurs in venous obstruction or the raised central venous pressure of heart failure).

Volume

The vascular compartment is the 'central player' in fluid and electrolyte physiology because it is the vehicle by which solutes and oxygen reach the tissues and waste is removed. Its composition determines the composition of the interstitial compartment and, indirectly, the intracellular compartment. It is small, about 5.5 litres, two-thirds of which is in the venous circulation and one-third in the arterial circulation. The all-important part of the system is the arterial circulation because it maintains oxygen delivery. Even transient disruption of arterial oxygen supply can have catastrophic consequences.

Since the circulation is a closed system, cardiac function depends upon venous return as well as on an intact myocardium. The veins are the 'capacitance' vessels, which can absorb extra fluid volume or 'top up' the circulation in states of volume depletion. The single most important term in understanding fluid balance is

volume, and this can be subdivided conceptually into venous and arterial volume. The terms **volume depletion** and **volume overload** will be used here to discuss disease and clinical management in preference to 'dehydration' and 'overhydration', because disease usually affects sodium and water homeostasis rather than water alone. Figure 47 illustrates the vascular system schematically and shows how it changes in different pathological conditions.

Homeostatic mechanisms

Haemorrhagic shock is the most extreme example of volume depletion. Arterial baroreceptors activate the sympathetic system leading to:

- vasoconstriction to divert blood away from skin, intestine and kidneys and maintain arterial volume (pale, clammy, oliguric)
- venoconstriction to maintain venous return from the reserve volume in the capacitance vessels
- tachycardia to maximise cardiac output.

In health, homeostatic mechanisms have to compensate for variations in the intake of fluid and dietary sodium and loss through the kidneys, skin, intestinal tract and lungs. Two mechanisms operate: thirst, which regulates water intake, and the endocrine system, which regulates renal water and electrolyte handling. The sensation of thirst is controlled by hypothalamic osmoreceptors. There are several endocrine mechanisms.

Antidiuretic hormone

ADH is primarily secreted in response to changes in plasma osmolality sensed by the hypothalamic osmoreceptors; in states of volume depletion, the arterial baroreceptors increase ADH secretion, irrespective of osmolality, to 'preserve volume at all costs'. ADH increases water absorption in the collecting duct (p. 175).

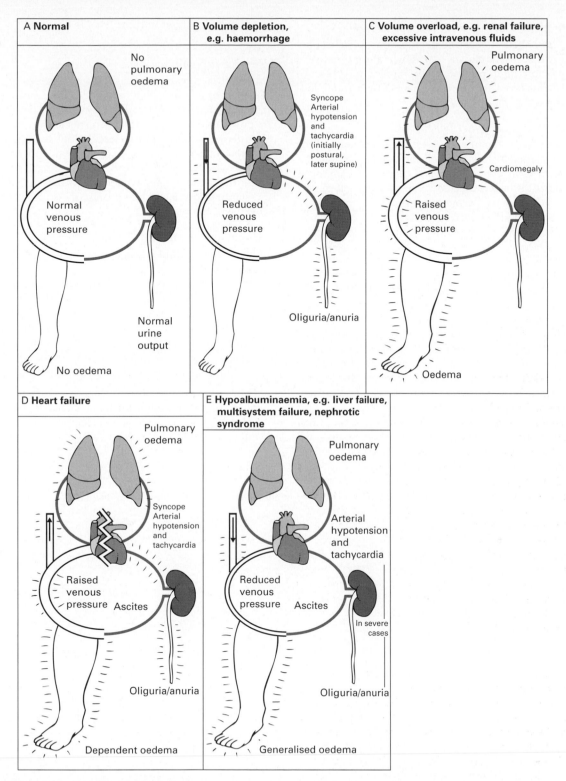

Fig. 47 Fluid physiology in health and disease.

Aldosterone

This is the end-product of the renin–angiotensin–aldosterone system. Aldosterone is released in response to secretion of renin determined by renal perfusion (i.e. afferent arteriolar blood-flow) as sensed by the juxtaglomerular apparatus; it increases sodium/water reabsorption (in exchange for potassium) in the distal tubule.

Atrial natriuretic peptide (ANP)

This is controlled by atrial stretch receptors and increases renal sodium/water loss; ANP and aldosterone have opposing effects.

Measurement of fluid–electrolyte balance

Having described the various compartments, it is now possible to discuss the clinical assessment that must always be done before attempting to interpret abnormal electrolyte biochemistry. Three compartments can be independently assessed at the bedside.

The interstitial compartment

An increase in interstitial fluid causes **oedema**. If the increase is caused by raised venous pressure (heart failure), the oedema is in dependent parts. If caused by venous obstruction, it is in the affected venous territory. If caused by increased capillary permeability or hypoproteinaemia, it is generalised. Remember that lymphatic obstruction also causes oedema by preventing drainage from the interstitial compartment.

The venous compartment

The 'window' into the venous compartment is the jugular venous system. Significant volume overload increases jugular venous pressure and volume depletion reduces it. Dogmatic rules taught about cardiovascular examination ('2 cm above the sternal angle at 45°') obscure the simple fact that bedside examination allows an estimate of central venous pressure by relating the height of the jugular venous pulse to the surface anatomy of the right atrium. If the pulse cannot be seen with the patient lying at 45°, it can be made visible by asking the patient to lie flat. Likewise, a very high venous pressure can best be assessed by sitting the patient upright. This is illustrated in Figure 48.

The arterial compartment

This is affected by cardiac disease and degrees of volume depletion or overload that cannot be compensated for by venous capacitance. Arterial overload is rare because there are powerful homeostatic mechanisms to prevent it. Likewise, depletion of the arterial circulation only occurs when the capacitance vessels are empty. It causes hypotension and tachycardia, initially only on standing. The way to assess the arterial compartment is to measure the lying and standing pulse and blood pressure (pulse is the more sensitive of the two).

Volume depletion

Reduced urine output is a sign of volume depletion, which begins as the homeostatic mechanisms operate at the stage of venous volume depletion. It proceeds to oliguria/anuria when there is significant arterial volume depletion.

One of the greatest disservices done to medical students by conventional teaching is the concept of 'dehydration' and physical signs such as increased skin turgor and sunken eyes. These are indeed signs of reduced total body water, but more often mislead than help because:

- They are insensitive. Body water rarely changes in isolation from sodium, so changes in vascular volume occur long before there is a detectable reduction of interstitial fluid volume.

A **Normal**

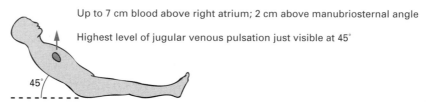

Up to 7 cm blood above right atrium; 2 cm above manubriosternal angle

Highest level of jugular venous pulsation just visible at 45°

45°

B **Increased venous pressure**

>7 cm blood above right atrium; >2 cm above manubriosternal angle

Jugular venous pulsation may extend up to ears
Sit patient up if highest level of venous pulsation cannot be seen

45°

C **Volume depletion**

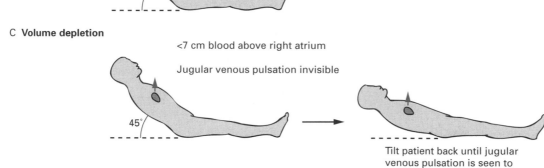

<7 cm blood above right atrium

Jugular venous pulsation invisible

45°

Tilt patient back until jugular venous pulsation is seen to confirm diagnosis of volume depletion

Fig. 48 Assessing venous pressure.

- They are not specific. Skin turgor is affected by ageing, and dryness of the mouth by the respiratory rate.
- They are notoriously difficult to assess accurately.

The only reliable conclusion that can be drawn from these tissue signs is that the patient with a moist tongue and/or moist axilla is unlikely to have serious volume depletion.

While careful physical examination is the key to clinical management, there may also be symptoms. Headache is an early symptom of volume depletion. Others do not occur until the *arterial* circulation is depleted; they are fatigue, lightheadedness, dizziness and syncope (particularly on standing), and oliguria. Symptoms of volume overload arise from the systemic and pulmonary *venous* circulation; they are breathlessness and oedema.

Fluid physiology in disease

Figure 47 relates the physiological principles discussed above to common disease states. Box 11 lists causes of volume depletion and overload. Heart failure and hypoproteinaemia are two disease states that deserve special mention because they present with mixtures of volume depletion and overload and can be understood by applying exactly the same principles.

Heart failure

Cardiac disease causes *effective* arterial volume depletion. There is reduced renal perfusion to which the homeostatic response is increased aldosterone secretion causing salt and water retention. The combination of pump failure and fluid retention increases venous volume. Heart failure is, therefore, a combination of effective arterial volume depletion and venous volume overload.

Box 11: Causes of volume depletion and overload

Volume depletion
- Excessive loss
  - Skin: sweating, as in fever, burns
  - Lungs: tachypnoea, as in asthma
  - GI tract: vomiting, diarrhoea, fistulae
  - Kidneys: salt-losing kidney, diabetes mellitus and other causes of osmotic diuresis, hypoadrenalism
- Inadequate intake
  - Severe illness
  - Anorexia
  - Neglect

Volume overload
- Insufficient loss
  - Renal failure
  - Heart failure
  - Steroid excess: Conn's syndrome, Cushing's syndrome, steroid therapy
- Excessive intake
  - Excessive saline therapy

Hypoproteinaemia

Hypoproteinaemia occurs in nephrotic syndrome and hepatocellular disease and may also be seen in severe illness when increased capillary leakage acts together with hypoproteinaemia to reduce the osmotic pressure difference between plasma and the interstitial fluid. The vascular colloid osmotic pressure is reduced and the interstitial fluid volume expanded at the expense of the vascular compartment. Patients may have symptoms and signs of volume depletion together with oedema.

The treatment of volume depletion and overload

Extracellular volume is primarily determined by the total body content of sodium, which itself determines water content. Volume depletion is treated by replacing salt and water (orally or intravenously). Volume overload is treated by removing salt and water. This is done with dietary restriction, diuretics and — in extreme cases — dialysis or haemofiltration.

The treatment of heart failure is more difficult and consists of:

- optimising cardiac function (e.g. correction of dysrhythmias), inotropic therapy, reducing cardiac work and increasing efficiency by reducing ventricular overload and 'stretch' with arterial and venous vasodilators
- interrupting the upregulated renin–angiotensin–aldosterone system with an ACE inhibitor/ angiotensin receptor antagonist
- removing salt and water with diuretics.

The physiological principles discussed above explain the major limitation of the treatment of heart failure; effective arterial volume is already reduced so diuretics and vasodilators that reduce it further can cause syncope and impair renal perfusion, leading to an increased plasma urea concentration. The treatment of severe heart failure consists of 'tight-rope walking' between the effects of treatment on the different compartments.

The management of hypoproteinaemia has been discussed under nephrotic syndrome (p. 184).

Disorders of sodium and osmolality

The biochemistry laboratory can only measure *concentrations* and *osmolalities*, which are uninterpretable unless *volume* in the compartments has been estimated at the bedside. So, for example, a patient with severe burns can have massive salt and water loss and circulatory collapse without any immediate effect on the plasma urea and electrolyte concentrations; only as the homeostatic mechanisms and reduced urine flow have their effects will the biochemistry become abnormal.

Since 'water follows sodium' (because sodium, the major extracellular cation, determines osmolality and 'draws' water), the plasma concentration is not a reliable marker of total body sodium content. It can only reflect the relative amounts of sodium and water in the extracellular fluid. Therefore, a low serum sodium concentration is caused by an excess of water relative to sodium; total

---

Box 12: Causes of hyponatraemia

Water overload
- Psychogenic polydipsia
- Excessive i.v. dextrose
- SIAD (syndrome of inappropriate antidiuresis)
  - Carcinoma of the bronchus
  - Inflammatory lung diseases
  - Hypothyroidism
  - Hypoadrenalism
  - Idiopathic
  - Drugs: chlorpropamide, carbamazepine, syntocinon, phenothiazines, tricyclics
  - Hypothalamic disease: meningitis, encephalitis, tumour or granuloma

Homeostatic response to volume depletion
- Any cause of volume depletion (e.g. diuretic therapy) if patient has access to water

Heart failure

---

body sodium might be normal or low. Likewise, a high serum sodium is caused by *relative* water depletion, usually in the context of a low total body sodium.

Hyponatraemia

Hyponatraemia has a number of causes (Box 12).
Water overload may be caused by:

- excessive water drinking or i.v. dextrose treatment (e.g. postoperative)
- a primary abnormality (syndrome of inappropriate antidiuresis (SIAD); see below) in which there is excessive ADH secretion and impaired water excretion.

In both cases, total body water is increased and total body sodium normal. In excessive water drinking, the urine is very dilute but the capacity of the kidneys to excrete water is overwhelmed. In SIAD, the urine is very concentrated. Thus, measurement of urine osmolality distinguishes between them.

Hyponatraemia may also be caused by **volume depletion** (e.g. from diuretic therapy) **with continued water drinking**; hyponatraemia is caused by homeostatic ADH secretion in response to volume depletion. In this case, total body sodium is low.

The distinction between SIAD and hyponatraemia associated with volume depletion is made by assessing venous and arterial volume, measuring urea (if increased, this is a sign of volume depletion) and considering the patient's history. A fuller list of causes of hyponatraemia is shown in Box 12. In severe heart failure, hyponatraemia is caused by increased ADH secretion and thirst, caused by effective arterial volume depletion and often made worse by diuretic therapy.

Syndrome of inappropriate antidiuresis (SIAD)
Box 12 lists causes of SIAD; the syndrome may be idiopathic, drug-related, caused by ectopic ADH secretion or caused by disease of the chest or hypothalamus. It may

be the presentation of hypothyroidism or hypoadrenalism. Water retention lowers plasma osmolality and causes non-specific malaise and neurological problems including confusion, personality change and fits/coma owing to cerebral oedema (particularly likely at a serum solution <125 mmol/l). Apart from a low serum sodium and normal or low urea, plasma osmolality is low and urinary osmolality high (because excess ADH prevents the formation of a dilute urine). In mild cases, the treatment is water restriction, allowing loss through the lungs, skin and bowel to clear excess water. If the problem is prolonged, demeclocycline may be given to induce nephrogenic diabetes insipidus. In emergencies (e.g. uncontrolled fitting) hypertonic saline is given with a loop diuretic (to prevent volume overload and increase free water clearance). Correcting hyponatraemia too quickly (at a rate over 1 mmol/l per hr) can cause neurological complications, so this should only be done under expert supervision.

Hypernatraemia
Because 'water follows salt' and the osmoreceptors trigger thirst and ADH secretion when osmolality rises, hypernatraemia is unusual and can really only occur if the patient

- is very old, very young or neurologically disabled and has lost perception of thirst
- is too ill to drink
- has an osmotic diuresis (e.g. caused by glycosuria) and loses water disproportionately to sodium.

'Hyperosmolar dehydration' may arise with severe and prolonged hyperglycaemia (hyperosmolar non-ketotic diabetic coma) or other causes of osmotic diuresis. It may also be caused by diabetes insipidus, in which there is uncontrolled renal water loss. Since water is lost from both the extra- and intracellular fluid, patients rarely become hypernatraemic in this disease because they develop life-threatening water depletion with florid thirst before there is a major change in plasma sodium concentration.

Investigations are directed towards the underlying cause, and treatment consists of volume repletion, sometimes with judicious use of hypotonic saline or 5% dextrose.

Disorders of potassium

Since potassium is predominantly intracellular, major changes in total body potassium can occur with only minor changes in the plasma concentration. An important factor affecting plasma potassium concentration is pH, since potassium and hydrogen ions exchange with one another between the intracellular and extracellular compartments. So, for example, **acidosis** can *increase* plasma potassium by displacing it from the intracellular compartment and **alkalosis** can *lower* it without any change in total body content. Likewise hydrogen ion takes the place of potassium lost from cells, so hypokalaemia is accompanied by alkalosis. Catecholamines shift potassium into cells, as does insulin and any drug/disorder with a sympathomimetic effect.

Hypokalaemia

Hypokalaemia is the most common electrolyte disorder. It causes nerve and muscle dysfunction (particularly at a concentration <2.5 mmol/l) so its effects are:

- weakness
- ileus
- cardiac dysrhythmias.

Chronic hypokalaemia can also induce nephrogenic diabetes insipidus (p. 305) and cause thirst and polyuria.

The most common cause of hypokalaemia is renal loss through diuretic therapy. Box 13 lists others. Measurement of potassium excretion in a 24-hour urine sample is the main investigation. It is increased if the primary problem is renal loss and reduced in all other cases.

Management consists of correcting the cause of loss and replenishing the pool. Remember that potassium has to pass through the small extracellular pool to reach the intracellular fluid, so over-rapid potassium replacement can cause potentially fatal hyperkalaemia. Highly concentrated potassium solutions should never be given intravenously. The rate of replacement should not exceed 30 mmol/hr, even in severe hypokalaemia. Potassium replacement is best done orally.

Box 13: Causes of hypokalaemia and hyperkalaemia

Hypokalaemia
- Excessive loss
  - Renal: potassium-wasting diuretics, potassium-losing kidney, renal tubular acidosis (types 1 and 2)
  - Steroid excess: steroid therapy, Conn's syndrome
  - Osmotic diuresis: diabetes mellitus
  - Liquorice addiction
  - GI tract: persistent vomiting, diarrhoea, villous adenoma of the rectum, enterostomies, purgative abuse
- Inadequate intake
  - Malnutrition
  - Prolonged i.v. therapy without added potassium
- Shifts
  - Metabolic alkalosis
  - Insulin therapy
  - Severe illness (e.g. myocardial infarction)
  - Theophylline and sympathomimetic therapy
  - Poisoning: aspirin, theophylline

Hyperkalaemia
- Insufficient loss
  - Renal: potassium-conserving diuretics, ACE inhibitor therapy, renal failure
  - Steroid deficiency: Addison's disease, congenital adrenal hyperplasia
- Excessive intake
  - Excessive i.v. potassium
- Shifts
  - Metabolic acidosis
  - Insulin deficiency (diabetic ketoacidosis)
  - Cellular injury: burns, rhabdomyolysis, cytotoxic therapy

---

Hyperkalaemia

The causes, effects and treatments of hyperkalaemia are the mirror image of hypokalaemia. Renal failure and potassium-conserving drugs are the most common causes, and these are potentially lethal in combination. Hyperkalaemia may be asymptomatic or may present with muscle weakness. A serum potassium over 7 mmol/l is a medical emergency because it can cause cardiac arrest. Cardiographic signs of hyperkalaemia are 'tented' T waves, loss of P waves and widening of the QRS complex progressing to a 'sine wave' pattern. Management is shown in the emergency box.

Clinical Box: Emergency treatment: management of severe hyperkalaemia

- Give 50% dextrose 50 ml and soluble insulin 10 units; **this shifts potassium from the extracellular fluid into cells**
- Do an ECG
- Give 10–20 ml 10% calcium gluconate if there are signs of severe hyperkalaemia: tented T waves, loss of P waves and widening of the QRS complex; **this antagonises the effects of hyperkalaemia on the myocardium**
- Call for senior help
- Repeat plasma potassium and bicarbonate
- Prescribe calcium resonium orally or rectally; **this increases potassium excretion**
- Assess the patient's fluid status; give i.v. fluids if volume-depleted to increase potassium excretion; consider giving isotonic (1.4%) bicarbonate if volume-depleted and acidotic (bicarbonate shifts potassium into cells)
- Resistant hyperkalaemia may be an indication for dialysis in renal failure or unresponsive cases

---

4.6 Acid–base disorders

Learning objectives

At the very least, you should:

- understand the terms *respiratory* and *metabolic acidosis* and *alkalosis*
- understand that these changes may be primary or compensatory
- be able to interpret arterial blood gas measurements in those terms
- know the common diseases that affect acid–base balance
- understand the main principles of management.

Case Study

An elderly patient inappropriately prescribed metformin despite stage 4 chronic kidney disease is admitted moribund. From her measured plasma sodium of 134 mmol/l, bicarbonate 5 mmol/l and chloride

95 mmol/l, it is calculated that she has an increased anion gap of 34 mmol/l. Since she has no ketones in her urine, metformin-induced lactic acidosis looks the most likely diagnosis.

If fluid–electrolyte physiology seems complex, acid–base homeostasis and its disorders can seem even more so. However, you will encounter a limited range of these disorders as a newly qualified doctor and an even more limited range without senior supervision, so this discussion picks out only salient points relevant to management.

Mechanisms and terminology

Respiration affects acid–base balance because excess carbon dioxide combines with water to form carbonic acid. This is termed **respiratory acidosis** and may be an effect of respiratory disease or a homeostatic mechanism to maintain a normal pH in the face of **metabolic alkalosis**. Likewise, a reduced partial pressure of carbon dioxide (Pco_2) causes **respiratory alkalosis**, which may be primary (caused, for example, by hyperventilation) or to compensate for **metabolic acidosis**. The biochemical marker of respiratory acidosis and alkalosis is a change in Pco_2.

Metabolic acidosis may be caused by:

- increased intake of hydrogen ions, as in salicylate overdosage
- increased production of hydrogen ions, as in lactic acidosis or ketoacidosis (p. 324)
- decreased renal excretion of hydrogen ions (as in renal failure)
- a shift of hydrogen ions out of cells, as in hyperkalaemia.

The biochemical marker of metabolic acidosis is a fall in plasma bicarbonate. Normally there is a difference of about 10–15 mmol/l between the sum of plasma sodium plus potassium (the main cations) and bicarbonate plus chloride (the main anions). This is termed the **anion gap** and is 'filled' by unmeasured organic anions. If acidosis is caused by excess lactate, ketoacids or other unmeasured anions (particularly drugs), the anion gap is increased.

The marker of metabolic alkalosis is a rise in plasma bicarbonate. It is caused by either excess intake of alkali or excess loss of hydrogen ions through the kidneys or into the intracellular fluid.

Investigations

To obtain a true measurement of acid–base and blood gas status, pH and partial pressures of oxygen and carbon dioxide (Pao_2 and $Paco_2$, respectively) must be measured in arterial blood; venous blood cannot be used because it is affected by local tissue metabolism. Bicarbonate is ideally measured in arterial blood but venous bicarbonate approximates closely enough to arterial bicarbonate to be used for the diagnosis of metabolic alkalosis and acidosis. Chloride can be measured in venous or arterial blood.

Causes and differential diagnosis

Table 46 shows the four main patterns of abnormality described above. Note how the patterns of pH, $Paco_2$ and

---

Box 14: Causes of disordered acid–base biochemistry

Respiratory acidosis
- Respiratory failure
  - Airway obstruction
  - Mechanical problems of ventilation
  - Neuromuscular disease

Respiratory alkalosis
- Hyperventilation
  - Primary
  - Secondary to
    Alveolar disease
    Right–left shunting
    Salicylate poisoning

Metabolic acidosis
- Normal anion gap
  - Renal tubular acidosis
  - Bicarbonate loss from GI fistula

- Increased anion gap
  - Lactic acidosis
    Septic shock
    Tissue anoxia
    Liver disease
    Drugs: e.g. metformin
  - Ketoacidosis
    Diabetes
  - Poisoning
    Salicylate
    Ethanol
    Methanol
  - Renal failure
  - Liver failure

Metabolic alkalosis
- Ingestion of alkali
- Hypokalaemia
  - Gastric acid loss (pyloric stenosis)

---

bicarbonate differ between the four disorders. Box 14 lists their causes.

Clinical presentation

The symptoms and signs are usually those of an underlying disease, except that patients with metabolic acidosis characteristically have deep sighing (Kussmaul) respiration.

Management

The treatment of respiratory acidosis and alkalosis is directed at the underlying respiratory disease. Metabolic alkalosis rarely needs treatment in its own right. The treatment of acidosis is directed primarily at the underlying disease. Intravenous sodium bicarbonate is used to correct severe metabolic acidosis but must be given judiciously for several reasons:

- It is a solute load and contraindicated if the patient is already volume-overloaded.

Table 46 Interpretation of acid/base biochemistry

	Metabolic acidosis	Respiratory acidosis	Respiratory alkalosis	Metabolic alkalosis
pH	↓	↓	↑	↑
Paco$_2$	(↓)	↑	↓	(↑)
Bicarbonate	↓	(↑)	(↓)	↑
Chloride	↑*	(↓)	(↑)	↓

↓, fall; ↑, rise; () indicates compensatory as opposed to primary changes.
*Except where there is an excess anion such as lactate or ketoacids, in which case chloride is normal or low and the anion gap is increased.

- Hypertonic bicarbonate solutions are extremely damaging to peripheral veins.
- Abrupt correction of acidosis can cause acute, severe and potentially fatal hypokalaemia as potassium shifts into cells.
- It can temporarily worsen cerebral acidosis because it immediately corrects plasma acidosis and reduces the compensatory respiratory alkalosis but takes time to diffuse into the central nervous system.

Oral bicarbonate is occasionally given to compensate for chronic bicarbonate loss, as in renal tubular acidosis.

Four

Self-assessment: questions

Any or all of each set of five statements may be true or false. Choose your answers and see the reasoning behind the correct answer on page 205.

Multiple choice questions

1. Acute renal failure is a likely complication of the following:
   a. Sepsis (or sepsis syndrome)
   b. Polycystic kidney disease
   c. Major arterial surgery
   d. Retroperitoneal tumours
   e. Cardiogenic shock

2. The following are true:
   a. Serum urea is a more reliable measure than creatinine for the diagnosis of renal failure
   b. Diuretic therapy of heart failure can increase serum urea
   c. Serum creatinine may be misleadingly low in wasted patients with renal failure
   d. Plasma creatinine is primarily influenced by glomerular filtration not urine flow
   e. The urinary urea concentration provides useful information in the investigation of suspected renal failure

3. The following are causes of chronic renal failure:
   a. Gout
   b. Atherosclerosis
   c. Analgesic abuse
   d. Non-insulin-dependent diabetes
   e. Hypothyroidism

4. The following are true of renal dialysis and transplantation:
   a. Maintenance haemodialysis gives a better long-term quality of life than renal transplantation
   b. Transplantation is ideally suited to elderly patients with renal failure
   c. Pericarditis is an indication for dialysis in acute renal failure
   d. Acute dialysis can correct metabolic acidosis
   e. Maintenance dialysis gives people with chronic renal failure a normal life expectancy

5. The following may be associated with the nephrotic syndrome:
   a. Minimal change disease
   b. Treatment with beta-blockers
   c. Rheumatoid arthritis
   d. Diabetes mellitus
   e. Renal cell carcinoma

6. The following are true of the investigation of renal disease:
   a. No patient should go on to dialysis without having had a renal biopsy
   b. Intravenous urography (IVU) may worsen renal failure
   c. Urine microscopy can give valuable information as to the cause of renal failure
   d. Renal venography may be indicated in the investigation of nephrotic syndrome
   e. Retrograde pyelography is usually needed to diagnose urinary obstruction

7. Renal cell carcinoma:
   a. May be bilateral
   b. May present as a pyrexia of unknown origin (PUO)
   c. May present with pulmonary metastases
   d. Commonly causes hypertension
   e. Is extremely radiosensitive

8. Renal artery stenosis:
   a. Is invariably caused by atherosclerosis
   b. May cause renal failure in patients given ACE (angiotensin-converting enzyme) inhibitor therapy
   c. Can be reliably diagnosed by auscultating for renal bruits
   d. May be suggested by ultrasound as a unilateral small kidney
   e. Is a cause of hypertension

Single best answer multiple choice questions

For each numbered question, only ONE of the options lettered a–e is correct.

1. In patients presenting with acute renal failure:
   a. Sodium bicarbonate should be given routinely
   b. They are >90% likely to need long-term dialysis
   c. Skin turgor is a reliable guide to the need for i.v. fluid therapy
   d. Urinary catheterisation is sometimes indicated to monitor the response to therapy
   e. Intravenous pyelography is the investigation of choice to exclude urinary obstruction

2. The following are features of urinary infections in elderly people:
   a. Patients usually complain of dysuria
   b. A bacterial count of $>10^5$/ml is required for diagnosis
   c. They may present with constipation
   d. Sterile pyuria is most likely caused by tuberculosis

e. Investigation for anatomical abnormalities is always indicated

3. Which of the following statements about renal physiology and anatomy do you most strongly agree with?

   a. Glomerular filtration is a passive process determined by the balance between capillary hydrostatic, tubular and plasma oncotic pressures

   b. Epithelial tight junctions regulate the diffusion of albumin into Bowman's space

   c. The kidneys are 8–13 cm in length and the left is 1–2 cm lower than the right

   d. 30–50% of glomerular filtrate must obligately be reabsorbed in the proximal renal tubule to prevent circulatory collapse

   e. The kidneys are able to autoregulate glomerular filtration for diastolic pressures ranging from 20 to 120 mmHg

Extended matched questions

EMQ 1

Theme: Possible treatments in renal disease

Options

1. 10% dextrose
2. 0.9% sodium chloride
3. Hartmann's solution
4. 5% potassium chloride
5. 1.4% sodium bicarbonate
6. 5% dextrose
7. Dextrose saline
8. 0.45% sodium chloride
9. Water for injection
10. 8.4% sodium bicarbonate
11. Cross-matched blood
12. 1.8% saline

For each of the following patients that a house officer might be called to see, select the best treatment (more than one may be correct). Each item can be used once, more than once or not at all.

A. A 75-year-old man with chronic renal failure and acute gastroenteritis admitted after collapsing on the way to the toilet. He is not volume-overloaded; his urea is 35 mmol/l and his creatinine is 200 µmol/l.

B. A 69-year-old diabetic patient admitted semi-conscious and severely volume-depleted who has received 3 litres of saline: sodium 160 mmol/l, urea 40 mmol/l, glucose 50 mmol/l and bicarbonate 22 mmol/l.

C. A 62-year-old woman with acute renal failure and volume depletion who is dyspnoeic: sodium

138 mmol/l, potassium 7.2 mmol/l and bicarbonate 8 mmol/l.

D. A 58-year-old smoker with a hilar mass in resistant status epilepticus: sodium 108 mmol/l and urea 1.9 mmol/l.

E. A 23-year-old student with type 1 diabetes 8 hours after starting treatment for diabetic ketoacidosis, currently receiving 0.9% saline: glucose 10 mmol/l, sodium 139 mmol/l and urea 7.2 mmol/l.

EMQ 2

Theme: Possible tests for patients with renal disease

Options

1. Nephrostomy and antegrade pyelogram
2. Computed tomography
3. Micturating cystogram
4. Renal biopsy
5. Isotope renogram
6. Cystogram
7. Intravenous urogram
8. Renal arteriogram
9. Renal venogram
10. Duplex/Doppler ultrasound scanning

For each of the following patients with renal disease shown to have normal renal tracts on ultrasound scanning (unless indicated otherwise), select the most appropriate test (more than one may be correct). Each item can be used once, more than once or not at all.

A. A woman with ovarian cancer who has been admitted anuric with bilateral hydronephrosis and advanced renal failure.

B. A diabetic patient with no retinopathy who has proteinuria and microscopic haematuria.

C. A 62-year-old smoker with intermittent claudication, taking an angiotensin-converting enzyme (ACE) inhibitor and with mild renal failure.

D. A 70-year-old man with nephrotic syndrome whose renal function and leg swelling abruptly worsen.

E. A patient with pyrexia of unknown origin (PUO), sterile urine and a suspected renal mass.

Objective structured clinical examination (OSCE) stations

OSCE 1

This is a 5-minute station on volume assessment with a normal volunteer on a couch.

Examiner: Please show me how you would assess this patient with renal failure for volume depletion or overload.

OSCE 2

Examiner: I would like you to imagine you have been called to see the patient you examined in the last station because some abnormal laboratory results have just been phoned through. He is in his fifth postoperative day after major abdominal surgery and is just starting to take fluids by mouth but is still on a drip. You find him to be euvolaemic and he seems to be recovering quite well from his operation. His urea and electrolytes were normal immediately before surgery but now they are as follows:

Sodium	122 mmol/l
Potassium	3.1 mmol/l
Bicarbonate	28 mmol/l
Urea	2.3 mmol/l

  a. How do you interpret those results?
  b. What action would you take?

Case history questions

Case history 1

A 74-year-old man who has always had excellent health has been increasingly lethargic and short of breath for 3 months before he is admitted to hospital. He is found to have a serum urea of 58 mmol/l and a creatinine of 900 μmol/l.

1. In seeking a cause of his renal failure, name three particularly important points to be sought in his clinical history and examination.
2. What investigation would you request first to elucidate the cause?

He is found to have an enlarged bladder with bilateral hydronephrosis.

3. How should he be managed?

Despite relief of his hydronephrosis, his serum urea and creatinine remain high.

4. What other treatable factors might be contributing to his renal failure?

Case history 2

A 23-year-old single female shop assistant presents to you as her GP complaining of frequent micturition and a 'burning sensation' when she passes water. She has never had this problem before. She is otherwise fit and well and you last saw her 9 months previously.

1. Which of the following are appropriate courses of action?
   a. Refer her to a urologist
   b. Send her urine for culture and microscopy

   c. Treat her empirically with a broad-spectrum oral antibiotic
   d. Examine her, looking particularly for genital herpes
   e. Enquire about a new sexual partner and/or recent sexual activity

In the event you prescribe amoxicillin for 5 days and tell her to return if the problem is not better. She returns with the same symptoms 5 days later.

2. What should your course of action be now?
   a. Refer her to a urologist
   b. Send her urine for culture and microscopy
   c. Re-treat her with another oral antibiotic
   d. Examine her, looking particularly for genital herpes
   e. Refer her to a genitourinary medicine department

This time you take urine for culture and microscopy and then prescribe oral trimethoprim. She is advised to drink plenty of fluids and to urinate immediately after intercourse. She reports back in 7 days with improved symptoms but now complaining of 'irritating itchiness down below' and increased vaginal discharge. The urine result showed >100 white cells per high-power field and a culture of 10^6/ml *Escherichia coli* resistant to ampicillin and cefradine but sensitive to trimethoprim, gentamicin and norfloxacin.

3. Your course of action now is to:
   a. Refer her to a urologist
   b. Examine her and take a vaginal sample for *Candida* and *Trichomonas* and a cervical sample for *Chlamydia* and *Neisseria gonorrhoeae*
   c. Treat her empirically with a third oral antibiotic
   d. Treat her empirically for vaginal candidosis
   e. Refer her to a genitourinary medicine department

Key features questions

1. A middle-aged man with nephrotic syndrome and mild chronic renal failure due to glomerulonephritis has been lethargic and anorexic since he caught a bug on holiday a month ago. He is fully conscious, is cognitively intact and has no breathlessness or chest pain. His lying blood pressure is 110/60 mmHg. His lying pulse rate is 80 beats/min, rising to 112 beats/min when he stands up. His jugular venous pulse cannot be seen when he lies flat and his lungs are clear. He has no oedema. His temperature is normal. His investigations are as follows:

Sodium	132 mmol/l
Potassium	6.4 mmol/l
Creatinine	480 μmol/l
Estimated GFR	15 ml/min

Urea	45 mmol/l
Venous bicarbonate	16 mmol/l
Random glucose	6.3 mmol/l
ECG	Mild changes of ischaemic heart disease only
Chest radiograph	Cardiomegaly; clear lung fields
Urine dipstick	Heavy proteinuria and blood
Haemoglobin	88 g/l – normochromic picture

Identify the three most important points in his immediate management:

a. Infuse isotonic (5%) dextrose

b. Infuse isotonic bicarbonate

c. Infuse hypertonic bicarbonate

d. Infuse hypotonic saline

e. Infuse isotonic (0.9%) saline

f. Infuse hypertonic saline

g. Infuse albumin

h. Infuse synthetic colloid solution

i. Transfuse blood

j. Give i.v. glucose and insulin

k. Give i.v. calcium gluconate

l. Request urgent haemodialysis

m. Request urgent peritoneal dialysis

n. Haemofiltrate

o. Request a renal ultrasound scan

p. Request an intravenous urogram

q. Request a renal computed tomogram

r. Request a renal magnetic resonance scan

s. Request an isotope renogram

t. Request urine microscopy and culture

2. A 38-year-old woman who had recurrent urinary tract infections and a micturating cystogram showing vesico-úreteric reflux in childhood returns to the UK after living abroad for some years because her health is slowly deteriorating. She has had no recent urinary tract infections. Her blood pressure is 158/94 mmHg and she is apyrexial. She is not breathless and has no oedema. She is on no treatment. Results of investigations are:

Estimated GFR	26
Potassium	5.3 mmol/l
Calcium	1.89 mmol/l
Phosphate	2.4 mmol/l
Alkaline phosphatase	210 IU/l
Haemoglobin	740 g/l

Identify two treatments that it would be most appropriate to prescribe when she first attends the renal clinic:

a. Calcium lactate (phosphate-binding agent)

b. Sevelamer (phosphate-binding agent)

c. Parathyroid hormone

d. Colecalciferol

e. Alendronate

f. Calcium resonium (potassium-binding agent)

g. Doxazosin

h. Lisinopril

i. Bendroflumethiazide

j. Furosemide

k. Bumetanide

l. Verapamil

m. Amoxicillin

n. Trimethoprim

o. Nitrofurantoin

p. Gentamicin

Data interpretation questions

1. Table 47 shows biochemical findings for five patients. Suggest an interpretation (referring to Table 1 (p. 5) for those analytes for which you do not know the reference range).

Table 47 Biochemical data for patients 1–5

	1	2	3	4	5
Na$^+$ (mmol/l)	138	130	160	114	124
K$^+$ (mmol/l)	6.8	2.8	4.9	3.8	7.2
Urea (mmol/l)	43.0	16	58	2.1	8.8
Creatinine (μmmol/l)	780	118	400	86	120
HCO$_3^-$ (mmol/l)	15	32	24	26	19

2. Comment on the following biochemical findings in a patient with chronic renal failure. What management would be appropriate? Calcium 1.90 mmol/l, phosphate 2.1 mmol/l, alkaline phosphatase 450 IU/l.

3. Comment on the biochemical findings in patients 6–9 in Table 48.

Table 48 Arterial blood data for patients 6–9

	6	7	8	9
Pco_2 (kPa)	7.8	3.1	6.8	3.6
(mm Hg)	58	23	51	27
pH	7.2	6.9	7.6	7.5
HCO$_3^-$	32	5	36	18

4. Patients 10–15 in Table 49 had dysuria and/or frequency. Classify their disease appropriately and suggest a single course of action (e.g. treat with antibiotics, renal ultrasound, etc.).

Table 49 Microbiological and clinical data for patients 10–15

	10	11	12	13	14	15
Urine (white cells per high-power field)	>100	30	80	50	10	80
Culture result (cfu/ml)	10^4	$<10^2$	$>10^5$	$<10^4$	10^4	$<10^2$
Culture identification	Mixed flora		Proteus mirabilis	Mixed flora	E. coli	
Age	78	82	22	26	79	43
Sex	F	M	M	F	M	M

Picture question

The ultrasound scan in Figure 49 is of the left kidney of a 50-year-old woman with advanced ovarian cancer. She has recently lost over 1 stone in weight and complains of back pain. She is admitted vomiting, with a serum urea of 50 mmol/l and creatinine 1020 μmol/l.

1. What does the scan show?
2. What is the likely cause of this appearance?
3. How should she be managed?

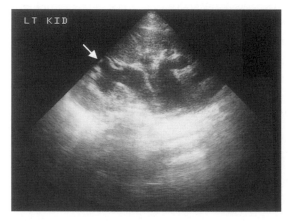

Fig. 49 An ultrasound scan of the left kidney.

Self-assessment: answers

Multiple choice answers

1. a. **True.** Commonly caused by prerenal factors such as sepsis syndrome.
    b. **False.** Polycystic kidneys cause chronic rather than acute renal failure.
    c. **True.** Major arterial surgery can cause renal ischaemia and acute tubular necrosis.
    d. **False.** Postrenal disease uncommonly causes *acute* renal failure, and retroperitoneal pathology is particularly unlikely to do so because it would need to involve both ureters simultaneously.
    e. **True.** Cardiac disease can critically impair renal perfusion.

2. a. **False.** Serum urea may be increased by protein catabolism and reduced urine flow as well as by renal failure. Serum creatinine is the more reliable marker.
    b. **True.** Poor cardiac output may increase serum urea by decreasing urine flow. Diuretic therapy can exacerbate the situation, in which case serum urea rises disproportionately to creatinine.
    c. **True.** Patients with reduced muscle bulk may have a normal serum creatinine even in the presence of renal failure because muscle bulk determines creatinine production.
    d. **True.** Creatinine is a marker of glomerular filtration.
    e. **True.** In renal failure, the kidneys are unable to excrete urea so the urinary urea concentration is low. This distinguishes renal failure from, for example, volume depletion, in which plasma urea is high but the kidneys retain the capacity to concentrate urinary urea.

3. a. **True.**
    b. **True.** As a result of extrarenal or intrarenal obstruction to the renal arterial circulation.
    c. **True.**
    d. **True.** Both insulin-dependent and non-insulin-dependent diabetes cause renal failure.
    e. **False.**

4. a. **False.** A successful transplant gives a better quality of life.
    b. **False.** The elderly tolerate immunosuppression poorly and are particularly susceptible to cardiovascular disease; they are treated with haemodialysis or peritoneal dialysis.
    c. **True.**
    d. **True.**
    e. **False.** Even if treated with renal replacement, there is increased mortality from cardiovascular disease in patients with renal failure.

5. a. **True.** This is the characteristic disease associated with nephrotic syndrome, particularly in children.
    b. **False.**
    c. **True.** It may be caused by amyloid associated with rheumatoid arthritis or by drugs used to treat the disease (gold or penicillamine).
    d. **True.** Up to 25% of patients with diabetic nephropathy have nephrotic range proteinuria.
    e. **False.**

6. a. **False.** There are limited indications for renal biopsy; usually in patients with mild-to-moderate parenchymal renal disease of uncertain aetiology or unexplained acute renal failure.
    b. **True.** Particularly in elderly patients and those with diabetes or myeloma, particularly if they are volume-depleted.
    c. **True.**
    d. **True.** Renal vein thrombosis may cause or exacerbate nephrotic syndrome.
    e. **False.** Renal ultrasound is the first-line investigation.

7. a. **True.**
    b. **True.** Renal cell carcinoma is prone to cause systemic symptoms.
    c. **True.** Both bony and pulmonary metastases occur.
    d. **False.**
    e. **False.**

8. a. **False.** Fibromuscular hyperplasia (10%) and radiation fibrosis are two other pathologies which can cause renal artery stenosis, although atherosclerosis is the most common pathology (90%).
    b. **True.**
    c. **False.** A renal bruit may be present but absence of a bruit is an unreliable way of excluding renal artery stenosis.
    d. **True.** Hypoperfusion causes reduction in renal size.
    e. **True.**

Single best answer multiple choice answers

1. **d is correct.** It is important to measure urine flow in the fluid management of acute renal failure. Not all patients have severe enough metabolic acidosis to need bicarbonate, and bicarbonate therapy could critically lower serum potassium if the patient were not hyperkalaemic. Bicarbonate therapy is used

only in selected cases. Acute renal failure (acute tubular necrosis) usually improves over 4–8 weeks and return to baseline renal function is usual. Skin turgor, like eyeball pressure, is a poor guide to blood *volume*. (See page 192 for reliable signs of volume depletion and overload.) Urinary obstruction should be excluded in all cases but pyelography is a poor method because visualisation of the kidneys depends on renal function to excrete the dye. The dye is nephrotoxic and may worsen renal failure. Ultrasonography is non-invasive, sensitive and specific for urinary obstruction.

2. **c is correct.** Or constipation may be coexistent, perhaps reflecting anorexia and dehydration. Falls or confusional states are other common presentations. Many urinary tract infections in elderly people are subtle in their presentation and may be relatively asymptomatic. Typically, the patient presents with 'going off their feet', confusion, anorexia or nocturia/incontinence. Fever is uncommon. Urine culture is an essential investigation in unwell elderly people. A bacterial count of 10^4/ml is sufficient for diagnosis. Sterile pyuria could be caused by tuberculosis, but there are more likely causes such as incompletely treated infection, urinary tract disease, etc. In women elasticity of the urethra is reduced postmenopausally and this can lead to infection. In men, urinary retention and catheterisation may lead to infection.

3. **a is correct.** Albumin does not normally diffuse into Bowman's space, and it is certainly not a regulated process. The right kidney is lower than the left, displaced by the liver. Over 90% of glomerular filtrate must obligately be reabsorbed. A kidney would not be expected to filter at a diastolic pressure of 20 mmHg.

Extended matched answers

EMQ 1

A. **2.** There are several clues that he is volume-depleted. His collapse may be syncope from volume depletion induced by gastroenteritis, and his urea is disproportionately raised compared with the serum creatinine. You are told that he is not volume-overloaded. Volume repletion with 0.9% saline would be appropriate.

B. **8.** It is good practice to give at least some of the i.v. fluid for diabetic hyperosmolar non-ketotic coma as 0.45% saline.

C. **5.** She is acidotic, hyperkalaemic and volume-depleted. It is logical to replace volume for her with 1.4% bicarbonate, which will also improve both her acidosis and hyperkalaemia.

D. **12.** He appears to have the syndrome of inappropriate antidiuresis (SIAD) caused by carcinoma of the bronchus. If his conscious level were normal, he could be treated by fluid

restriction. As it is, he needs i.v. twice-normal saline to bring his serum sodium slowly up towards normal.

E. **6 or 7.** The aim at this stage in the management of ketoacidosis is to 'hold' plasma glucose a little above normal with 5% dextrose, with added potassium and an insulin infusion. Use of dextrose saline would also be correct.

EMQ 2

A. **2 or 1.** She is likely to have bilateral ureteric obstruction caused by retroperitoneal spread of her cancer. CT will confirm the diagnosis; if she is thought fit for treatment, nephrostomy will treat her renal failure, and antegrade pyelography may delineate the site of the obstruction.

B. **4.** Diabetic patients with obvious nephropathy are not usually subjected to renal biopsy. Both the presence of haematuria and absence of retinopathy are atypical for diabetic nephropathy so a renal biopsy is indicated.

C. **8 or 10.** The diagnosis is likely to be renal artery stenosis.

D. **9 or 10.** The clinical history suggests renal vein thrombosis.

E. **2.** The history suggests a renal cell carcinoma, for which CT is an appropriate investigation.

Responses to OSCE stations

OSCE1

You are expected to examine the 'tissue', venous compartment and arterial compartment for signs of volume. It would be inappropriate to ask the volunteer questions, not just because you have been asked to examine but also because symptoms are less sensitive and specific than signs in this situation.

Assess tissue signs Check if the tongue and axillae are moist; if they are, the patient is unlikely to be significantly volume-depleted. Check the ankles and sacrum for oedema — its presence would suggest that the patient either is volume-overloaded or has vascular leakage, which is allowing salt and water to escape into the tissues.

Examine the jugular venous pressure
- Visible pulsation up to 2 cm above the manubrio-sternal angle suggests the patient is normovolaemic.
- If you cannot see venous pulsation, lie the patient flat to see when it appears, and assess the degree of central venous hypotension.
- If the pressure is raised, sit the patient up to see if you can identify the highest level of pulsation, and assess the degree of central venous hypertension.

Examine the arterial compartment Measure the pulse and blood pressure with the patient lying flat. Stand them up, then measure again after 2 minutes standing.

OSCE 2

The result shows low sodium and potassium concentrations with a (low) normal urea and (high) normal bicarbonate.

a. Interpretation. Although it would be very poor practice to have taken the blood from the same arm as his drip, an examiner would want you to suggest that as one possible cause for the abnormality, if only to dismiss it. This hyponatraemic patient is euvolaemic and has quite a low blood urea. This seems to be 'dilutional hyponatraemia'. It could be due to the syndrome of inappropriate antidiuresis but a more common cause in a postsurgical patient would be over-treatment with 5% dextrose. The low potassium could be due to insufficient potassium replacement to make up for ongoing losses in the perioperative period, again an iatrogenic problem.

b. Action. To confirm the diagnosis:
- Check who took the blood and where they took it from.
- Examine the patient's fluid and prescription charts to establish what fluids were given.
- Check what fluid the patient is currently receiving.
- Measure urinary osmolality and sodium concentration, both of which are likely to be low as the patient clears an excessive water load.
- It would be reasonable, also, to measure the urinary potassium concentration, which you would expect to be low if the fluid regimen had contained insufficient potassium.
  Management. Assuming the diagnosis of dilutional hyponatraemia due to excessive 5% dextrose is confirmed:
- Restrict oral water intake.
- Give no more 5% dextrose.
- Give 0.9% saline with added potassium.
- Observe the patient closely and repeat U&Es 12–24-hourly, expecting the abnormality gradually to normalise.

Case history answers

Case history 1

1. A common cause of renal failure in elderly men is prostatic disease. The history should concentrate on symptoms of prostatism and he should have a rectal examination and abdominal examination for bladder enlargement. Arterial disease is another likely cause. Symptoms and signs of cardiac and peripheral vascular disease should be sought. A full drug history should be taken. Ask for symptoms of urinary or systemic infection.

2. Immediate abdominal ultrasound to exclude urinary obstruction and assess renal size.

3. Urethral catheterisation. It is normal practice to clamp the catheter after 1–1.5 litres of urine has been drained because abrupt relief of pressure may precipitate severe polyuria and volume depletion.

4. He may be volume-depleted or overloaded and should be treated accordingly. His urine should be cultured because stasis predisposes to urinary infection and this may worsen renal function. Any nephrotoxic drugs (e.g. non-steroidal anti-inflammatory drugs) should be stopped.

Case history 2

1. a. **False.** She has the classical symptoms of acute uncomplicated cystitis. Referral is unnecessary.
   b. **True.** However, over 80% of cystitis infections are caused by *Escherichia coli* and most respond to antibiotics if treated empirically.
   c. **True.**
   d. **False.** The symptoms are so suggestive of a urinary infection that examination is probably unnecessary.
   e. **True.** Cystitis in young women often follows sexual activity and these are sensible questions.

2. a. **False.** This is unnecessary.
   b. **True.** Now it is imperative to send a culture as she has failed therapy. If one had already been sent, a result to guide treatment would be available.
   c. **True.** She has the same symptoms and failed therapy with the first-line antibiotic. In fact, amoxicillin and ampicillin are poor empirical choices for urine infections as only about 40% of *E. coli* are susceptible in the UK. Trimethoprim or ofloxacin would be better.
   d. **True.** More justification now, to exclude vulval disease, but the problem is still very likely to be cystitis.
   e. **False.** Unnecessary for uncomplicated cystitis.

3. a. **False.** Urinary symptoms have improved.
   b. **True.** The symptoms are typical of vaginal candidiasis (p. 423) and she has a good precipitating cause: two courses of antibiotics. However, if she has (or had) a new partner (or an unfaithful regular partner) she could well have a sexually transmitted disease and examination and culture are important.
   c. **False.** New symptom complex not suggestive of cystitis.
   d. **True.** See (b) above.
   e. **True.** Now an appropriate course of action, particularly if you are not equipped to take appropriate cultures for sexually transmitted diseases *and* she has had a new partner.

Key features answers

1. **e, o, t are correct.** The scenario makes it very clear that the patient is volume-depleted. It is likely he has developed acute-on-chronic renal failure due to the illness a month ago. Intravenous fluid could

reverse the situation and may be all that is needed. Isotonic saline would be the most appropriate fluid, given in generous quantity (perhaps 5 litres or more in the first 24 hours). There is no indication that hypoalbuminaemia is the cause of his volume depletion since he has no oedema and he is not in left ventricular failure, so it would not be appropriate to infuse albumin. Nor would it be appropriate to transfuse blood because he is neither shocked nor severely anaemic, and a blood transfusion might worsen his hyperkalaemia. Given the normal ECG, his hyperkalaemia does not need urgent therapy and is likely to improve quite quickly as he is volume-replaced. He does not need acute dialysis. An abdominal ultrasound scan should be requested to exclude obstruction and a midstream urine should be sent for microscopy and culture, particularly given the presence of haematuria (though it could be due to the glomerulonephritis). It would not be wrong to give an antibiotic in this case, but it would be reasonable to hold off pending the result of a urine culture. This case illustrates the old adage that, when you see acute renal failure, you should think of the three common, reversible causes: *volume depletion*, *obstruction* and *infection*. He certainly has the first of those three, and you need to exclude the second and third. He is not severely ill, and the most appropriate treatment is to restore circulating volume with saline and see if his renal function improves.

2. **b, h are correct.** She is in chronic renal failure. There is evidence of renal bone disease; she needs a phosphate-binding agent, and one that does not contain calcium would be the best choice. She might also be treated with a vitamin D analogue, but not colecalciferol which is the only vitamin D preparation on the list. She is hypertensive and controlling her blood pressure is a high priority. ACE inhibitors are the class of drug on the list of options for which there is clearest evidence of a beneficial effect on the progress of chronic renal failure, though any drug that lowers her blood pressure will be of some benefit. She might benefit from long-term antibiotic therapy if she had recurrent/persistent urinary infection, but no evidence of active urinary infection is given. She would benefit from iron and perhaps erythropoietin therapy but they are not on the list of options.

Data interpretation answers

1. Patients with data in Table 47.

    Patient 1 Typical biochemistry of severe renal failure with very high creatinine and urea, hyperkalaemia and metabolic acidosis.

    Patient 2 There are multiple abnormalities. Plasma urea is high but creatinine is normal, suggesting volume depletion or impaired renal perfusion resulting in reduced urine flow. Plasma

sodium is slightly low, implying water retention as a result of increased antidiuretic hormone (arginine vasopressin) secretion. There is also a hypokalaemic alkalosis. These abnormalities could best be explained by heart failure, the hypokalaemic alkalosis being caused by treatment with a loop diuretic. Volume depletion from vomiting is another possibility.

Patient 3 Hypernatraemia is uncommon because it usually causes extreme thirst; this patient has an extremely high plasma urea and moderately high creatinine. This suggests volume depletion with secondary renal failure. This picture is seen in diabetic non-ketotic hyperosmolar coma; note the *absence* of acidosis. The patient is drowsy and either unaware of the hyperosmolality or too ill to drink. Plasma glucose in this case was 76 mmol/l.

Patient 4 Plasma sodium is low. This may be because of excessive water retention or water retention in compensation for severe volume depletion. The latter is unlikely because urea is low–normal. This picture is seen in severe water intoxication resulting from psychogenic polydipsia or the syndrome of inappropriate antidiuresis.

Patient 5 The most striking abnormality here is the high serum potassium. Serum sodium is low and urea high, suggesting volume depletion with compensatory ADH secretion and water retention. This is characteristic of hypoaldosteronism, as seen in Addison's disease. Note the mild acidosis. Serum chloride, in this case, will be increased in compensation for the reduced bicarbonate.

2. This is a typical picture of renal bone disease; serum phosphate is high because of renal phosphate retention and calcium is low. Alkaline phosphatase is high, suggesting secondary hyperparathyroidism with bone disease. The patient may have bone pain, weakness and malaise. Management is with phosphate-binding agents by mouth (calcium carbonate) and a vitamin D analogue.

3. Patients 6–9 with data in Table 48.

    Patient 6 Respiratory acidosis. (low pH with a raised Pco_2); there is a compensatory metabolic alkalosis. This picture is seen in, for example, an exacerbation of chronic obstructive pulmonary disease.

    Patient 7 The acidosis here is **metabolic** because bicarbonate is low; there is compensatory hyperventilation and a reduced Pco_2.

    Patient 8 This alkalosis (raised pH) is **metabolic** because bicarbonate is high; there is a compensatory respiratory acidosis (hypoventilation).

    Patient 9 Again, alkalosis (high pH); in this case it is **respiratory** because Pco_2 is low; there is a compensatory metabolic acidosis.

4. Patients 10–15 with data in Table 49.

    Patient 10 A 'sterile pyuria' in an improperly collected sample contaminated from the vulva with some faecal contents. Repeat sample in a few days.

Patient 11 Also mild 'sterile pyuria'. Consider fastidious organisms, tuberculosis, antibiotic treatment, etc. If no prior antibiotics, consider tuberculosis, especially if Asian. However, mild pyuria is common in elderly people. Repeat.

Patient 12 A complicated urinary tract infection in a young man; possibly related to a stone. Needs a renal ultrasound and a antibiotic in first instance.

Patient 13 Acute urethral syndrome if symptomatic. Urine findings similar to those of bacterial vaginosis but symptom complex different. Treat with prolonged (e.g. 14 days) antibiotics.

Patient 14 Normal urine in an elderly patient: consider prostatic hypertrophy or bladder/prostate cancer. Rectal examination and prostate-specific antigen.

Patient 15 Sterile pyuria. Repeat. If same, take early morning urine for mycobacterial culture and microscopy. Check for analgesia abuse or other causes of papillary necrosis.

Picture answers

1. Pelvi-calyceal dilatation.
2. The ultrasound appearance could result from distal ureteric obstruction or from vesico-ureteric reflux.

The patient is in renal failure and has an intra-abdominal malignancy. Hypercalcaemia is one possible explanation for her renal failure and back pain might indicate bone involvement, but in this case the renal ultrasound appearance would be normal. The ultrasound appearance, in this context, suggests obstruction. For her to be in this degree of renal failure, the obstruction is likely to be bilateral. She might have bladder outflow obstruction but the most likely explanation is retroperitoneal spread of malignancy with bilateral ureteric obstruction. Her back pain fits that diagnosis.

3. She needs further investigation by ultrasound and/or computed tomography to assess the state of her pelvic tumour and retroperitoneum. Assuming her general condition justifies it, her obstruction must be relieved. If the problem were bladder outflow obstruction, the treatment would be bladder catheterisation. If she has ureteric obstruction, she needs a percutaneous nephrostomy, which can be sited under ultrasound/fluoroscopic guidance, or a ureteric stent, which is a longer-term solution.

Neurological disease

5.1 Clinical aspects

Learning objectives

You should be able to:

- link neuroanatomy to neurological problem-solving
- use your knowledge of the major diseases affecting the nervous system to place them appropriately in your differential diagnoses
- describe some of the other, less common, neurological diseases
- set out the principles of investigation and management of the major neurological diseases.

Case Study

Joan Whiting has been worrying the surgical nurses since this morning and they have asked you to help. Joan has been doing funny things like not putting her pyjama top on her right arm and putting toothpaste on to her finger when she is washing. The staff nurse is convinced that Joan is confused, but you think that Joan's speech is more nonsensical and she has difficulty in obeying your commands.

One of the keys in dealing with a neurological problem is using your knowledge of the anatomy of both the central and the peripheral nervous system. In this chapter, neuroanatomy and physiology are linked with the clinical problems.

Terminology

In neurology there are many different terms that are easy to confuse and which can distract you from understanding of a clinical problem. One common difficulty is the use of the prefixes 'a' and 'dys'. In precise terms, the former means the complete absence of the function (e.g. aphasia), whereas the latter simply implies impairment (e.g. dysphasia). In practice they can be used interchangeably. Similarly hemiparesis (weakness) and hemiplegia (complete paralysis) are used without distinction. Here is a list of definitions/explanations for terms which are particularly difficult.

Dyspraxia This is the inability to carry out voluntary purposeful movement correctly despite apparently normal motor, sensory and coordinative functions. It can be thought of items of a planning failure in a sequence of discrete motor actions. Dyspraxia is usually seen in left cerebral hemisphere damage.

Agnosia This is a failure to recognise some object despite the sense by which it is normally recognised remaining intact (e.g. visual agnosia, sensory agnosia). This is different from nominal dysphasia where an object is recognised but cannot be named; so in nominal dysphasia, a patient may not be able to name a pen, but can show how it is used. In dyspraxia, the patient would not recognise the pen. Agnosias occur with either left or right hemisphere damage.

Neglect/inattention/denial These more commonly occur in right hemisphere damage. The person shows less attention to one side of their body or space. Mild degrees need bilateral stimulation to be apparent (visual/sensory extinction). In severe forms, patients deny that one side of the body belongs to them.

Dysphasia This is a problem with *language*, not simply speech. One important aspect is that if a patient has a marked expressive dysphasia then some receptive problems will be present. A common misconception is that the patient 'understands everything that is said to them'.

Dominance Another common misunderstanding is the term **dominant hemisphere**; this refers to dominance for language and is almost always the left hemisphere (including 80% of left-handed people). Dominance does not mean the most important.

Impairment, disability and handicap It is important to know the definitions of and relationship between impairment, disability and handicap. If you think of a person with a stroke:

Impairment Impairments are the direct neurological consequences of the underlying pathology. You can think of them in terms of the 'symptoms and signs' you use to diagnose a stroke. Examples are dysphasia, hemiparesis and hemianopia.

Disability A stroke causing impairment will usually affect a person's behaviour or function. Examples of disabilities include difficulty in walking, dressing or cooking. The relationships between impairments and disabilities are complex, with other influences such as the local environment (ward, house, work) and the person's psychological state (dependency, depression). In stroke, difficulty in dressing might be caused by impairment of movement (hemiparesis), coordination (limb ataxia), sensation (hemisensory loss) or planning movement (dyspraxia).

Handicap Even more complex are the relationships between handicap and impairment/disability. Handicap refers to the social consequences of pathology (i.e. a stroke), which arise at the level of the person's own roles and activities. Examples of handicap include loss of a job or breakdown of a relationship. One important aspect is that handicap can arise as a consequence of an impairment without any disability. An example would be the loss of a heavy goods vehicle (HGV) licence as a consequence of a hemianopia (impairment but no disability).

Other disease Impairment/disability/handicap can also be considered in terms of diseases in other systems. Examples would be the social stigma (handicap) attached to a positive test for human immunodeficiency virus (HIV), or the change in working practice for a surgeon who is found to be hepatitis B antigen-positive. These illustrate that handicap can result from a disease process without any impairment.

Common symptoms

In neurological practice, there are certain symptoms that you must be able to evaluate and either link to particular disease processes *or* discount so that the patient is reassured that there is no serious problem. One important pitfall to avoid is dismissing something you do not understand as being 'hysterical, psychosomatic, supratentorial' or some other demeaning label. As in all branches of medicine, someone with more experience may be able to make sense of the clinical picture. When in doubt — ask!

There are a number of crucial questions that you should ask yourself when taking a history from someone with possible neurological disease.

What is the age of the patient? An old person is unlikely to have recent-onset multiple sclerosis. A young person is unlikely to have Parkinson's disease.

What is the time course of the symptoms? Abrupt onset is likely to be vascular or epileptic but could result from hypoglycaemia. Onset over a few hours may be infective, though occasionally viral meningitis has an abrupt onset. Progression over several weeks may point to a tumour. Years of gradual decline are likely to be degenerative.

What is the pattern of the symptoms with time? If it is a constant decline, then a degenerative condition is

probable. If the pattern is relapsing and remitting, then an inflammatory condition such as multiple sclerosis may be responsible.

Is the problem a global one such as loss of consciousness or confusion? If so, then causes outside the brain may be responsible, such as hypoglycaemia or arrhythmia.

Are there focal neurological symptoms or signs? If yes, can they be placed at one site or do they cover more than one site?

Is there any relevant family history for vascular or degenerative disease? Do not simply enquire what the patient's parents died from, but ask for detail — such as whether there is a 'family peculiar walk' or foot deformity suggestive of a spinocerebellar syndrome. You need to be able to construct a family tree.

Headache

Everybody gets a headache from time to time. The aim is, first, to separate out headache caused by underlying disease from the remainder. If you use headache as a model for the questions above, a template for sorting out the problem starts to develop. If a headache has an abrupt onset, particularly if it is severe with neck stiffness, then subarachnoid haemorrhage should be suspected. A headache that has been present for years ('never free from it') is unlikely to be caused by neurological disease. One that comes and goes and is associated with flashing lights/ visual disturbance is likely to be migraine, but recent onset in an older person might suggest temporal arteritis. If the headache is global ('like a band round the head'), this suggests a tension headache, whereas an intense retro-orbital pain might suggest periodic migraine/cluster headache. If the headache is associated with focal neurological signs, a more sinister cause is likely, possibly a tumour. You should also consider other head and neck problems such as sinusitis. Remember, most headaches are not indicative of serious disease, but you need to be able to identify the small number that are.

Blackouts/funny turns

Many patients will present with a 'funny turn'. The causes can be thought of as brain (e.g. fits) or non-brain (e.g. cardiac dysrhythmia).

The first question is whether the person did, or did not, lose consciousness. This can be difficult to be sure of as patients may fill in gaps in their memory ('I must have tripped'). One clue may be the extensive facial bruising suggesting a fall without any protective outstretching of the hands.

What was the person doing immediately before? A blackout in a hot crowded room whilst standing up suggests a simple vasovagal attack. Were there any prodomal features or, if the person did not lose consciousness, how did they feel during the episode? Palpitations would suggest a disturbance in cardiac rhythm (**Stokes–Adams attack**). An odd feeling prior to the event might be caused by the **aura** of epilepsy.

For any patient presenting with a blackout, you should seek out a witness to the event. They can describe what happened, which is important for the diagnosis of epilepsy.

A key feature is how the person felt following the attack. If it was caused by cardiac dysrhythmia, recovery is characteristically quick. Similarly, recovery following a vasovagal event (a 'faint') is rapid once the person lies down (never hold them up). There are often symptoms of excessive vagal activity (e.g. nausea). In contrast, a person is commonly confused and drowsy after a fit, wishing to sleep for several hours.

Unfortunately, the aetiology of the blackouts may not be clear, and your examination (neurological and general) may not be helpful. Investigations may then be appropriate.

Cardiac causes

A 12-lead electrocardiograph (ECG) is most useful for revealing stable abnormalities, e.g. left axis deviation with right bundle branch block (bifascicular block), which predispose to bradyarrhythmias. A 24-hour ECG recording is often requested, but the yield from these is *small* and the test should only be done if frequent attacks are present.

Drop attacks

Occasinally, elderly patients describe drop attacks in which they suddenly feel that their legs are giving way and they fall to the ground (sometimes hurting themselves). Afterwards, they may complain of difficulty in getting up, such that they have to crawl to an object they can use to climb back into an upright position. The hallmark of drop attacks is that the person does *not* lose consciousness at any stage. The attacks can come in clusters, then may settle. Sometimes, head turning appears to precipitate them. The aetiology is complex and a number of different conditions can cause similar attacks, but in many patients the cause of drop attacks remains unknown. Identified causes of attacks include **narcolepsy** in younger people and **carotid sinus hypersensitivity** in older patients. In the latter condition, stimulation of the carotid sinus leads to bradycardia, hypotension or both. Sometimes, hypersensitivity is a cause of syncope (loss of consciousness). A useful investigation is the **tilt table**, which stresses the carotid sinus.

Neurological causes

An electroencephalograph (EEG) is frequently ordered but is of limited value. It may show a potential epileptic focus with spike activity. A normal EEG does *not* rule out epilepsy. Computed tomographic (CT) and magnetic resonance (MR) scans are other common investigations that are requested but seldom add much.

The message is that careful histories from the person *and* witnesses are the most important steps to take in the diagnostic process.

Confusion

Chronic confusion is discussed under Dementia (p. 233). Acute confusional states occur at all ages, not just in elderly people. The features include a disturbance of conscious level (**delirium**), with disorientation in place and time. Patients may be agitated or withdrawn. As with any organic brain syndrome, *visual* hallucinations are common and the symptoms may vary over time. There are many causes of acute confusion and you should think of them in broad categories:

- brain problems: stroke, infection, trauma
- metabolic and electrolyte disturbance: e.g. hypoglycaemia, hyponatraemia
- toxins: alcohol, drugs
- infections: pneumonia, urinary tract infection
- others: e.g. myocardial infarction (brain perfusion).

Focal neurology

The key diagnostic questions you need to address in a patient with a focal deficit are:

- Can the deficit result from a single lesion or must there be more than one site involved?
- At what level is the lesion: cerebral hemisphere, brainstem, spinal cord, peripheral nerve, motor endplate or muscle?
- What is the time course, e.g. sudden (vascular/fit) or gradual deterioration (degenerative)?

The clinical diagnosis can often be made from the answers to these questions. For example, a rapid deterioration in visual acuity with a previous history of ataxia and urinary difficulties in a young person suggests multiple sclerosis (multiple sites, affected at different times). In contrast, an episode of fleeting loss of vision in one eye in an older person (**amaurosis fugax**) is suggestive of a platelet embolus from the carotid artery (single site).

A further guiding rule is to try to place the lesion as peripherally as possible. For example, sensory loss should be considered first as a peripheral nerve problem. If this does not fit the clinical picture, then move up through the spinal cord towards the integrating centres in the parietal lobe until all the sensory features can be accounted for. In another example, a hemiparesis could be anywhere from the high cervical cord upwards, but an exaggerated jaw jerk would place the damage above the level of the pons; dysphasia would place it in the cerebral hemispheres. Without these other signs, little precision can be achieved.

Cranial nerve abnormalities

Damage to the cranial nerves must be diagnosed on the basis of the common symptoms and examination findings.

Optic nerve/visual disturbance

A common presenting symptom is visual difficulty. You must know the important elements of the visual pathway so that you can determine the cause and pathophysiological process involved (Fig. 50). Lesions along this pathway cause particular visual disturbances (Table 50).

You must also know the path involved in the light reflex (Fig. 51). The other pupillary reflex is **accommodation**, in which the pupils constrict, the eyes converge and ptosis occurs on looking at an object close up. In an **Argyll–Robertson** pupil, the light reflex is lost but accommodation is preserved. Characteristically, the pupils are small, irregular and unequal. In the past, the most common cause was neurosyphilis, but now diabetes mellitus is a common cause of pupillary abnormalities. The **Holmes–Adie** pupil

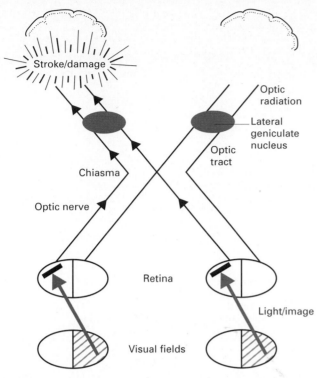

Fig. 50 The visual pathway. Damage on one side of the brain (e.g. stroke) causes a homonymous hemianopia on the opposite side.

is typically seen in young women, in whom the pupil is large and responds to light sluggishly. There is an association with limb areflexia.

Horner's syndrome

In Horner's syndrome there is damage to the *sympathetic* supply to the orbit. The pathway involved has a long course, starting in the hypothalamus, running down through the brainstem and flowing out through T1 in the spinal cord. Fibres then run back into the skull as a plexus round the carotid artery and into the orbit. Damage anywhere along this route can cause a Horner's syndrome. Important causes are cerebrovascular disease and tumours growing in the apex of the lung damaging the brachial plexus (**Pancoast's tumour**), though most cases are idiopathic. There are four cardinal signs of Horner's syndrome:

- meiosis (constricted pupil)
- partial ptosis
- enophthalmos (eye shrunken into socket)
- anhydrosis (lack of sweating on ipsilateral side of face).

Oculomotor nerves

The third, fourth and sixth cranial nerves act together to produce smooth visual fixation and tracking. You must know the direction of the prime action of the muscles

Table 50 Visual symptoms arising from damage to the visual pathway, site of damage and common pathological processes

Visual symptom	Site of damage	Common pathologies*
Fleeting loss of vision in one eye (amaurosis fugax): 'Like a curtain coming up/down'	Central retinal artery	Microemboli, often from carotid artery
Monocular blindness: 'Can't see at all out of one eye'	Optic nerve, eye	Trauma, infection, bleeding (diabetes), central retinal artery thrombosis, temporal arteritis
Field defects in one eye (scotomas): 'I seem to have a blind spot'	Retina, branch of retinal arteries, part of optic nerve	Glaucoma (arcuate scotoma), retinal artery thrombosis, MS, CMV retinitis in AIDS
Bitemporal hemianopia: 'Can't see things to the side'	Chiasma; if upper part, lower fields lost, and vice versa	Tumour: pituitary, craniopharyngioma (child)
Homonymous hemianopia: 'Can't see to the left (right)'	Optic tract Optic radiation Occipital cortex	Tumours, vascular damage: stroke
Sudden bilateral visual loss: 'Struck blind'	Occipital cortex: cortical blindness (Anton's syndrome), patient may not complain of blindness	Vascular
Flashing lights/zigzag lights (fortification spectra): loss of part of visual field	Occipital cortex	Migraine

MS, multiple sclerosis; CMV, cytomegalovirus; AIDS, acquired immunodeficiency syndrome.
*In the UK the most common causes of blindness are diabetes mellitus, glaucoma and senile macular degeneration.

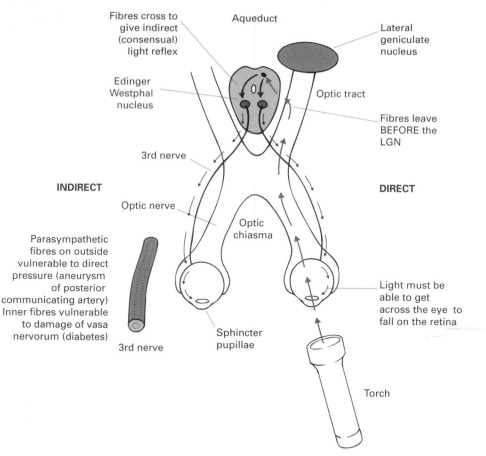

Fig. 51 Pathway for light reflex; LGN, lateral geniculate nucleus.

involved (Fig. 52). In trying to unravel diplopia it is useful to remember three simple rules:

- Diplopia is maximal on looking in the direction of the prime action of the muscle.
- The false image is always displaced furthest in the direction of action of the muscle affected.
- The false image is always the least distinct.

Third cranial nerve palsy. This is commonly caused by either an aneurysm or diabetes and it results in:

- complete ptosis
- the eye turned down (unopposed action of superior oblique muscle) and out (lateral rectus)
- a large pupil that is non-reactive to light (Fig. 51).

Fourth nerve palsy This is very rare in isolation. It causes diplopia when looking down and away from the affected side (eye adducted).

Sixth nerve palsies These are relatively common, either from vascular lesions or as a false localising sign in raised intracranial pressure where the nerve is trapped as it crosses the falx cerebri.

Visual movements Other problems with visual movements are described on page 227.

Fifth nerve

The fifth nerve supplies sensation to the face, including the cornea, through the ophthalmic branch. The mandibular

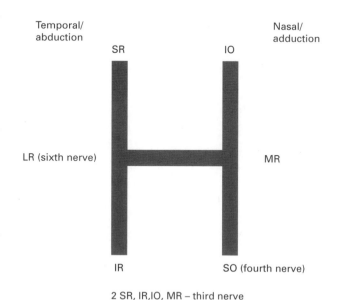

2 SR, IR, IO, MR – third nerve

Fig. 52 Primary action of extrinsic ocular muscles and their innervation. SR, MR, LR and IR, superior, medial, lateral and inferior rectus muscles, respectively; IO and SO, inferior and superior oblique muscles, respectively.

division supplies the muscles of mastication (temporalis, masseter and pterygoids). An important element in examining trigeminal function is the corneal reflex (efferent arc: facial nerve). An absent or diminished corneal reflex may be an early sign of an **acoustic neuroma** (pressure on the fifth nerve in the cerebello–pontine angle). Divisions of the fifth nerve are commonly affected by herpes zoster.

Trigeminal neuralgia. This is an important clinical problem affecting the fifth nerve. It is a condition of unknown aetiology that runs a relapsing and remitting course. It is very rarely bilateral. Typically the age of onset is 60–70 years. Patients describe *lancinating* pain, which may be precipitated by stimulating a *trigger zone* or by activities such as yawning or brushing teeth. On examination there are *no* physical signs and investigations (if done) are normal. The main treatment is carbamazepine.

Seventh nerve

The most common cranial nerve lesion you will see in practice is a facial nerve palsy. You must be able to draw the diagram in Figure 53 in order to understand how facial nerve damage manifests. An important additional detail is that the upper part of the face is *bilaterally innervated*. What this means is that each motor cortex (left and right precentral gyrus) sends fibres to the facial nucleus on both sides. Consequently:

- an upper motor neurone lesion (e.g. caused by a stroke), affecting the pathway from only one cortex, will spare the upper part of the face

- a lower motor neurone lesion (damage to the nucleus or the nerve) will cause complete paralysis of one half of the face.

Facial weakness often results from damage to the facial nerve. In trying to pinpoint where the damage is located, you need to know the information in Figure 53. For example, an acoustic neuroma (eighth nerve) may compress the facial nerve as it runs towards the internal auditory meatus and all function may be lost, whereas damage in the facial canal — for example, in **Bell's palsy** — will spare the greater superficial petrosal nerve and hence lacrimation.

Ramsay–Hunt syndrome A complete facial palsy may be caused by geniculate herpes zoster. Some vesiculation may be observed around the ear canal. Prognosis for recovery is much worse than in Bell's palsy.

Eighth nerve

In neurological practice, the most important diagnosis is the rare acoustic neuroma, which is discussed on page 224.

Ninth and tenth nerve

The ninth nerve is sensory to the palate, fauces and upper pharynx with branches to the carotid sinus (monitoring blood pressure) and carotid body (monitoring arterial oxygen partial pressure). It also supplies the stylopharyngeal muscle which, with the palatopharyngeus muscle (vagus) elevates the palate. The vagus nerve is motor to the palate including the pharyngeal constrictors. Weakness of

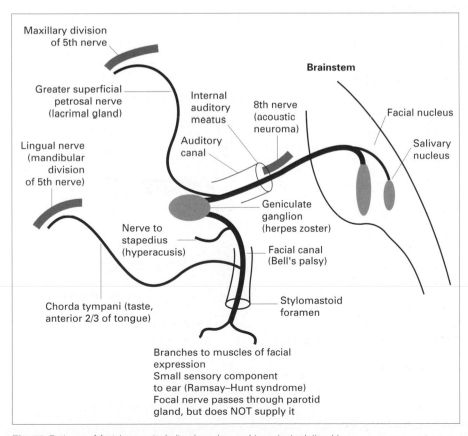

Fig. 53 Pathway of facial nerve, including branches and important relationships.

one side of the palate causes the uvula to be drawn *away* from the affected side. The principal effect of damage to the nerves/nuclei, e.g. in the medulla (vascular, motor neurone disease) or around the jugular foramen, is **dysphagia**. Swallowing is a complex act requiring coordination between a number of different centres. Three stages are recognised:

- Oral/preparatory: lip closure (seventh nerve), mastication (fifth nerve), manipulation by the tongue (twelfth nerve) and presentation of the bolus to the pharynx.
- Pharyngeal (ninth and tenth nerve): the soft palate lifts together with the larynx, and the pharyngeal constrictors assist the bolus through to the upper end of the oesphagus.
- Oesophageal (discussed on p. 117).

The presence or absence of the gag reflex (sensory ninth nerve, motor tenth nerve) is of no use in predicting aspiration. All patients who are drowsy should be considered at risk. In making an assessment of swallowing, the main features of dysphagia are a 'wet' voice and coughing on taking a small amount of fluid. In neurological dysphagia, unlike obstructive dysphagia, the greater problems are with thin liquids rather than solids because of difficulty in controlling the former.

Twelfth nerve

Tongue function can be affected by bulbar (i.e. medullary) damage or pseudobulbar damage. In a unilateral lesion, the tongue will point *towards* the affected side. Bulbar weakness, caused by ischaemia, encephalitis, motor neurone disease or **syringobulbia** (very rare, caused by a cavity in the middle of the brainstem), will cause wasting of the tongue with fasciculation, dysphagia and dysarthria.

Pseudobulbar palsy This is caused by *bilateral* damage of the pyramidal tract system (e.g. stroke, motor neurone disease). It causes dysphagia, *emotionalism* (inability to control emotions with crying at inappropriate times or excessively) and a tongue which appears small and 'stuck' to the floor of the mouth. The dysarthria is likened to talking with a mouthful of marbles.

Basic investigations

Examination of cerebrospinal fluid

The brain is covered by the meninges, which consist of the thick dura mater externally, the arachnoid, lining the dura, and the pia mater, adherent to the brain and spinal cord. The arachnoid and the pia bound the subarachnoid space, which is filled by the cerebrospinal fluid (CSF). The CSF is produced at a constant rate of about 450 ml/day by the **choroid plexuses** of the lateral (most important), third and fourth ventricles. Flow is from the lateral ventricles into the third ventricle and then the fourth ventricle by way of the aqueduct. Foramina allow drainage from the fourth ventricle into the pontine cistern and cisterna magna. Blockage along this route may cause a **non-communicating hydrocephalus**. Causes include tumour or blood within the ventricular system.

The CSF flows through the cisternal spaces and over the cerebral hemispheres. Absorption into the dural venous sinuses is through the **arachnoid villi**. Block here, e.g. by blood from a subarachnoid haemorrhage, may cause a **communicating hydrocephalus**.

Rarely a **normal pressure hydrocephalus** occurs in elderly people. In this, slow pressure waves can be demonstrated by continous monitoring (these gradually dilate the ventricles), but isolated pressure readings are normal. Patients have a triad of dementia, gait dyspraxia and urinary incontinence. It is important to make the diagnosis because around one-third of patients will respond to insertion of a ventricular shunt.

Another rare condition is **benign intracranial hypertension**, where there is an overproduction of CSF. The disease is most common in young women and is associated with the oral contraceptive pill, pregnancy and obesity. Presentation is with headaches, an enlarging blind spot and progressive visual failure that can be permanent if not diagnosed early. Papilloedema is found on examination. A CT or MR scan will show slit-like ventricles and effacement (compression) of the sulci of the cerebral hemispheres. A lumbar puncture will show a greatly elevated CSF pressure (≥ 20 cmH$_2$O) and repeated lumbar punctures may improve the symptoms. Again, it is important to make the diagnosis, as patients can respond to acetazolamide or corticosteroids. Sometimes neurosurgical intervention is needed to decompress the brain.

The CSF volume is around 80–200 ml (i.e. will turn over 3–4 times each day) with a recumbent pressure of 8–18 cmH$_2$O. It is important to know the approximate normal values for CSF constituents as this is essential to make decisions on the results of an urgent CSF specimen. Key values are given in Box 15.

The indications for a lumbar puncture are suspected:

- meningitis
- encephalitis
- subarachnoid haemorrhage (if CT scan negative)
- benign intracranial hypertension.

The main contraindications to lumbar puncture are focal signs, evidence of raised intracranial pressure, a space-occupying lesion on CT scan or a significant bleeding tendency. The patterns of abnormalities found in the CSF with different disease processes are the keys to synthesising the information into a differential diagnosis (Table 51).

Box 15: Normal values for CSF constituents

- Protein: 0.25–0.50 g/l
- Glucose[a]: 2.5–5.5 mmol/l
- White cells: $<5 \times 10^6$ white cells/l
- Red cells[b]: 0

[a]This is dependent on the blood glucose value (should be 50–70% of the blood values: N.B. diabetes mellitus).
[b]Should be zero. However, a 'bloody tap' may contaminate the fluid. If some red cells are present in all specimen samples, this suggests subarachnoid haemorrhage. If decreasing values in successful samples, this suggests a 'bloody tap'. One white cell is allowed for every 1000 red cells.

Table 51 Relevant tests and abnormalities in CSF with disease processes

Disease process	Pressure	Cells	Glucose	Protein	Microbiology	Special notes
Bacterial meningitis	May be increased	High neutrophils (95–100%)	Very low or undetectable	High or very high	Gram stain or culture positive	Partially treated: may be culture negative
Viral meningitis	Usually normal	High lymphocytes (10–100%); early disease: neutrophils	Low	Normal or slightly high	PCR useful	Common
Viral encephalitis		Mild increase in lymphocytes	Low	Normal or slightly raised	PCR useful	May be red cells in herpes simplex
Brain abscess/ parameningeal focus	May be increased	High neutrophils (60–100%)	Normal or low	High	Culture and Gram stain negative (75%)	Check CT scan carefully
Fungal meningitis	May be increased	High lymphocytes	Low or normal	Normal or raised	India ink stain culture positive, cryptococcal antigen positive (95%)	Usually AIDS or other immunocompromised patient
Tuberculous meningitis	May be increased	Lymphocytes, usually 100%	Low	High or very high	ZN stain (10–20%) and culture (30%)	Uncommon
Malignancy	Variable	Malignant cells on cytology	Low	Some increase	Negative	Rare
Guillain–Barré syndrome	Normal	Slight increase in lymphocytes in early stages	Normal	Raised after first week	Negative	
Multiple sclerosis	Normal	Slight increase in lymphocytes in relapse	Normal	Mild rise	Negative	May have oligoclonal protein bands (but take blood for protein electrophoresis at same time)
Subarachnoid haemorrhage	May be raised	Red cells increased	Normal	High	Negative	Xanthochromia (red cell pigment) present

PCR, polymerase chain reaction; ZN, Ziehl–Neelsen; CT, computed tomography; AIDS, acquired immunodeficiency syndrome.

Imaging techniques

CT and MR imaging techniques have revolutionised neurological practice. When looking at a CT or MR scan, go through a set routine:

- Orientate yourself: left/right; anterior/posterior.
- Was contrast given? If not, then on a CT scan any dense white areas in the brain are either blood or (less common) calcium.
- Describe any obvious abnormality in terms of its position, size, shape and any effects on surrounding brain tissue (compression: midline shift).
- Look for other abnormalities which may be more subtle and present in other areas of the brain.

The use of CT/MR scanning is discussed within the common neurological problems described below.

Electroencephalography

Though now regarded as an 'old' investigation, EEG is still useful as a tool for unravelling a neurological problem but it has limitations. Approximately 5% of the population have an 'abnormal' EEG, particularly young people. Therefore, it cannot be used to 'diagnose' epilepsy; it is there as an adjunct to careful history and examination. In certain cases, 24-hour recordings or telemetry can be useful.

There are certain conditions in which an EEG can yield characteristic findings (Table 52). In most other conditions in which abnormalities are seen (for example, drug toxicity or cerebral oedema) the findings are non-specific (for example, generalised or localised slow waves).

Nerve conduction tests and electromyography

You do not need to know the detail of the specialised nerve conduction tests and electromyography (EMG). What you must know are the clinical problems for which you should request these investigations and you should understand what the results will tell you.

Nerve conduction studies determine the *conduction velocities* within the nerves and will be impaired if the myelin sheath is damaged. Therefore, conditions such as **Guillain–Barré syndrome** show marked slowing of con-

duction. Diseases that attack the axons or nerve bodies, such as **motor neurone disease**, will show minimal impairment of conduction but a reduced number of motor units (amplitude of signal). Nerve conduction studies can show localised areas of demyelination resulting from pressure, such as in the carpal tunnel syndrome (wrist) or ulnar nerve palsies (elbow).

EMG is useful for showing changes in the innervation of muscles or disorders of muscles themselves. Therefore, acute/subacute denervation, such as in motor neurone disease, will show fibrillating potentials. Problems at the motor endplate, such as in **myasthenia gravis** or **Eaton–Lambert syndrome**, will produce characteristic changes, as can inflammation in the muscles (**myositis**) or an intrinsic abnormality such as **dystrophia myotonica**.

Common drugs

The most common drugs used in neurological practice are for epilepsy (p. 237) and for Parkinson's disease. These are dealt with below. The use of hypnotics and neuroleptics is outside the scope of this book. Analgesia is dealt with elsewhere (p. 346). Occasional use of corticosteroids and immunosuppressives is discussed in the context of the relevant disease.

5.2 Infection

Case Study

The gradual onset of headache over 4 days, culminating in him taking to his bed, characterised the presentation of this previously well 23-year-old PhD student. In accident and emergency he was mumbling but had not been drinking. He had not vomited. He had mild neck stiffness but nil else on examination. A CT scan of his head was normal. A lumbar puncture showed 22 white cells (≈60% lymphocytes), protein of 0.6 mg/l and a normal CSF/blood glucose ratio. There was extensive discussion about whether aciclovir was appropriate or sufficient therapy.

Table 52 Characteristic electroencephalography (EEG) abnormalities with disease processes

Disease processes	Notes on EEG abnormality
Petit mal epilepsy	3/s spike and wave activity
Partial epilepsy	May be no abnormality; may have 'focus' with spike activity
Hepatic encephalopathy	Triphasic waves
Herpes simplex encephalitis	Temporal lobe abnormality (30–50%)
Creutzfeldt–Jakob disease (prion disease)	Slow background (1–2/s) repetitive spikes

Bacterial meningitis

Pathogenesis and epidemiology

Bacteria enter the meningeal space either directly because of a hole in the dura or via the bloodstream. The two most common organisms causing meningitis in adults are *Neisseria meningitidis* and *Streptococcus pneumoniae*. Both of these enter the body through the nasopharynx. Why *Strep. pneumoniae* causes pneumonia in some individuals and meningitis in others is unclear. Likewise why *N. meningitidis* causes meningococcal septicaemia (p. 413) or meningitis is not understood.

N. meningitidis infection is more common in young adults and teenagers; the incidence of *Strep. pneumoniae* meningitis increases with age.

Clinical presentation

The onset of bacterial meningitis is usually abrupt and rapidly progressive. The time from first symptom to death is frequently as short as 48 hours and sometimes as little as 24 hours. Therefore bacterial meningitis *must* be treated as a medical emergency. The symptoms that should lead to suspicion of meningitis are:

- headache
- vomiting
- fever
- impaired consciousness.

Patients may also complain of photophobia, chills, sore throat, rash and painful or stiff neck.

Clinical evaluation and emergency management

Your evaluation of the patient with possible meningitis should be rapid and focused so as not to delay therapy. Apart from the above symptoms, seek information about immunocompromising factors and allergies. Your examination should look for neck stiffness, papilloedema/ absence of pulsation in retinal veins, focal neurological signs, ear disease, rash, signs of pneumonia and ventilatory status. If neck stiffness is present, together with the above symptoms (especially if consciousness is impaired), you should make a presumptive diagnosis of meningitis.

Clinical Box: Emergency treatment: management of meningitis

In general practice/community
1. Administer benzylpenicillin 1.2 g i.v. or i.m.
2. Arrange emergency transport to hospital

In hospital
1. Prescribe cefotaxime 2 g or ceftriaxone 4 g i.v. (if none available use benzylpenicillin 1.2 or 2.4 g) and dexamethasone 10 mg i.v. and ask nurses or colleague to prepare drugs immediately
2. Take blood for blood culture, serology, full blood count, creatinine, urea, electrolytes and glucose
3. Set up an i.v. infusion
4. Give antibiotics and dexamethasone
5. Do a lumbar puncture (LP) *before an urgent CT* if:
   - Not immunocompromised
   - No fits
   - No papilloedema (or normal retinal vein pulsation)
   - No focal neurological signs
   - No major impairment of consciousness
   - No coagulopathy.
   An LP is very important in getting antimicrobial therapy right.
6. If CT scan is done first and is normal, do an LP; if CT shows focal disease, seek senior guidance
7. Do blood gases and administer oxygen if necessary
8. Take complete history and do full physical examination
9. Speak to consultant microbiologist or infectious disease physician about case and decide empirical antibiotic regimen, in particular the need for vancomycin to cover penicillin-resistant *Staph. pneumoniae*
10. Transfer to single room or intensive care

At this stage in hospital practice the emergency treatment outlined in the box should be initiated. You should endeavour to ensure that all patients with meningitis receive antibiotics within 30 minutes of arriving in the hospital. Delay will worsen outcome.

Differential diagnosis

If the patient is hospitalised, alcoholic or immunocompromised, altdiolie other causes of meningitis should be considered. Examples include *Listeria monocytogenes*, Gram-negative organisms or the fungus *Cryptococcus neoformans*. The lumbar puncture is *critical* for these patients; otherwise treatment is likely to be wrong. In addition, penicillin resistance in pneumococci is an increasing problem and optimum therapy for these patients can only be decided if the organism is cultured. The lumbar puncture also distinguishes viral from bacterial meningitis and allows herpes simplex encephalitis to be diagnosed with confidence (p. 222). If the patient is young and acutely ill with the typical purpuric rash of meningococcal disease, a lumbar puncture adds little to a blood culture and need not be done.

Management

Dexamethasone (10 g 6-hourly for 4 days), given before or with antibiotics, reduces mortality in pneumococcal meningitis from 34% to 14%, without apparent side-effects. These drugs slightly reduce neurologic sequelae in meningococcal meningitis.

Antibiotics are usually given for 7–10 days. Avoid giving too much fluid; keep patients slightly sodium- and water-depleted to reduce cerebral oedema. Isolation is required for 24 hours for meningcococcal disease only.

Prognosis and complications

The mortality of meningococcal meningitis is around 10% and of pneumococcal meningitis is 25%, rising to 60% in elderly people, if treated only with antibiotics. Bacterial meningitis, especially pneumococcal, carries a high rate of neurological sequelae if the patient survives, although this is reduced from 52% to 26% with dexamethasone. Deafness is the most common deficit. Memory deficits, motor disability and more complex problems are quite common.

Prevention

All forms of meningitis are notifiable diseases (p. 429). Household contacts or those who have given mouth-to-mouth resuscitation to patients with meningococcal meningitis or septicaemia require antibiotic prophylaxis (p. 410).

Brain abscess

Pathogenesis and epidemiology

Most brain abscesses are related to chronic ear disease, but dental, sinus, pulmonary and cyanotic congenital heart disease are also predisposing factors. In many patients, no underlying cause is found. An increasing number of cerebral abscesses occur in immunocompromised patients. In these patients, opportunistic pathogens such as *Nocardia*, *Aspergillus* or *Toxoplasma* are more frequent than bacteria. For this reason, you should always try to ascertain the immune status of the patient. About half the cases occur in young adults.

Clinical presentation

Typically patients have symptoms for 1–2 weeks before admission and diagnosis. Chronic ear infection is found in 40%. Nausea and vomiting with drowsiness are common. However, the clinical findings are not distinctive:

- Headache is the most common symptom (75%).
- Only 10% of patients are unconscious.
- Fever is only present in 30%.
- Focal signs are found in 70%.
- Neck stiffness is found in only 15%.

Investigations

Radiological findings

The typical CT appearance (with contrast) is an area of central necrosis, with ring enhancement surrounded by oedema. Frequently there is midline shift. The appearances are usually sufficiently distinctive to distinguish a brain abscess from tumour. Abscesses are found throughout the brain and are multiple in about 25% of patients. MR scanning is more sensitive, especially in immunocompromised patients.

Management

If the patient has acquired immunodeficiency syndrome (AIDS), empiric therapy for toxoplasmosis is given without confirmation of the diagnosis. In all other patients, aspiration of the lesion or excision is the next step. As anaerobic organisms are common, rapid transport of the specimen to the laboratory is crucial. In over one-third of patients, four or more bacteria are grown from the abscess. Antibiotic management is then directed against the appropriate pathogens. Empirical therapy of brain abscess always includes metronidazole and should include an antistreptococcal agent (such as penicillin or ampicillin) and a broad-spectrum Gram-negative agent (such as cefotaxime), all in large doses.

Prognosis

If managed appropriately, the overall mortality from brain abscess should be <10%, with all deaths occurring in patients presenting unconscious. The mortality from brain abscess in immunocompromised patients is much higher, especially with *Aspergillus*.

Tuberculous meningitis

You must be able to distinguish the common treatable forms of lymphocytic meningitis (e.g. tuberculous meningitis) from viral meningitis, primarily using the CSF results (Table 51).

Epidemiology

Tuberculous meningitis is an uncommon cause of meningitis in the UK but is the most common cause worldwide of subacute meningitis in non-AIDS patients. About 3–10% of all patients with tuberculosis have meningitis.

Clinical presentation

Symptoms increase in severity over 2–6 weeks prior to presentation. In the UK, most cases occur in patients from the Indian subcontinent. Vomiting, headache and anorexia are the most common features (50–75%). Drowsiness is seen in a third of patients. More severely affected patients, usually those who present late, may be unconscious or have cranial nerve palsies, hemiparesis or other localising features. Fever is not common. Examination shows

- neck stiffness (90%)
- papilloedema (30%)
- focal neurological signs (25%, in severe cases).

In the UK, a previously well Asian patient with a 2-week history of vomiting and headache is likely to have tuberculous meningitis. If there is also neck stiffness, the diagnosis is highly likely.

Investigations

Key investigations are:

- chest radiograph: to seek evidence of concurrent or prior pulmonary or miliary tuberculosis
- tuberculin skin test
- CT or MR scan of brain (to visualise tuberculomas and rule out other brain abscess or tumour)
- CSF examination (see below and Table 51).

The typical CSF specimen shows many white cells — usually $100–400 \times 10^6$ cells/l — which are predominantly or exclusively lymphocytes, a very high protein content (e.g. >1.0 g/l) and a low glucose content. This picture is characteristic and clinically useful, as acid-fast bacilli are seen in the CSF in only a minority and culture is positive in only 25–50% of patients. Therefore, confirmation of the diagnosis is difficult. The usual problem is that the CSF is consistent with tuberculous meningitis but no confirmatory data (such as a strongly positive tuberculin skin test) are available. In these circumstances, you should seek expert advice.

Tuberculous meningitis can be relatively silent in patients with AIDS, typically presenting in Africans.

Management

Treatment for tuberculous meningitis is similar to that for other forms of tuberculosis. Four drugs should be given initially, as this disease has such a poor outlook if under-treated; resistance is an increasing problem (p. 78). Dexamethasone should be used as treatment is started if there is impaired consciousness.

Outcome

The mortality of tuberculous meningitis is about 15–50%, depending on how delayed treatment is. Neurological sequelae, such as diplopia, deafness, hemiparesis and mental retardation, are common in survivors (20–25%). A significant proportion of patients (10–20%) develop hydrocephalus (headache or declining mental status) and require a ventricular shunt.

Fungal meningitis

Cryptococcal meningitis

The most common cause of fungal meningitis is *Cryptococcus neoformans*. In the UK, there are about 40 cases each year, mostly in AIDS and other immunocompromised patients.

Cryptococcus is acquired through inhalation and can cause pneumonia or lung nodules. However, 85% of patients have meningitis. It presents subacutely, rather like tuberculous meningitis. CSF examination will show a lymphocyte predominance, and in non-AIDS patients a raised protein and low glucose. Yeasts (by India ink examination) are seen in 75% of patients and cryptococcal antigen is usually positive, as is culture.

Treatment is with amphotericin B and flucytosine followed by fluconazole. If treatment is initiated promptly the outcome is good, especially in AIDS.

Viral meningitis

Epidemiology

Overall, viral meningitis is more common than bacterial meningitis. The widespread use of mumps vaccine has reduced the number of cases substantially. There are many causes of non-bacterial meningitis, some of which require specific therapy. To make things easier for you, Table 53 includes all major infectious causes of a lymphocytosis in the CSF.

Clinical presentation

Viral meningitis presents with headache and neck stiffness, without impairment of consciousness (see Viral encephalitis). The headache is often severe, coming on gradually over 1–6 hours. Occasionally it has a sudden onset, and then you should think first of subarachnoid haemorrhage. Occasionally, there are associated features such as parotitis or orchitis in mumps or cranial nerve herpes zoster, or other features of primary HIV infection (p. 383). Headache is a common feature of influenza and atypical pneumonia, so also consider these diagnoses.

Table 53 Infectious causes of lymphocytic CSF

Cause	Treatment required
Viral	
Enteroviruses*	No
Mumps virus	No
Adenovirus	No
Lymphocytic choriomeningitis virus	No
Varicella zoster virus	No
Herpes simplex virus	Yes
Human immunodeficiency virus	Yes
West Nile virus	No
Other	
*M. tuberculosis**	Yes
*Mycoplasma pneumoniae**	Yes
Lyme disease	Yes
Leptospirosis	Yes
Syphilis	Yes
Cryptococcus spp.	Yes
Coccidioidomycosis	Yes
Brucellosis	Yes

*Most common in UK.

Often, there are no useful clinical features to make an aetiological diagnosis.

Investigations

Lumbar puncture is useful. The total cell count is elevated with a neutrophil predominance (up to 90%) in most patients in the first 2 days or so, but a lymphocyte predominance thereafter. The glucose is usually normal; in about 10% of patients it can be slightly low but it is never extremely low. The protein may be mildly elevated (up to about 0.8 g/l) but is rarely above 1.0 g/l (Table 51). Virus detection by polymerase chain reaction (PCR) is the most sensitive means of making the diagnosis.

The most useful tests for the enteroviruses (the commonest cause) are CSF, throat and stool viral cultures and PCR. Mumps virus can be grown in the urine. HIV is best identified by requesting a blood HIV viral load test, as seroconversion can be delayed. If HIV is identified, this would be an indication to treat early with antiretroviral therapy (p. 387). All forms of meningitis are notifiable diseases.

Management

Viral meningitis is usually a benign illness that is self-limiting in normal people. Bed rest and symptomatic relief for headache are all that is required. If deterioration in the level of consciousness occurs, then the diagnosis is probably a meningoencephalitis (or other non-viral disease) with implications for management (see below).

Viral encephalitis

Epidemiology

Around 1000 documented (and many more undocumented) cases of viral encephalitis occur in the UK each year. There are several causes of viral encephalitis, which generally present in the same way. Most cases of encephalitis in the UK are caused by common viruses present worldwide. These include Coxsackie virus and echoviruses (enteroviruses), adenovirus, mumps, measles, varicella zoster, Epstein–Barr virus and others.

Clinical presentation

Encephalitis is characterised by the acute onset of a febrile illness, with mental status abnormalities with or without fever. Any or all of the following features can occur:

- headache
- altered level of consciousness
- behavioural and speech disturbance
- neurological signs
- seizures, which may be focal or generalised.

Many patients with viral encephalitis have neck stiffness and cells in the CSF, and the term meningoencephalitis is often used. The cardinal features distinguishing viral encephalitis from meningitis are alterations in consciousness and behavioural changes.

Differential diagnosis

The differential diagnosis of viral encephalitis is broad. It includes bacterial infections of the central nervous system (CNS) (including *Listeria* and tuberculosis), cryptococcal meningitis, Lyme disease, drug overdoses, vascular disease, carbon monoxide poisoning, systemic lupus erythematosus and heterozygous ornithine transcarbamylase deficiency. The diagnosis can be established with reasonable certainty by excluding structural lesions on CT and MR scanning, lumbar puncture with PCR, serology and repeated careful observation. In addition, stool, urine and throat swabs may grow the virus.

Investigations

The lumbar puncture is of value provided the CSF findings are interpreted correctly (Table 51). Rarely, if ever, is the CSF entirely normal in encephalitis. Typically, white cells are increased but may be only just abnormal, e.g. 7×10^6 cells/l. Red cells are often increased in herpes simplex encephalitis. The glucose is normal, except in some cases of mumps meningoencephalitis, when it is slightly low. The protein may be normal, or more commonly slightly elevated. As with viral meningitis, PCR diagnosis on CSF is the most sensitive and rapid way to determine the aetiology. Other conditions can usually be excluded by measuring carbon monoxide, autoantibodies, toxins and serum ammonia.

The EEG is not specific enough to establish with certainty the aetiology of encephalitis, although a temporal focus suggests herpes simplex encephalitis (Table 52).

CT and MR scans are principally of use in excluding other diseases. Occasionally a focus of haemorrhagic necrosis or inflammation is identified, but the specificity of such findings is poor.

Management

The treatment of encephalitis is mostly supportive but may include admission to the intensive care unit if the

Table 54 Glasgow Coma Scale*

Category	Score
Eye opening	
Spontaneous	4
To speech	3
To pain	2
None	1
Best verbal response	
Orientated	5
Confused	4
Inappropriate	3
Incomprehensible	2
None	1
Best motor response	
Obeying commands	5
Localising	4
Flexing	3
Extending	2
None	1

*The scores are added up to give an overall rating between 3 and 14; minimum score is 3.

Glasgow Coma Score is low (Table 54). Treatable infectious causes are:

- herpes simplex or herpes zoster encephalitis, which is treated with aciclovir i.v. for 10 days
- mycoplasma meningoencephalitis, treated with i.v. clarithromycin or tetracycline
- primary infection with HIV, which should be treated with triple therapy (seek advice).

New drugs are in development for enteroviruses.

Prognosis

Encephalitis is an extremely unpredictable disease. Some patients are ill for only a few days and make a complete recovery. Most are unwell for 2–6 weeks and then make a slow recovery. Many never regain their full mental faculties and short- or long-term memory loss is common. In the UK, the mortality is low. Encephalitis is a notifiable disease.

Post-infective encephalomyelitis

Encephalitis may appear after a generalised viral infection (most commonly measles, varicella, influenza and mumps) has resolved. The onset is often abrupt with seizures and reduced consciousness or memory change, but the prognosis usually good.

Rabies

A 'rabies scare' following a dog bite among travellers in rabies-endemic areas is not rare (2% of all UK travellers to the 'tropics' or outside the developed nations); hence the need for you as a practising doctor to have some knowledge of the disease and immunisation.

Pathogenesis and clinical features

Rabies is an RNA virus that is transmitted to humans by an animal bite, almost always from a dog. The virus is present in the saliva of the animal. A break in the skin is necessary to transmit the virus. The virus then enters unmyelinated nerves and travels gradually up the axon until it reaches the spinal cord. It disseminates rapidly through the CNS causing an illness with characteristic stages, ending in death. The incubation period is very variable, from 2 weeks to 11 years. The earliest symptoms are pain or paraesthesia at the wound site together with malaise, fever and anorexia. CNS disease is manifest as intermittent hyperactivity, hallucinations, bizarre behaviour and convulsions. Later pharyngeal spasms occur on swallowing.

Management of a bite

Following a dog bite in a rabies-endemic country, three actions are appropriate if the skin was broken:

- washing the wound with soap and water for 5 minutes and leaving unsutured
- instillation of rabies immunoglobulin locally around the wound and systemically
- active immunisation (five injections over a month).

Immunoglobulin and vaccine should be administered within 48 hours if possible, but certainly within 5 days. If followed, this regimen has been 100% effective.

Prion disease

Prion diseases are associated with the accumulation in the brain of an abnormal partially protease-resistant isoform of a host-encoded glycoprotein called prion protein (PP). Human prion disease causes dementia and is known as Creutzfeldt–Jakob disease (CJD). It has been transmitted from human tissue to human via:

- corneal transplantation
- human growth hormone injections derived from pituitary glands collected from cadavers.

Fortunately there are only about 50 cases in the UK annually. Most occur in middle age and are sporadic. The incubation period is a mean of 12 years (range 4–40). In 1996 a new variant of CJD called vCJD was described in younger people. It is now proven to be caused by the same agent that causes bovine spongiform encephalopathy (BSE) in cattle. It has an incubation period exceeding 10 years. Only those humans and cattle homozygous for PP codon 129 polymorphism (valine to methionine change) are susceptible: 38% of the Caucasian population. Transmission occurs by consumption of contaminated food.

Clinical presentation

Memory loss, diminished intellect and poor judgement are typical presenting features of CJD. Florid psychiatric symptoms including visual and auditory hallucinations are common. Myoclonus and/or muscle fasciculation and wasting are typical but may not be present initially. Cerebellar forms also occur with ataxia and incoordination, followed later by dementia and myoclonus.

vCJD presents with behavioural change, often prompting psychiatric referral. Dysaesthesiae and ataxia are early features, whereas dementia and myoclonus are late.

Investigations

EEG is helpful late in CJD but not vCJD disease (Table 52). CT scanning and other imaging contributes little to the diagnosis, which is essentially clinical. vCJD can be diagnosed by tonsillar or appendix biopsy. Cerebral biopsy and/or postmortem is required for diagnosis of CJD. If biopsy is undertaken, all surgical instruments have to be discarded afterwards as there is no known way to 'sterilise' them.

Prognosis

All patients with CJD or vCJD die, usually over a period of 12–18 months in vCJD and with a more rapid decline in CJD.

Tetanus

Although only 5–15 cases of tetanus occur annually in the UK, hundreds of cases occur in most developing countries. Tetanus is almost completely preventable by immunisation, but as *Clostridium tetani* is a soil organism, all immunisation programmes will have to continue indefinitely.

Clinical presentation

The cardinal features of tetanus are:

- trismus: involuntary clenching of the jaw (100%)
- muscle spasms
- dysphagia.

Common presenting features include back pain and an infected wound.

Management

Management must be in an intensive care unit, with specific treatment including wound excision, metronidazole, antitetanus immunoglobulin intramuscularly and intrathecally and, in severe cases, tracheostomy and paralysis.

Prognosis

The mortality is about 10% in the UK but much higher abroad. Tetanus is a notifiable disease.

5.3 Tumours

Learning objectives

You should be able to:

- describe the natural history of tumours
- discuss how they are diagnosed
- state how the different pathological types influence natural history and diagnosis.

Five

Joe Gallagher has been increasingly vague and 'not quite right' for the last couple of months and he seems to be quite bemused by his wife's 'fussing'. When you examine him, he seems to be ignoring his left side and there is also a mild left-sided weakness, with increased reflexes. In his basic investigations, the only abnormality is 4 '+' of blood in his urine.

Rare tumours such as chordomas, dermoid tumours or haemangioblastomas are outside the scope of this book.

Epidemiology and clinical presentation

Cerebral tumours (40% are metastatic) account for approximately 10% of all tumours. Three modes of presentation predominate:

- focal neurological deficit as the tumour invades and compresses surrounding tissue
- focal epilepsy, which may become generalised from the outset
- signs of raised intracranial pressure: somnolence, headache, vomiting.

Headache on its own is a *very rare* presentation of a brain tumour.

Benign tumours

Meningioma

Meningiomas commonly arise in the parasagittal region around the falx, or over the cerebral hemispheres, the wing of the sphenoid bone or the olfactory groove. They are slow-growing tumours that often calcify and account for approximately 15% of all brain tumours with increasing incidence with age. They produce symptoms by imitating the cortex (epilepsy) and compressing the brain (producing focal or genalised symptoms) or the cranial nerves. The overlying bone may either erode or become hyperostotic. A CT scan shows a homogeneous, space-occupying lesion that densely enhances after contrast media. A similar appearance with enhancement is seen on MR scans. Surgical removal can be curative but is often difficult and the tumour may regrow and become locally invasive.

Cerebello–pontine angle tumour

Acoustic neuromas (**schwannomas**) arise from the eighth cranial nerve (vestibulo-cochlear). They slowly grow and may invade the surrounding tissue. As they enlarge, progressive deafness occurs as well as damage to the other nerves in the cerebello–pontine angle. Therefore, patients may have facial sensory loss (fifth nerve: particularly loss of corneal reflex) and facial weakness (seventh nerve: lower motor neurone), together with ipsilateral cerebellar signs. Eventually, hydrocephalus develops. Plain skull radiographs may show erosion of the internal auditory meatus, but an MR scan is the investigation of choice, showing a mass that enhances with contrast media. A CT scan is also useful, but bone may interfere with the image. If the tumour is not invasive, complete surgical removal is feasible.

Malignant tumours

Pathology

Primary tumours arise from glial cells (hence glioma) with most originating from astrocytes and oligodendrocytes. There is a spectrum of malignancy amongst astrocytomas (graded I–IV). Grade I is very slow-growing with patients surviving many years with little deficit as the brain has time to adapt and deform as the tumour increases in size. At the other extreme is **glioblastoma multiforme** (grade IV), which is rapidly growing; patients rarely survive more than 1 year. The tumour invades surrounding tissue and may cross the corpus callosum to the contralateral hemisphere. Gliomas rarely metastasise.

Brain metastases from distant tumours are common, particularly from bronchus, breast and kidney. In some patients, the location of the primary tumour remains unknown. Lymphomas may also affect the CNS, including the spinal cord. This is particularly common in AIDS (p. 388).

Clinical presentation

The most common presentation is an insidious progressive neurological deficit over weeks or months. Some patients present with fits (focal or generalised). Later symptoms and signs of raised intracranial pressure supervene with headache, vomiting and somnolence. When you see a person with a focal deficit such as a monoparesis, hemisensory loss or limb ataxia, your main differential diagnosis will be with a stroke. The main questions to ask are the length of the history and the onset. A stroke happens quickly, then, in most cases, there is some recovery. In tumour, the progression lends to be relentless. Occasionally, bleeding takes place into the tumour with a sudden deterioration in the neurological deficit. In these cases, clinical differentiation from a stroke is difficult, though a CT or an MR scan will clarify.

Investigations

Neuroimaging (either CT or MR with contrast) is the key to diagnosis. On plain scanning, an irregular, heterogeneous mass may be seen compressing the surrounding brain with a mass effect giving:

- effacement of cerebral sulci
- obliteration of the ipsilateral ventricle
- midline shift
- dilatation of the contralateral ventricle.

Slow-growing, grade I astrocytomas may show small areas of calcification. Rapidly growing tumours often have large areas of surrounding oedema, which appear on a CT scan as very low-density (black) regions. Irregular enhancement is seen after contrast. It may be very difficult to distinguish a solitary metastasis from a primary brain tumour, although metastases are often multiple.

Management

In malignant brain tumours, the treatment is predominantly palliative, including control of seizures. The overall prognosis has changed very little despite improvements in imaging, surgery, chemotherapy and radiotherapy. Almost all patients with glioblastoma multiforme are dead within 3 years. Surgical removal is usually not feasible. Lymphomas may temporarily respond to chemotherapy. For palliation of metastatic disease, radiotherapy may be of help. For all patients, you should consider referral to an oncologist or radiotherapist. A significant proportion of patients may obtain benefit lasting several weeks to months from high-dose dexamethasone, which reduces the surrounding oedema. Side-effects from the high steroid dose are common, particularly with myopathy, hyperglycaemia and hypokalaemia.

5.4 Cerebrovascular disease

Learning objectives

You should be able to:

- establish the diagnosis of stroke and describe the neurological impairment
- advise people on the prognosis for survival and disability in strokes
- assess risk factors for stroke
- put into practice the principles of rehabilitation, including working in a multidisciplinary team
- discuss the pathophysiology, presentation and management of subarachnoid haemorrhage.

Case Study

You are being given a hard time in the Medical Admissions Unit by Anne Wallis, who is 57 years old and a 'senior executive'. She has had a brief episode of left-sided clumsiness. On examination, you have found her pulse to be 70 beats/min irregular and blood pressure 188/78 mmHg. You now know that the CT scan was normal and carotid artery scan shows 60% stenosis on the right and 95% on the left. She is keen to go home.

Strokes are common and, as a house physician, you will be dealing with one or two new strokes per week.

Vascular anatomy and neuroanatomy

The brain is supplied by four arteries (two carotid and two vertebral). It is important to realise that, although these feed the circle of Willis, sudden occlusion of a major vessel *cannot* be compensated for by collateral flow because the circle is usually incompletely formed. If the reduction in blood flow takes place over several weeks or more, then there can be some compensation as the circle opens up.

The circulation should be considered in terms of the **carotid** (anterior) and the **vertebrobasilar** (posterior) circulation. The common carotid bifurcates into the external and internal carotid arteries. The bifurcation is one of the most common sites for atheroma. The main branches of the internal carotid artery (none outside the cranium) are:

- the **ophthalmic artery**, which is important because platelet emboli originating in the carotid bifurcation cause **amaurosis fugax** (Table 50)

- the **middle cerebral artery**, which supplies most of the parietal, temporal and some of the lateral surface of the frontal lobe; occlusion causes massive damage, i.e. hemiparesis (arm > leg), dysphasia (left hemisphere), neglect (right hemisphere) and hemianopia
- the **anterior cerebral artery**, which supplies the anterior pole of the frontal lobe and the medial surface; occlusion causes hemiparesis (leg > arm), dysphasia (left hemisphere), urinary incontinence and personality changes
- the **anterior communicating artery**, which joins the arteries on either side and is one of the sites for berry aneurysm (see Subarachnoid haemorrhage, p. 230).
- the **posterior communicating artery**, another major site for a berry aneurysm. Expansion of this can cause a painful third nerve palsy with a large pupil owing to compression of the parasympathetic fibres running on the outside of the nerve. Berry aneurysms cause approximately one-third of third nerve palsies (the other major cause being diabetes mellitus). The posterior communicating artery joins the posterior cerebral artery.

The vertebrobasilar system is formed by the two vertebral arteries (one may be rudimentary or absent) joining to form the basilar artery. The vertebrobasilar system supplies the brainstem and midbrain. After giving off several branches, including the **posterior inferior cerebellar artery** (PICA; see Lateral medullary syndrome, p. 227), it terminates in the posterior cerebral arteries, which supply the occipital lobes. These are predominantly concerned with vision. Unilateral damage causes a hemianopia, in which the macula may be spared (Table 50), and bilateral damage can result in cortical blindness.

Stroke

Stroke is the preferred term rather than cerebrovascular accident or CVA. You should take care in diagnosing and describing a stroke. In describing the stroke, you should refer to the side of the brain affected. Thus a left stroke would describe a left cerebral hemisphere infarct leading to a right hemiparesis and dysphasia. You will find it helpful to ask the patient (or a witness) the following questions.

How quickly did it happen? Sudden onset is classically seen in an embolic stroke, but thrombotic occlusion or haemorrhage may progress over a few hours. A longer time course (>24 hours) would be against the diagnosis of stroke.

Are there focal neurological symptoms or signs? Many strokes, but not transient ischaemic attacks (TIAs) (see below), lead to impaired consciousness, but lack of focal signs is against the diagnosis.

Have the symptoms persisted for longer than 24 hours? By definition *complete* recovery within 24 hours is diagnostic of a TIA and is not a stroke.

Epidemiology

Cerebrovascular disease is the third most common cause of death in the UK. It consumes approximately 6% of the NHS budget, mainly in long-term care/nursing costs.

The incidence rises exponentially with age. In an average health economy of 250 000, the incidence is 200–300 new strokes each year with a prevalence of 600–700 people disabled by stroke.

Pathology

Strokes can be divided into two main pathophysiological types: infarction and haemorrhage.

- **Infarction** is caused by sudden occlusion of an artery by either thrombosis or embolus from a distant source; damage to the neurones occurs as a result of ischaemia with subsequent disruption of function and death.
- **Haemorrhage** is caused by bleeding, often originating from penetrating vessels deep within the brain substance. Damage occurs as the blood tracks between neurones and fibres causing pressure and occlusion of supplying and draining vessels. Small aneurysms (**Charcot–Bouchard**) found with hypertension are associated with this bleeding. Another source is from vessels weakened by amyloid deposition, which is associated with age.

It is useful to know the relative frequencies of the different pathologies. In every 100 strokes, approximately 80 will be caused by infarction secondary to thromboembolism. It is now thought that an embolus is more important than thrombosis in situ, because atheroma is relatively uncommon in the intracerebral vessels. The common sources of emboli are shown in Figure 54.

Clinical presentation

A stroke can affect any part of the brain and may be very small or very large. There is a huge number of possible permutations of symptoms and signs. You do not need to know all of these; what you must be able to do is assess a patient and document accurately the neurological impairment at the time you see them. The picture will change over time.

Strokes may be silent: that is, no symptoms were noticed, yet on a CT or MR scan there is evidence of old damage. In these patients, questioning may elicit an 'odd' episode.

Once you have diagnosed that the patient has had a stroke, the next question is, what is the nature of the stroke? As stated above, infarction is the commonest pathology. It is *not* possible to differentiate reliably at the bedside between haemorrhage and infarction; a CT or MR scan is needed.

The third stage is to decide on the site and extent of the stroke. Many patients present with a hemiparesis, but remember that the path of the pyramidal tract starts in the precentral gyrus then runs down through the cerebral peduncles and the midbrain, before decussating low down in the brainstem. Consequently, unilateral weakness tells you very little about the site of the stroke and you need to ask about other symptoms and seek out other signs. The main divisions in stroke are between:

- cerebral hemisphere
- lacunar
- brainstem.

The location of major functions is shown in Figure 55. Dysphasia, dyspraxia and neglect have been described and can be used to locate the site of a stroke.

Anterior circulation (carotid) ischaemia

It is useful to think of these locations as either **total anterior circulation infarcts** (TACI) or **partial anterior circulation infarcts** (PACI).

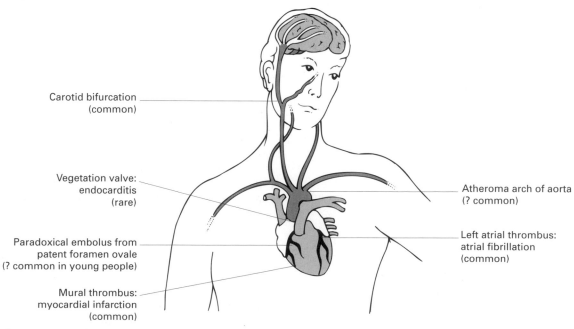

Carotid bifurcation (common)

Vegetation valve: endocarditis (rare)

Paradoxical embolus from patent foramen ovale (? common in young people)

Mural thrombus: myocardial infarction (common)

Atheroma arch of aorta (? common)

Left atrial thrombus: atrial fibrillation (common)

Fig. 54 Possible sources of emboli to the brain.

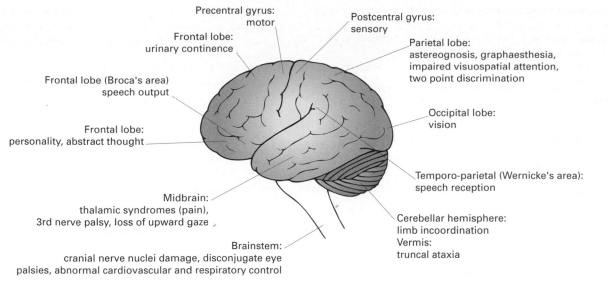

Precentral gyrus:
motor

Frontal lobe:
urinary continence

Frontal lobe (Broca's area)
speech output

Frontal lobe:
personality, abstract thought

Postcentral gyrus:
sensory

Parietal lobe:
astereognosis, graphaesthesia,
impaired visuospatial attention,
two point discrimination

Occipital lobe:
vision

Temporo-parietal (Wernicke's area):
speech reception

Midbrain:
thalamic syndromes (pain),
3rd nerve palsy, loss of upward gaze

Brainstem:
cranial nerve nuclei damage, disconjugate eye
palsies, abnormal cardiovascular and respiratory control

Cerebellar hemisphere:
limb incoordination
Vermis:
truncal ataxia

Fig. 55 Anatomical localisation of important brain functions.

TACI. A TACI is a huge stroke caused by occlusion of either the internal carotid or the middle cerebral artery on one side. Virtually all of one hemisphere is damaged, so the complete picture can comprise:

- drowsiness/unconsciousness
- complete hemiparesis
- hemisensory loss
- dysphasia (left) or neglect (right > left)
- incontinence
- hemianopia and forced deviation of the eyes towards the side of the stroke.

In summary, this stroke causes gross brain damage and has a poor prospect for survival or good recovery.

PACI A PACI is a smaller event, with a wedge-shaped infarct caused by blockage of one of the small arteries supplying the cerebral hemispheres. The symptoms and signs will vary according to where the lesion is, but there may simply be, for example, an expressive dysphasia. Patients have a good probability of recovery, but have a significant risk of a further stroke.

Lacunar strokes (LACI) These are small discrete infarcts (occlusion of small penetrating arteries) around the internal capsule, thalamus and basal ganglia. They are often multiple. Patients present with one of the following:

- isolated hemiparesis
- pure hemisensory loss
- hemiparesis with limb ataxia (clumsy).

Prognosis for survival and recovery is very good. There is a strong association with hypertension.

Posterior circulation (vertebrobasilar) infarction (POCI) Patients present with symptoms and signs of brainstem damage. Features include:

- severe truncal ataxia (midline vermis lesion)
- limb clumsiness (signs ipsilateral to cerebellar hemisphere damage)
- gaze palsies

— *conjugate* (involuntary, '*forced*', parallel deviation of the eyes away from the site of the stroke)
— *disconjugate* (where the eyes do not act together)
- respiratory rhythm disturbance
- hemiparesis (contralateral).

Mortality is high because of damage to vital centres, but, if the patient survives, prospects for functional recovery are good with a low probability of recurrence.

Lateral medullary syndrome This is caused by an infarction in the territory of the posterior inferior cerebellar artery. Classical symptoms are ipsilateral facial paraesthesia or pain (spinal nucleus of fifth nerve), severe vertigo and vomiting, dysphagia, dysphonia, ataxia and contralateral limb sensory impairment. On examination, a Horner's syndrome may be present, with ipsilateral facial loss of pain and temperature and contralateral limb spinothalamic sensory impairment. However, in many cases the symptoms and signs vary.

Investigations

In accident and emergency, one of the main decisions is choosing the investigations that will make a difference to the immediate management. These vary according to the presentation and your assessment of the patient. Table 55 summarises the important ones to consider both as urgent and non-urgent tests. In general, patients who are very unlikely to survive (e.g. deeply unconscious: Glasgow Coma Scale 3, see Table 54) should not be subjected to investigations.

Prognosis

It is important that you are aware of the prognosis following a stroke in terms of survival, recovery and risks of further events, so that you can advise patients and carers appropriately. Up to half of all patients who are admitted will die in hospital. Early deaths result from compression/ damage to major structures: for example, the respiratory

Table 55 Main investigations in stroke, with indications for urgency

Investigation	When to perform	Reason
Blood sugar (BM stix)	All patients, on admission	Hypoglycaemia can cause focal signs; missing it can cause irreversible damage
Chest radiograph	Some patients, on admission	Semi-conscious, may have or be at risk of aspiration pneumonia
	All patients, non-urgent	To exclude neoplasia
Full blood count	All patients, non-urgent	To exclude erythrocytosis, thrombocythaemia
Urea and electrolytes	Some patients, on admission	May have or be at serious risk of water depletion; if electrolyte disturbance suspected
	All patients, non-urgent	To exclude renal impairment and to help to manage fluids
CT or MR brain scan	Some patients, on admission	1. Those on anticoagulants 2. Suspected **cerebellar haematoma**: only indication for surgical intervention 3. Suspicion of abscess, meningitis or subarachnoid haemorrhage
	Most patients, within 7 days	1. Considering anticoagulants, aspirin 2. Still uncertain of diagnosis 3. Determine nature of stroke
Erythrocyte sedimentation rate (ESR)	On admission Non-urgent	If temporal arteritis suspected To exclude vasculitis
ECG	Some patients, on admission, All patients, non-urgent	If recent myocardial infarction suspected For rhythm (particularly atrial fibrillation) left ventricular hypertrophy (LVH), old infarction
Duplex colour flow Doppler studies of carotid artery	Within 7 days unless severe stroke	Candidate for carotid endarterectomy
Echocardiography	Non-urgent	Suspicion of a cardiac source of emboli (e.g. valve lesions, replacements)
Venous to arterial circulation shunt test (VACS)	Non-urgent	Young patient – possible paradoxical embolus
Other tests: e.g. blood culture	Some patients, on admission	If septicaemia/meningitis/endocarditis suspected
Other tests: cholesterol, *Treponema pallidum* haemagglutination (TPHA), rheumatoid factor (RF), antinuclear factor (ANF), etc.	Some patients, non-urgent	1. Young, strong family history of vascular disease 2. Suspected neurosyphilis 3. Suspected vasculitis

centre in the brainstem. Subsequent brain swelling leads to further deterioration, with coning of the hemispheres into the posterior fossa and the brainstem through the foramen magnum. Unlike in myocardial infarction, those stroke patients who die do so within a few days rather than the first few minutes.

Deaths in the next few weeks are often caused by pulmonary emboli or pneumonia. Late deaths are commonly caused by further stroke or myocardial ischaemia.

On admission, the single most unfavourable prognostic sign is a reduced conscious level. If the patient has a Glasgow Coma Scale of 3 (Table 54), then the chances of survival and good recovery are very slim. Other bad prognostic signs are complete hemiparesis, urinary incontinence and forced deviation of the eyes.

Of the 50–70% who survive, half will make a very good recovery. The remainder will be left with significant disability and handicap. In relation to stroke type:

- TACI: poor prognosis (survival or disability)
- PACI: recover well, but have a high chance of early recurrence
- LACI: do reasonably well but have a risk of recurrence
- POCI: high mortality but may do well if they survive.

Management

The management of stroke patients can be divided into early and late phases.

Early stages

In the immediate aftermath of a stroke thrombolysis will improve outcome if given *within 3 hours of onset* of symptoms in an ischaemic stroke. Using tissue plasminogen activator, the number needed to treat (NNT) for one patient to have a good outcome is 8 and only 3 for an improved outcome. However, these benefits reduce if treated between 3 and 6 hours following onset of stroke and disappear beyond this time frame. The challenge (which is greater than with myocardial infarction) is to improve the system (and public education) so that a patient who is likely to benefit is transported, admitted, assessed, scanned and thrombolysed within 3 hours of onset of symptoms.

Apart from this specific treatment, overall management is directed at preventing complications. Patients are at risk of deep vein thrombosis and pulmonary emboli. Low molecular weight heparin therapy may be needed, but care should be taken beforehand to exclude haemorrhage as a cause of the stroke. Pyrexia should be managed by exclusion of infection, paracetamol and fans. Pressure sores may develop, unless the patient is assessed as being at risk and correctly nursed.

High blood pressure may be noted in the first few hours following a stroke. This should not be treated unless **hypertensive encephalopathy** is diagnosed (very rare; p. 46). Otherwise lowering blood pressure is more likely to do harm as **autoregulation** of cerebral blood flow is lost.

In an insulin-dependent diabetic patient, any major event may precipitate ketoacidosis. Hyperglyaemia in any patient is risk factor for a poor outcome. This should be managed in the standard way, avoiding hypoglycaemia.

All stroke patients must be screened for dysphagia before being given anything orally. The screening should include:

- conscious level
- postural control (it is almost impossible to swallow lying down)
- control of oral secretions (cough, 'wet' voice)
- simple water test — coughing on small amounts of fluid
- measurement of nutritional status (e.g. body mass index).

Where doubt exists, a modified barium swallow or fibreoptic endoscopic evaluation (FEES) is useful for assessing dysphagia. If patients cannot meet their fluid requirements, intravenous or subcutaneous fluids should be started. Modified diet (e.g. thickened fluids) and attention to posture may help to overcome dysphagia. If patients are unable to swallow, a nasogastric tube should be inserted early to provide nutrition. Longer-term, nutrition may be supplied using a percutaneous endoscopic gastrostomy.

Late stages

The late management of stroke is based on active rehabilitation and reducing the risk of further events. Of the survivors, approximately one-quarter will make a rapid recovery and one-quarter will make a very poor recovery requiring long-term care. The remainder (half) benefit from admission to a specialist stroke rehabilitation service. This is associated with:

- lower death rate
- shorter hospital stay
- less disability on discharge
- greater chance of going home.

Overall, for every 12 patients treated in a dedicated stroke unit, one will benefit.

Most recovery will take place in the first few months; by about 6 months the patient may have *plateaued*. Patients with significant *right* (non-dominant) hemisphere damage tend to have a worse prognosis. However, most patients will walk again, possibly using aids, though many of these will be severely restricted (disability and handicap). Recovery of hand function is often poor, particularly if there is no movement at all by 7 days. Speech can go on improving for more than a year.

Prevention

Prevention of strokes is very important, both for the individual and for society. Since the early 20th century, the incidence of both cerebral haemorrhage and infarction has been declining. This *predated* any medical advances — for example, antihypertensives — but the continuing decline *may* be influenced by medical intervention.

For the decline in stroke incidence to continue, the major factors causing stroke need to be known, together with any means whereby these can be altered. Schemes can be implemented to reduce stroke by targeting either the *whole population* or *individuals*. The approach can be further refined by aiming at **primary** prevention for the person who has had no previous vascular episodes (including TIAs) and **secondary** prevention for the person who has had an event.

A key concept in prevention is the *risk* of something happening. This can be divided into:

- **absolute** risk: applies to an individual without any external reference, e.g. a 70-year-old man has a 12% absolute stroke risk over 10 years (1 in 8 chance)
- **relative** risk: refers to the chances of an event occurring relative to something else, e.g. in a woman taking the oral contraceptive pill, the *relative* risk of stroke is increased several fold, but the *absolute* risk remains extremely small in young women.

For primary prevention, in any patient, vascular risk factors should be treated if the absolute risk is >30% over 10 years. It is assumed to be greater than this for secondary prevention.

In relation to stroke and specific treatments:

- If a person has a TIA or stroke, the absolute risk of a future stroke is approximately 13% in the first 3 months then 5–10% per annum.
- A person following a stroke also has an *absolute* risk of 8%/year of having a myocardial infarction; this is the most common cause of death.
- The biggest risk factor is hypertension; this accounts for at least half of all strokes. The ideal blood pressure is <140/85 mmHg (<130/80 in diabetic patients). Treatment is usually as a combination to achieve best control (e.g. an ACE inhibitor such as perindopril and a calcium antagonist such as amlodipine).
- Carotid disease is an important risk factor (emboli); if a patient has had a TIA and has >70% stenosis on the relevant side, then a carotid endarterectomy can be

Five

beneficial (*secondary* prevention). There is limited evidence for operating on asymptomatic patients.

- Aspirin (75 mg) is beneficial in *secondary* prevention; it reduces the risk of a stroke by 30% and vascular death by 15% (*relative* reduction). In a recent stroke, aspirin should be combined with dipyridamole. If a patient is intolerant of aspirin, clopidogrel can be used.
- In a person with atrial fibrillation, particularly with valvular heart disease, *anticoagulation* will reduce the relative risk of a stroke by two-thirds (the change in absolute risk, if the person had a stroke/TIA, is from 12%/year to 4%/year).
- Treating elderly hypertensive people, because of their high *absolute* risk, is more beneficial than in younger people (more strokes prevented).
- Hormone replacement therapy is associated with a relative increase in risk of 30%.
- Cholesterol-lowering with a statin is associated with a 21% relative reduction in risk (but you have to treat 156 patients for 1 year to prevent 1 stroke). Guidelines suggest reducing total cholesterol to less than 5 mmol/l (though some advocate treatment regardless of level).
- Smoking reduces life expectancy by an average of 10 years (65% of life-long non-smokers (male doctors) were alive at age 80 years compared with 32% of life-long smokers).

Subarachnoid haemorrhage

The pathophysiology and presentation of subarachnoid haemorrhage (SAH) are different to those of stroke. Most SAHs are caused by bleeding from **berry aneurysms** around the circle of Willis. These classically occur at the bifurcations, commonly at the origins of the middle cerebral, anterior cerebral and the anterior and posterior communicating arteries. SAH occurs in young people, but the risk increases with age. There is also an association with polycystic kidneys. There is a small familial risk but no evidence for benefit of screening first-degree relatives. Most aneurysms are in the anterior circulation (75%) and a small proportion are multiple (20%). A minority of SAH (10%) is caused by bleeding from an arterio-venous malformation. In some patients (10%) a site is never identified.

Clinical presentation

The classical presentation of SAH is with a severe headache. The person may say that they thought that 'someone had hit them on the head with a hammer'. They may remember a severe headache a few days/ weeks earlier (**herald bleed**) but the frequency of this has been over-emphasised in the past. There is a very high risk (20–40%) of rebleeding within the first 3 weeks. If bleeding extends into the brain, there may be focal signs, rapid loss of consciousness and death. An aneurysm on the posterior communicating artery may cause a third nerve palsy. Blood in the CSF causes meningeal irritation (neck stiffness, headache, photophobia). Another problem is vascular spasm, which particularly affects the artery where the aneurysm

is situated. Large bleeds promote spasm, which, in turn, may cause widespread brain infarction. Occasionally, aneurysms present through a mass effect causing compression of adjacent tissues (e.g. third nerve palsy).

Investigations

Because of the high mortality and risk of rebleeding, it is vital that the diagnosis is established early and a referral made to a neurosurgical centre. The investigation of choice is a CT scan to demonstrate the blood within the subarachnoid space (sensitivity >90% in the first 24 hours). MR scanning is not of sufficient sensitivity. If the scan is negative (10% of SAHs) and there is no evidence of raised intracranial pressure, a lumbar puncture should be done. Blood-stained fluid will be obtained and, after 24 hours, xanthochromia (almost 100% sensitivity) develops because of breakdown of haemoglobin, which persists for 1–2 weeks. For patients in whom surgery would be considered (<65 years, not deeply unconscious), angiography should be performed. Due to the high levels of catecholamines, ECG abnormalities are often present (myocardial ischaemia/infarction).

Management

The initial management is stabilisation and support of the circulation and ventilation. Very high blood pressure and raised intracranial pressure are treated. All patients should be given **nimodipine** (a calcium antagonist) to reduce the risk of spasm, which is greatest in young patients with large bleeds. In those patients fit enough, early surgery to clip accessible aneuryms is advised, given the high risk of early rebleeding. Other endovascular techniques are now available (e.g. coils). In a patient who deteriorates, you should consider rebleeding, spasm or hydrocephalus. A CT scan can help to distinguish between these.

Prognosis

The mortality from SAH is high, with as many as a third of patients dying within a few hours and a further third dying in the first month.

Arterio-venous malformations

Bleeding is often less pronounced in arterio-venous malformations, compared with berry aneurysms, with episodes over a number of years producing mild neurological deficits. Epilepsy is common (50% of presentations). An enhanced CT scan may be abnormal and an MR scan may be diagnostic, though the definitive investigation is angiography. Surgery or embolisation of feeding vessels is sometimes undertaken but may be technically difficult with a high risk.

Subdural haematoma

Acute extradural (arterial) and subdural (venous) bleeds usually occur as a result of trauma. Chronic subdural haematoma is mainly a problem of elderly people and alcoholics. In the history, there may be a story of a minor head injury. The patient presents with a fluctuating level of consciousness with or without focal signs (e.g. hemiparesis) over several weeks/months. The condition is caused by oozing from damaged subdural veins. Osmotic changes in the haematoma cause it to expand and contract. A CT scan will usually show a characteristic abnormality of a localised rim of hypodensity between the brain and the skull (sometimes bilateral). The patient should be referred to a neurosurgical unit.

5.5 Degenerative conditions

Learning objectives

You should be able to:
- construct a framework for describing degenerative conditions of the nervous system
- set out the differences between Parkinson's disease and parkinsonism
- describe the features of Parkinson's disease
- set out the principles of its management
- discuss the features of Alzheimer's and multi-infarct dementia and understand how these conditions differ
- set out the principles of the management of dementia and the value of multidisciplinary teamwork
- describe the features of motor neurone disease
- state how you would exclude other (potentially treatable) causes of the patient's problem.

Case Study

Simon Leahy has been deteriorating for several months. His son says that Simon has not been the same since the death of his wife a year ago. Socially, he has become withdrawn and has stopped playing bridge because of difficulty with scoring. Recently bills have been left unpaid, but some have been paid twice. His son says that his father has become much more forgetful, such as not remembering the names of his grandchildren. There has been a recent argument because he keeps phoning his son but cannot remember doing so.

The central and peripheral nervous system is affected by many different degenerative conditions. You will find it useful to divide them into inherited and acquired conditions.

Inherited conditions

Spinocerebellar ataxias

The spinocerebellar ataxias are a complex set of disorders. They range from very rare pure cerebellar disorders seen in childhood through spinocerebellar disorders to hereditary **spastic paraparesis** (autosomal dominant) affecting the corticospinal tracts, which usually is diagnosed in middle age.

Friedreich's ataxia

The typical spinocerebellar disorder is Friedreich's ataxia, which is inherited as an autosomal recessive with the gene located on chromosome 9 (unstable repeat expansion gene). In this disorder, three CNS systems are affected:

- cerebellum
- spinocerebellar tracts
- corticospinal tracts.

In addition, all patients have degeneration in the cells of the dorsal root ganglia, resulting in loss of joint position sense (posterior columns) and a sensory neuropathy. In the late stages, the neuropathy is sensorimotor.

Patients usually present in late childhood/early adulthood with an ataxic syndrome, nystagmus, dysarthria, spastic paraparesis and extensor plantars with *absent* reflexes. Other features include a cardiomyopathy (and conduction problems), diabetes mellitus and low intelligence. Life expectancy is reduced, with death from cardiac failure/dysrhythmias around the fourth decade. **Formes frustes** are seen, that is affected family members may be only slightly affected, e.g. 'funny' walks or being bad at games.

No specific treatment is available. Management is supportive.

Huntington's disease

Huntington's disease is a rare autosomally dominant inherited condition. It typically presents in the fifth or sixth decade of life with a progressive basal ganglia movement disorder (chorea, parkinsonism) and dementia. There are no specific abnormalities on imaging. Specialist counselling services are available and, as with most inherited conditions, genetic testing looking for the abnormal CAG repeat sequence on chromosome 4 is now available. Because of the late onset, counselling is complicated, given the implications of being positive for a progressive, untreatable condition (which usually occurs after the age that people have children).

Wilson's disease

Wilson's disease arises as a disorder of copper metabolism inherited as an autosomal recessive syndrome (p. 146). Heterozygotes have no clinical features. In the CNS, copper deposition in the basal ganglia and elsewhere causes dyskinesias (chorea, athetosis) and parkinsonism together with a progressive dementia. In the eye, copper deposition at the margin of the cornea causes a **Kayser–Fleischer** ring, which is best seen on slit lamp examination. Onset is often insidious. The condition needs to be diagnosed early and treated with copper chelators for any chance of remission.

Benign essential tremor

Benign essential tremor is one of the commonest movement disorders and is seen either as a sporadic disorder or running in families (50% of cases) with an autosomal dominant inheritance. It may present at any time in adult life and worsens over the years. It is a positional tremor, often mild and worsened by emotion. The quality of life of affected patients is often significantly affected (employment socialising). CT and MR scans are normal. The tremor is helped by alcohol and responds to **propranolol**.

Five

Acquired degenerative disorders

Parkinson's disease

Aetiology

The most important concept you need to grasp is that **Parkinson's disease** refers to degeneration of the neurones of the substantia nigra of unknown aetiology that causes progressive akinesia, rigidity and a tremor, whereas **parkinsonism** refers to the same symptoms and signs but occurring secondary to some other condition. The most common causes of parkinsonism are antidopaminergic drugs (metoclopramide, neuroleptics) and cerebrovascular disease (see Vascular dementia, p. 234). Other rare causes include carbon monoxide poisoning, exposure to a 'designer' drug (MPTP) and, with other signs, Huntington's disease and Wilson's disease.

Epidemiology and pathophysiology

The prevalence of Parkinson's disease increases with age, affecting around 1 in 200 people over the age of 65 years. The aetiology is not clear but may involve exposure to some environmental toxin. The symptoms start to appear after the loss of at least 80% of the neurones of the substantia nigra, which show depigmentation. These dopaminergic neurones project to the basal ganglia where other neurotransmitter abnormalities and receptor changes are found. Microscopically, **Lewy bodies** are found in the residual nigral neurones. If Lewy bodies are found more widely in the cerebral hemispheres, cognitive impairment (dementia) may be significant (see below). There are no specific features on CT or MR scans.

Clinical presentation

You need to look for the following:

- tremor
- bradykinesia
- rigidity (cogwheel/lead pipe)
- flexed posture
- postural instability.

Symptoms commonly start in the sixth decade of life, but there is a wide variation. Even with treatment, the life expectancy is reduced, with the disease taking approximately 10 years to run its course. The symptoms and signs are often asymmetrical. You will find that diagnosing Parkinson's disease in the early stages is difficult. The symptoms are vague and signs minimal.

Tremor Initially, the patient may complain only of *tremor*. This is coarse (4–6 Hz) and starts in the thumb and fingers (often one side initially and remains asymmetric); as the disease progresses it may worsen to affect the hand, arm and trunk. It disappears at rest (e.g. while watching television) and is made worse by holding a posture and by anxiety.

Bradykinesia and rigidity Reduction in movement may be noticed by people close to the patient. Gradually, there is a slowness and difficulty in initiating and changing any voluntary movement. Accompanying the bradykinesia is an increase in tone. This rigidity is present throughout passive movement of a limb and is described as **lead pipe** (cf. the 'clasp knife' increase in tone seen in

pyramidal tract disorders). The superimposition of the tremor on the hypertonia leads to **cogwheel rigidity**.

Posture Observing the patient you will notice a **flexed posture** with a shuffling gait (**festinant**) and loss of arm swing. Falls are frequent because of loss of postural control. Other features are loss of facial expression, dysphagia and dribbling of saliva. The voice is reduced in amplitude (**dysphonia**) with little intonation and a tendency to peter out. As the disease progresses, the dopamine transmission starts to become inconsistent, with sudden freezing of movement (**on-off phenomena**), and gross difficulty in starting movement and stopping walking.

Other symptoms Parkinson's disease is also associated with marked cognitive slowness and impairment. In some patients, Lewy bodies, which are usually confined to damaged neurones in the substantia nigra, are found much more widely in the cerebral cortex (**Lewy body dementia**, see below). Alzheimer's disease is also more common in patients with Parkinson's disease.

Overall management

Your role in the management of Parkinson's disease involves much more than simply prescribing drugs. One important aspect is counselling patients and their families/carers about the effects of a progressive neurological condition leading to a premature death. You must recognise that anxiety and depression go with this but may be amenable to therapy. Other disciplines may help: physiotherapists with mobility, occupational therapists with activities of daily living, speech and language therapists with communication and swallowing, and social workers with financial worries and social support.

Drug treatment

The main defect is failing dopamine transmission in the basal ganglia. Therapy is aimed at preserving transmission for as long as possible. Dopamine cannot cross the blood–brain barrier so the precursor **L-dopa** is used, which is then converted to dopamine within the substantia nigra. An alternative approach is to use a direct dopamine agonist like ropinirole. In general, agonists are often used rather than dopamine replacement therapy in the early stages of the disease, particularly in younger patient, because this may delay the onset of some of the more troublesome late phenomena (see below).

For many years, prior to the introduction of L-dopa, anticholinergic drugs such as **benzatropine** were used. Their main action is on tremor rather than bradykinesia and rigidity. They are often used in patients with parkinsonism secondary to neuroleptic drugs, in whom dopamine receptor stimulation must be avoided to prevent exacerbating the mental disturbance.

The main aims of currently available therapy are:

- to preserve independence for as long as possible
- to achieve smooth duration of effect
- to create minimum side-effects.

Achievement of these is dependent on tailoring therapy to individual patients and involving them in decision-making. As the disease progresses, a combination of treatments is often employed, but, as in epilepsy, therapy should be kept simple.

Table 56 Major drugs used in Parkinson's disease, mode of action and side-effects

Drug	Action	Side-effects	Notes
L-Dopa	Dopamine replacement	Postural hypotension, nausea, confusion. High doses: chorea (peak dose effect)	Need a peripheral decarboxylase inhibitor: prevents peripheral breakdown. Short half-life: give frequent doses (over four times a day). Slow-release preparations available
Ropinirole, pramipexole, pergolide	Dopamine agonist	Nausea, postural hypotension, confusion, psychosis	Use first in younger patients
Apomorphine	Dopamine agonist	Nausea, postural hypotension	High efficacy, used in end-stage disease; has to be given subcutaneously
Selegiline	Monoamine oxidase type B inhibitor		Give once a day; well tolerated; mild antiparkinsonian and mood-uplifting effect; need to reduce L-dopa dosage (blocks metabolism); minor place in treatment
Entacapone	COMT inhibitor		Blocks breakdown of levodopa – patients need to be on L-dopa (more available for transport across blood–brain barrier)
Benzatropine	Cholinergic antagonist	Blurred vision, urinary retention, dry mouth, confusion	Main effect is on tremor; not very effective

COMT, catechol-O-methyl transferase.

Various phenomena may be observed with disease progression:

- *Peak dose effect*: choreiform movements are observed approximately 30 minutes after taking L-dopa and result from excessive stimulation of dopamine receptors.
- *On-off phenomena* are caused by fluctuations in dopamine concentrations within the basal ganglia.
- *End of dose effect* is because of the effect of L-dopa wearing off prior to the next dose being taken.

The main approach to limiting these effects is to employ small frequent doses of L-dopa; this reduces the peaks and troughs found with larger, less frequent doses. The different modes of action of the drugs used and the common side-effects are summarised in Table 56.

Dementias

Dementia is a chronic failure of cognitive function. It must be differentiated from an acute or subacute confusional state (delirium), though it predisposes to the development of these.

Epidemiology

The prevalence of dementia increases rapidly with advancing age; 20% of those aged 85 years have at least a mild form; 5% are severely affected. The majority of these result from Alzheimer's disease. This is predominantly seen in old people, but it can occur before the age of 65 years.

The other major cause of dementia is cerebrovascular disease, but this is less common than Alzheimer's disease. The prevalence of vascular dementia increases exponentially with age and is related to the known risk factors for vascular disease, such as hypertension.

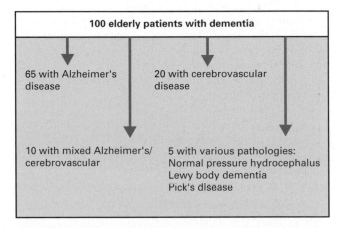

Fig. 56 The prevalence of dementia from different pathological causes. Lewy body dementia may account for some cases of apparent Alzheimer's disease and may be a more important cause than indicated here.

In clinical practice, you will find it useful to keep in mind the relative frequencies of the different causes of dementia (Fig. 56).

Alzheimer's disease
Pathophysiology

The histological hallmarks of Alzheimer's disease are **neuronal plaques** and **neurofibrillary tangles**, with widespread cortical loss of neurones. Some of these features are found in the brains of elderly people without dementia, but not to the same extent.

Within the cortex and the subcortical connections/projections, there are abnormalities in most transmitter systems, but a deficit in acetylcholine transmission is most closely linked to clinical features. Genetic factors are important; the dementia is inherited as an autosomal dominant in a small number of families but more than 90% of cases are sporadic and onset is >60 years. Furthermore, patients with Down's syndrome have a very similar dementia, but it develops much earlier. Most research is now focused on lipoprotein E-epsilon 4 genotype, abnormal expression of β-amyloid protein and microvascular changes.

Clinical presentation

Typically, patients present with an insidious decline in memory and other cognitive functions. There is increasing disruption of cortical function with fragmentation of language, disorientation in time, difficulty with intellectual tasks such as money matters, personality changes including disinhibition, and wandering. The memory loss is marked with failure to retain or recall important information. Over a period of months and years, cortical function becomes progressively disrupted until the patient is aphasic, incontinent (in the early stages urination/defaecation may occur inappropriately because of disinhibition) and immobile, and fails to recognise even close relatives. Weight loss can be marked.

Diagnosis

When faced with a patient with possible Alzheimer's disease you must understand two things.

- *There is no diagnostic test.* A CT or MR scan may show 'cerebral atrophy', but it does so in many normal elderly people. The diagnosis is based mainly on the clinical history outlined above with use of psychological tests in some patients. There are no focal neurological signs.
- *It is difficult to differentiate between Alzheimer's disease and vascular dementia.* Important features to look for in the latter are hypertension, previous strokes (or CT scan evidence), stepwise deterioration with some improvement/plateau after each event and focal neurological signs.

A mini-mental state examination (MMSE) is a useful adjunct to clinical assessment. It is scored out of 30, and a score of <20 is a strong indicator of cognitive impairment.

Management

Palliative treatments for Alzheimer's disease are starting to appear. Some anticholinesterases such as donepezil produce an improvement in cortical function by improving the deficit in acetylcholine transmission in patients with mild-to-moderate disease. Memantine (an N-methyl-D-aspartate (NMDA) antagonist) may also give some benefit. However, managing patients involves much more than offering specific treatment. The key is working as part of a multidisciplinary team looking at all aspects of support, including that of the carer. Many house officers find it difficult to find their own role within this team. Your main responsibilities are:

- The diagnosis and management of any medical problems: acute illness (e.g. infection, myocardial infarction) and its treatment can cause an **acute on chronic confusional state**. Diagnosis of an acute

illness may be difficult because of the lack of a clear history from a demented patient, but correct and prompt treatment may make a large difference in functional outcome.

- The judicious use of drugs such as the atypical antipsychotics (e.g. alanzapine, quetiapine) in patients who are very agitated, aggressive or have a gross disturbance of sleep pattern.
- Being aware that depression (particularly in the early stages) is common and can be treated.
- Adopting a behavioural approach to management: caring for patients in a familiar environment with familiar people using a consistent approach.
- Coordinating the plans of the different agencies involved after an acute illness so as to ensure smooth discharge.
- Making time available for talking with the carers.

Prognosis

Alzheimer's disease can progress at different rates, usually with death after several years.

Vascular dementia

Pathophysiology

The mechanisms involved in vascular dementia are different to those of Alzheimer's disease. It can be conceptualised as the summative effects of lots of small strokes causing a stepwise deterioration in overall brain function. Occasionally, though, a single stroke in the deep structures around the basal ganglia can cause a permanent confusional state. In other patients, chronic ischaemia damages the white matter (axonal connections) at the junction with the cerebral hemispheres (**Biswanger's disease**).

Clinical presentation

Typically, the patient will have a history of several strokes: some minor and some major. The progression is in steps, with acute deterioration caused by the stroke being followed by a period of partial recovery and a new (lower) functional plateau. There is commonly a history of hypertension or other vascular risk factors such as atrial fibrillation or diabetes.

On examination, as well as impaired cognition, there will be focal signs: for example, brisk reflexes and an upgoing plantar response.

Investigations

The investigation of vascular dementia is similar to that of stroke (Table 55). A CT or MR scan may show multiple areas of infarction. An ECG may confirm the presence of atrial fibrillation.

Management

The general management of vascular dementia is the same as that for Alzheimer's disease. Although there is no firm evidence that it influences the course of the disease, the consensus is that the known vascular risk factors should be treated and the patient prescribed aspirin.

Lewy body dementia

Lewy body dementia is being increasingly recognised as an important cause of chronic cognitive impairment. It was first described in relation to Parkinson's disease, but in some patients, the dementia is the dominant early feature. The characteristics of Lewy body dementia are:

- progressive dementia
- marked fluctuations in cognitive function, including excessive drowsiness and reduced alertness
- visual hallucinations
- parkinsonian motor symptoms and signs
- marked sensitivity to neuroleptic drugs (e.g. haloperidol). These can cause severe Parkinson-like side-effects, including rigidity, immobility and being unable to communicate.

Currently, there is no specific licensed treatment.

Motor neurone disease

Epidemiology

Motor neurone disease (amyotrophic lateral sclerosis) affects males much more than females and commonly presents in middle age, but it occurs over a wide age range. In a small number of cases, the condition is familial.

Clinical presentation

The diagnosis should be considered in any patient with progressive motor symptoms and signs. An important aspect is to exclude other, potentially treatable problems, such as cervical spondylosis. *Any* sensory signs rule out the diagnosis of motor neurone disease.

The disease affects both upper and lower (anterior horn cells) motor neurones, so the symptoms and signs depend on the relative involvement of different neuronal groups. Segments C8 and T1 may be affected with weakness, wasting and fasciculation of the small muscles of the hand (particularly 1st dorsal interossei). Another pattern is involvement of the pyramidal tract neurones innervating the lower limbs, causing weakness, spasticity and hyper-reflexia. As the disease progesses, a mixture of signs are seen, e.g. arreflexia in the lower limb with extensor plantar responses. Impact on the bulbar musculature is frequently severe, with dysphagia, aspiration and dysarthria. The oculomotor neurones are usually spared, as are those controlling bladder and bowel function.

Investigations

Diagnosis is clinical, supported by electrophysiological studies. EMG will show a subacute denervation pattern with fibrillation, large motor unit and polyphasic/potentials. Nerve conduction studies show only minimal slowing.

Management

As with dementia, there is no effective treatment and the principles of management, including multidisciplinary teamwork, are similar. Riluzole may have a modest effect on survival. Unlike in dementia, the patient is not cognitively impaired, even though communication may be difficult. A major challenge is to give support through the illness. Spasticity may be helped by baclofen or tizanidine. You should also be vigilant for evidence of depression, which you can treat. Management often involves speech and language therapists, physiotherapists, occupational therapists, social workers and nurses, as well as referral to specialist clinics such as for seating/wheelchairs and also for alternative feeding methods (e.g. percutaneous endoscopic gastrostomy (PEG)).

Prognosis

As with many degenerative conditions, the time course can vary, but death usually occurs within 5 years.

5.6 Epilepsy

Learning objectives

You should be able to:

- state how you would make a diagnosis of epilepsy
- discuss how to classify seizures
- describe the appropriate investigations to request and how to interpret these
- outline a management plan, including the advantages and disadvantages of the drug options, taking into account lifestyle and occupation.

Case Study

Fozia has had two blackouts in the last 6 weeks. Both have occurred when she was alone at home. Her partner found her asleep on the floor and she seemed dazed when he tried to wake her. All Fozia can remember is a strange feeling passing over her and then her partner talking to her. She is concerned, as she has recently started work delivering for a supermarket and also she and her partner are trying for a family.

A fit (seizure) is a symptom. It may be the first symptom of a brain tumour, cerebrovascular disease or encephalitis. Sometimes it is a manifestation of a metabolic disturbance or a reduced seizure threshold (e.g. caused by alcohol or other drugs). Epilepsy is a continuing liability to seizures.

Epidemiology

Seizures are common, with a lifetime probability of approximately 1:20 of having a fit at some time. In adult life, the prevalence of epilepsy increases with age. The prognosis, though, is much better than is generally perceived. On treatment, two-thirds of people with epilepsy become fit-free and, eventually, two-thirds do not require any medication.

Diagnosis

You must evaluate the diagnosis of a fit on clinical grounds using the patient's account and, most important of all, the account of a witness. There are two main questions that you should consider:

- Is it a fit? Differentiate from other causes of blackouts and funny turns (p. 211)
- What type of fit is it? Seizures are classified into two categories: *generalised* and *partial* (Fig. 57).

Examples of generalised fits are **grand mal** and **petit mal** (predominantly in childhood). In a grand mal seizure,

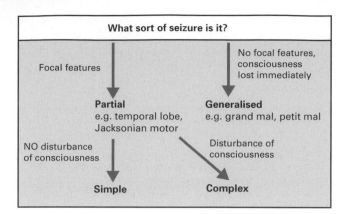

Fig. 57 Types of epilepsy. Partial fits may generalise, causing a grand mal seizure.

there is no aura, consciousness is lost from the outset and tonic clonic movements are observed for a short time. An important point is that if someone has *bilateral* shaking and is fully conscious, then it is *not* epilepsy. Tongue biting and urinary incontinence may be observed. Following the fit, in the **post-ictal** stage, the patient is drowsy.

In partial epilepsy, there is a focus that discharges periodically. Consequently, there are focal symptoms or signs depending on the location of the focus. In the temporal lobe, this may manifest as an aura (e.g. an odd feeling starting in the stomach and 'washing' over the patient), new surroundings being intensely familiar (déjà vu), failure to recognise familiar surroundings (jamais vu), or odd smells can be experienced (e.g. 'burning rubber'). If the focus is in another part of the brain, there may be shaking of a limb (Jacksonian epilepsy).

Partial epilepsy can be divided into **simple partial epilepsy** with no disturbance of consciousness at any stage and **complex partial epilepsy** where consciousness is disturbed.

Many patients with epilepsy are referred to accident and emergency after a seizure. In your assessment, you should consider whether the patient is a known epileptic and if this represents a typical event, or whether it is a manifestation of another disease process.

A careful examination should be carried out looking for focal signs and meningism. Fits can cause a fever and abnormalities in the CSF (raised white cells) so, at times, the picture can be confusing.

Status epilepticus

Status epilepticus is defined as a series of fits without regaining consciousness. Continued epileptic activity leads to exhaustion and cerebral damage, so you must take urgent action. The mortality is 10–30%. Maintenance of airway, breathing and circulation is extremely important. Intravenous (or rectal) diazepam and a loading dose of phenytoin are used. If the seizures continue, senior colleagues must be consulted.

Investigations

The diagnosis of epilepsy is based on the history *not* on EEG findings (p. 218). The use of an EEG (Table 52) is both

for identifying a focus and for showing the characteristic abnormalities of certain types of epilepsy.

An MR or CT scan looking for a structural brain lesion is indicated in anyone with either focal signs on examination or partial epilepsy. It is not of great value in diagnosing epilepsy. An MR or CT scan is indicated in late-onset epilepsy (>60 years), but you should note that most cases are *not* caused by a tumour but by a cerebrovascular disease.

Management

You must manage the patient in the context of their life. Does the diagnosis of epilepsy have major consequences for employment or recreational activities such as driving a car? The most common difficulty is with driving. In the UK, patients must let the Driver and Vehicle Licensing Agency (DVLA) and their insurance company know about *any* change in their health status that may affect their ability to drive. Your obligation is to inform patients of this requirement and to advise any driver who you regard as a danger to themselves or other road users not to drive (and note your advice in the medical records).

A person with epilepsy who holds a *standard* driving licence cannot drive until seizure-free for 1 year, on *or* off treatment. After this time, they can resume driving, providing there is 'no ongoing liability to have seizures', e.g. an astrocytoma. An exception to this rule is a person who only has nocturnal (during sleep) seizures. They can drive even though they are still having fits, providing the pattern has been established for 3 years. The law for those holding a heavy goods or public service vehicle licence is more stringent. The person can only drive these vehicles if free from seizures for 10 years, on no antiepileptic drugs for 10 years and has been examined by a specialist.

Drug treatment

When talking to patients about their future, important points are:

- Patients who have had a single seizure may not require preventative anticonvulsant therapy. This should be a joint decision between the patient and the physician, based on discussion of the likelihood of recurrence, the effectiveness of therapy and the potential adverse effects.
- Approximately 80% of patients (less with partial epilepsy) will obtain acceptable control with a single drug.

There are different mechanisms of action of anticonvulsants (Box 16); some drugs exert their effects through multiple mechanisms (and some mechanisms are unclear).

Recommended drugs are:

- sodium valproate and lamotrigine for both generalised and partial epilepsy (carbamazepine and phenytoin are effective, but have greater toxicity)

Monitoring of drugs Plasma level monitoring of drugs is generally not routinely used, apart from checking on compliance in patients whose seizures are not controlled. When treatment is started, the dose is increased gradually until either toxic effects supervene or seizure control is

Box 16: Mechanism of action of anticonvulsant drugs used in epilepsy

Sodium channel blockers
- Carbamazepine
- Phenytoin

Calcium current inhibitors
- Phenytoin

GABA enhancers
- Clobazam
- Clonazepam
- Vigabatrin
- Gabapentin

Glutamate blockers
- Lamotrigine

Unkown/multiple
- Sodium valproate (GABA, sodium)
- Topiramate (sodium, GABA, glutamate)
- Levetiracetam

GABA, gamma-aminobutyric acid.

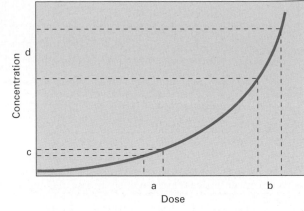

Fig. 58 Relationship between phenytoin dosage and plasma concentration, showing that the same increase in dose (a,b) can produce markedly different changes in plasma concentrations (c,d) dependent on saturation of the metabolic pathway.

obtained. The only exception to this approach is for phenytoin (see below).

Continuing therapy Once seizure control is obtained, an important question is when to stop treatment. In 60% of adults who have had no fits for 2 years, it is usually possible to withdraw drugs over 2–3 months without a recurrence. However, there are other considerations, such as occupation and driving.

Specific drugs

Clonazepam It is particularly used in myoclonic seizures, but is also effective in generalised and partial epilepsy. The main drawbacks are development of tolerance (clobazam similarly) and somnolence. It can be used in emergency treatment of status epilepticus.

Topiramate It is a highly effective anticonvulsant that is used either as a single therapy or as an additional treatment in resistant epilepsy. The most common side-effects involve cognition, including impaired concentration, somnolence, mood disturbance and confusion. It can also cause ataxia and fatigue. As with lamotrigine, it is best introduced at a low dose, then slowly increased.

Levetiracetam Like topiramate, this is a potent anticonvulsant and is well tolerated, with the most common side-effects being somnolence and dizziness. It can be used in patients with liver or renal impairment, so is particularly useful in elderly patients.

Sodium valproate This is used in generalised or partial seizures. Its biological half-life (i.e. prevention of seizures) is longer than its physical half-life. Major side-effects in adults are weight gain (appetite stimulant), hair thinning, thrombocytopaenia and tremor (high doses).

Carbamazepine You must increase the dose of carbamazepine gradually to allow it to induce its own metab-

olism. Major side-effects are dizziness, nausea, headache, drowsiness, hyponatraemia and a rash (5–10%). As an enzyme inducer, carbamazepine reduces the efficacy of sodium valproate, lamotrigine, theophylline, warfarin and the oral contraceptive pill.

Phenytoin Above a certain level, the metabolism of phenytoin becomes saturated. Consequently, a small increase in dose can cause markedly different changes in plasma levels, dependent on which part of the curve the patient lies (Fig. 58). There is also the potential for dangerous drug interactions, e.g. with cimetidine (an enzyme inhibitor). Phenytoin has a long half-life and should be given once per day. Side-effects include gum hypertrophy, hirsutism and facial coarsening. Toxicity includes sedation, ataxia and nystagmus.

Vigabatrin It is occasionally used in resistant partial seizures. Side-effects are visual problems, drowsiness, fatigue, irritability, weight gain and psychosis. Any patient commencing vigabatrin therapy should have their vision carefully checked before starting and during follow-up.

Lamotrigine Side-effects include rashes (5%), headache, blood dyscrasias and sleep disturbance. It needs to be introduced at a low dose, then slowly increased. Lamotrigine is increasingly being used as a first-line drug because of its effectiveness and tolerability (if slowly titrated).

Gabapentin It is excreted unchanged in urine and the dose should be reduced in renal impairment. Side-effects are somnolence, dizziness and ataxia.

Epilepsy and pregnancy

If any of your patients are pregnant or are considering starting a family it is important for them to know about the likely risks. Even without drug therapy, the relative risk of fetal malformation or fetal loss in an epileptic patient is increased by 25%; taking drugs doubles this. Abnormalities occur with *all* the main drugs; most are minor anomalies, such as odd facial appearance.

The main abnormalities are shown in Table 57. The risk increases with number and dosage of antiepileptic drugs used. The principle is to treat with a single drug.

Five

Table 57 Examples of teratogenic effects of antiepileptic drugs

Drug	Effect
Carbamazepine	Spina bifida (1%), hypospadias
Sodium valproate	Spina bifida (1.5%), hypospadias and craniofacial and skeletal anomalies
Phenytoin	Congenital heart disease, cleft palate

After delivery, most drugs are excreted in breast milk but concentrations are low, so breast feeding is acceptable.

Seizure control In pregnancy, drug levels may fall, leading to loss of control. This is mainly because of increased clearance by the maternal liver and reduced protein binding because of a fall in albumin concentration.

Contraception Carbamazepine and phenytoin induce hepatic microsomal enzymes, so the combined or progesterone-only pill is unreliable as a contraceptive. (A way round this is to increase the dose of estradiol in the combined pill.) Valproate and the newer drugs, gabapentin, lamotrigine and vigabatrin, do *not* induce enzymes.

Prognosis

A single seizure has a much better prognosis for future recurrence compared with a series of fits. A different 'population' of newly diagnosed epileptics is seen within specialist clinics compared with primary care; most patients have already had a series of fits and the prognosis is one of definite epilepsy.

5.7 Inflammatory conditions

Learning objectives

You should be able to:
- recognise Guillain–Barré syndrome in a patient presenting with progressive paralysis
- assess the possibility of multiple sclerosis in a young person with neurological symptoms
- discuss the principles of management of multiple sclerosis.

Case Study

In accident and emergency you see Isobel, who tells you that, a week ago, she noticed a funny feeling in a spot on her chin and this has now spread over all the left side of her face. She is adamant that the top of her head and her neck are unaffected and that her ear feels normal. She does remember that she was admitted about 6 years ago because her left leg had gone 'funny' and was giving way, but it got better.

There are a number of conditions affecting the nervous system that have, as a central feature, evidence of a disordered defence/immune mechanism. One example of an acute problem is Guillain–Barré syndrome. A recently described 'mimic' of Guillain–Barré syndrome is West Nile virus infection. An important example of a chronic problem is multiple sclerosis.

Guillain–Barre syndrome

It is important that you consider a diagnosis of Guillain–Barré syndrome in any patient with an acute progressive paralysis as survival and recovery depend on appropriate management. The condition occurs at all ages. In at least half, a minor illness ('viral') precedes the onset and triggers the immune response against myelin.

Pathology

There is intense demyelination of the peripheral nerves. The brunt of the damage is to the most heavily myelinated and longest fibres. It is due to an immunological reaction directed against myelin.

Clinical presentation

The first symptom may be back pain or altered sensation in the feet, followed by progressive, ascending paralysis. The diagnosis is mainly based on the clinical history and physical signs, including arreflexia. Other patterns occur with involvement of the bulbar musculature and, importantly, the respiratory muscles. The natural history is progression over a 2–3 weeks to a nadir (it may be faster), then slow recovery as remyelination takes place.

Investigations

CSF examination will show evidence of disordered immune response with a mild pleocytosis in the first week, followed by a rise in protein (Table 51). Nerve conduction studies demonstrate the demyelination. Request PCR for West Nile virus in appropriate cases.

Management

When assessing a patient, the main concern is to identify the need for respiratory support by monitoring and arterial blood gases. A rising Pco_2 is an indication for ventilation. Repeated plasmaphoresis modifies the disease process, with fewer patients requiring ventilation, and it also improves the outcome; it is contraindicated in West Nile virus infection. An alternative is intravenous gammaglobulin.

A major cause of death is the gross autonomic disturbance in patients with complete paralysis, who experience large swings in blood pressure together with dysrhythmias.

More than 75% of patients have very good or full recovery, and mortality is less than 5%.

Multiple sclerosis

Multiple sclerosis is more common in young people and is very rare after the age of 60 years. It is a disease of temperate climates and, in the UK, increases in frequency from south to north. The risk is associated with a childhood spent within these zones. These clues point to a continuing disordered immune reaction initially triggered by an infection acquired as a child.

Pathology

Multiple sclerosis is a dynamic condition with areas of demyelination (plaques) often occurring, but a smaller number leading to symptoms. The pathological process produces plaques of demyelination in the CNS (myelin produced by oligodendrocytes rather than Schwann cells). These plaques occur at different times and places but do have a predilection for certain areas, such as the visual pathway and the cervical posterior columns. In the initial demyelination, there is surrounding oedema and inflammation changes, with subsequent shrinkage and maturation of the plaque. Hence, the clinical picture is a focal neurological impairment with subsequent (partial) recovery as involution takes place.

Clinical presentation

It is often difficult to make the diagnosis in the early stages. Hallmarks are disturbance of visual acuity and micturition. By the time the disease is established, over 90% will have urinary frequency, urge incontinence, urinary retention, etc. As with motor neurone disease, the pattern of symptoms and signs depends on where the lesions are. Patients may have, for example, cerebellar signs, proprioceptive loss, spasticity or weakness. Fatigue is a common symptom.

Factors associated with a poor outcome (disability and survival) are:

- male gender
- onset at a later age
- predominant motor signs
- frequent relapses
- constant decline with no remission.

When talking to patients, you should remember that

- a substantial number do well with no/few further attacks
- most slowly deteriorate over 5–25 years but remain active and not grossly disabled for much of this time
- a small number deteriorate rapidly and die (<5 years).

It is also useful to think of the types of multiple sclerosis divided into:

- Relapsing remitting multiple sclerosis, which often terminates in secondary progressive disease. It is in the treatment of relapsing remitting disease that most progress has been made.
- Primary progressive multiple sclerosis.

Investigations

The clinical diagnosis is made on the basis of acute neurological deficits separated not only neuro-anatomically but also over time, with no other clear cause (e.g. cerebral toxoplasmosis in AIDS). Investigations, up to relatively recently, were focused on supporting this, e.g. disordered visual evoked potentials in patients with spinal cord symptoms and signs. Other investigations provided evidence of disturbance of CNS immunology, with oligoclonal immunoglobulin bands in the CSF (but not the blood) indicating intrathecal production. Unfortunately,

these investigations have limited sensitivity in a person with early, rather than established, multiple sclerosis.

The principal investigation now is **MRI**, which shows the distribution of the plaques of demyelination, both recent (using gadolinium enhancement) and old. In typical cases the high T2 signal plaques are seen in the periventricular area and the corpus callosum, as well as the white matter in the optic tracts, spinal cord and brainstem.

When considering the possibility of multiple sclerosis, you must bear in mind treatable diseases. One important example would be spinal cord compression in a patient presenting with a paraparesis.

Management

A team approach to the management is very important. Patients may need help and advice with their urinary difficulties; some will practise intermittent self-catheterisation. They may have to be registered as partially sighted (through an ophthalmologist). You should also monitor for depression.

High-dose corticosteroids reduce the duration of relapse but do not have any effect on the ultimate outcome. Beta-interferons and glatiramer acetate have been shown to decrease the number and severity of the relapses. It is still unclear what long-term impact they have on the course of the disease.

5.8 Coma

> ### Learning objectives
>
> You should be able to:
> - use the Glasgow Coma Score to assess patients
> - assess the likely cause of coma

Case Study

Fred Levendowski has collapsed in the garden at home. His wife tells you that he has been well all his life apart from his diabetes. Now, his breathing is laboured, pulse 48 beats/min, blood pressure 210/104 mmHg and oxygen saturation 90%. He does not respond when you are examining him; the right side is flaccid and his eyes are looking to the left. The left pupil is dilated.

In the evaluation of a patient with impaired consciousness, you must know and use the Glasgow Coma Scale (Table 54). Always contact senior colleagues. The principles of management are:

1. resuscitation with checks of airway (A), breathing (B) and circulation (C), then
2. consideration of cause and treatment.

A history is crucial and should be sought out from any witness; it will help to determine the cause as the list of possible aetiologies is huge (Box 17). One important differentiating factor is the presence of focal neurological signs and a major consideration is identifying treatable

Box 17: Causes of coma/disturbed conscious level

Without focal signs (mostly non-CNS pathology)

- Hypoglycaemia
- Subarachnoid haemorrhage (may be focal signs)
- Electrolyte disturbance, e.g. hyponatraemia
- Menignitis or encephalitis
- Drugs: particularly taken in overdose; may be specific antagonists or therapies (e.g. narcotics, benzodiazepines, lithium)
- Epilepsy
- Trauma (extradural, subdural, concussion)
- Encephalopathy: hepatic
- Respiratory failure: acute rise in carbon dioxide
- Carbon monoxide poisoning
- Hypothermia (<35°C)

With focal signs (mostly intracranial pathology)

- Stroke (haemorrhage and infact)
- Tumour: very late
- Brain abscess: look for other evidence
- Epilepsy
- Trauma
- Hypoglycaemia (check blood sugar in all unconscious patients immediately)

factors. The management is dependent on the accurate diagnosis and, for specific disorders, is described elsewhere.

5.9 Diseases of the spinal cord

Learning objectives

You should be able to:
- outline the structure of the spinal cord and its blood supply
- describe the common patterns of abnormal sensation.

Case Study

Three years ago, Claire Fuller had treatment for breast cancer and is on anastrozole. Now she is very distressed with lower thoracic back pain, which has been getting steadily worse over the past month, and for the last week her legs have been giving way. Today, it all got 'too much' when she could not go to the toilet.

Anatomy

You will find it useful to be able to visualise the cross-sectional layout of the spinal cord (Fig. 59). Certain key points should be noted:

- Sensory fibres enter the spinal cord through the **posterior** (**dorsal**) roots; motor fibres leave through the **anterior** (**ventral**) roots.

- The cell bodies for the posterior column lie in the **dorsal root ganglia**, their axons synapse in the cuneate and gracilis nucleus and, from here, the fibres decussate and ascend in the **medial lemniscus**

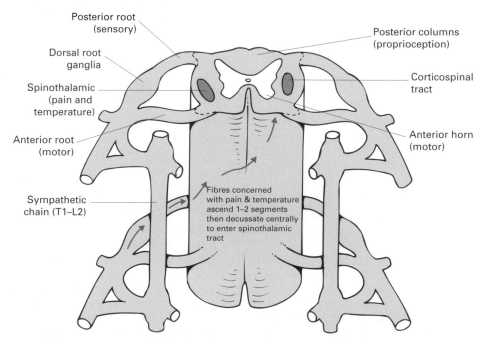

Fig. 59 Cross-sectional layout of the spinal cord.

through to the thalamus and then the postcentral gyrus.

- In the posterior column, fibres from the lowest segments of the spinal cord lie *medially* and hence will be damaged by an expanding central cord lesion.
- The fibres joining the **spinothalamic tracts** ascend the cord for a few segments before crossing; a central lesion, by interrupting this decussation, can cause a *suspended* (normal sensation above and below) loss of pain and temperature over part of the trunk.
- Fibres from the lower limbs lie close to the surface of the spinothalamic tracts and are susceptible to extrinsic pressure.
- The **corticospinal tracts** decussate in the pyramids and run in the lateral part of the cord.

Common patterns of abnormal sensation

Unilateral loss of all modalities Usually results from a lesion in the thalamus or the posterior part of the internal capsule.

Loss of pain/temperature on one side of face and opposite side of body Usually caused by a lateral medullary syndrome (p. 227).

Bilateral loss of all forms of sensation below a definite level ('sensory' level) Caused by compression of the cord (or transverse myelitis). Upper level may be indicated by zone of hyperaesthesia. Note that the bony level does not correspond to cord segment level (i.e. the cord ends at the L1/L2 disc).

Hemisection (Brown–Séquard) of the cord Results in paralysis and loss of proprioception/vibration on the same side of the body with loss of pain/temperature on the contralateral side, apart from a thin band of analgesia at the level of the damage (Fig. 59). It is more common to get incomplete forms.

Impairment of pain/temperature sensation over several segments Indicates an intrinsic lesion of the cord, near the centre involving crossing fibres. Common in syringomyelia (cavity in the centre of the cord) and intrinsic cord tumours.

Loss of sensation of 'saddle' type Impairment of all sensory modalities over the lowest sacral segments. Often accompanied by loss of leg reflexes and sphincter control. It is caused by a **cauda equina** lesion.

Sacral 'sparing' Can occur with extrinsic cord compression caused by the fibres from the lower cord segments lying medially in the posterior column away from the pressure. This pattern is often seen with extradural tumours, with sparing of the saddle area.

Blood supply of the cord

Anterior spinal artery syndrome

The cord has a poor blood supply relying on penetrating arteries at multiple levels. The anterior spinal artery supplies all of the spinal cord *except* the posterior column. The artery is heavily dependent on a branch of the aorta entering at around the 12th thoracic vertebra. When blocked by atheroma or during repair of an aortic aneurysm, an anterior spinal artery syndrome can occur, with weakness below T10–T12 and loss of pain/temperature sensation but *not* light touch (sparing of posterior columns).

Spinal strokes

Spinal strokes can occur; because of the poor collateral supply, these often affect the cord in a patchy manner, with several segments being affected asymmetrically.

Subacute combined degeneration of the spinal cord

Subacute combined degeneration of the spinal cord (SACD) is now a rare condition caused by vitamin B_{12} deficiency. There are usually concomitant haematological changes (p. 269). The main features in an established case are a combination of:

- posterior column loss: impairment of proprioception
- corticospinal damage: weakness in lower limbs
- peripheral neuropathy: loss of reflexes, stocking loss of sensation.

It was commonly seen in patients with pernicious anaemia and is treated with vitamin B_{12} injections, which will prevent further damage.

5.10 Peripheral nervous system

Learning objectives

You should be able to:
- use your detailed knowledge of the dermatomes and myotomes in diagnosis
- examine a patient to diagnose damage to peripheral nerves
- discuss the investigations in and management of peripheral neuropathies.

Case Study

Alan's feet have been troubling him for several months and have been getting worse with burning pain. You can feel the pulses in his feet, but there is a distal sensory loss in his legs, slightly worse on the right than the left. Alan finds the sensation unpleasant over his shins and cannot feel anything on his feet. Both knee and ankle jerks are absent.

Dermatomes and myotomes

In order to detect sensory impairment, you need a detailed knowledge of dermatomes. When examining the patient, place them in the anatomical position (palms facing anteriorly). Important points are:

- C2 supplies the back of the scalp up to the vertex.
- C3 and C4 include the neck and upper part of the shoulder.
- C5–C8: C5 area is the outer aspect of the shoulder and upper limb; C6, the lateral aspect of the forearm to the thumb and index; C7, a strip down the centre of the forearm to the middle finger; C8, the inner side of the forearm and the ring and little

Five

fingers; T1, the medial aspect of the upper arm to the axilla.

- On the chest wall, C4 and T2 are adjacent; the nipple is at T5, the rib margin at T8, umbilicus at T10 and symphysis pubis at T12.
- The anterior aspect of the thigh is supplied by L1–L3, the medial aspect of the calf by L4, and the lateral aspect and dorsum of the foot by L5; the sole and little toe are supplied by S1.
- The perineum is supplied by concentric rings of S3–S5.

Similarly a knowledge of **myotomes** is essential:

- diaphragm: C4
- shoulder muscles and flexors of elbow: C5, C6
- triceps and extensors of wrist and fingers: C7
- flexors of wrist and fingers: C7, C8
- hand muscles: C8, T1
- intercostals and lumbar/abdominal muscles: T2–L3
- quadriceps and adductors: L3, L4
- ilio-psoas: L1–L5
- glutei: L4, L5
- hamstrings: L4–S1
- muscles controlling ankle: L5, S1
- foot muscles: S1, S2
- bladder, anal sphincter: S2–S4.

There are a few key points that you must know about the cervical roots and the brachial plexus:

- It is the C5 and C6 roots that are most likely to be affected by cervical spondylosis (loss of biceps and supinator jerks).
- The medial cord (T1 and C8) is vulnerable to pressure from a cervical rib or infiltration from a bronchial carcinoma (**Pancoast's syndrome**).

Medial cord damage causes weakness and wasting of the intrinsic muscles of the hand (T1). A **Horner's syndrome** is also likely to be seen (T1 sympathetic outflow). Appropriate initial investigations would be chest and cervical spine radiographs.

Peripheral nerves

Examination of the arm should enable diagnosis of damage to the radial, ulnar and median nerves. The nerve supply to important muscles and sensory distribution are summarised in Table 58.

Upper limb

Radial nerve The radial nerve can be damaged at two main places:

- If pressure is applied in the axilla — for example, by using a crutch — this will cause weakness of the triceps (elbow extension); neoplastic infiltration of the axilla may cause a similar problem.
- A *Saturday night palsy* is caused by pressure on the radial nerve in the spiral groove of the humerus. Examination shows normal triceps power with weakness of the wrist and finger extensors; this causes the typical **wrist drop**.

In radial nerve palsies there is very little sensory loss.

Ulnar nerve Commonly the ulnar nerve is damaged at the elbow as it passes behind the medial epicondyle, resulting in weakness of the intrinsic muscles of the hand. Wasting and guttering will be seen, affecting the interossei and the hypothenar eminence. A key diagnostic feature is the deformity of the hand. If the lumbricals are paralysed, then the long extensors of the metacarpophalangeal (MCP) joints can pull these joints into hyperextension; because of this, the proximal interphalangeal (PIP) and the distal interphalangeal (DIP) joints go into flexion and a **claw hand** is produced. For an ulnar nerve lesion, this affects the little and ring fingers (sparing the lateral two lumbricals: median nerve) with only a slight deformity of the middle and index fingers (**ulnar claw hand**). However, if the damage is at T1 then all the lumbricals are affected, causing a **true claw hand.**

Median nerve The median nerve is commonly damaged at the wrist in a **carpal tunnel syndrome**. Often the condition is idiopathic, but there are many specific causes: for example, obesity, pregnancy, hypothyroidism and rheumatoid arthritis. The characteristic symptom of a carpal tunnel syndrome is pain in the sensory distribution of the nerve, though this may spread up the forearm. The pain is worse at night and the patient may relieve the pain by shaking the hand. On examination, other than detecting any sensory loss, the main focus should be looking for wasting of the thenar eminence and weakness of *abductor pollicis brevis* and *opponens pollicis*.

Table 58 Important (not all) muscles supplied by the three main nerves of the upper limb and the sensory distribution

Radial nerve	Ulnar nerve	Median nerve
Motor		
Triceps	Interossei (finger abduction/adduction)	Abductor pollicis brevis
Wrist extensors	Medial lumbricals (3 and 4) (flex metacarpophalangeal (MCP) joints)	Opponens pollicis
Finger extensors	Hypothenar eminence: little finger	
	Adductor pollicis: only muscle in thenar eminence supplied by ulnar nerve	Lateral lumbricals (1 and 2)
Sensory		
Back of hand only between thumb and index finger	Little finger and medial part of ring finger	Thumb, index, middle and lateral part of ring finger

Investigation and management For all nerve lesions, your clinical assessment will form the basis of diagnosis. Confirmation can be sought through nerve conduction studies (p. 218).

Radial nerve palsies (Saturday night or crutch) Relief of pressure will usually lead to recovery. A wrist splint should be used to support the hand in the neutral position whilst this takes place.

Ulnar nerve entrapment/damage at the elbow Surgical freeing of the nerve is sometimes required.

Carpal tunnel syndrome Treatment of the underlying condition may help as can local injection of corticosteroids. Commonly, surgical release is needed.

Lower limb

Femoral nerve Damage to the the femoral nerve will result in weakness of knee extension and consequent difficulty in getting up from a chair or climbing stairs. Quadriceps wasting will be seen with loss of the knee jerk. **Femoral amyotrophy** is seen in poorly controlled diabetics and is often associated with pain, depression and weight loss. It is treated by improving diabetic control (converting to insulin).

Lateral popliteal nerve The other important nerve lesion in the lower limb is damage to the lateral popliteal nerve as it winds round the head of the fibula. A foot drop occurs because of weakness of dorsiflexion. Again, a mononeuritis from diabetes may be the cause, but it is also seen following prolonged pressure, such as by a plaster cast or in an unconscious patient.

Peripheral nerve disease

Mononeuritis and mononeuritis multiplex

Mononeuritis and mononeuritis multiplex have complex aetiologies with a common factor being a vasculitic process affecting the vasa nervorum. Patients present with either a single nerve (often cranial nerve) or a mixture of nerve lesions. It may be painful. Mononeuritis occurs in, amongst other conditions, aggressive rheumatoid disease, systemic lupus erythematosus (SLE) and polyarteritis nodosa. Sudden-onset flaccid weakness with fever suggests West Nile virus infection. Treatment is directed towards the underlying problem.

Peripheral neuropathy

The hallmark of a peripheral neuropathy is a *symmetrical glove and stocking loss*, which is unlike the asymmetry seen in mononeuritis multiplex or other local nerve damage. There are hereditary sensorimotor neuropathies such as **peroneal muscular atrophy** (Charcot–Marie–Tooth syndrome: autosomal dominant). Among acquired causes diabetes mellitus is the commonest; others include AIDS, drugs (amiodarone, nitrofurantoin) and pellagra (pyridoxine deficiency) and neoplasia. Most cases are idiopathic.

Early features are of dyaesthie/paraesthesiae in the feet ('like walking on cotton wool'), although many patients have no symptoms at all. On examination, the ankle jerks are lost and some distal wasting and weakness may be found, but the dominant feature is often symmetrical sensory impairment with a zone of impaired sensation

giving way to numbness more distally. Occasionally, the neuropathy can be painful.

Investigations

Diagnosis is made on clinical grounds, supported by nerve conduction studies. If the pathological process is damaging myelin, the nerve conduction pattern will be different (i.e. marked slowing) to one causing axonal/neuronal loss. You should target investigations to the probable/possible cause(s) identified in the history and examination. The tests may include blood sugar (diabetes), rheumatoid factor (rheumatoid disease/amyloid), antinuclear factor (SLE), chest radiograph (neoplasia), full blood count (vitamin B_{12}, folate deficiency), erythrocyte sedimentation rate (ESR)/plasma viscosity (inflammatory disease), immunoglobulins (paraproteinaemia) biochemical profile (uraemia) and possibly HIV status (AIDS).

Management

Management is aimed at the underlying cause. Care must be taken about footwear and chiropody to prevent any ulceration/infection, which may result in gangrene, particularly if vascular supply is affected.

Non-metastatic manifestation of malignancy

A peripheral neuropathy can be seen as a **paraneoplastic syndrome**. Non-neurological manifestations are discussed elsewhere (p. 81), but malignancy may present or be associated with a primary cerebellar degeneration, a myasthenic-like syndrome (see below), a primary motor neuropathy or a myositis. Malignancy should always be considered in any patient with an odd neurological syndrome.

5.11 Muscle disease

Learning objectives

You should be able to:
- describe the common causes of muscle disease
- list the common clinical presentations
- discuss the investigation of a patient with possible muscle disease.

Case Study

Edna has been seeing double for about 10 weeks, but it seems to vary. At times, she is seeing double on looking to the left and right, which seems worse when she is watching TV in the evening. When you examine her, her eye movements are normal, but she does have difficulty in getting on to the couch. From her first outpatient assessment, you know that low levels of acetylcholine receptor antibodies have been detected.

Structure of muscle

The functional unit of muscle is the motor unit, which comprises a single motor neurone innervating, via its axon, a variable number of muscle fibres. Muscle fibres are divided using histology and biochemistry into:

Five

- Type I fibres: smaller than type II, larger numbers of oxidative enzymes and mitochondria; they contract and relax relatively slowly, being important in postural control.
- Type II fibres: have a higher content of glycogen and are geared for anaerobic metabolism; these are **fast twitch** fibres.

Clinical presentation

The major features of muscle disease are weakness and fatigability. An inflammatory myopathy (and some metabolic syndromes) may be painful. Wasting or even hypertrophy is sometimes apparent and it is important that you document its distribution as it may help in diagnosis. The reflexes are usually preserved, unlike in a peripheral neuropathy.

Muscle disease can be divided into inherited disease (you should take a careful family history) and acquired disease.

Investigations

Initial investigations of suspected muscle disease should include chest radiography (malignancy, thymic tumour), full blood count, ESR (inflammatory/connective tissue process), rheumatoid factor, antinuclear factor, creatine phosphokinase (muscle enzyme: may need measurement of the skeletal muscle isoenzyme MM). Electromyography may show evidence of disordered muscle function. A muscle biopsy is sometimes indicated, with enzymatic assays, histological stains and electron microscopy.

Inherited disease

Many inherited diseases are rare conditions seen only in specialist clinics or in paediatric practice. The muscular dystrophies are genetically determined conditions that produce progressive destruction of the skeletal muscles. The classification is based on the clinical picture (distribution of affected muscle groups) and the mode of inheritance (Table 59).

X-linked dystrophies

The X-linked dystrophies are caused by an abnormal membrane-associated protein (**dystrophin**) coded at Xp 21. The protein has a major role in maintaining membrane stability (sarcolemmal) during muscle contraction. It is absent in Duchenne and reduced in Becker muscular dystrophy.

Duchenne muscular dystrophy

More patients are surviving to young adulthood with Duchenne dystrophy, though by this stage, they are usually immobile with muscle contractures, severe kyphoscoliosis, frequent chest infections and dysrhythmias. The condition presents with delayed motor development and then causes progressive weakness. Diagnosis is based on the clinical picture and an elevated creatine kinase (indicating muscle cell necrosis). If there is doubt, then EMG and muscle biopsy (absence of dystrophin) are used. There is no effective treatment.

Carrier detection is very important to patients and their families.

Becker muscular dystrophy

Becker dystrophy presents later and patients often can walk until their third or fourth decade. Like patients with Duchenne dystrophy, they often have muscle hypertrophy.

Dystrophia myotonica

Dystrophia myotonica is a rare, but important, muscle disease. It is inherited as an autosomal dominant, with the gene located on chromosome 19. Males, particularly those born to affected females, are more severely affected and the severity is linked to increasing numbers of **repeat sequences** within the abnormal gene. Physiologically, myotonia is caused by instability in the sodium and chloride channels of the muscle membrane, resulting in repetitive discharges following a short period of contraction.

Myotonia (delayed relaxation) is the characteristic feature, which worsens in the cold. Wasting of temporalis and masseter muscles is observed, together with some distal muscle atrophy. Ptosis occurs. Dystrophia myotonia is a multisystem disorder associated with cataracts, frontal balding, diabetes, cardiomyopathy and gonadal atrophy. Sleep apnoea is common.

The condition presents in the third or fourth decade and life expectancy is reduced. The myotonia may be helped by procainamide and phenytoin.

Acquired disease

Myasthenia gravis

Myasthenia gravis occurs in adults of all ages, being slightly more common in females. It is more often associated with a thymoma in older people. The symptoms and signs result from failure of neuromuscular transmission because of blockade of the acetylcholine receptor on the muscle endplate by receptor antibodies. Characteristic symptoms are:

- diplopia
- weakness and fatigability: increasing weakness for repetitive tasks (e.g. brushing hair, using screwdriver) or at the end of a day.

On examination, you may demonstrate the weakness by asking the patient to make repeated movements. A key point is that the weakness is variable. Ptosis is often present

Table 59 Muscular dystrophies

Mode of inheritance	Type of dystrophy
X-linked recessive	Duchenne Becker
Autosomal dominant	Fascioscapulohumeral Limb girdle (some families) Scapuloperoneal (some families) Myotonic
Autosomal recessive	Limb girdle (some families) Scapuloperoneal (some families)

and the patient may complain of diplopia in all directions. Unlike peripheral nerve damage, reflexes are preserved.

Investigations

A chest radiograph (postero-anterior and lateral) and a thoracic CT scan should be performed looking for a thymic tumour. Blood should be taken for acetycholine receptor antibodies. If there are none, it is unlikely that the patient has the disease. An EMG will show diagnostic features and can be used to differentiate true myasthenia gravis from the much rarer **Eaton–Lambert syndrome**. The latter is a paraneoplastic syndrome with many of the features of myasthenia, except that the weakness *improves* on rapid repetition.

Injection with the short-acting anticholinesterase edrophonium can confirm the diagnosis by showing immediate and dramatic improvement. The peak expiratory flow rate (PEFR) can be used to demonstrate the change objectively.

Management

For many years, the only treatment available for myasthenia was an anticholinesterase such as **neostigmine** or **pyridostigmine**. These have to be given frequently because of their short half-lives (3–4-hour dose interval) and can produce excessive cholinergic stimulation. They do not alter the underlying disease process. More recently, the aim has been towards disease modification through immune modulation. Thymectomy has been shown to be a safe procedure that will produce a remission over several months and will last a long time in those patients *without* a thymoma. Corticosteroids can also be beneficial; these have to be introduced in a low dose as they can temporarily produce a worsening of the condition. Sometimes other immunosuppressives (e.g. **azathioprine**) are used. Plasmapheresis can be used as a short-term measure.

As a medical house officer, you need to be able to recognise a crisis in a patient with known myasthenia. If the person is receiving anticholinesterases, then the differential diagnosis lies between a **myasthenic crisis** and a **cholinergic crisis**. There may be clues to the correct diagnosis in the history: for example, poor compliance with medication or treatment with aminoglycoside antibiotics, which have a curare-like (competitive antagonism) effect. Usually, it is very difficult to differentiate between the two different crises. Much more importantly, you should assess ventilation with PEFR, vitalograph and blood gases. A specialist opinion should be sought with a view to ventilation. An edrophonium test can be used to diagnose a myasthenic crisis but this may cause respiratory paralysis if given to a patient who is overtreated with anticholinesterases. The test should *only* be done in an intensive care unit.

Myopathies

A number of conditions result in a myopathy. Almost always this affects the **proximal musculature**, resulting in difficulties with rising from a chair, lifting the arms high or climbing stairs. Wasting may occur, but it may not be obvious.

Conditions causing a proximal myopathy include endocrine disease such as Cushing's disease, acromegaly and thyrotoxicosis. Toxins such as alcohol may be important, and binge drinking may cause acute muscle necrosis. A myopathy may be seen as part of a non-metastatic manifestation of malignancy (paraneoplastic syndrome). One of the most important causes of a proximal myopathy is treatment with corticosteroid at doses above 10 mg of prednisolone per day.

Myositis

Particularly in connective tissue disease (Ch. 8), the skeletal musculature may be affected by vasculitis and inflammation. When this is chronic and mild, pain may not be a feature and the presentation is that of a proximal myopathy. The hallmark is a raised creatine phosphokinase.

In a small percentage of patients, a characteristic rash with a heliotrope (red-purple) discoloration of the skin over the dorsum of the MCP joints and around the eyelids may be apparent: **dermatomyositis**.

As with many neurological syndromes, myositis may be a marker for a malignant process. This is now known to be less common than previously thought. Management is of the underlying condition, but high-dose steroids are often used to suppress the inflammatory process.

Self-assessment: questions

Any or all of each set of five statements may be true or false. Choose your answers and see the reasoning behind the correct answer on pages 254–255.

Multiple choice questions

1. The following are true:
   a. There is weakness of elbow extension in a crutch palsy
   b. Wasting of the hypothenar eminence occurs in the carpal tunnel syndrome
   c. Abduction of the thumb is impaired in an ulnar nerve lesion
   d. The index finger is hyperextended at the metacarpophalangeal (MCP) joint in an ulnar nerve lesion
   e. Sensation is lost over the whole of the back of the hand in radial nerve damage

2. In a patient treated for epilepsy the following are true:
   a. Drug levels of carbamazepine are very useful in the management
   b. Sodium valproate is useful and safe during pregnancy
   c. A patient with epilepsy who has been fit-free for 4 years and who stops their medication must not drive for a further 2 years
   d. Respiratory depression is associated with clomethiazole infusions for status epilepticus
   e. The use of sodium valproate makes the combined oral contraceptive pill unreliable

3. The following are true:
   a. A cerebellar vermis lesion will result in a marked intention tremor
   b. Macular sparing is a characteristic of lesions affecting the optic tract
   c. In a patient with marked visuo-spatial inattention, the lesion is most likely in the left cerebral hemisphere
   d. Agnosia means inability to plan and execute motor tasks
   e. Dyscalculia is a feature of Alzheimer's disease

4. The following are true of stroke risk:
   a. Following a transient ischaemic attack (TIA), most patients will have a stroke within 3 years
   b. Carotid endarterectomy is of proven value in preventing strokes in patients with severe stenosis who have had recent events (TIA, minor stroke) in that territory
   c. Treating hypertension is of proven value in patients up to the age of 80 years
   d. Anticoagulation will reduce the risk of a stroke in patients in sinus rhythm

   e. The benefit of an intervention for a patient depends on the absolute risk

5. Features of a right sixth nerve palsy include:
   a. Convergent strabismus
   b. Diplopia worse on looking to the right
   c. False image parallel to the true image
   d. False image occurring further to the left than the true image
   e. Images becoming increasingly separated on looking to the left

6. Pressure on the facial nerve at the internal auditory meatus by an acoustic neuroma may cause:
   a. Loss of taste
   b. Loss of ability to blink
   c. Loss of supply to the parotid gland
   d. Loss of sensation to the cheek
   e. Loss of sweating over the cheek

7. Parkinson's disease is associated with:
   a. Loss of dopamine transmission
   b. Cogwheel rigidity
   c. Tardive dyskinesia
   d. Intention tremor
   e. Festinant gait

8. The following are true of myasthenia gravis:
   a. An equal sex incidence
   b. Diplopia and papilloedema are the main ocular signs
   c. Usually a loss of tendon reflexes
   d. A deficiency of acetyl cholinesterase
   e. Fasciculation often occurs

9. A 19-year-old girl presents with a 12-month history of repeated falls. A diagnosis of epilepsy is supported by the fact that:
   a. There are abnormal sensations prior to the attack
   b. They only occur in the presence of the mother
   c. They only occur when watching television
   d. There have been feelings of increased anxiety over the last year when on a bus or in shops
   e. They only occur when standing upright

10. The following are more suggestive of dementia than of depression:
    a. Several episodes of antisocial behaviour
    b. Mutism
    c. Duration of symptoms less than 1 month
    d. Worsening of symptoms during the early morning
    e. Marked impairment of concentration

11. The following are causes of predominantly lymphocytic meningitis:
    a. Enteroviruses
    b. Sarcoidosis
    c. *Cryptococcus neoformans*
    d. Tuberculosis
    e. Herpes simplex virus

12. With respect to lumbar puncture:
    a. Coagulopathy is a contraindication
    b. Papilloedema is an absolute contraindication
    c. The procedure may cause meningitis
    d. The less CSF is removed, the less likely coning is to occur
    e. Post-lumbar puncture headache is related to the size of the needle used

13. The following diagnoses should be considered when a patient presents with a combination of fever and impaired conscious level:
    a. Pneumonia
    b. Tuberculous meningitis
    c. Malaria
    d. Viral meningitis
    e. Pontine haemorrhage

14. Outcome from bacterial meningitis relates to:
    a. Age of patient
    b. Time to first administration of antibiotic
    c. CSF concentration of antibiotic
    d. Development of antibiotic resistance during therapy
    e. The causative organism

Single best answer multiple choice questions

For each numbered question; only ONE of the options lettered a–e is correct.

1. A 19-year-old student is brought to the accident and emergency department by ambulance. Her flatmate panicked and dialled 999 when the student collapsed. The history is that the student had been practising lacrosse that afternoon and had been hit hard on the side of the head by the ball. She had blacked out for a few seconds then had been dazed, but had carried on. However, when she got back to the flat with her friend, she could not remember anything about the match. When watching TV, she vomited then became very drowsy. On examination in accident and emergency, her Glasgow Coma Score is 7 and her right pupil is dilated. What is the most likely diagnosis?
    a. Intracerebral haematoma
    b. Subarachnoid haemorrhage
    c. Acute extradural haematoma
    d. Chronic subdural haematoma
    e. Intraventricular haemorrhage

2. A 27-year-old woman is seen in the outpatient department because of headaches, which have been present over a couple of months and seem worse in the morning. There is no past medical history of note and the only medication is the oral contraceptive pill. On examination, her body mass index (BMI) is 30 kg/m² and, in the central nervous system, there is swelling of the optic discs. What is the most likely diagnosis?
    a. Temporal arteritis
    b. Optic neuritis
    c. Glioblastoma multiforme
    d. Benign intracranial hypertension
    e. Migraine

3. A 31-year-old woman is seen in the accident and emergency department because of a severe headache. It came on suddenly that morning and is described as the 'worse she has ever had'; since then it has eased just a little. On examination, there is some neck rigidity and photophobia. What is the best initial investigation?
    a. Computed tomogram (CT) with contrast
    b. CT scan
    c. Magnetic resonance imaging
    d. Lumbar puncture
    e. Doppler scan of her carotid arteries

4. A 39-year-old woman is seen on the medical admissions unit because of weakness in her legs and numbness. It started with some back pain a week previously, then she has noticed that her legs have got gradually weaker. She also feels that her hands might be affected. On examination, her reflexes are absent and there is weakness and sensory loss in her legs and hands. What is the most likely diagnosis?
    a. Poliomyelitis
    b. Anterior spinal artery occlusion
    c. Lumbar disc protrusion
    d. Metastatic disease
    e. Guillain–Barré syndrome

5. A 60-year-old woman is seen in the accident and emergency department because of increasing confusion. She had been to her regular neurology outpatient review appointment a week earlier, when she seemed fine, apart from concerns about the frequency of her fits. On examination in the accident and emergency department, there are no abnormalities, apart from the confusion. In her investigations:

Urea	5.7 mmol/l
Creatinine	69 µmol/l
Sodium	121 mmol/l
Potassium	4.5 mmol/l

   Which drug is the most likely cause of her confusion?

a. Carbamazepine

b. Sodium valproate

c. Lamotrigine

d. Gabapentin

e. Topiramate

6. In a young adult with fever, headache and neck stiffness:

   a. Regardless of any rash, a lumbar puncture is certainly indicated

   b. Penicillian i.v. or i.m. is almost always the best treatment

   c. An HIV test should be done in almost all cases

   d. Even if a sore throat preceded headache, lumbar puncture is indicated

   e. It is essential to get clotting test results before doing a lumbar puncture

7. Which of the following best describes 'meningoencephalitis'?

   a. Headache, neck stiffness and confusional state

   b. An aseptic meningitis with a normal CT or MR brain scan

   c. An aseptic meningitis with a confusional state with or without focal neurological signs

   d. An abnormal CSF with lymphocyte predominance, in which tuberculosis and fungal meningitis are ruled out

   e. An acute confusional state with fever and neck stiffness

8. Acute flaccid paralysis:

   a. Is a feature of HIV infection

   b. Is a feature of acute human T-cell lymphotrophic virus type 1 (HTLV 1) infection

   c. Is a feature of West Nile virus infection

   d. Is not a feature of acute intermittent porphyria

   e. Is typical of lead poisoning

Extended matched questions

EMQ 1

Theme: Possible neurological diagnoses

Options

1. Alzheimer's disease

2. Cerebral glioma

3. Drug-induced parkinsonism

4. Guillain–Barré syndrome

5. Parkinson's disease

6. Mononeuritis multiplex

7. Motor neurone disease

8. Multiple sclerosis

9. Myasthenia gravis

10. Sensorimotor neuropathy

11. Stroke

For patients A–E select the most likely diagnosis. Each option can be used more than once.

A. A 59-year-old man has increasing difficulty at work over several months. He is finding it very difficult working with spreadsheets and finances. His wife says that he can no longer do the crossword, which he was very good at. On examination, the only findings are that he cannot complete 'serial 7 s' and is unable to recall a sentence completely.

B. A 32-year-old man presents with increasing unsteadiness over a few days. He had one odd episode of weakness of his right hand 12 months previously, which got better over a few weeks. On examination, you find truncal ataxia and nystagmus in looking to the right and left.

C. A 76-year-old woman presents with falls. She has been started on treatment for some paranoid ideas a couple of months ago. On examination, she has a generalised increase in tone; there is no tremor, but movements are slow. Fine finger movements are impaired.

D. A 51-year-old woman has been dropping things for about 6 months. This has been getting worse and she now says that her left foot tends to trip her up when she walks. On examination, there is asymmetrical wasting of the intrinsic muscles of the hands; reflexes are absent in the arms but brisk in the legs. There is weakness of dorsiflexion of the left foot. There are no abnormal sensory signs.

E. A 43-year-old man gives a 4-week history of increasing difficulty in using his left hand. In the last few days, he has noticed that his left leg is not working properly. On examination, there is weakness and an increase in reflexes and tone in his left arm and leg.

EMQ 2

Theme: Neuroanatomical tracts

Options

1. Left corticospinal tract in the internal capsule

2. Right corticospinal tract in the internal capsule

3. Left cerebellar-spinal tract

4. Right cerebellar-spinal tract

5. Left spinothalamic tract in the cord

6. Right spinothalamic tract in the cord

7. Posterior columns

For each patient, select the tract most likely to be involved. Each option can be used more than once.

A. A patient presents with incoordination of her left hand with past-pointing and impaired finger-nose test on the left side.

B. A patient with loss of joint position and deep pain sensation in both lower limbs, but intact pinprick sensation.

C. A patient with loss of fine movement in his left hand, reduced power in elbow extension and increased reflexes in his left arm. The tone in the arm and leg is normal.

D. A patient with an area of hyperaesthesia over his left trunk and loss of pinprick sensation in his right leg, but with preserved light touch.

E. A patient with clumsiness of both hands and slow writhing (athetoid-like) movements in his fingers with his arms outstretched and his eyes closed.

EMQ 3

Theme: Confusion
Options

1. Alzheimer's disease
2. Chronic subdural haematoma
3. Gliobastoma multiforme
4. Iatrogenic
5. Hypoglycaemia
6. Lewy body dementia
7. Post-ictal
8. Transient ischaemic attack
9. Urinary tract infection
10. Vascular dementia
11. Viral encephalitis

For each patient with confusion, please select the most likely diagnosis.

A. A 78-year-old woman has been intermittently confused over a couple of weeks. During these episodes, her husband has also noticed that her right side appears weaker. She is known to be in atrial fibrillation and is treated with warfarin. In the past medical history, she has osteoarthritis and her mobility is poor. She has a history of falls.

B. A 67-year-old man is admitted with confusion and visual hallucinations. Examination shows a bilateral increase in tone with some tremor of his right hand. Generally he seems slow and is quietly spoken. Investigations are normal. Following admission, the confusion fluctuates and at times he appears sleepy. At other times he complains of seeing birds flying around the ward.

C. An 83-year-old woman has been very upset since the death of her husband 2 months ago. She has not been sleeping or eating well and has been very tearful, saying that she does not see any future. Her daughter took her to her mother's GP a few days ago. Since then she has become increasingly confused and agitated. On examination, apart from the confusion, there are no other physical signs. All investigations are normal.

D. You see a 36-year-old man in the accident and emergency department. The ambulance has brought him after a passerby saw the patient lying on the pavement with blood coming from his mouth and incontinent of urine. When you see him, he is confused and drowsy, with trauma to his tongue. He smells strongly of alcohol. All tests are normal, including an urgent CT scan, and he slowly recovers over several hours.

E. A 57-year-old woman is seen in the outpatient department. She is unable to give a clear history, but her husband says that she has been increasingly 'strange', doing things like putting her trousers on back to front and putting the electric kettle on the gas hob. This has been worsening over several weeks. On examination, her speech is limited to brief phrases and few words. There is a right-sided weakness. A general examination is normal and basic tests, including chest radiograph, do not show any abnormalities.

Objective structured clinical examination (OSCE) stations

OSCE 1

This is an interview with a simulated carer.

Examiner: You are the house officer on call for medicine. You have just admitted a 73-year-old man who has had a transient ischaemic attack (TIA). His wife has arrived and he has asked you to explain the problem to her. Please tell her what the problem is.

OSCE 2

You enter the station and a young woman is sitting with the examiner, who explains that Kate Cartwright has been troubled with blurred vision and a previous episode of unsteadiness. She has seen a neurologist, who has referred her for an MRI. Ms Cartwright has come to see her GP, as she is not sure what the test entails. Your GP tutor asks you to explain the test to Kate.

Case history questions

Case history 1

A 57-year-old man with known diabetes presents to his general practitioner following an episode lasting a few minutes during which 'a curtain descended over my left eye'. Following this he was fine. He had one similar episode 2 weeks previously when his speech was 'garbled' as well as his vision 'going funny'. This lasted a few minutes.

1. What are the diagnoses and where are the lesions?
2. What tests, if any, would you request?
3. How would you treat him?

Unfortunately, 2 weeks later he develops sudden onset of right-sided weakness, starts to talk 'rubbish' and is noticed to be looking constantly to his left. He is admitted to hospital where his conscious level deteriorates over the next 8 hours. He develops constant urinary incontinence.

4. What tests would you do as an emergency?
5. What is the likely diagnosis and prognosis?
6. Assuming he survives, how should he be managed?

Case history 2

A 27-year-old woman feels unwell and feverish. She has vague urinary symptoms and was given trimethoprim. Ten days later she develops unsteadiness in walking and tingling in her feet. She complains of stiffness in her legs and ill-defined low back pain. Over the next few days she notices increasing leg weakness.

1. Discuss the differential diagnosis.

Case history 3

A 55-year-old man presents with a 1-year history of progressive dysarthria and trouble swallowing, with recurrent chest infections. Some wasting of the muscles of his hands is apparent. Nerve conduction studies in the legs show a conduction velocity of 42 m/s (normal 50 m/s) and EMG shows some fibrillatory potentials and giant motor units. The creatine phosphokinase measurement is normal.

1. What is the diagnosis?
2. If the patient had sensory disturbance, how would this change the diagnostic possibilities?
3. Outline a management plan.

Case history 4

A 19-year-old male Asian student is brought in to accident and emergency drowsy but communicating. He is accompanied by his flatmate. Staff nurse tells you he has a fever of 38.5°C, blood pressure of 100/60 mmHg and a pulse of 110 beats/min. He complains of headache and vomiting of about 36 hours' duration. He looks ill.

1. The following actions are appropriate immediately:
   a. Check his travel history in detail
   b. Do an urgent blood count
   c. Send him to a ward where you will see him very soon
   d. Arrange an urgent chest X-ray immediately
   e. Examine his skin while completing the history

You learn that he was previously well and never admitted to hospital before. He was born in the UK, has not travelled anywhere for 2 months and is not allergic to any antibiotics that he knows of. He has marked neck stiffness but no rash and no focal neurological signs on examination of his cranial nerves, limbs or cerebellum. His chest is clear to auscultation and he has not coughed during the examination.

2. The following actions are appropriate:
   a. Administer i.v. antibiotics and dexamethasone
   b. Do a lumbar puncture immediately after taking blood and inserting an i.v. line
   c. Do a lumbar puncture after getting his platelet count
   d. Do a CT scan first (there is an on-call emergency CT scan service in the hospital)
   e. Give loading doses of phenytoin to prevent fits

Two hours later, the patient has had a lumbar puncture, CT scan and his first dose of antibiotic and he has been admitted to the ward. The microbiologist telephones to say that the CSF is consistent with bacterial meningitis and Gram-negative cocci are seen intracellularly, consistent with *Neisseria meningitidis* in the CSF.

3. Now you should:
   a. Put the patient in a side room
   b. Wear a mask when visiting him
   c. Administer rifampicin prophylaxis to his flatmate, the staff nurse in accident and emergency, the ambulancemen and yourself
   d. Inform the consultant responsible for communicable disease control now, by telephone, that the patient has been admitted
   e. Reassure his parents that he is likely to make a full recovery

Key features questions

1. A 47-year-old woman has a 9-month history of progressive left-sided deafness, with tinnitus and a feeling of dizziness. On examination, hearing is diminished on the left side, Rinne's test is normal on both sides and Weber's test lateralises to the right. Cranial nerve testing showed a diminished corneal reflex on the left side. Formal audiograms shows a high-frequency deafness for both air and bone conduction on the left side.

What investigation would you do next and why?

2. On the medical admissions unit, you see Fred Parker, a 34-year-old man with multiple sclerosis. He is paraplegic and uses a wheelchair to get around the house. He has an indwelling catheter that was first put in 3 years ago. One of Fred's carers called the ambulance because she found him fitting. In the last few days, Fred has not been very well and was complaining of feeling hot and cold, with pain in his back just underneath his ribs on the left side. When you see him, he is rousable and appears to be post-ictal. His temperature is 39°C, the chest is clear and there is no neck stiffness. He does have some tenderness in his left renal angle.

How would you manage him and why?

3. A 32-year-old woman was playing tennis and had a sudden pain in the right side of her face and neck. Following this, she notices that her left side is weak and she cannot see on that side. Examination shows a right Horner's syndrome and moderate weakness of her left arm and leg.

What would be the definitive investigation?

4. A 62-year-old woman is seen in the outpatient department. She gives a 4-month history of feeling that she is slowing up and is also having trouble getting going when she wants to walk. She also says that it has been difficult turning over in bed at night and she wakes with some aches and pains. Her husband says that her voice has become softer and she does not smile as much. He has also noticed a tremor in her left hand, particularly when she is upset.

What would you expect to find on examination?

Data interpretation questions

1. In a patient with a presumed diagnosis of Guillain–Barré syndrome, comment on the sequences of spirometry and blood gases given in Table 60.

Table 60 Respiratory parameters measured in a patient with a presumed diagnosis of Guillain–Barré syndrome

	Monday a.m	Monday p.m.
FEV$_1$ (litres)	1.7	1.1
FVC (litres)	2.5	1.7
pH	7.32	7.30
Pao$_2$ kPa (mmHg)	10.7 (80)	9.3 (70)
Paco$_2$ kPa (mmHg)	5.7 (43)	6.3 (47)
HCO$_3$ (mmol/l)	27	29

FEV$_1$, forced expired volume in 1 sec; FVC, forced vital capacity; Pao$_2$ and Paco$_2$, arterial partial pressure of oxygen and carbon dioxide, respectively.

2. Table 61 gives information on CSF in patients with fever, impaired mental status or headache, or a mixture of these. Give the most likely diagnosis for patients A–F.

Table 61 Data obtained for CSF in patients A–F

	A	B	C	D	E	F
Red cell count (hpf)	150	20	23 000	22	12	20
White cell count (hpf)	9	8	14	1700	450	180
Polymorphs (%)	20	0	50	99	70	10
Protein (g/l)	0.58	0.69	0.9	1.2	0.51	0.9
Glucose (CSF) (mmol/l)	3.2	4.2	3.8	0.2	3.4	1.1
Blood glucose (mmol/l)	5.6	6.4	5.9	6.2	5.8	4.8

hpf, high-power field: ×10^6/l.

Picture questions

1. You see a 46-year-old-man in accident and emergency. He has a 4-week history of left-sided weakness. A CT scan is done the following day (Fig. 60). During examination, the patient is asked to draw a clock face (Fig. 61).

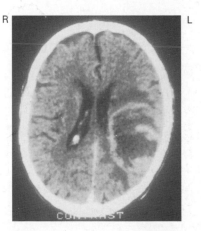

R   L

Fig. 60 A CT scan for a man with left-sided weakness.

a. What do you want to know about the history of the weakness?
b. List three abnormalities shown on the scan.
c. What is the differential diagnosis?
d. Why has he drawn the clock (Fig. 61) this way?
e. What day-to-day problems might he have because of this problem?

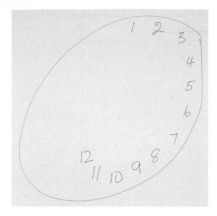

Fig. 61 A clock face drawn by a man with left-sided weakness.

2. A 54-year-old woman is admitted through accident and emergency complaining of a severe headache. A CT scan is performed within 24 hours (Fig. 62A). A second scan is done at 2 weeks because of concerns (subsequently proved unfounded) about the diagnosis (Fig. 62B).

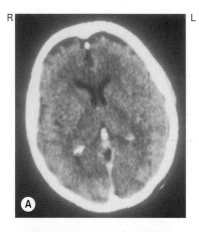

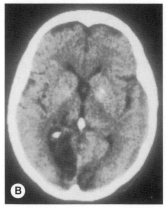

Fig. 62 CT scans of a woman with a severe headache. **A** The first scan. **B** A further scan 2 weeks later.

a. Describe the abnormalities on the scan shown in Figure 62B.
b. Why are these not present in Figure 62A, given that her condition has not changed?

c. What symptoms would she be complaining of other than her headache?
d. What artery supplies the area of abnormality?

3. A 73-year-old man is brought to accident and emergency. He is drowsy. The history from his wife is that he is on long-term anticoagulants because of atrial fibrillation and a previous stroke. He suddenly deteriorated on the day of admission. Figure 63 is a CT scan of the patient.

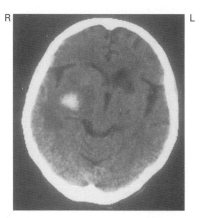

Fig. 63 A CT scan in an elderly patient.

a. Why was an urgent CT scan requested?
b. What does the scan show?
c. What should you do now?

4. You are asked to see a 33-year-old woman in accident and emergency; she is drowsy and unable to give a history. Her temperature is 37.5°C and she has neck rigidity. An urgent CT scan is carried out (Fig. 64).

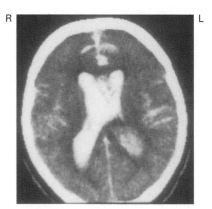

Fig. 64 A CT scan in a drowsy patient with neck rigidity.

a. Describe two abnormalities on the scan.
b. What should you do now?
c. If she survives, what neurological problems might she develop?

5. You are looking after a 34-year-old woman with Friedreich's ataxia who is confined to a wheelchair and is complaining of left-hand weakness.

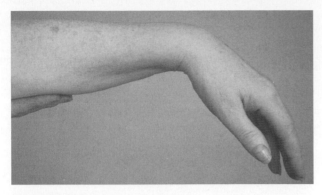

Fig. 65 Friedreich's ataxia.

a. What does Figure 65 show?

b. What particular features would you look for on examination?

c. Why has she developed this problem?

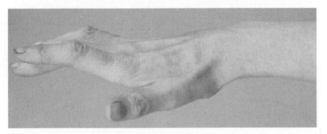

Fig. 66 A patient complaining of slowly developing right-hand weakness.

6. A 63-year-old man in the outpatient department complains of right-hand weakness which has developed over 5 months (Fig. 66).

a. Describe the abnormality.

b. Where is the neuroanatomical lesion likely to be?

c. Name one possible cause.

Short notes

1. The daughter of a patient who has been diagnosed clinically as having Alzheimer's disease wants to ask what tests you are doing, what treatment can be offered and what will happen in the future. Consider what you would do if the daughter became angry and aggressive (would be a suitable question for a viva).

2. What would be your immediate management, including pertinent questions in the history, examination findings, investigations and treatment?

a. In a patient with three seizures over 30 minutes with no recovery of consciousness in between.

b. In a patient with known myasthenia who is generally weak and drowsy.

3. In a patient with one of the following symptoms, where is the lesion likely to be and name a common pathological process?

a. Reduction in visual acuity over several hours with impaired colour vision (blurred and colours 'washed out').

b. Loss of the left visual field with macular sparing.

c. Loss of both temporal fields starting with the lower fields.

d. Loss of left temporal vision in one eye in a 35-year-old man with progressive weight loss.

4. A 59-year-old man enters outpatients complaining of dizziness and almost immediately has a grand mal seizure. Moments after recovery from this, his pulse rate is 38 beats/min. Discuss your management of him, both diagnostic and therapeutic, from this moment.

5. How would you examine a patient whom you suspect of having a space-occupying lesion in the right cerebral hemisphere.

6. Discuss the drugs used in Parkinson's disease with specific reference to control of symptoms and side-effects.

7. An ambulance team brings a comatose middle-aged woman into the accident and emergency department. How would you assess her level of consciousness and what causes of her condition would you consider?

Self-assessment: answers

Multiple choice answers

1. a. **True**. The triceps is affected in a crutch palsy.

   b. **False**. It is the median nerve (**thenar** eminence) that is commonly damaged.

   c. **False**. The little and ring fingers are affected.

   d. **False**. There is no deformity of the index finger (lumbrical supplied by median nerve).

   e. **False**. There is little sensory loss.

2. a. **False**. Drug levels are used simply to assess overall compliance.

   b. **False**. All the main drugs are associated with some teratogenicity.

   c. **False**. You must know the medico-legal position on epilepsy (p. 236): for an ordinary car licence in the UK, it is the fit-free period that counts (1 year), not withdrawal of treatment.

   d. **True**. It should only be used in a high-dependency unit.

   e. **False**. Sodium valproate is *not* an enzyme inducer (unlike carbamazepine and phenytoin).

3. a. **False**. A vermis lesion will result in gross *truncal* ataxia.

   b. **False**. Macular sparing is a feature of occipital lobe damage.

   c. **False**. Visuo-spatial inattention can occur with left-sided lesions, but it is more common with *right* hemisphere problems.

   d. **False**. Agnosia is a problem with interpretation of sensory information (see agnosia and dyspraxia, p. 210).

   e. **True**. Remember other higher cortical functions, e.g. dysphasia, dyslexia.

4. a. **False**. After a TIA, the absolute risk of stroke is 5–10% per year.

   b. **True**. In symptomatic patients with 70–99% stenosis (not occluded) endartectomy is beneficial.

   c. **True**. Treating elderly hypertensive people is cost-effective because of their high absolute risk.

   d. **False**. Anticoagulation is of proven benefit for those in *atrial fibrillation*.

   e. **True**. If the patient's absolute risk of something happening is extremely small, they are not going to get much benefit from an intervention.

5. a. **True**. Complete paralysis of the lateral rectus leaves the medial rectus unopposed, thus producing a convergent strabismus, though mostly the paralysis is only brought out when the eye is abducted.

   b. **True**. Diplopia is maximal on looking in the direction of the primary action of the muscle.

   c. **True**. Unlike a superior oblique palsy.

   d. **False**. False image is always displaced furthest in the direction of action of the muscle: in this case, looking to the right.

   e. **False**. Images become increasingly separated looking to the right.

6. a. **True**. The chorda tympani runs along the facial nerve.

   b. **True**. The facial nerve supplies the orbicularis oculi muscle, which closes the eye. In addition, an absent or diminished corneal reflex may be an early sign of an acoustic neuroma.

   c. **False**. Logical though it might be, the facial nerve does *not* supply the parotid gland; the glossopharyngeal nerve does.

   d. **False**. Many patients with a facial nerve palsy will say that their face feels 'funny', but on examination there will not be any sensory signs.

   e. **False**. Sweating is controlled through sympathetic fibres (impaired in Horner's syndrome).

7. a. **True**. Although the mechanism is unclear, it does involve loss of dopaminergic neurones.

   b. **True**. Cogwheel rigidity is a superimposed tremor on the 'lead pipe' increase in tone.

   c. **False**. Patients with tardive dyskinesia have slow stereotypic movements such as 'tromboning' of the tongue. It is associated with neuroleptic (e.g. haloperidol) treatment causing a blockade of dopamine receptors, which become supersensitive (upregulated).

   d. **False**. Intention tremor is a sign of cerebellar disease.

   e. **True**. To festinate means to hurry/accelerate — always trying to catch up with the centre of gravity.

8. a. **False**. It is slightly more common in females.

   b. **False**. Papilloedema and loss of pupillary reflexes are *not* features, but over 90% have ocular involvement (diplopia).

   c. **False**. In muscle or neuromuscular disease, tendon reflexes are usually preserved, unlike in a peripheral neuropathy.

   d. **False**. There is blockade of the acetylcholine receptor on the muscle endplate by antibodies.

   e. **False**. Fasciculation is brief spontaneous contraction of muscle fibres causing a flicker of movement under the skin; it is often associated with motor neurone disease. In myasthenia gravis, fasciculation would imply overtreatment with anticholinesterases.

9. a. **True.** An aura would suggest partial epilepsy.

   b. **False.** This suggests attention-seeking behaviour.

c. **True.** A stroboscopic effect is known to occur when watching TV or playing video games, and in clubs.

d. **False.** This is indicative of agoraphobia, although this is unusual in a young person.

e. **False.** This suggests a vasovagal attack.

10. a. **True.** Antisocial behaviour is more in keeping with the personality change of dementia.

b. **False.** Mutism can occur in depression.

c. **False.** Short duration of symptoms suggests depression.

d. **False.** Diurnal variation suggests depression.

e. **False.** Poor concentration can also occur in depression.

11. a. **True.** Polio, Coxsackie virus and enterovirus all cause viral meningitis. Early in viral meningitis, up to 90% of the white cells may be polymorphs, changing to lymphocytes over the next few days.

b. **True.** Although it is a rare cause and virtually always associated with other (e.g. pulmonary, skin) manifestations of disease and cerebral lesions on CT scan.

c. **True.** It is relatively common in patients with AIDS or lymphoma and in transplant recipients; also occasionally occurs in non-immunocompromised patients.

d. **True.** The most common cause worldwide of *chronic* lymphocytic meningitis; early in disease neutrophils may predominate in CSF.

e. **True.** However, it usually causes viral encephalitis with few cells in the CSF. Impaired consciousness is a hallmark of encephalitis.

12. a. **True.** However, if correctable (e.g. haemophiliac) and the indication for lumbar puncture is strong enough, then it should be corrected and the lumbar puncture carried out.

b. **False.** It is the presence of a mass lesion and displacement of the ventricular system that leads to papilloedema which is the contraindication. It is essential to do a lumbar puncture in some circumstances — for example, in benign intracranial hypertension for diagnostic and therapeutic reasons — despite papilloedema.

c. **False.** Given the number of lumbar punctures done for myelograms and other investigations, the incidence of meningitis following lumbar puncture is exceptionally rare.

d. **False.** Coning (the brainstem being forced down into the foramen magnum) is *not* related to the amount of CSF removed. It is related to a mass lesion *and* high intracranial pressure. In fact, after a lumbar puncture is done, much more CSF leaks out from the dural hole than is removed during the procedure. So you should try to take at least 5 ml of CSF for diagnostic purposes.

e. **False.** Most post-lumbar puncture headache is not related to anything other than entering the epidural space. A small minority of cases are related to continued leakage of CSF through the dura. A blood patch procedure is helpful if post-lumbar puncture headache persists beyond 5 or 7 days.

13. a. **True.** Many infections lead to a confusional state and/or drowsiness, including pneumonia. Remember to check the arterial gases if conscious level is poor, or if there is a raised respiratory rate or chest signs and/or chest radiograph infiltrate.

b. **True.** Classical presentation with neck stiffness, often with focal neurological signs.

c. **True.** Cerebral malaria is common in late presentations (e.g. after 3–5 days of illness) and there may be few parasites in the peripheral blood.

d. **False.** If conscious level is impaired, then it is *not* simply viral meningitis. If the problem is intracranial, it may be bacterial meningitis, viral encephalitis, fungal meningitis, brain abscess, subdural empyema or a vascular event. Urgent admission and investigation is absolutely necessary.

e. **True.** With other typical features, e.g. sudden onset, pinpoint pupils.

14. a. **True.** Mortality is highest in elderly people.

b. **True.** Delays lead to increased mortality and morbidity.

c. **True.** The CSF concentration of antibiotic needs to exceed by 20-fold the minimum inhibitory concentration of the infecting organism. This is the primary reason why i.v. therapy is necessary in meningitis.

d. **False.** Apart from rare Gram-negative meningitis, this does not happen. However, there is an increasing problem of penicillin resistance in *Streptococcus pneumoniae*, which would necessitate therapy with vancomycin.

e. **True.** *Neisseria meningitidis* has a lower mortality than *Strep. pneumoniae* meningitis. Furthermore about 5% of community-acquired cases are caused by other organisms, such as *Listeria monocytogenes*. *Listeria* is intrinsically resistant to all cephalosporins, which are now the most common first-line treatment for meningitis.

Single best answer multiple choice answers

1. **c is correct.** The history of trauma, brief loss of consciousness and apparent lucidity followed by collapse is typical. She needs an urgent scan and neurosurgical review.

2. **d is correct.** The history is suggestive of raised intracranial pressure. Although this might be due to a brain tumour, the BMI and oral contraceptive pill point to benign intracranial hypertension, which needs immediate admission and investigation (MR scan initially) because of the risk to vision.

3. **b is correct.** The history and examination findings are highly suggestive of a subarachnoid haemorrhage. It is typical that the headache is severe and is most intense at onset. A plain CT scan is best for showing blood in the subarachnoid space.

4. **e is correct.** The history could be due to spinal compression (disc, tumour) in the lumbar or thoracic region, but the back pain (at the onset), then progressive paralysis of the legs and hands with sensory disturbance, is consistent with Guillain–Barré syndrome.

5. **a is correct.** The history of confusion soon after a neurology review suggests that her treatment was altered. The blood tests show significant hyponatraemia, which causes confusion and is a known side-effect of carbamazepine.

6. **d is correct.** Meningococcal and viral meningitis is often preceded by sore throat. Streptococcal sore throat can cause neck stiffness (as can *Shigella* and *Salmonella* gastroenteritis, without meningitis); hence the question. Answer a is nearly true, except that in classical meningococcaemia with a purpuric rash, the diagnosis is not in doubt and resistance in *Neisseria meningitidis* is not a problem. b is false. Not only are several rarer organisms causing meningitis intrinsically resistant to penicillin (i.e. *Mycobacterium tuberculosis*, *Listeria monocytogenes*, *Haemophilus influenzae* and *Escherichia coli*) but there is increasing resistance in *Strep. pneumoniae*. c is nearly true. If the final diagnosis is bacterial meningitis, an HIV test is not indicated for this reason alone. If it is aseptic or viral meningitis, then yes, it is indicated in most cases (in adults) as primary HIV infection is a cause of viral/aseptic/lymphocytic meningitis. e is false. Clotting test results are needed only if a history of bleeding or bruising is present. This only delays the procedure and reduces the microbiological yield of the lumbar puncture.

7. **c is the best answer.** a is false. These are necessary components of 'meningoencephalitis' but could describe bacterial meningitis (which in reality is usually a bacterial meningoencephalitis, but this is not a term in current usage). b is false. This describes an aseptic or viral meningitis or tuberculous or cryptococcal meningitis. d describes aseptic or viral meningitis. e is false as there is an ever broader differential including staphylococcal sepsis or necrobacillosis, for example.

8. **c is the best answer.** West Nile virus mimics polio and, like polio, is usually asymmetrical. a is false. Neurological features of primary HIV infection include an aseptic meningitis, meningoencephalitis and transverse myelitis; late-stage HIV includes infection, peripheral neuropathy, dementia and autonomic neuropathy, but not an acute flaccid paralysis. Few clinical syndromes are associated with acute HTLV 1 infection but long-term infection may cause tropical spastic paraparesis. d is nearly true. Acute intermittent porphyria presents as a

confusional state or 'crisis', often with severe pain, which impairs movement and includes absent reflexes. Acute lead poisoning leads to an acute encephalopathy, chronic lead poisoning to reduced mental acuity and a peripheral neuropathy, but not acute flaccid paralysis.

Extended matched answers

EMQ 1

A. **1.** The history is vague but points towards a general decrease in cognition, particularly affecting calculation. The examination findings and the memory impairment confirm this.

B. **8.** The truncal ataxia is consistent with a midline cerebellar vermis lesion. The previous episode is likely to have involved the corticospinal tract. The age of the patient with two episodes affecting different parts of the central nervous system makes multiple sclerosis very likely.

C. **3.** The patient has signs of parkinsonism. In view of the absence of a tremor, the symmetrical signs and treatment of paranoid ideas it is most probably caused by treatment with a neuroleptic drug.

D. **7.** This patient has a progressive problem that is characterised by asymmetrical signs involving both upper and lower motor neurones.

E. **2.** The main differential diagnosis is between a stroke and a tumour. The progressive history over a few weeks makes the latter highly probable.

EMQ 2

A. **3.** The cerebellum and its connections are not crossed, so incoordination on the left side implies impairment on that side.

B. **7.** Deep pain is transmitted via the posterior columns (tested in the lower limbs by squeezing the Achilles tendon — but only do it after explaining to the patient!). Light touch is transmitted by both the spinothalamic and the posterior columns.

C. **2.** Changes in tone are not mediated by the pyramidal (corticospinal) tracts; many patients with strokes (and other conditions) have normal or low tone.

D. **5.** Pain and temperature fibres entering the cord ascend for a few segments, before crossing over. Hence, external compression gives rise to a band of abnormal sensation on the side of the compression and loss of pinprick sensation below this on the opposite side of the body.

E. **7.** Patients with marked posterior column dysfunction in the cervical cord (often multiple sclerosis) lose all joint position in their hands and fingers. When their eyes are closed, their fingers move to try to provide some information on their position in space (pseudo-athetosis).

EMQ 3

A. 2. The history of atrial fibrillation and right-sided weakness might indicate transient ischaemic attacks, but the intermittent confusion, falls and warfarin point to a subdural haematoma. She needs an urgent CT scan.

B. 6. The examination findings are consistent with Parkinson's disease. The combination of fluctuation with visual hallucinations is typical of this type of dementia (p. 234).

C. 4. The history of bereavement and distress points to her GP prescribing either an antidepressant or an anxiolytic to help. The time course is suggestive of the confusion dating from this visit. All tests are normal, which is against another cause such as an infection.

D. 7. The history of drowsiness, confusion, tongue biting and incontinence suggests that this patient has had a seizure. A normal CT scan excludes other causes such as a intracranial bleed.

E. 3. The progressive neurological symptoms with dysphasia, dyspraxia and right-sided weakness indicate a space-occupying lesion in the left cerebral hemisphere. The general examination findings and the basic investigations do not suggest metastatic disease.

Responses to OSCE stations

OSCE 1

This station could have a different introduction without the clear steer from the examiner that the patient has given permission for you to speak to his wife. OSCE stations can be designed to address attitudes and other important ethical and medico-legal issues. Many students simply address the medical content of a station (TIA and what facts need to be conveyed) and ignore other professional behaviours.

This station is not constructed to test your ability to 'break bad news', e.g. the unconscious patient with a severe stroke who is unlikely to live or regain independence. However, many of the same principles apply (warning shots, clear simple language, listening and observing how the person responds, offering to come back to explain again).

You would be assessed against the following criteria:

- Did you introduce yourself and give your post (e.g. house officer, foundation trainee)?
- Did you consider where you might talk to the person (at the bedside, office)?
- Did you explain about a TIA using simple language (questioning people understand the terms: artery, ischaemia, etc.)?
- Did you explain what will happen next (investigations, risk of stroke)?
- Did you give the person good opportunities to ask questions ('Is there anything you would like to ask me?')?

Suggestions for further practice Take any opportunity to sit in on/observe a junior doctor (and senior) talking to carers/relatives. Concentrate on the communication skills being used rather than the medical content. Consider how the carer reacted and was involved.

OSCE 2

The criteria for marking this station would probably include:

- MRI stands for magnetic resonance imaging.
- There is no risk to the patient (and the test is also safe in pregnancy) nor any after-effects.
- It uses magnetic waves to build a picture of the body.
- It involves lying down on a stretcher that goes into a tunnel. Some patients can find it claustrophobic.
- It can be noisy — so you may be offered ear plugs.
- You cannot wear anything metal (e.g. jewellery, watches, rings, earrings).
- Patients cannot usually be scanned if they have pacemakers or metal implants.

The examiner would also want you to demonstrate:

- introduction
- clarification of what the patient understands about the test already (so as to start at an appropriate baseline)
- giving opportunities for the patient to express concerns and responding to these empathically with clear information.

Case history answers

Case history 1

1. The patient describes left amaurosis fugax and a left cerebral hemisphere transient ischaemic attack.

2. Major risk factors that can be targeted are hypertension, cardiac emboli in atrial fibrillation and carotid stenosis. In addition, a basic screen can be justified, which should include a full blood count (thrombocythaemia, polycythaemia rubra vera), erythrocyte sedimentation rate (ESR) (vasculitis), lipids, urea and electrolytes (renal impairment; hypertension) and chest radiograph (cardiomegaly). A 12-lead electrocardiogram (ECG) as well as careful cardiovascular examination will determine the rhythm and whether there is evidence of serious heart disease (valve, muscle). An echocardiogram may be required (valves, left ventricular function, hypertrophy). The presence or absence of a **carotid bruit** is not of value (high false-positive and false-negative rates); the patient needs ultrasound examination of his carotid arteries. A CT or MR scan is now recommended in most protocols.

3. The treatment will depend on the risk factors identified. Advice on lifestyle (smoking, weight, diet, etc.) is important. Remember that he is diabetic and, as such, is at greater absolute risk of a vascular event. At the very least, he should be started on low-dose aspirin (75 mg) and his blood pressure checked (target 130/80 or less). If he is in atrial fibrillation, he

should be given anticoagulation therapy unless there is a strong contraindication. A statin should be started to lower cholesterol to less than 5 mmol/l. If he has a 70% or greater stenosis of his left common or internal carotid artery (but not occlusion), carotid endarterectomy should be advised, whilst counselling him about the small risk of the operation resulting in a major stroke or death (2% upwards, depending on the surgeon).

4. The emergency tests for a patient with an acute stroke are outlined in Table 55.

5. He has had a major stroke: probably total anterior circulation infarction (TACI), either from occlusion of the middle cerebral or the internal carotid artery, though it is possible that he has had a major haemorrhage. The outlook is very bleak. The vast majority of patients who are unconscious at 24 hours following their stroke will die and most of the survivors will be very disabled.

6. If he survives, then the initial management will be to avoid complications. Major ones are deep-vein thrombosis (CT scan within 7 days would exclude a cerebral haemorrhage and allow the use of prophylactic heparin therapy) and aspiration pneumonia; impairment of swallowing is very common. If these are present, the patient should have fluid and nutrition by another route. Other complications to consider are epilepsy, shoulder subluxation and urinary tract infection (particularly with use of a catheter). He should be assessed by a specialist for possible transfer to a stroke rehabilitation unit, but it is likely that he will remain dependent and will require long-term nursing care.

Case history 2

1. The history is a subacute progressive illness with probable paralysis of her legs. This is consistent with Guillain–Barré syndrome, which often has a prodromal minor infection and back pain. Other possibilities would be a spinal cord compression, possibly caused by an epidural abscess, but this is rare and usually there would be more systemic disturbance. Polio is now exceedingly uncommon and, in this case, the sensory symptoms are against the diagnosis. In a young woman, the symptoms may be the first manifestation of multiple sclerosis causing impairment of bladder function. Appropriate investigations should be done (including MR scan).

Case history 3

1. The diagnosis is motor neurone disease. The patient has dysarthria, which implies problems with articulation. This may be caused by cerebellar disease or damage to the bulbar musculature, at the level of either upper or lower motor neurones. The difficulty in swallowing and recurrent chest infections imply repeated aspiration, again pointing to impaired function of the bulbar musculature. The

time course is relatively long and the disease is progressive; neither fits with cerebrovascular disease. The electrophysiological studies show denervation but relatively normal conduction velocities, implying that the damage is to the axons of the α-motor neurones rather than demyelination. The abnormalities in the legs demonstrate a widespread disease process.

2. All of the features point to motor neurone disease. However, if sensory disturbance was present, the diagnosis becomes untenable. Another diagnostic possibility would be a non-metastatic manifestation of malignancy. Myasthenia gravis or Eaton–Lambert syndrome could be considered, but the electrophysiological studies are against these. With sensory abnormalities around the face, the very rare possibility of syringobulbia (a cavity or **syrinx** in the medulla) might be considered.

3. The initial situation is one of breaking bad news, given that the patient has an incurable progressive disease that is going to cause paralysis (but not loss of cognition) and eventual death. The key to longer-term management is multidisciplinary (p. 235). In this case, immediate issues are communication and swallowing problems. An assessment by a speech and language therapist is needed and, the patient may need videofluoroscopic examination of swallowing. In anarthria, alternative communication aids are needed and, if swallowing is severely disturbed, then a percutaneous endoscopic gastrostomy (PEG) may be inserted endoscopically.

Case history 4

1. a. **False.** The travel history is important but there are other immediate priorities; however, you do want to know about recent travel.

   b. **True.** When you take blood, but blood culture and CSF are more important.

   c. **False.** Absolutely the wrong action. He represents your first priority in the whole hospital because he probably has an acute life-threatening infection and time is of the essence. If a crash call came just as you were assessing him, you should still ensure he is given antibiotics immediately.

   d. **False.** Should be done, but not yet as it will not alter your immediate management.

   e. **True.** Very important to act swiftly. You should undress him so you can carefully inspect his skin for petechiae typical of meningococcal disease. Look especially around his wrists, ankles, sides of trunk and conjunctivae. Also look immediately for neck stiffness.

2. a. **True.** As quickly as possible in a large dose, e.g. 2 g cefotaxime and 10 g dexamethasone.

   b. **True.** While he is being given his first dose of antibiotics.

   c. **False.** Although coagulopathy is a contraindication to lumbar puncture, he does not have any features suggestive of disseminated intravascular coagulation or a history of haemophilia.

d. **False.** No need as no focal neurological features. If you did the CT scan first, you would be practising defensive, not good, medicine.

e. **False.** Anticonvulsants are not indicated routinely in patients with meningitis, unless they are already taking them or have had a fit.

3. a. **True.** You should have him put in a side room, as quiet is important for these patients with severe headache, and because of the risk of transmission. With the incidence of penicillin-resistant pneumococci increasing, this is more and more important. Ideally, these patients should be admitted to an infectious disease unit.

b. **True.** For 24–48 hours, depending on your hospital's policy.

c. **False.** Only to those sharing the same house and/or bed. The only hospital staff who require prophylaxis are those who have given mouth-to-mouth resuscitation.

d. **True.** Very important, as there could be an evolving outbreak requiring public health measures immediately. **Telephone** notifications are required for meningococcal disease, typhoid and viral haemorrhagic fever.

e. **True.** On balance he will survive (90% chance) but there is still a risk of unilateral or bilateral deafness or other deficit. However, you should be cautious on your first discussion of outcome, until it is clear how he is responding to treatment.

Key features answers

1. MR scan. The patient has a left acoustic neuroma. A key feature is the left sided sensorineural deafness (Weber's and Rinne's tests). The diminished corneal reflex (sensory-trigeminal and motor-facial nerves) is a 'hard' neurological sign, which in this context localises the problem to the left cerebellar-pontine angle. A CT scan can be helpful, but due to the proximity of bone, an MR scan is a better imaging technique. The management is surgical removal.

2. Presumed left pyelonephritis. Patients with multiple sclerosis can develop epilepsy as the disease progresses. However, it is important to search for a trigger for seizures. In this case, the prodromal symptoms suggest an infection. A patient may have a pyrexia following a seizure, but 39°C suggests that it is due to another cause. The next question is the source of the infection. An indwelling catheter predisposes the patient to an ascending urinary tract infection and the pain suggests a pyelonephritis. The management will involve investigations (full blood count, urea and electrolytes (kidney function), blood cultures) and fluids, oxygen and antibiotics (e.g. cefuroxime — a broad-spectrum covering Gram-negative organisms). Culture and microscopy of the urine is likely to be unhelpful, as white cells and organisms will be present. However, if the patient does not respond, then it may help in choice of antibiotic. An ultrasound would also be indicated (drainage of the kidneys, abscess, perinephric collection).

3. MR angiography. The patient presents with sudden onset of left-sided signs, including a probable left homonymous hemianopia, which is consistent with a left partial anterior cerebral stroke (PACS). This is unusual in a woman of this age (you would want to know more from her history, including contraception), but also the onset was during (strenuous) exercise, the patient has facial and neck pain and she has a left Horner's syndrome. This points to a dissection of the left carotid artery, which can occur spontaneously or following trauma. The sympathetic fibres run up around the artery to re-enter the skull; if they are damaged, this will result in a Horner's syndrome. MR angiography will show an occluded carotid possibly with a false lumen or clot.

4. Asymmetrical signs, lead pipe rigidity, stooped posture, festinant gait, bradykinesia, pill-rolling tremor, micrographia. Parkinson's disease can be difficult to diagnose in the early stages. Patients often complain of just slowing up. The difficulty in turning over in bed (with subsequent aches and pains) is characteristic. Similarly, dysphonia (loss of volume of voice) may be noticed. Unlike parkinsonism, Parkinson's disease is usually asymmetrical, particularly in the early stages.

Data interpretation answers

1. The data show impending respiratory failure. The patient has a deteriorating hypoxia, hypercarbia (ventilatory failure: type 2) and a respiratory acidosis. The immediate management would be to ask a consultant in intensive care to see the patient with a view to ventilation. Action should have been taken on the first set of results.

Patient A Consistent with herpes simplex encephalitis; consider subarachnoid haemorrhage.

Patient B Typical of viral encephalitis, possibly herpes simplex, and would still be treated with aciclovir for 10 days or until diagnosis clear. Rule out HIV infection (primary), West Nile virus and enterovirus infection (defined in Table 51).

Patient C Most likely a subarachnoid haemorrhage or a bloody tap. Key information is missing here: namely, whether xanthochromia is present or not. If it is, subarachnoid haemorrhage is most likely.

Patient D Bacterial meningitis.

Patient E Viral meningitis (up to 90% of white cells may be polymorphs; in bacterial meningitis over 99% are polymorphs, with the sole exception of *Listeria* meningitis).

Patient F Tuberculous meningitis. Often the protein is higher than this. It could be fungal meningitis or, rarely, sarcoidosis.

Picture answers

1. a. The most important question is whether the weakness developed suddenly and is now improving (suggesting a vascular cause — stroke) or whether it is progressive. If it is the latter, it should lead to suspicion of a tumour.

   b. The patient has an irregular large lesion in the right temporo-parietal region. It is predominantly low-density (black) with enhancement by contrast. The surrounding brain tissue is also low-density (high water content — oedema). There may be some compression of the right lateral ventricle, but there is no displacement across the midline.

   c. The appearances are caused by a tumour. The differential diagnosis is between a primary brain tumour and a solitary metastasis. When the mass is solitary, it is impossible to decide between the two diagnoses. You should consider common causes of metastatic disease, such as a bronchial carcinoma (chest radiograph).

   d. The clock face shows left-sided neglect. This is caused by the tumour in his non-dominant hemisphere. Less commonly, neglect is seen in left (dominant) hemisphere lesions.

   e. The drawing test points to a problem that is likely to have a major impact on his day-to-day function. He may deny any neurological problems (anosagnosia) and may try to walk regardless of his paralysis. He may injure his left side because of not attending to it when doing things. He may fail to register objects/people in his left visual field. Food may remain uneaten on the left-hand side of his plate. The left side of his body may not be dressed. The message is that visuospatial problems (neglect) cause a greater disability/handicap than simply weakness down one side.

2. a. The CT scan (Fig. 62B) shows areas of low attenuation (hypodensity) in both the left (most) and right occipital cortices.

   b. She has had infarction in both the occipital lobes. A scan done very early (<24 hours: Fig. 62A) following infarction will be normal, as the changes take time to develop. In haemorrhage, the high density (owing to the blood) is visible immediately but then becomes isodense and eventually hypodense. Therefore, a CT scan should be done immediately to diagnose haemorrhage but delayed a few days to diagnose infarction. In a stroke, the compromise is to arrange a scan at around 3 days.

   c. Bilateral occipital lobe damage will result in loss of vision. Patients often do not complain of profound visual loss because the 'receiving'

station has been damaged and so they are unaware that they should be seeing things.

   d. The occipital lobes are supplied by the posterior cerebral arteries, which are the final branches of the vertebrobasilar system. The posterior cerebral artery gives off some penetrating vessels to the posterior limb of the internal capsule (anterior fibres, motor; posterior, sensory).

3. a. The patient is on anticoagulants and has become drowsy. The concern is that he has intracerebral bleeding and you may have to reverse his anticoagulation. A scan will demonstrate this.

   b. The scan (Fig. 63) shows an area of high attenuation surrounded by a rim of low attenuation deep in the left cerebral hemisphere adjacent to the basal ganglia. These appearances are caused by a cerebral haemorrhage.

   c. You should measure his prothrombin time (International Normalised Ratio) and discuss the problem with the haematologist urgently. The patient may need factor concentrate and the reversal of anticoagulation, with vitamin K. The problem with the latter is that it makes it very difficult to re-establish the patient on anticoagulation therapy for several days.

4. a. The CT scan (Fig. 64) shows extensive blood in the ventricular system (lateral ventricles) and also in the subarachnoid space ('brightness' around the sulci). The appearances are caused by a large subarachnoid haemorrhage with ventricular extension. More commonly, blood will be seen in the subarachnoid space.

   b. You should contact the nearest neurosurgical unit to discuss transfer. Given the severity of the bleed, her prognosis is very poor.

   c. The three complications of subarachnoid haemorrhage that you should consider are: risk of re-bleeding; development of vasospasm, which may produce focal neurological deficits (particularly in the territory where the aneurysm is situated); and, with extensive blood in the subarachnoid space and ventricular system, a communicating or non-communicating hydrocephalus. This is likely to present with drowsiness and vomiting owing to increasing intracranial pressure. Management is by insertion of a shunt.

5. a. The patient has a left wrist drop owing to a radial nerve lesion.

   b. You should demonstrate her inability to extend her wrist. If the lesion is in the axilla (crutch palsy), then triceps will be involved and she will have weakness of elbow extension. If the damage is to the radial nerve in the spiral groove of the humerus (Saturday night palsy), then triceps is spared. When examining the rest of the hand, fixate the wrist on a flat surface; otherwise the intrinsic muscles of the hand will appear weak and you will erroneously diagnose median and ulnar nerve palsies.

c. Most likely she has developed this problem because of pressure on the radial nerve from the wheelchair rest as the arm hangs over the side.

6. a. He has a true 'claw' hand with hyperextension of the metacarpophalangeal joints and flexion of the interphalangeal joints.

b. It is caused by weakness of the intrinsic muscles of the hand with consequent unopposed action of the long extensors of the metacarpophalangeal joints. It is probably caused by a T1 lesion rather than combined ulnar and median nerve palsies. It is not caused by an ulnar nerve lesion alone as this causes clawing that is confined to the fourth and fifth fingers.

c. Possible causes are a dumb-bell tumour of the T1 nerve root (schwannoma — neurofibromatosis), cervical rib, syringomyelia or Pancoast tumour.

Short notes answers

1. Breaking bad news is always difficult. Here, you are being asked to provide more information to a relative, when the diagnosis has already been disclosed. Sketch out your answer using the framework in the question. The first task would be to go over what Alzheimer's disease is. Alongside this, explain that the diagnosis is based on clinical findings, but if in doubt, you might ask for a detailed psychological assessment. The daughter may have heard of donepezil (anticholinesterase). Research studies have shown its usefulness in mild-to-moderate Alzheimer's disease. Whilst explaining about the drug treatment, emphasise the support that is available from the different agencies. In a general medical unit, involve the old-age psychiatrists. As well as support, they can advise on the use of donepezil (or another anticholinesterase). An important principle is to try not to remove hope. Whilst Alzheimer's disease is progressive, for many patients the course is relatively slow over a number of years.

   People may feel very angry about serious illness — partly related to the apparent injustice of the condition 'picking out' either them or one of their close relatives. The anger may focus on you or on the health services in general. Acknowledge people's right to anger in the situation they find themselves in and do not react to it personally. You should remain calm, responding reasonably to questions and issues. At the end of the interview, you should offer to see the person again.

2. a. This patient is, by definition, in status epilepticus and requires senior help. The first task is to go through the 'ABC' routine: airway, breathing, circulation. The second is to control the fits; the usual treatment is with intravenous or rectal diazepam. The next step (which should start immediately) is to gather information. Is the patient a known epileptic? If yes, has there been

any change in the medication or compliance? In a patient who is not a known epileptic (and even in a patient with epilepsy), the major causes are:
- intracranial, e.g. infection, trauma, vascular, tumour, etc.
- systemic, e.g. overdose (tricyclic antidepressants), hypoglycaemia (diabetes) and metabolic disturbance (e.g. hyponatraemia).

   Your **history-taking** (witnesses, carers, etc.), examination and initial investigations should be done keeping this framework in mind.

   Management is governed by your diagnostic list and your overall assessment of the patient's condition, e.g. fluid balance, ventilatory status. In a person who has not been previously diagnosed as being epileptic, you will probably need to start prophylactic anticonvulsants. A *loading dose* (much higher than maintenance dose) of phenytoin can be given i.v. (i.m. doses are very poorly absorbed). The patient may need admission to the intensive care unit, with the fitting controlled by a clomethiazole or thiopental infusion. Some patients are managed by paralysis and ventilation.

b. The patient is probably in crisis: either myasthenic or cholinergic. You must consider other causes, e.g. infection (or treatment with aminoglycosides). As with the patient (2a) above, your first task is to check ABC. In a person with myasthenia, the 'B' of the assessment is very important. You must measure and record the peak flow rate and arterial blood gases. Ask for senior help/advice; be very careful with a patient who might be tiring and will rapidly deteriorate into ventilatory failure.

3. a. In neurological disease, the first question to ask is 'where is the anatomical site of the problem?' In this case the symptoms point to the retina/optic nerve. The second question relates to the time course. If the problem was vascular, then the history would be of a sudden onset; here it is more gradual and would suggest something evolving. The description best fits with optic neuritis, probably caused by multiple sclerosis.

b. The description is of a left homonymous hemianopia. In the optic tracts and radiation this is usually complete, but in the occipital cortex, the macula may be spared.

c. The bitemporal hemianopia is characteristic of damage around the chiasma. When the problem starts with the *lower* fields, it relates to compression from *above* (think of opposites), possibly because of a craniopharyngioma.

d. The history is consistent with cytomegalovirus retinitis in AIDS. The retinal appearances are characteristic, with white exudates and haemorrhage: 'cottage cheese and ketchup' or 'pizza' (p. 389).

4. In the initial description, there are a number of facts that put the case into context. In a man of this age, think of the common pathologies: for example, ischaemic heart disease. The dizziness followed by a seizure implies cerebral anoxia, especially when coupled with the bradycardia after the event. Going down this path, the description is in keeping with a **Stokes–Adams attack** (p. 27). Another possibility would be a dysrhythmia/reduction in cardiac output in association with an acute myocardial infarction. The initial management would be to obtain a 12-lead ECG (not simply a rhythm strip) and consider monitoring on the coronary care unit. Troponin measurement may be helpful. The second path is to think about intracranial causes and examine for focal neurological signs. In a patient with raised intracranial pressure, a bradycardia may occur in conjunction with rising blood pressure. Acutely, this could be caused by bleeding; longer-term, the patient may have an intracranial tumour, either primary or secondary.

   You should obtain more information. Is the patient a diabetic? In any case, a blood glucose measurement must be done. Is the patient a known epileptic? Has the patient taken an overdose? Tricyclic antidepressants usually cause a tachycardia, but digoxin could cause heart block.

5. The question is asking you to focus your examination on the particular signs that you might expect. The answer is not a 'full neurological examination'. You need to check for evidence of raised intracranial pressure: drowsiness, loss of retinal vein pulsation, papilloedema, bradycardia, hypertension. Damage to the right hemisphere is going to cause symptoms on the left side of the body: hemiparesis, hemisensory loss, hemianopia. Particular problems with the right (non-dominant) hemisphere would be inattention and neglect of the left side (visual/sensory). In association with this, the patient may deny any problems (anosagnosia) and may have problems with dressing. Is the patient right- or left-handed? If left-handed then, in 20% of patients, there might still be impairment of language. If the lesion is in the parietal lobe, there may be particular problems (does not depend on the side of the lesion). Check for arm drift, **astereoagnosis** (inability to integrate the sensory and motor systems to identify an object in the hand), **graphaesthesia** (inability to identify numbers drawn on the hand) and impaired **two-point discrimination**.

   You should also consider the rest of the patient. Is this a brain abscess or a tumour? Are there any clues to the aetiology on general physical examination?

6. Details for this question are given on page 232 and in Table 56. Remember that anticholinergic drugs are used to ameliorate the tremor (limited effect). Side-effects include blurred vision, dry mouth, urinary retention and constipation (blockage of cholinergic receptors). The main aim of therapy is to preserve/boost transmission at the dopamine receptor either by using L-dopa or a dopamine agonist (in the later stages these may be combined). The side-effects are listed in Table 56. Discuss the pharmacokinetics of the drugs in relation to the dosage regimens: for example, the phenomena of **on-off** and **peak dose effects**.

7. The question is emphasising the importance of being able to assess conscious level using the Glasgow Coma Scale (Table 54). Terms such as semiconscious, stuporose, etc. mean different things to different people and you should not use them. The number of possible causes are huge. Consider two steps: first, division into 'brain' causes and 'non-brain' causes; second, filter these by incidence, i.e. causes in a middle-aged woman; see Box 17.

Haematology

6.1 Background

Learning objectives

You should:
- know what to ask about in the haematological history and what to look for on examination
- know when to measure and how to interpret a full blood count, film and erythrocyte sedimentation rate (ESR)
- understand the other main haematological investigations and when to carry them out
  - haematinics: iron and total iron-binding capacity, ferritin, vitamin B_{12}, folate and red cell folate
  - coagulation tests: international normalised ratio (INR), prothrombin time (PT), activated partial thromboplastin time (APTT), plasma fibrinogen, D-dimer, tests for inherited thrombophilia
  - investigation of haemoglobinopathy, including sickle screen and haemoglobin electrophoresis
- know the indications for, and the information that can be gained from bone marrow examination and lymph node biopsy
- know which situations commonly confront a house officer and understand how to manage them
- know enough about the other major haematological diseases to recognise them, make appropriate and timely referrals and explain them to your patients.

Case Study

An elderly woman has lived alone and done her own shopping and housework until she is admitted with angina. Her conjunctivae are pale. Non-pathological lymph nodes can be felt in the axillae and groins, but her liver and spleen are impalpable. She has a haemoglobin of 40 g/l, mean cell volume of 120 fl and platelet count of 50×10^9/l. Her blood film shows hypersegmented neutrophils. It seems she may have pernicious anaemia.

This chapter is structured around disorders of:

- red cells
- white cells
- platelets
- coagulation.

Remember, however, that individual diseases commonly affect more than one element.

Physiology

The marrow is a large organ, approaching the size of the liver. In adults, most of it is in the flat bones, including the sternum, pelvis and vertebrae. White blood cell precursors form 75% of the marrow and most of the rest consists of erythroid precursors. Megakaryocytes (from which platelets are formed) are scattered throughout. It may seem surprising that so much of the marrow is devoted to the white cell series, given that there are 500 times as many red cells as white cells in the circulation. However, erythrocytes have a mean life of 120 days whereas white cells have a circulating lifespan measured in hours. Even in health, marrow is an extremely active tissue which is able to respond to sudden stresses like haemorrhage and infection. All blood cells are derived from multipotent, uncommitted stem cells. These differentiate into the lines of committed stem cells from which red cells, platelets, monocytes, granulocytes and lymphocytes are formed. The processes of differentiation and proliferation are controlled by growth factors, including interleukins, colony-stimulating factors and erythropoietin.

Clinical assessment

A clinical assessment begins as the patient walks into the room or you go to the bedside:

- What is the colour of their skin?
  - Are they pale?
  - Do they have a plethoric complexion?
  - Is their skin bruised?
- Are they in pain?
- Are there any obvious swellings of the neck or face?

- Is the patient unkempt or thin, and is there a smell of alcohol?
- What is the patient's racial origin and gender?

History

Specific symptoms

Anaemia The symptoms include:

- tiredness
- breathlessness
- chest pain
- ankle swelling.

Tiredness is thought of as the classical symptom of anaemia but most tired people are not anaemic and some patients (particularly elderly ones) have few symptoms despite profound anaemia. That is usually because the anaemia has developed slowly and their lifestyle does not make heavy demands for oxygen. Apart from tiredness, impaired oxygen delivery causes breathlessness, light-headedness and faints. It worsens angina and can precipitate heart failure, especially if it is superimposed on coronary artery disease.

Red cell excess (erythrocytosis) The symptomatology is covered on page 273.

Leucopenia The symptoms of leucopenia (more specifically neutropenia) include:

- mouth ulceration
- infective symptoms.

White cell excess (leukaemia and lymphoma) The symptomatology is relatively specific to individual diseases, which are covered on pages 276–280.

Platelet/coagulation disease Symptoms include:

- easy bruising
- bleeding
- thromboses.

Thrombocytopenia causes petechial haemorrhages and bruising. When it is severe, it also causes bleeding from the gums, into the gut or, most seriously, into the brain. Impaired coagulation more commonly causes bleeding into soft tissues than overt external bleeding. Haemophilia may cause prolonged bleeding from minor injuries and surgery but often presents with bleeding into joints. Other hereditary clotting disorders are rare, apart from von Willebrand's disease, which most often causes skin and mucous membrane bleeding because the abnormality results in a defect of platelet function. A detailed history is the most important part of the investigation of a bleeding disorder. Remember to ask about menorrhagia and bleeding problems after dental extractions and surgery. Thrombophilia is a term used to describe an increased tendency to thrombosis (usually venous).

General history

You should take a detailed drug history from every patient. Remember not just the prescription drugs but also medicines bought over the counter. Take a family history if the patient has haemolytic anaemia, a bleeding tendency or thrombophilia and construct a family tree if it is positive. Take a dietary and alcohol history. Note the length of

history and take particular note if the symptoms suggest that more than one aspect of haematological function is affected (e.g. symptoms of infection, bruising *and* anaemia). Be alert to symptoms of systemic disease, such as weight loss, dyspepsia, change in bowel habit, night sweats and pruritus.

Examination

Your examination (Fig. 67) should include

- a thorough and systematic examination of the skin
- careful palpation of all groups of lymph nodes (including deep palpation of the abdomen)
- inspection of the conjunctivae and mouth
- palpation of the spleen and liver
- a thorough search for signs of infection including body temperature.

Red cell disorders

The physical signs of anaemia are extremely subjective. Examine the conjunctivae, which are less affected by variations in capillary blood flow than the skin or nail beds. *Definite* conjunctival pallor is relatively specific for moderate-to-severe anaemia. Examine the sclerae carefully for jaundice (not detectable until serum bilirubin is raised to

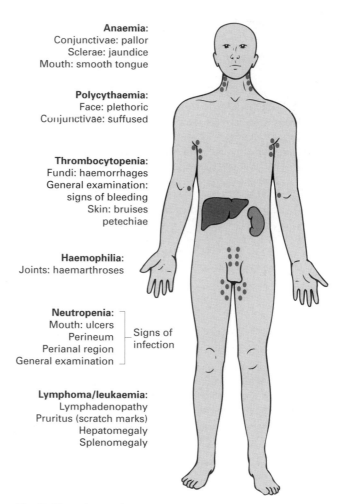

Anaemia:
Conjunctivae: pallor
Sclerae: jaundice
Mouth: smooth tongue

Polycythaemia:
Face: plethoric
Conjunctivae: suffused

Thrombocytopenia:
Fundi: haemorrhages
General examination:
signs of bleeding
Skin: bruises
petechiae

Haemophilia:
Joints: haemarthroses

Neutropenia:
Mouth: ulcers
Perineum
Perianal region   Signs of infection
General examination

Lymphoma/leukaemia:
Lymphadenopathy
Pruritus (scratch marks)
Hepatomegaly
Splenomegaly

Fig. 67 Physical signs of haematological disease. Uncommon signs are omitted.

three times normal); it is present in haemolytic but not other types of anaemia. Look at the patient's face; a plethoric complexion with suffusion of the conjunctivae may be a sign of erythrocytosis. Examine the abdomen for splenomegaly, which is a prominent feature of chronic extravascular haemolysis, and is a key finding in polycythaemia vera.

White cell disorders

Neutropenia should be considered in any patient with severe oral ulceration/candidiasis. Examination for lymphadenopathy requires skill, not just in knowing where and how to palpate but in interpreting the findings. If there are palpable lymph nodes, note:

- whether they are hard, firm or soft
- whether they are tender or non-tender
- their approximate size
- whether they are mobile and discrete or matted together.

Minor lymphadenopathy is commonly found in normal people, particularly if they have a history of injury or infection. Pathological lymph nodes are larger and sometimes coalescent or matted. Lymph nodes that are enlarged because of infection are smaller than those of lymphoma (usually less than 2 cm) and more likely to be discrete. The distribution of lymphadenopathy in Hodgkin's and non-Hodgkin's lymphoma (NHL) is considered on page 279. Assess the size of the spleen and liver and search for abnormal masses in the abdomen. Mild splenomegaly may be caused by an infection or portal hypertension but moderate or massive splenomegaly in the UK suggests lymphoma, myelofibrosis or chronic leukaemia. Hepatomegaly may be found in myeloproliferative diseases. Tissue infiltration (particularly of the gums) occurs in some leukaemias.

Platelet and coagulation disorders

Petechial haemorrhages are a sign of thrombocytopenia. They are characteristically seen first over the lower legs, where capillary pressure is highest. Later they become generalised, and may coalesce as bruises (ecchymoses), particularly over the arms. Inspect the gums for bleeding and the fundi for retinal haemorrhages, which should be taken very seriously as a sign of impending cerebral haemorrhage. Joint swelling caused by bleeding (haemarthrosis) is an important feature of haemophilia and other coagulation disorders.

Thrombocytosis and other hypercoagulable states have no specific physical signs other than those of arterial or venous thrombosis.

Investigations

There are a large number of investigations in haematology, some routine and some for more specialised parameters. Box 18 lists the more common tests and the abbreviations for these tests.

Blood count and film

When you take blood, you can affect the result by:

- Excessive cuffing: a prolonged increase in venous pressure artificially increases the haematocrit.

> **Box 18:** Investigations in haematology
>
> **Blood count and film**
> - Full blood count; **including haemoglobin (Hb)** white cell count (WCC), platelet count and mean cell volume (MCV)
> - Blood film
> - Differential white cell count
> - Erythrocyte sedimentation rate (ESR)
>
> **Haematinics**
> - Iron and total iron-binding capacity
> - Ferritin
> - Vitamin B_{12}
> - Folate and red cell folate
>
> **Coagulation**
> - International normalized ratio (INR)
> - Prothrombin time (PT)
> - Activated partial thromboplastin time (APTT)
> - Plasma fibrinogen
> - Fibrin degradation products (FDPs)
> - D-dimer
>
> **Bone marrow aspirate**
>
> **Bone marrow trephine biopsy**
>
> **Lymph node biopsy**

- Being slow to put blood in the tube or not mixing it thoroughly: coagulation in the tube gives a falsely low platelet count and abnormal coagulation results.

Automated counters measure concentrations (per unit volume) of red cells, haemoglobin, platelets and leucocytes (lymphocytes, monocytes, neutrophils, eosinophils and basophils). They also measure the percentage of red cells present as reticulocytes (newly released cells) and calculate indices which describe the size of red cells and platelets and the degree of haemoglobinisation. Normal values for adults are shown in Table 1 (p. 5). In addition, a dried and stained blood film can be inspected to assess the morphology of the cells and detect abnormal cells. Some of the terms you will come across on blood film reports are given in Table 62.

Interpreting the haemoglobin and red cell indices

Anaemia is diagnosed when there is a reduction in the concentration of haemoglobin caused by a reduced number of red cells or a reduced amount of haemoglobin within the cells. An *increase* in haemoglobin concentration resulting from an increased number of red cells per unit volume is termed erythrocytosis.

Whenever you are told that a patient is anaemic, you should ask for the mean cell volume (MCV), by which anaemias are classified (explained further on page 267). The cell counter also tells you how similar the red cells are to one another in size. This is expressed as the red cell distribution width (RDW). A low RDW signifies a normal,

Table 62 Terms used to describe abnormalities of red blood cells

Term	Description
Hypochromia	Defective haemoglobinisation, as in some anaemias
Anisochromia	Variable haemoglobinisation, as in haemolysis
Polychromasia	Bluish tinge to the red cells, reflects increased erythropoiesis
Microcytosis	Small size (p. 267)
Macrocytosis	Large size (p. 267)
Anisocytosis	Variable size, as in iron deficiency
Poikilocytosis	Abnormal shape, as in myelofibrosis (p. 278)
Erythrocytosis	Increased number of red cells
Spherocytosis, elliptocytosis	Abnormal shape resulting from congenital or acquired cell membrane defect
Sickle cells	Abnormal shape resulting from abnormal haemoglobin
Target cells	Increased surface:volume ratio; as in liver disease
Fragmented or damaged cells	Trauma to red cells (p. 272)
Inclusions	
Basophilic stippling	Immature cells resulting from accelerated haemopoiesis
Iron granules (siderocytes)	Seen with special stain in sideroblastic anaemia
Howell–Jolly bodies	Nuclear remnants seen after splenectomy

homogeneous population of cells. An increased RDW signifies heterogeneity in cell size as a result of:

- active haemopoiesis, because immature red cells (reticulocytes) are large
- treatment of iron deficiency, resulting in a mixture of microcytic and normocytic cells
- mixed deficiency, giving both small and large diseased cells.

Reticulocytes can be counted automatically and are expressed as an absolute value.

White cells and platelets

Changes in cell counts are diagnosed by the automated counter. Examination of the film gives an accurate differential count and detects cells such as leukaemic blast cells. It also detects morphological changes such as the degree of lobulation of the neutrophil nuclei. In infection, neutrophils are relatively immature and may appear as bands rather than having the normal multilobulated appearance: a 'left shift'. Conversely, the neutrophils are hypersegmented ('right-shifted') in megaloblastic anaemia because vitamin B_{12} or folate deficiency impairs haemopoiesis (p. 268). There may also be cytoplasmic abnormalities, e.g. vacuolation or heavy granulation of neutrophils during

bacterial infection. Abnormalities of neutrophils, such as hypogranularity, are seen in myelodysplasia.

Platelets

A simple platelet count is the clue to most platelet diseases.

Erythrocyte sedimentation rate

The erythrocyte sedimentation rate (ESR) is a very crude test which measures the rate (in mm/hr) at which red cells sediment. Abnormal proteins in inflammatory conditions and myeloma cause rapid sedimentation. The ESR is, therefore, a non-specific marker of infection, inflammation and neoplasia. It may be non-specifically raised in anaemia and some non-inflammatory diseases such as uraemia. In some hospitals, blood viscosity or **acute-phase proteins** are measured as more reliable markers of inflammation.

Haematinics

The blood count must always be checked before measuring haematinics because it is unlikely that a patient has significant iron, vitamin B_{12} or folate deficiency if the count is normal. An extremely high index of suspicion (e.g. suspected subacute combined degeneration of the cord, p. 241) would be needed to justify these extra measurements in the face of a normal blood count. Similarly, it is wasteful to measure serum iron or ferritin if the diagnosis of iron deficiency is obvious from the clinical context and blood count. With those provisos, measure:

- vitamin B_{12} and folate in patients with macrocytic anaemia
- iron in patients with microcytosis
- all three in a patient with anaemia and a normal MCV but a high RDW (to exclude a mixed deficiency).

The diagnosis of iron, vitamin B_{12} and folate deficiencies is considered on page 269.

Tests of coagulation and fibrinolysis

These are discussed on page 282.

Bone marrow examination

Bone marrow can be examined either as an aspirate from the sternum or iliac crest or as a trephine biopsy from the iliac crest. Marrow aspirate is useful for detailed cytology, cell counts and assessment of iron stores. Trephine biopsies are useful for judging cellularity, detecting tumour and diagnosing myelofibrosis (p. 278).

Remember that marrow examination is not infallible in detecting tumour deposits because they may be absent from the area sampled. Marrow aspiration is an uncomfortable procedure which should not be done without good indications. These include:

- to confirm iron deficiency or megaloblastic anaemia, if the diagnosis is in doubt or the patient does not respond to treatment
- to investigate unexplained anaemia
- to investigate suspected leukaemia, myeloma or other haematological malignancy
- to monitor response to the treatment of leukaemia

- to diagnose cancer, where there is circumstantial evidence of marrow involvement
- to investigate agranulocytosis or thrombocytopenia
- to stain and obtain cultures for suspected tuberculosis, histoplasmosis and leishmaniasis.

In some conditions — notably myelofibrosis and malignant infiltration of the marrow — bone marrow aspiration may be unsuccessful. A 'dry tap' is pathological and of diagnostic value.

Lymph node biopsy

Lymph node biopsy is the definitive investigation to diagnose lymphoma and identify its histological type. It is also used to diagnose disseminated cancer and other causes of lymphadenopathy. The features of lymph nodes that make them 'suspicious' are described on page 278, and other clinical features suggesting lymphoma are described on page 279. Which node should be biopsied is partly a surgical decision and partly determined by their 'feel'. Lymph node biopsies are usually taken under general anaesthesia. The specimen will be ruined for some analyses if it is put straight into formalin. It should be promptly handled by a skilled histology technician. Remember to request culture if tuberculosis is suspected.

6.2 Red cell disorders

Learning objectives

You should:
- understand the range of diseases that cause anaemia and how they do so
- know how to diagnose and treat anaemias
- know the indications for blood transfusion and how to avoid complications
- know what polycythaemia is, what can cause it and how it causes symptoms and signs.

Case Study

A man in his sixties who has smoked since he was a teenager has end-stage chronic obstructive pulmonary disease with type 2 respiratory failure. He has a plethoric complexion and a haemoglobin concentration of 188 g/l. His white cell and platelet counts are normal and he has no splenomegaly. His chronic hypoxia has caused secondary polycythaemia.

Erythropoiesis:

- is controlled by erythropoietin, which is secreted by the kidneys
- is stimulated by hypoxia
- requires an adequate supply of folic acid, vitamin B_{12} and iron
- is inhibited by poor nutrition, systemic disease and local disease within the marrow.

Anaemias

Think of anaemias in terms of:

- decreased red cell production
- increased loss.

This classification is expanded in Table 63. Note that the commonest form, iron deficiency anaemia, often results from a combination of both. The MCV is central to the diagnosis of anaemia. Remember that:

- iron deficiency causes microcytosis
- vitamin B_{12} and folate deficiency cause macrocytosis (other causes are covered on p. 269)
- the anaemia of marrow suppression is often normocytic.

Exceptions to these rules are discussed under individual diseases. Given the haemoglobin and MCV, white cell count, platelet and reticulocyte counts and a description of the blood film, you can make a working diagnosis in most cases.

Iron deficiency anaemia

Iron deficiency anaemia is the most common and, to the generalist, most important anaemia because it:

Table 63 A classification of the anaemias

	Decreased production	Increased destruction/ loss
Acute haemorrhage		+
Haematinic deficiency		
Iron deficiency	+	±
B_{12} deficiency	+	+
Folate deficiency	+	+
Hypoplastic anaemias		
Idiopathic	+	
Secondary	+	
Anaemia of chronic disease	+	
Marrow replacement		
Leukaemias	+	
Myeloma	+	
Other tumours	+	
Congenital haemolysis		
Spherocytosis and elliptocytosis	±	+
Sickle cell disease		+
Thalassaemia		+
Glucose-6-phosphate dehydrogenase deficiency		+
Acquired haemolysis		
Autoimmune		+
Microangiopathic		+
Hypersplenism		+

Six

- is a significant public health problem
- may be the presentation of an occult gastrointestinal (GI) carcinoma at a curable stage
- is eminently treatable whatever its cause.

Iron deficiency is caused by an imbalance between dietary availability and blood loss, so much of the population is iron-deficient in areas of the developing world where GI parasites are endemic. Active growth, pregnancy and lactation increase the demand for iron and may unmask deficiency. The prevalence of depleted iron stores in women of menstrual age may be as high as 20% and that iron deficiency can persist into the postmenopausal years if they have a poor diet and do not replete their iron stores. Iron deficiency is much less prevalent in adult men and is likely to be due to occult bleeding, most often from the GI tract.

There are sizeable iron stores in the liver, reticuloendothelial system and marrow, as well as in the erythrocytes themselves, so negative iron balance must exist for some time before anaemia develops. For the same reason, replenishment of iron stores takes longer than the restoration of haemopoiesis, and iron treatment should be continued after the haemoglobin has returned to normal.

Causes

These are:

- blood loss
- dietary deficiency
- malabsorption.

Iron may be malabsorbed as a result of small intestinal disease or after gastrectomy.

Sources of blood loss, in order of frequency, are:

- menstruation
- the GI tract (Ch. 3)
- the urinary tract.

In practice, it may be difficult to decide whether menorrhagia is the sole cause of blood loss. If in doubt, suspect another disease.

Common causes of GI blood loss are:

- gastritis, peptic ulcer or oesophagitis, particularly in patients taking aspirin, non-steroidal anti-inflammatory drugs (NSAIDs) or steroids
- diverticular disease
- carcinoma of the stomach, caecum or colon
- angiodysplasia of the colon, an increasingly recognised cause in elderly people
- oesophageal varices.

A less common cause is Meckel's diverticulum.

Although only a small minority of iron-deficient patients have GI tumours, it is worthwhile identifying them because diagnosis at the stage of a predominantly mucosal lesion may allow curative surgery.

Clinical and haematological signs

Symptoms and signs were covered earlier and in Figure 67. An early sign on the blood film is variability in size and shape of the red cells. In established iron deficiency, they are hypochromic and microcytic and 'pencil cells' may be seen.

Diagnosis and further investigations

Iron deficiency is overwhelmingly the most common UK cause of microcytosis but it also occurs in thalassaemia and, sometimes, in the anaemia of chronic disease. If there is doubt, iron deficiency is diagnosed by measuring serum iron and total iron-binding capacity. These are measured together because binding protein deficiency may lower the serum iron concentration without signifying true iron deficiency; <10% saturation of iron-binding capacity is diagnostic of iron deficiency. Measurement of serum ferritin is a better reflection of iron stores (particularly to detect iron overload, as in haemochromatosis). Absence of stainable marrow iron stores and a significant improvement in the blood count with iron replacement are definitive evidence of iron deficiency.

Stool samples are often tested for occult blood to confirm or exclude the GI tract as the site of blood loss, but they may be falsely positive or negative. Dietary assessment and tests for malabsorption (p. 127) may be indicated. The investigations are not complete until a patient with unexplained iron deficiency has had gastroscopy and colonoscopy to look for a site of blood loss.

Management

There is little to choose between the many formulations of oral iron. Ferrous sulphate is usually prescribed. It may cause nausea, abdominal pain, diarrhoea or constipation, in which case the dose should be reduced or a different iron salt given. A response should be seen within 1 week of starting treatment and a rise in haemoglobin of 10 g/l each week is to be expected. Treatment is continued for 3 months after the haemoglobin has returned to normal to replenish iron stores.

Megaloblastic anaemias

Vitamin B_{12} (cobalamin) and folic acid are coenzymes for cellular metabolism, particularly haemopoiesis. Deficiency affects DNA synthesis in all marrow cell lines and the red cell precursors develop 'megaloblastic' morphological changes. Ineffective erythropoiesis reduces the production of mature red cells and they are enlarged (macrocytic). Formation of platelets and granulocytes is also impaired.

Vitamin B_{12} and folate deficiency are not the only causes of macrocytosis; other common causes, in approximate order of frequency, are:

- alcohol abuse
- liver disease
- active haemopoiesis (immature red cells are large): haemolytic anaemias, acute blood loss

Less common causes include:

- myelodysplasia
- acute myeloid leukaemia
- aplastic anaemia
- antifolate drugs: methotrexate, phenytoin.

However, vitamin B_{12} and folate deficiency are the only common conditions to produce the typical megaloblastic bone marrow appearances. They have identical haematological features but differ in their causes and non-haematological manifestations. This section will first present the common features and then the differences between them.

Clinical and haematological features

Patients typically present with symptoms of anaemia and malaise. These develop insidiously and the anaemia may be very severe by the time the diagnosis is made. Elderly people, in particular, may tolerate it surprisingly well until they present with heart failure or angina resulting from tissue hypoxia. There may be:

- mild jaundice caused by haemolysis of the defective red cells
- fever
- glossitis
- splenomegaly (very unusually).

Although moderate neutropenia and thrombocytopenia are common, they are not usually symptomatic. Vitamin B_{12} deficiency may, uncommonly, present with its neurological complications (Ch. 5). There may be features of an underlying GI disease in vitamin B_{12}, folate or a mixed deficiency anaemia.

Whatever the cause, the blood film shows:

- pancytopenia
- macrocytosis: large oval red cells
- hypersegmentation of the neutrophil nuclei (termed a 'right shift')
- megaloblasts in peripheral blood in severe cases.

This haematological picture is so characteristic that the diagnosis can generally be made without bone marrow examination, the definitive way of demonstrating megaloblastic change.

Vitamin B_{12} deficiency

Vitamin B_{12} is present in meat and dairy produce. It is absorbed as a complex with intrinsic factor (IF) produced by the gastric parietal cells. Pure dietary deficiency is exceptionally rare because there are large hepatic stores but can occur in alcoholics and vegans. More commonly, deficiency is caused by

- autoimmune damage to the gastric parietal cells: pernicious anaemia
- destruction of vitamin B_{12} by bacterial overgrowth in diverticulae, blind loops or fistulae
- disease of the terminal ileum where the B_{12}–IF complex is absorbed: usually Crohn's disease
- pancreatic exocrine deficiency
- gastrectomy.

Pernicious anaemia

Pernicious anaemia is an organ-specific autoimmune disease caused by antibodies to gastric parietal cells and intrinsic factor.

- It is commoner in women than men.
- It may develop from adolescence onwards but is most common in middle to old age.

It is associated with:

- blood group A
- failure of gastric acid secretion
- an increased risk of gastric carcinoma
- an increased incidence of the other organ-specific autoimmune diseases, including vitiligo, diabetes mellitus, hypothyroidism and Addison's disease.

The diagnosis is made by demonstrating a reduced serum vitamin B_{12} concentration and IF antibodies. It is confirmed by the Schilling test, in which radiolabelled B_{12} is given on two occasions, first on its own and then with oral IF. Urinary excretion of the label is measured. In pernicious anaemia, there is malabsorption which is correctable by IF. Other causes of malabsorption are not correctable.

Neurological effects of B_{12} deficiency

Full blood counts are now so widely available that B_{12} deficiency is usually recognised and treated before it has any significant neurological effects; however, some individuals may develop neurological effects with little or no anaemia. These include:

- optic atrophy
- dementia
- subacute combined degeneration of the cord (Ch. 5).

Management

One simple rule is that folate and vitamin B_{12} should always be given together in megaloblastic anaemia, at least until the haematinic results are known, because folate treatment alone can increase haemopoiesis in patients with pure vitamin B_{12} deficiency and actually precipitate neurological complications. Patients with vitamin B_{12} deficiency should be given injections of vitamin B_{12} weekly for 6 weeks and then 3-monthly indefinitely thereafter. The reticulocyte response should be checked after 7 days. Potassium supplements are needed in some cases, as well as iron and folate, because cellular anabolism requires potassium. Whether or not patients with severe megaloblastic anaemia should be transfused is controversial because even careful transfusion can precipitate heart failure. If it is done, it should be slow and with diuretic cover and should not aim to restore haemoglobin immediately to normal.

Folate deficiency

Folate is absorbed in the upper small intestine. The body stores are relatively small so folate deficiency develops earlier in malabsorption syndromes than does iron or vitamin B_{12} deficiency. For the same reason, folate deficiency is more likely to have a purely dietary cause, to develop during pregnancy or to be precipitated by active haemopoiesis in haemolytic states. Folate metabolism is vulnerable to a wide range of drugs and is actually the target of some chemotherapeutic agents, e.g. methotrexate. These are the main causes of folate deficiency:

- dietary, e.g. in
  — alcoholism
  — elderly or neglected people

Six

- increased demand
  - pregnancy
  - active haemopoiesis, e.g. haemolytic anaemia
- malabsorption
  - coeliac disease
  - pancreatic insufficiency
  - postgastrectomy
  - Crohn's disease
- drugs which interfere with folate absorption
  - phenytoin
- drugs which interfere with folate metabolism
  - methotrexate
  - phenytoin
  - trimethoprim.

Investigation of the cause of folate deficiency will depend on the context in which it is diagnosed. If there is a clear dietary or drug cause, no further investigation is needed. Otherwise, investigation for malabsorption is indicated.

Diagnosis
A low serum or red cell folate concentration confirms the diagnosis. Of the two, red cell folate more accurately reflects total body folate stores.

Prevention and management
Pregnant women are routinely given prophylactic oral folate. Alcoholic or poorly nourished patients should be given folate as part of their rehabilitation. Proven folate deficiency is treated with oral folic acid. As explained above, this must never be given alone in macrocytic anaemia unless vitamin B_{12} deficiency has been excluded. If there is evidence of iron deficiency, oral iron should also be given.

Aplastic/hypoplastic anaemia
Aplastic anaemia is a rare condition which may be congenital or acquired. It may be primary (no cause identified) or secondary to:

- drugs, e.g. chloramphenicol, chemotherapy, zidovudine, ganciclovir, phenylbutazone
- irradiation
- chemicals
- infection, e.g. viral hepatitis
- autoimmune disease.

There is usually leucopenia and thrombocytopenia as well as anaemia, although pure red cell aplasia may occur. The aplasia may be *transient* or *chronic*, and *partial* (hypoplastic) or *complete* (aplastic). The symptoms and signs depend on the relative degrees of anaemia, thrombocytopenia and neutropenia. The red cells are usually macrocytic. The marrow trephine biopsy is hypoplastic. The differential diagnosis is with other causes of pancytopenia, particularly marrow replacement/fibrosis. Severe aplastic anaemia has a high mortality. A significant number of patients respond to antilymphocyte globulin or other immunosuppressive treatments, but the best chance of cure lies in bone marrow transplantation from a human leucocyte antigen (HLA)-identical sibling donor. Androgens and corticosteroids have occasionally been effective.

Supportive care of the neutropenic patient (p. 275) and transfusions of platelet and red cells are needed. With time, platelet and red cell antibodies develop and may complicate management.

Leucoerythroblastic anaemia
Leucoerythroblastic anaemia is used to describe a condition in which the blood film shows immature leucocytes and erythroblasts. Essentially, it reflects stress on the bone marrow. It has many causes, notably marrow infiltration with a solid tumour, myeloma, lymphoma, leukaemia or myelofibrosis. It is investigated by marrow aspiration/biopsy.

Anaemia of chronic disease
Anaemia caused by chronic disease is, second to iron deficiency, the most common anaemia you are likely to encounter. Common causes are:

- chronic infection
- renal failure
- liver disease
- malignancy
- autoimmune disease.

The typical pattern is a normocytic or microcytic anaemia with reduced serum iron and total iron-binding capacity, intact marrow iron stores and reduced erythroblast haemosiderin. It is usually caused by suppressed erythropoiesis, although other mechanisms such as haemolysis may contribute. The anaemia is often relatively mild. The anaemia of renal failure, however, is often very severe because the kidney is the site of production of erythropoietin. Injections of recombinant forms of erythropoietin can successfully treat the anaemia of renal failure and, sometimes, other secondary anaemias.

Haemolytic anaemias
Destruction of red cells by a disease process either intrinsic or extrinsic to the cell causes:

- shortened red cell survival
- increased erythropoiesis
- anaemia if erythropoiesis cannot keep pace with red cell destruction.

There may be morphological changes in the red cells, giving a clue to the cause of haemolysis.

In most haemolytic anaemias, red cells are removed by macrophages of the reticuloendothelial system, chiefly in the spleen. This process is termed **extravascular haemolysis**. Breakdown of haemoglobin increases the plasma level of unconjugated bilirubin, causing clinically overt jaundice in severe haemolysis. Splenomegaly and pigment gall stones may occur.

When there is rapid breakdown of red cells within the circulation (**intravascular haemolysis**), haemoglobin is liberated. Initially, it is bound to plasma proteins called haptoglobins. When the binding capacity of haptoglobins is exceeded, free haemoglobin is filtered in the kidneys and converted to haemosiderin in renal tubular cells. Haemosiderin can be detected in urine.

The haemolytic anaemias are a heterogeneous group of disorders which can be classified into congenital and acquired forms. Congenital haemolytic anaemias include:

- haemoglobinopathies
  — sickle cell disease
  — thalassaemia
- membrane defects
  — spherocytosis
  — elliptocytosis
- red cell enzyme defects
  — glucose-6-phosphate dehydrogenase deficiency.

Acquired haemolytic anaemias include:

- autoimmune
- non-immune
  — microangiopathic haemolytic anaemia
  — prosthetic heart valve
  — drug- or toxin-induced
  — paroxysmal nocturnal haemoglobinuria.

Diagnosis

The clinical features of haemolytic anaemias are those of the anaemia, the sequelae of haemolysis and any underlying cause. In addition to haematological features, patients with chronic haemolytic anaemia are prone to leg ulceration as well as pigment gall stones.

Laboratory features of haemolysis are:

- evidence of increased erythropoiesis: reticulocytosis, polychromasia, erythroid hyperplasia of bone marrow
- evidence of increased red cell breakdown: increased plasma unconjugated bilirubin and urinary urobilinogen, reduced plasma haptoglobin.

Congenital haemolytic anaemias

The only congenital haemolytic anaemias covered here are those that you might expect to encounter as a house officer.

Sickle syndromes Sickle syndromes are caused by a recessively inherited amino acid substitution in the haemoglobin A molecule, which causes it to become insoluble and cross-link under hypoxic conditions. This causes haemolysis, stickiness and microvascular occlusion.

Africans are most often affected, so heterozygotes are common in areas with a high African population. They may develop symptoms after surgery or during any situation that causes hypoxia.

'Sickle trait' can be diagnosed by the in vitro 'sickle test' and by haemoglobin electrophoresis.

Homozygotes are more severely affected. They have a chronic haemolytic anaemia and may have sickling crises precipitated by:

- hypoxia
- dehydration
- infection
- other systemic stresses.

During crises, microvascular occlusion causes infarcts of bone and soft tissues. Patients experience severe pain, fever and malaise. Splenic infarcts lead to hyposplenism and an increased risk of pneumococcal septicaemia. *Sal-monella* osteomyelitis occurs in areas of infarcted bone. There may be soft tissue complications, including retinopathy, acute renal papillary necrosis, acute pulmonary syndrome and leg ulcers. Pigment gall stones are common. Pregnancy is hazardous. Prophylactic penicillin is required to prevent pneumococcal septicaemia.

Sickling crises are treated by:

- keeping the patient warm
- oxygen
- intravenous fluids
- opiate analgesia
- antibiotics.

The thalassaemias The thalassaemias are a group of congenital haemolytic anaemias caused by mutations or gene deletions affecting the α- and β-globin chains (α- and β-thalassaemia, respectively). They vary in severity from a chance finding in an asymptomatic individual to a disease that is incompatible with life. Synthesis of abnormal haemoglobin causes 'ineffective erythropoiesis'. There is microcytosis and the cells are irregular in size, shape and degree of haemoglobinisation.

Heterozygotes (thalassaemia trait) usually remain asymptomatic but may become mildly anaemic during intercurrent infection or pregnancy. Remember thalassaemia trait in the differential diagnosis of microcytic anaemia. Thalassaemia major is not considered further here.

Acquired haemolytic anaemias

Autoimmune haemolytic anaemia Autoimmune haemolytic anaemia (AIHA) is most commonly idiopathic but may be caused by:

- autoimmune disease, e.g. systemic lupus erythematosus (SLE)
- neoplasia, e.g. chronic lymphocytic leukaemia
- infection, e.g. infectious mononucleosis, *Mycoplasma*
- drugs, e.g. methyldopa.

The anti-red cell antibody involved may cause haemolysis at body temperature ('warm AIHA': usually IgG) or only at temperatures well below 37°C ('cold AIHA': usually IgM) and the clinical picture varies accordingly.

Cold AIHA (cold haemagglutinin disease) Haemolysis is mediated by complement and usually intravascular, classically causing episodes of dark urine (haemoglobinuria) after cold exposure. At the same time, agglutination of red cells in peripheral capillaries may cause peripheral cyanosis, Raynaud-like symptoms and even gangrene. Cold AIHA may occur as a transient problem after infectious diseases such as infectious mononucleosis or *Mycoplasma* pneumonia. Red cell agglutinates can be seen on a blood film at room temperature.

Warm AIHA Haemolysis is usually extravascular, particularly in the spleen, and leads to jaundice and splenomegaly. The blood film shows spherocytosis.

Direct antiglobulin test In either case, the definitive test for AIHA is the direct antiglobulin test, in which antibodies are demonstrated on the red cell surface by the addition of anti-human globulin, which will cause agglutination.

Management of warm AIHA Warm AIHA can be treated with:

Six

- steroids
- splenectomy
- immunosuppressive therapy.

Management of cold AIHA Patients with cold agglutinins should be kept warm; they respond less well to steroids and splenectomy. Blood transfusion may be needed for haemolytic crises, but cross-matching can be difficult.

Non-immune acquired haemolytic anaemias The non-immune acquired haemolytic anaemias are caused by:

- fibrin deposited in the microcirculation, as in disseminated intravascular coagulation (DIC) (p. 285)
- platelet aggregates in the microcirculation — thrombotic thrombocytopenic purpura (TTP)
- heart valves or other mechanical prostheses
- toxic causes, including uraemia, lead poisoning and some drugs
- paroxysmal nocturnal haemoglobinuria, a rare condition in which deficiencies of membrane proteins make the red cells susceptible to the lytic actions of serum complement.

In the case of DIC and mechanical red cell damage, schistocytes (fragmented red cells) are seen on the blood film.

Blood transfusion

There are two quite distinct indications for blood transfusion:

- to restore volume after acute blood loss
- to restore the red cell mass in a patient with anaemia and a normal blood volume (compensated anaemia).

An excellent, 'official' guide is available at www.transfusionguidelines.org.uk

Acute blood loss

Acute blood loss is caused by trauma, haemorrhage, usually from the GI tract, and surgery. If haemorrhage is severe, there is circulatory collapse. The physical signs are from the blood loss itself and from volume depletion (p. 194).

You should transfuse red cells (with other fluids, if needed) as quickly as necessary to restore the circulation, monitoring the pulse, blood pressure and urine output. Remember that the haemoglobin concentration is no guide to the severity of acute blood loss because it takes time for haemodilution to occur.

Transfusion for anaemia

In anaemia, plasma volume is normal despite lack of red cells. This process of compensation takes hours or days after acute blood loss. The indications for transfusion are less strong than after acute blood loss because:

- the patient is not shocked
- treating the underlying cause of anaemia is a more permanent (albeit slower) solution than transfusing red cells, which have a short lifespan

- transfusion increases blood volume and may cause volume overload (heart failure).

Transfusion may nevertheless be indicated to:

- relieve symptoms
- prepare anaemic patients for surgery
- increase the red cell mass in case of further bleeding.

As a rule of thumb, blood transfusion:

- is rarely indicated if the haemoglobin concentration is above 100 g/l
- may be indicated between 80 and 100 g/l
- is likely to be needed below 80 g/l.

In general, iron, vitamin B_{12} or folate deficiency should be treated with haematinics. Transfusion for anaemia is particularly hazardous if the patient is in heart failure, when red cells should be given with an i.v. loop diuretic and close observation of the patient's haemodynamic state. Blood transfusion is expensive and potentially hazardous. It should not be 'dished out' carelessly. In some circumstances treatment with erythropoietin is preferable to repeated red cell transfusion (e.g. renal failure, certain malignancies).

Blood groups

The main ABO system consists of two markers inherited as Mendelian dominant traits from the parents. The red cells of an individual may carry the A antigen (group A), the B antigen (group B), both (group AB) or neither (group O). The antigens are carried on many tissues other than red cells and individuals are exposed early in life to those antigens that they do not carry. Thus group A individuals have agglutinins to the B antigen and vice versa; group O individuals have agglutinins to both antigens and group AB individuals have agglutinins to neither. The importance of this system to blood transfusion is that donated cells may be lysed by host agglutinins; lysis of host cells by donor agglutinins is not usually a problem. Table 64 summarises the system and reminds you that group O subjects are 'universal donors' because their cells have neither antigen and will not be lysed if they are transfused into group A, B or AB recipients. Group AB subjects are 'universal recipients' because they have agglutinins against neither antigen.

The rhesus (D) blood group system is also conceptually very simple. About 85% of the Caucasian population (and a higher proportion of Asians) carry the D (or rhesus) antigen on their red cells. Those who are rhesus-negative may develop antibodies against the D antigen but only if exposed to it by blood transfusion or, in pregnancy, by placental leakage.

Cross-matching

After determining the patient's ABO and rhesus blood groups, donor red cells of an appropriate group are then cross-matched, both at room temperature and at 37°C against patient's serum, to detect cold and warm antibodies. Positive results in these tests mandate further investigation and a significant delay before compatible blood can be made available.

Table 64 The ABO and rhesus blood group systems

Blood group	Relative frequency (%) in Caucasians	Alleles	Agglutinins present	Plasma will agglutinate cell types	Comment
O	45	Null, null	Anti-A, anti-B	A, B, AB	Universal donor
A	40	A, A or A, null	Anti-B	B, AB	
B	10	B, B or B, null	Anti-A	A, AB	
AB	5	A, B	None	None	Universal recipient
Rh+	85	D+	None	None	
Rh-	15	D-	None or anti-D	None or Rh+	

Complications of transfusion

The major risks of HIV and hepatitis B and C infection can largely be eliminated by careful screening of donor blood. Other potential complications are:

- minor febrile reactions
- haemolytic reactions
- severe allergic reactions
- transfusion-related lung injury
- problems caused by massive transfusions
- chronic iron overload
- variant Creutzfeldt–Jakob disease (vCJD).

Minor febrile reactions

Minor febrile reactions are not uncommon, particularly in patients who have developed platelet and/or white cell antibodies from repeated transfusions. They have become much less common since most units of red cells have been leucodepleted.

Acute, severe haemolytic reactions

Severe acute haemolytic reactions are fortunately rare, invariably caused by ABO incompatibility (e.g. a group O recipient receiving group A blood) and almost always caused by elementary errors like the incorrect labelling of blood samples or incomplete pretransfusion checks. They are likely to lead to undefendable litigation. The patient may develop pyrexia and chest or abdominal pain and pass black urine, rapidly progressing to shock, acute renal failure and DIC. If a haemolytic reaction is suspected, you should:

- stop the transfusion immediately
- give intravenous hydrocortisone and chlorphenamine
- check the patient's identity and details of the donor blood
- return the blood to the transfusion laboratory with a fresh sample of the patient's blood
- call for senior help and resuscitate as needed.

Severe allergic reactions

Severe allergic reactions occur occasionally. Patients who are deficient in IgA (1 in 600) and produce anti-IgA antibodies are particularly at risk.

Transfusion-related acute lung injury

Acute lung injury can be caused by aggregation of neutrophils in lung capillaries precipitated by anti-white cell antibodies in donor plasma and usually results from transfusion of fresh frozen plasma; it may result in acute respiratory distress.

Massive transfusion

Massive transfusions may lead to particular problems. Hypocalcaemia can result from the chelating action of citrate, particularly if there is liver disease, which impairs citrate metabolism. Dilution of platelets and clotting factors by stored blood leading to an increased risk of bleeding is another potential complication.

Iron overload

Repeated blood transfusions in refractory anaemias can eventually lead to cardiac, liver and endocrine damage.

vCJD

The emergence of vCJD and its possible transmission by blood transfusion has been a major problem for blood transfusion services. It has led to the sourcing of all plasma for transfusion from non-UK donors, the banning of donations from individuals who have, themselves, received a transfusion within 10 years, and major investment into efforts to develop a screening test for the disorder. The risk is very small but the impact has been huge.

Polycythaemia

The term polycythaemia (increased number of red cells) is frequently used to mean erythrocytosis (increased haemoglobin concentration). Whilst not strictly correct, it has become accepted in medical parlance. Polycythaemia and erythrocytosis are therefore both defined as an increased red cell mass. You will recognise it on the blood count as an increased haemoglobin concentration, red cell count and haematocrit. It may be *absolute*, or *relative* to a reduced plasma volume.

Absolute polycythaemia may be:

- primary: termed polycythaemia vera
- secondary to increased erythropoietin.

Causes of secondary polycythaemia include:

- compensatory increased erythropoietin secretion as a result of
  — tissue hypoxia
  — lung disease

— cyanotic heart disease
— altitude
— hypoventilation (Pickwickian syndrome)
- non-compensatory increased erythropoietin secretion from
  — renal tumour or cysts
  — other tumours.

Only lung disease is a common cause of clinical polycythaemia.

Polycythaemia increases the oxygen-carrying capacity of blood but it also increases viscosity and impairs blood flow. Many of its clinical effects are the result of stasis and impaired tissue oxygenation.

Polycythaemia vera

Polycythaemia vera is a neoplastic stem cell proliferation which increases the formation primarily of red cells but also of leucocytes and platelets. Clinical manifestations result from:

- hyperviscosity
- tissue hypoxia
- vascular occlusive events resulting from stasis and thrombocytosis.

Paradoxically, patients may also bleed easily because their platelets are dysfunctional.

Clinical presentation

Patients may present with:

- systemic symptoms such as pruritus (particularly after a warm bath) or malaise
- an arterial or deep venous thrombosis
- neurological symptoms, including headache, tinnitus and visual disturbance
- cardiovascular symptoms, including angina and intermittent claudication
- dyspepsia or non-specific abdominal pain signifying GI mucosal ulceration
- episodes of epistaxis or GI haemorrhage
- gout.

On examination, there is plethora, cyanosis, injection of the conjunctivae and, in most cases, splenomegaly. There may also be hepatomegaly. The blood count shows a haematocrit in the range 50–70%, with leucocytosis and an increased platelet count. The red cell mass, measured isotopically, is increased. There is often iron deficiency with red cell microcytosis, and this may cause confusion by reducing the haemoglobin to normal. Bone marrow trephine biopsy shows hyperplasia of all elements. A mutation of the *JAK 2* gene on chromosome 9 can be detected in a high proportion of cases. Serum uric acid and vitamin B$_{12}$ are usually raised.

Management

Treatment is with:

- venesection to reduce hyperviscosity
- hydroxyurea or an alkylating agent to reduce stem cell proliferation
- occasionally P^{32} in elderly patients.

The aim is to reduce both the haematocrit and the platelet count. Life expectancy is reduced despite treatment, and the disease may transform into acute leukaemia or myelofibrosis.

Relative polycythaemia

Relative polycythaemia is far more common than polycythaemia vera. It is a disorder often seen in middle-aged hypertensive men who drink and smoke too much. The primary abnormality is a reduced plasma volume. The aetiology is unknown.

Faced with an apparently polycythaemic patient:

- measure the haematocrit more than once to be sure the apparent erythrocytosis is not a cuffing artefact
- consider the possibility of secondary polycythaemia, of which the common cause is chronic lung disease; measure the blood gases
- check that the patient is truly polycythaemic (i.e. exclude *relative* polycythaemia) by measuring the red cell mass.

If the patient has a leucocytosis, thrombocytosis or splenomegaly, the diagnosis is likely to be polycythaemia vera.

6.3 White cell disorders

Learning objectives

You should:

- understand the causes of neutropenia
- know what infections to be concerned about in the neutropenic patient and what to do if such a patient develops a fever
- know the diseases of white cell proliferation and how they are diagnosed and treated.

Case Study

The parents of a 12-year-old boy with anaemia and leucocytosis are told that he has leukaemia. Shocking though the news is, they are relieved to hear that there is a more than 50% chance that he can be cured. His treatment will include chemotherapy and radiotherapy.

A simple way of approaching white cell disorders is to think in terms of white cell numbers. They may be:

- reduced, increasing susceptibility to infection
- increased, signifying systemic disease or marrow proliferation.

Physiology

Granulocytes

Granulocytes are the most abundant white cells in peripheral blood.

Neutrophils

Most granulocytes are neutrophils, a key element of defence against most bacteria and some fungi. Most neutrophils in the normal person are present in the blood loosely adherent to the walls of vessels (marginating pool). When the appropriate stimulus comes along (such as a bacterial infection) they are released from the marginating pool and attracted to sites of inflammation by chemotactic factors, including complement. Once a neutrophil comes into contact with a microbe or foreign body it attaches itself, ingests it into a vacuole called a phagosome and kills it.

Eosinophils

These are the next most abundant form. They attack parasites which are too large to be phagocytosed, and also have a role in mucosal immunity.

Basophils

These are the least abundant form. They release histamine and other inflammatory mediators during immediate hypersensitivity reactions.

Monocytes

Monocytes are large non-granulated white cells that are released from the bone marrow, circulate for several days and then enter tissues to become the tissue macrophages, including pulmonary alveolar macrophages, osteoclasts and the Kupffer cells of the liver. They engulf and kill bacteria in tissues and, as antigen-presenting cells, play a key role in immunity.

Lymphocytes

Lymphocytes are derived from the same stem cells of the bone marrow as the other cell lines. During fetal development, they migrate out to populate the thymus, liver, spleen, lymph nodes and other lymphoid tissues. In adult life, some lymphocytes are formed in the marrow but most are formed in lymphoid tissues elsewhere. There are two distinct cell lines, morphologically identical but distinguishable by cell-surface markers. The B cells — plasma cells and memory cells — are responsible for humoral immunity. T cells are responsible for cell-mediated immunity and for activating B cells. The subtypes of T cells are not discussed further here but an understanding of them is crucial to an understanding of AIDS (p. 387).

Leucopenia

Leucopenia is a reduction in the number of white blood cells.

Lymphopenia is a common finding and often, in itself, of no great significance. It may be caused by:

- steroid therapy
- HIV infection
- autoimmune disease
- lymphoma
- irradiation.

Neutropenia is caused by:

- decreased production
  - primary or secondary (e.g. drugs, irradiation) aplasia
  - acute leukaemia
  - acute myeloid
  - acute lymphoblastic leukaemia
  - myelofibrosis
  - malignant marrow infiltration
  - myelodysplasia
  - viral infection
- increased consumption
  - hypersplenism
  - antineutrophil antibodies
  - overwhelming infection.

Severe neutropenia is relatively rare except in haematological malignancies and as a result of their treatment.

Management of neutropenia

The normal neutrophil count is around $2–5 \times 10^9$ cells/l. There is an increasing risk of infection when the count falls below 1×10^9 cells/l and the risk of invasive infections rises substantially when the count falls below 0.5×10^9 cells/l. A longer duration of neutropenia (e.g. more than 7 days) also puts the patient at substantially greater risk of life-threatening infection. Infections include:

- Gram-negatives, including *Pseudomonas aeruginosa*, which can be rapidly fatal
- Gram-positives, particularly *Staphylococcus epidermidis* (usually related to indwelling central venous lines and not immediately life-threatening)
- mucosal and invasive candidiasis
- invasive pulmonary aspergillosis
- herpes simplex virus (especially mouth ulcers).

A typical clinical scenario is that you are on call for haematology patients and summoned to the ward because a patient with no circulating neutrophils has developed a new fever 7–14 days after chemotherapy for leukaemia. You need to:

- assess whether there are any localising symptoms such as cough, rash, nasal symptoms, abdominal pain, etc.
- examine the mouth, chest, skin, rectal area and any other sites that are symptomatic
- assess whether the patient is in shock or going into respiratory failure
- order an urgent chest CT scan if the illness has any respiratory features
- check the notes and recent results for any positive microbiology
- take at least one blood culture and collect any other microbiological specimens that are indicated by the patient's symptoms
- start broad-spectrum i.v. antibiotics according to the policy of the unit; typically these will include coverage for *Ps. aeruginosa* and streptococcal infections as a minimum (e.g. tazocin, piperacillin)
- if there are any unusual features, the patient is very ill, or new fever or clinical features emerge while on antibiotics, you should contact a senior member of staff.

Expert microbiological advice is needed if the patient remains profoundly neutropenic and has persistent fever.

Monoclonal antibody treatments
- Anti-CD20, which is expressed on B cells, is used in the treatment of B cell non-Hodgkin's lymphoma.
- Anti-CD52, which is expressed on mature lymphocytes, is used in the treatment of chronic lymphocytic leukaemia.

Ceasing therapy
Antibiotics and antifungals can usually be stopped when the neutrophil count has risen above 0.5×10^9 cells/l.

Leucocytosis

Causes of leucocytosis include:

- neutrophilia
  — infection, usually bacterial
  — inflammation
  — connective tissue disease
  — myeloproliferative disease
  — non-haematological malignancy
  — corticosteroid therapy
  — diabetic ketoacidosis
- eosinophilia
  — parasitic infection
  — allergy
  — drug reaction
  — connective tissue disease, e.g. microscopic polyarteritis (Churg–Strauss syndrome)
  — cancer
- lymphocytosis
  — viral infection
  — post-splenectomy
  — lymphoproliferative disease
- basophilia: rare and usually caused by myeloproliferation
- monocytosis
  — infection, particularly during convalescence
  — connective tissue disease
  — myeloproliferative disease.

In many cases, the cause is obvious. In others, detailed haematological investigation is needed. Remember the common causes and remember that diabetic ketoacidosis and steroid therapy cause leucocytosis in the absence of infection.

The leukaemias, myeloproliferative disorders and lymphomas

These neoplastic diseases may seem hard to understand and remember but a few simple principles provide a framework on which the diseases hang:

- All of them are neoplastic clonal proliferations but they differ in their degree of malignancy.
- The more chronic diseases tend to become increasingly malignant with time.
- A distinction can be drawn between *lymphoproliferative* and *myeloproliferative* diseases.
- Myeloproliferation frequently involves more than one cell line.
- Other marrow tissues that are not derived from stem cells, such as fibroblasts, may proliferate

LYMPHOPROLIFERATION

Chronic lymphocytic leukaemia

Lymphoma – Hodgkin's
                   Low-grade non-Hodgkin's

Myeloma
High-grade non-Hodgkin's lymphoma
Acute lymphoblastic leukaemia

STEM CELL

Acute myeloid leukaemia
  including: monocytic
                  myelomonocytic   ⎤ Types
                  promyelocytic

Myelodysplasia
Chronic granulocytic leukaemia
Polycythaemia vera
Primary thrombocythaemia

Chronic myelofibrosis

MYELOPROLIFERATION

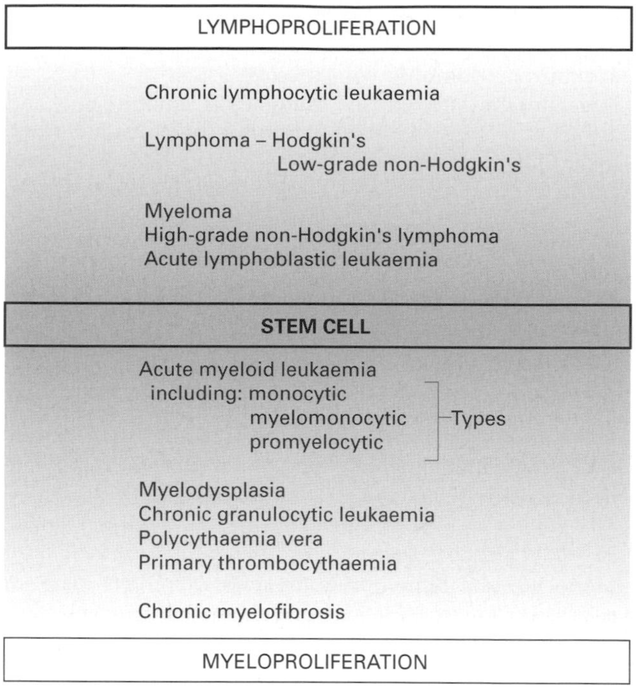

Fig. 68 Schematic represenation of the lymphoproliferative and myeloproliferative diseases. The darkest shading indicates the highest degree of malignancy.

reactively in myeloproliferation to produce myelofibrosis.

Figure 68 shows the relationship between the diseases. In general, the more malignant the disease, the more intense the treatment required and the higher the chance of cure. Low-grade diseases tend to be chronic and incurable.

The acute leukaemias
Classification and risk factors
There are two broad categories of acute leukaemia, **acute lymphoblastic leukaemia (ALL)** and **acute myeloid leukaemia (AML)**, the latter including several subtypes, shown in Figure 68. The incidence of ALL peaks in childhood. It is more common in males. AML is a disease of both children and adults, with a rapidly rising incidence in old age and no gender difference. Radiation exposure, genetic factors, viral infections and toxins, including chemotherapeutic drugs, have been implicated as risk factors for leukaemia, although the cause in an individual case is usually unknown.

Clinical and haematological features
Acute leukaemia may arise de novo or in patients with chronic myeloproliferative disease or myelodysplasia. The clinical manifestations result from marrow dysfunction and tissue infiltration. They include:

- symptoms and signs of anaemia
- bruising, bleeding and purpura (thrombocytopenia)
- increased susceptibility to infection (neutropenia).

Tissue infiltration may cause:

- bone and joint pain
- gum infiltration
- rashes.

There is occasionally hepatosplenomegaly and, in ALL, lymphadenopathy. The diagnosis is made on blood film and bone marrow examination. There is usually anaemia and thrombocytopenia. There may be leucopenia or a leucocytosis with blasts (primitive cells) in peripheral blood. The marrow is hypercellular and infiltrated with blasts. AML and ALL are distinguished and subclassified on morphological, cytochemical, immunological and cytogenetic characteristics. Rod-shaped cytoplasmic bodies, named Auer rods, are a virtually pathognomonic feature of AML.

Management

The treatment of ALL has been one of the success stories of oncology because two-thirds of children (fewer adults) are cured. Most forms of acute leukaemia are amenable to chemotherapy, but equally important is the intensive supportive treatment with antibiotics and blood products, and sympathetic management of the patient and his/her family. The aim is to eliminate the abnormal clone from blood, bone marrow and other sites and allow repopulation with normal haemopoietic cells. This is termed **remission**. A discussion of the specific drugs and regimens is beyond the scope of this chapter but treatment may include the following phases:

1. remission induction: elimination of neoplastic tissue, allowing recovery of normal marrow
2. consolidation of remission
3. prevention of recurrence in extramedullary sites (as in ALL) and maintenance of remission
4. treatment of relapses.

There are some important differences between the treatment of ALL and AML. More intensive myelosuppression is used in AML; consequently the risks of infection and bleeding are greater. In ALL, there is a high risk that systemic chemotherapy will not eradicate malignant cells from certain extra-medullary 'sanctuary' sites, including the brain, spinal cord and testes; therefore, additional local treatment (e.g. intrathecal chemotherapy) is given. Relatively low-dose maintenance therapy is often continued for 2–3 years in ALL, whereas induction in AML is followed by several further courses of very intensive chemotherapy over a much shorter period of time in an attempt to prevent relapse.

If a suitable donor is available (preferably an HLA-identical sibling), allogeneic bone marrow or peripheral blood stem cell transplantation may be performed in both AML and ALL, in an attempt to reduce the chance of relapse. This offers a 'graft-versus-leukaemia' effect, in addition to the benefits of the chemotherapy given, but may at the same time cause graft-versus-host disease, which has a significant morbidity and mortality. Alternatively, autologous transplantation, using the patient's own bone marrow or peripheral blood stem cells, collected during remission, may be employed. This avoids the risk of graft-versus-host disease but does not have the benefit of a graft-versus-leukaemia affect, and there is a chance that the transplanted marrow may still contain leukaemic cells.

Prognosis

Over 90% of children and 80% of adults with ALL achieve remission; the 5-year survival for children is over 60%, but unfortunately the majority of adults relapse and die of leukaemia. The remission rate with intensive chemotherapy in AML is over 70%, but the 5-year survival is only 20%. Many patients are elderly and not treated intensively, which results in a 5-year survival for all patients with AML of approximately 5%. Increasing age has an adverse prognostic effect on all types of leukaemia and a high white count at presentation predicts a bad outcome. Specific cytogenetic defects in the leukaemic cells are closely related to either a good (e.g. t(8; 21) in AML) or bad (e.g. t(9; 22) in ALL) prognosis.

There is increasing interest in directing specific treatments towards molecular genetic defects newly identified in haematological malignancies. A big success story in this regard has been the treatment of acute promyelocytic leukaemia, a subtype of AML that carries a high risk of early death from bleeding in DIC. The genetic abnormality (t(15; 17)) involves a retinoic acid receptor gene, and it has been found that complete remission can be achieved by administration of all-*trans*-retinoic acid. Intensive chemotherapy still has to be used, but the risk of early death and incidence of relapse have been markedly reduced; as a result, the cure rate is now approximately 70%.

Myelodysplastic syndrome

Myelodysplastic syndrome describes a group of disorders characterised by cytopenias of one or more cell lines with a cellular marrow and morphological abnormalities in both marrow and peripheral blood. Cytogenetic abnormalities can often be demonstrated. The cytopenias are presumed the result of ineffective haemopoiesis. Myelodysplastic syndrome progresses, at a variable rate, to AML. Management is supportive until leukaemia develops, when cytotoxic therapy may be indicated, although the outlook is poor at this stage. Many patients are elderly and unsuitable for intrusive treatment. Allogeneic bone marrow transplantation can be considered in younger patients.

Myeloproliferative diseases

Chronic granulocytic leukaemia

Chronic granulocytic leukaemia (CGL, also known as chronic myeloid leukaemia (CML)) is an uncommon disease which may occur at any age but peaks in the 50–60 age group. It is characterised by uncontrolled proliferation of myeloid progenitor cells, generally most noticeable in granulopoietic cells but also affecting red cells and platelets. The characteristic feature, present in >95% of patients, is the **Philadelphia chromosome**, resulting from a reciprocal translocation between the long arms of chromosomes 9 and 22 (t(9; 22)). This produces an abnormal fusion gene called *bcr/abl* which can be detected in virtually all cases, and codes for a protein which is an activated tyrosine kinase that leads to unregulated blood cell proliferation.

Six

These are the clinical features and some modes of presentation of CGL:

- Patients typically present with symptoms of anaemia, weight loss, fatigue, anorexia, drenching sweats or abdominal discomfort.
- There is palpable splenomegaly in 50%, which may be massive, and there may be symptomatic splenic infarction.
- There may be symptoms and signs of haemorrhage.
- The diagnosis may be made by chance on a blood count.

There is marked leucocytosis including neutrophils and myelocytes in particular and, in many cases, basophils and eosinophils. The platelet count is usually normal or raised at presentation. The bone marrow shows granulopoietic hyperplasia.

CGL can be distinguished from other causes of leucocytosis by:

- symptoms and signs
- blood film
- Philadelphia chromosome
- reduced leucocyte alkaline phosphatase score on a blood film.

CGL progresses after about 3 years to a more malignant phenotype, culminating in an accelerated phase. This may be marked by rapid transformation to acute leukaemia (AML or ALL), or more gradual deterioration involving such features as anaemia, massive splenomegaly, myelofibrosis, marked basophilia or thrombocytosis. Response to treatment is generally poor and the outlook is bleak.

During the chronic phase, the disease can be easily controlled by simple oral chemotherapy, usually hydroxyurea, but this does not eradicate the Philadelphia chromosome and, therefore, does not prevent malignant transformation. Alpha-interferon can produce occasional cytogenetic remissions but, until recently, the only treatment with a good chance of curing the disease has been allogeneic bone marrow or stem cell transplantation in those patients with a suitable donor who are fit enough to undergo the procedure. Management has been dramatically changed by the recent development of a drug called imatinib, which selectively binds to the *bcr/abl* adenosine triphosphate binding pocket and switches off downstream signalling. Cytogenetic remissions can be achieved in a high proportion of patients with chronic phase disease, with good responses in some patients with transformed disease. However, it is too early to know what proportion of those remissions will be sustained long-term and whether resistance will ultimately develop in the majority.

Polycythaemia vera and thrombocythaemia

Although polycythaemia vera and thrombocythaemia are myeloproliferative disorders, they are described in the red cell (p. 273) and platelet (p. 280) sections of this chapter because their clinical features are determined by the predominant cell type in peripheral blood rather than their progenitor cell.

Myelofibrosis

Myelofibrosis describes a disease in which proliferation of fibrous tissue in the marrow is the main feature. It may be the final result of other myeloproliferative diseases or may present as a primary disorder in middle-aged or elderly people. There is leucoerythroblastic anaemia with teardrop poikilocytosis in the peripheral blood (p. 270) and massive splenomegaly. It is usually impossible to aspirate marrow. Trephine biopsy shows extensive fibrosis. The treatment is supportive, sometimes with splenectomy to improve red cell, white cell and platelet survival. Myelofibrosis may progress to acute leukaemia.

Lymphoproliferative diseases

Hodgkin's disease

There are incidence peaks of Hodgkin's disease in early adulthood and old age. The two main clinical characteristics of lymphomas are lymphadenopathy and systemic symptoms.

A cardinal feature of Hodgkin's disease (which distinguishes it from NHL) is that, when more than one group of nodes is involved, they are always contiguous, suggesting lymphatic spread of malignant cells. The cervical nodes are most often involved. With disseminated disease, there may be hepatosplenomegaly and extralymphatic involvement. Systemic symptoms include pruritus, fever, night sweats and weight loss. Anaemia is common. There may be neutrophilia and eosinophilia. Impaired cell-mediated immunity predisposes to infection, most typically herpes zoster. Alcohol-induced pain at the site of the disease is a quite specific symptom.

The diagnostic feature on lymph node biopsy is the presence of multinucleated **Reed–Sternberg cells**.

There are several histological subtypes of Hodgkin's disease which vary, among other things, in the relative proportion of lymphocytes and reactive elements in the malignant tissue. Staging, however, is the most important determinant of treatment and prognosis. This is based on the Ann Arbor system which, in its simplest form, is:

- stage I: involvement of one group of lymph nodes only
- stage II: involvement of more than one group of lymph nodes on one side of the diaphragm
- stage III: involvement of lymph nodes on both sides of the diaphragm
- stage IV: presence of extra-lymphatic disease (e.g. bone marrow, liver).

The disease is also subclassified as:

- A: no systemic symptoms.
- B: presence of fever, night sweats or significant weight loss.

Staging therefore involves:

- a careful history and examination
- liver function tests
- CT scanning of chest, abdomen and pelvis
- bone marrow trephine biopsy.

Less favourable prognosis is associated with:

- lymphocyte-depleted histology
- higher stage
- B subtype symptoms
- increasing age
- very bulky lymphadenopathy (e.g. massive mediastinal enlargement).

Broadly speaking, treatment is with local radiotherapy for stages IA and IIA disease, and with chemotherapy, with or without radiotherapy, for higher stages. Depending on the above factors, Hodgkin's disease has a 50–90% 5-year survival.

Non-Hodgkin's lymphoma

NHL is a more heterogeneous group of disorders with varying malignancy and prognoses and may arise in a B-cell (commonest) or T-cell line. It differs from Hodgkin's disease in four ways:

- higher prevalence
- older mean age at diagnosis
- non-contiguous, multicentric spread
- extranodal involvement is more common.

Several types of NHL are known to be associated with viral infections, including Epstein-Barr virus in post-transplant lymphoma, human T-cell lymphotrophic virus-1 and HIV. Like Hodgkin's disease, NHL may present with lymphadenopathy and systemic symptoms, although the symptomology is more diverse.

Remember that lymphadenopathy must always be taken seriously. In younger people, it is more likely to be caused by infection than malignancy. In older people, there is a high likelihood of cancer (usually localised lymphadenopathy), lymphoma or chronic lymphocytic leukaemia (generalized lymphadenopathy). The diagnosis of NHL is made by biopsy. It is staged as for Hodgkin's disease.

There are two broad histological categories:

- **Low-grade NHL**: this is indolent, but may become more aggressive with time; it is essentially without cure but survival may be prolonged (>5 years).
- **High-grade NHL**: this form carries a much higher early mortality but is more responsive to treatment, with an approximately 30% 5-year disease-free survival.

Management Because NHL is usually more widespread than Hodgkin's disease at presentation, treatment is more often with chemotherapy, although localised disease is treated with radiotherapy. The use of the monoclonal antibody CD20 (rituximab) has significantly improved responses in some B-cell lymphomas. Stem cell or bone marrow transplantation is used in some patients.

Chronic lymphocytic leukaemia

Chronic lymphocytic leukaemia (CLL) is the least malignant of the leukaemias and is characteristically a disease of elderly people. It is more common in men than women. It may be a chance finding on a blood film or may present with lymphadenopathy or anaemia. Typically, there is hepatosplenomegaly. The blood film shows (sometimes massively) increased numbers of mature lymphocytes. Because the lymphocytes are abnormal B cells in over 95% of patients, there may be:

- a 'paraprotein' (see Myeloma, below)
- depression of normal immunoglobulins and increased susceptibility to infection
- autoimmune phenomena such as haemolytic anaemia or thrombocytopenia.

Many patients require no treatment, but cytotoxic therapy, corticosteroids or monoclonal antibody therapy may be indicated for symptomatic progressive disease. Progressive disease causes:

- worsening lymphocytosis
- increasing hepatosplenomegaly and lymphadenopathy
- eventually, bone marrow failure.

There is a 50% 5-year survival.

Multiple myeloma

Multiple myeloma is a malignant proliferation of plasma cells (B cells), which are relatively highly differentiated and secrete a monoclonal immunoglobulin. Myeloma is predominantly a disease of old people, although it may arise at any time in adult life. The plasma cells may secrete:

- IgG, with or without free light chains (50% of patients)
- IgA, with or without free light chains (25%)
- free light chains only (25%)
- other patterns of paraprotein (<1%)

The clinical features result from:

- plasma cell proliferation
- effects of the paraprotein
- impairment of normal haematological function.

There is bone destruction caused by local activation of osteoclasts by plasma cells without the normal osteoblastic response. This may cause diffuse osteopenia or, radiologically, punched-out lesions at the site of plasma cell deposits. Pathological fractures may result. Localised extra-medullary proliferations of plasma cells may produce plasmacytomas, tumours that can arise in any part of the body. Bone destruction mobilises calcium; consequently hypercalcaemia (p. 360) is a common complication of myeloma.

Renal failure is the other frequent complication of myeloma. It is most commonly precipitated by the nephrotoxic effect of free light chains but may also be caused by:

- hypercalcaemia
- hyperuricaemia and urate nephropathy
- infection
- amyloid deposition in the kidneys
- plasma cell infiltration of the kidneys.

Hyerviscosity is a possible problem in patients with high levels of serum paraprotein but this rarely occurs in myeloma. It is seen more often in Waldenstrom's macro-globulinaemia, a rare plasma cell proliferative disease with an IgM paraprotein.

The effects upon normal haematological function include:

- increased susceptibility to bacterial infection (typically septicaemia or pneumonia) as a result of neutropenia, defective T-lymphocyte function and reduced secretion of normal immunoglobulins
- anaemia or pancytopenia because of marrow replacement or suppression of haemopoiesis.

Clinical presentation

Patients may present with bone pain or fractures (particularly involving the spine and ribs), weight loss, anaemia, infective episodes and renal failure. Other typical symptoms include thirst, polyuria, nocturia (owing to hypercalcaemia and/or renal failure), constipation (from hypercalcaemia), lethargy and confusion.

The diagnosis is based upon finding:

- a high ESR (except in those with only light chain secretion)
- the paraprotein, by immunoelectrophoresis of blood and/or urine
- reduced concentrations of normal immunoglobulins (immune paresis)
- radiological evidence of generalised osteopenia or local bone destruction
- increased plasma cell numbers in a bone marrow aspirate.

Other laboratory features include:

- anaemia, thrombocytopenia and leucopenia
- renal failure
- hypercalcaemia.

It should be noted that the term **Bence–Jones proteinuria** is of historical interest only. It describes the behaviour of light chains in boiled urine, now superseded by immunoelectrophoresis of concentrated urine.

Management

Patients may become caught in a vicious spiral of hypercalcaemia, volume depletion and renal failure. The first step for such patients is i.v. fluid therapy (described under acute renal failure, p. 179). Infection should be sought and treated, pain controlled, and hypercalcaemia treated with i.v. bisphosphonate if fluid alone does not control it. Radiotherapy may be useful to treat severe localised pain and may be urgently indicated to relieve spinal cord compression by a plasmacytoma. Definitive treatment involves chemotherapy. The intensity of the regimen employed generally depends upon the age of the patient, varying from oral melphalan in elderly perrople to high-dose chemotherapy and stem cell transplantation in younger individuals. Thalidomide is also an effective treatment which is now used extensively and there is considerable optimism with regard to newer agents such as the immunomodulatory derivates (IMiDs) and proteosome inhibitors. Overall, the 50% survival is about 2 years but many patients live considerably logner. Most patients are

now also given long-term bisphosphonate therapy to delay the debilitating effects of myeloma bone disease.

6.4 Platelet disorders

Learning objectives

You should:
- be able to understand the clinical presentations of platelet disorders
- understand the indications for platelet transfusions
- understand how increased platelet numbers can cause thrombophilia.

Case Study

A 16-year-old girl develops a petechial skin rash soon after a viral infection. Her marrow shows active thrombopoiesis. The platelet count reaches a minimum of $20 \times 10^9/l$ but she has no serious bleeding. She recovers spontaneously without steroid therapy.

Physiology

The role of platelets is to 'plug' defects in damaged vessels, initiate coagulation and promote healing. They:

- adhere to the vessel wall
- become activated
- degranulate
- aggregate.

This can best be thought of as a cascade process, which becomes self-perpetuating as the elements activate one another.

The cascade may be triggered by:

- damage to the vessel wall, which exposes platelets to collagen and von Willebrand factor (vWF)
- blood coagulation, which leads to thrombin formation
- the activation of other platelets, which causes discharge of adenosine diphosphate (ADP), thromboxane A_2 and platelet-derived growth factor
- inflammation, which leads to release of platelet-activating factor from neutrophils and monocytes.

The process of adherence and aggregation is promoted by the prostaglandin thromboxane A_2. This is derived from arachidonic acid within platelets and held in check by prostacyclin, which is synthesised from arachidonic acid in the endothelium.

Adherence leads to platelet degranulation. The contents of the granules attract other platelets, cause platelet aggregation and trigger blood coagulation. Uncontrolled platelet adhesion and thrombosis are prevented by secretion of prostacyclin and activation of protein C (p. 282) from adjacent healthy endothelium.

Platelet numbers can easily be measured with an automated counter. Their function can be assessed crudely by measuring how long a patient bleeds after 'nicking' the skin (bleeding time) and more accurately by platelet aggregation tests in the laboratory.

Conceptually, platelet disorders are straightforward. Patients may have too many or too few platelets or platelets that do not work properly. Changes in platelet numbers are caused by increased or reduced thrombopoiesis or platelet consumption. Moderate thrombocytopenia (e.g. count < 50 × 10^9 cells/l) or decreased platelet function may result in easy bruising or excessive bleeding with surgery. Severe thrombocytopenia (e.g. count < 10 × 10^9 cells/l) can cause spontaneous mucosal or intracerebral haemorrhage, in which case urgent platelet transfusion is indicated. Transfused platelets have a short life and transfusions may need to be repeated daily. Thrombocytosis or increased platelet activity raises the coagulability of blood, causing arterial and venous thromboses. Thrombocytosis is treated with antiplatelet drugs or chemotherapy.

Thrombocytopenia

Decreased platelet production is usually caused by one of the major haematological diseases, i.e leukaemia, lymphoma, myelodysplasia, myeloma or aplastic anaemia. Other causes include:

- myelosuppressive chemotherapy
- metastatic bone marrow infiltration
- megaloblastic anaemia.

Increased platelet loss may be caused by:

- increased activity of the spleen, causing 'sequestration' of platelets
- entrapment of platelets in fibrin deposited in small vessels (see DIC, p. 285)
- immunity or autoimmunity.

The two immune mechanisms of platelet destruction are:

- antibodies formed against platelet antigens
- antigen–antibody complexes (e.g. precipitated by a drug), which bind to platelets and accelerate their destruction.

Idiopathic (immune) thrombocytopenic purpura, marrow suppression and DIC are the most important conditions to know about.

Idiopathic thrombocytopenic purpura

Idiopathic thrombocytopenic purpura may occur acutely, often in infants or young adults, sometimes soon after a viral infection and with a self-limited course which does not require treatment. It may also have a less acute presentation, typically in a young adult or middle-aged woman, and a chronic course.

The presentation is with purpura and bleeding, which may be severe. In its subacute form, it may be a chance laboratory finding. The disease is frequently benign but may lead to serious bleeding, such as GI or (rarely) cerebral haemorrhage. Platelet antibodies can be demonstrated in some patients and the marrow is active, signifying compensatory thrombopoiesis. Steroids, either immunosuppressive drugs or high-dose immunoglobulin infusions may be used. In the chronic form, steroid therapy may induce a lasting remission. If it does not and thrombocytopenia is severe, splenectomy may be effective by removing the site of platelet destruction.

Thrombocytosis

Thrombocytosis may result from decreased platelet consumption after splenectomy, although it is usually only transient. Increased production may be secondary to any marrow stimulus such as bleeding, haemolysis surgery or as a reaction to inflammation or malignancy. The one primary disease is **essential thrombocythaemia**, an uncommon myeloproliferative disease characterised by increased numbers of variably active platelets. As has been explained above, patients may either develop arterial/venous thromboses or bleed. It is characteristically a disease of middle or old age. The marrow shows megakaryocyte proliferation with other myeloproliferative features. Treatment is with antiplatelet drugs, chemotherapy, or anagrelide (a drug which inhibits platelet release from megakaryocytes). Leukaemic transformation or myelofibrosis may be late complications.

Antiplatelet therapy

Particularly in ischaemic heart disease and transient ischaemic attacks, antiplatelet therapy is of proven value in preventing arterial thromboses. It may also protect against venous thrombo-embolism. Aspirin is the most commonly used drug. It works by irreversible inhibition of cyclo-oxygenase, the key enzyme in prostaglandin synthesis. Since cyclo-oxygenase inhibition prevents synthesis of endothelial prostacyclin as well as platelet thromboxane, aspirin has prothrombotic as well as antithrombotic effects. These effects are dose-related and the balance can be shifted towards antithrombosis by giving lower doses. The main side-effects are dyspepsia, peptic ulceration and GI haemorrhage. Clopidogrel, a thienopyridine, is effective in acute coronary syndrome and stroke. It is used in patients who are sensitive to aspirin, or combined with aspirin in high-risk patients. Platelet glycoprotein receptor antagonists are also used in acute coronary syndrome.

Whether **antiplatelet** or **anticoagulant** therapy is more appropriate depends on the pathophysiology of the disease in question; platelet activation is central to the arterial thrombo-embolism of cerebrovascular (p. 230) and ischaemic heart disease (p. 11), so an antiplatelet agent is the treatment of choice to prevent them. Intracardiac thrombosis and venous thrombo-embolism are more dependent on the coagulation pathways and are, therefore, treated with anticoagulants.

6.5 Coagulation disorders

Learning objectives

You should:
- understand how coagulation defects are acquired
- know how warfarin and heparin work, when to use them, and their potential dangers
- understand the concept of hypercoagulability (thrombophilia) and its causes.

Case Study

The coroner is very critical of a doctor who prescribed warfarin for atrial fibrillation to an alcoholic man who later died of a massive cerebral haemorrhage. The risk of prescribing warfarin, in the view of the coroner, far outweighed its likely benefits.

Physiology

The functions of the coagulation and fibrinolytic system are to:

- maintain the fluidity of blood
- plug damaged vessels
- prevent the uncontrolled propagation of blood clot
- remove clot as healing proceeds.

Coagulation is a complex process, triggered by damage to tissue or the vessel wall. This exposes collagen or releases tissue thromboplastin, which activate the coagulation cascade, summarised in Figure 69. Platelet activation also triggers coagulation. The final result is conversion of fibrinogen to an insoluble fibrin plug. This is catalysed by thrombin formed from its precursor, prothrombin. Within the cascade, there are intrinsic and extrinsic systems. These converge on a common pathway that activates the final two steps of thrombin and fibrin formation. Calcium is essential to coagulation. The coagulation factors are synthesised in the liver; a number of them are dependent on vitamin K.

There are also mechanisms that restrain coagulation, notably the thrombin inhibitor antithrombin III. Protein C is another. This protein is activated by thrombin formation and feeds back to suppress the coagulation cascade. Protein S is a cofactor for that inhibitory pathway.

Once formed, clots are lysed by plasmin with the release of fibrin degradation products (FDPs). The conversion of plasminogen to plasmin is promoted by tissue plasminogen activator (tPA). The dynamic equilibrium between the formation of fibrin and its removal maintains haemostasis.

Warfarin prolongs coagulation by preventing the hepatic synthesis of vitamin K-dependent clotting factors (II, V, IX and X). Heparin potentiates antithrombin III. Fibrinolytic drugs include **streptokinase** and **recombinant tPA**, both of which potentiate plasmin formation and the breakdown of fibrin.

Fig. 69 The coagulation and fibrinolytic systems.

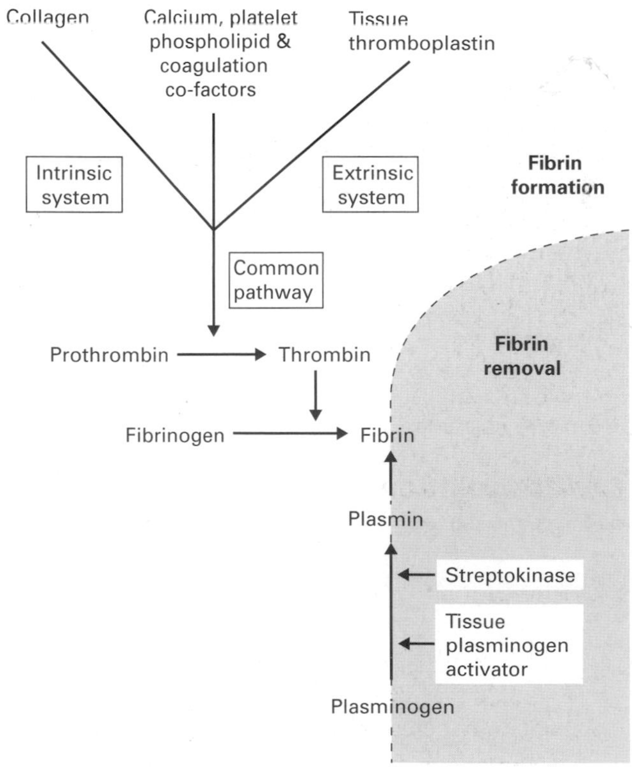

Tests of coagulation and fibrinolysis

Two tests are in general use (Fig. 70): the prothrombin time (PT) and activated partial thromboplastin time (APTT). The PT tests the extrinsic system, common pathway and fibrin formation. It is sensitive to deficiency of the vitamin K-dependent clotting factors and is prolonged by:

- malnutrition
- warfarin
- hepatocellular dysfunction
- fat malabsorption
- consumption of clotting factors, in DIC
- inherited deficiency of factor VII.

When the PT is used to measure the effect of warfarin, it is performed with standardised reagents (so that it is reproducible from one laboratory to another) and expressed as the international normalised ratio (INR).

The APTT tests the intrinsic system, common pathway and fibrin formation. It is affected by:

- liver disease
- circulating inhibitors of coagulation, including heparin
- DIC
- haemophilia A (factor VIII) and B (factor IX).

The APTT is prolonged by deficiency of the vitamin K-dependent clotting factors but less so than the PT. If prolongation of either the PT or APTT is caused by deficiency of a factor, or factors, it can be corrected in the laboratory by mixing normal plasma (replete with those factors) with the patient's plasma. If the prolonged PT or APTT is

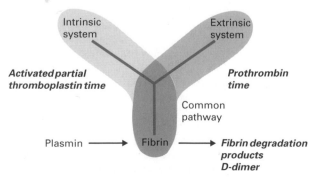

Fig. 70 Tests of coagulation and fibrinolysis.

caused by an inhibitor, it cannot be corrected in this way. The APTT is more sensitive than the PT to circulating inhibitors and is used to monitor heparin therapy.

There are two tests of fibrinolysis:

- measurement of D-dimer, a very sensitive test for the breakdown of cross-linked fibrin, used in the diagnosis of venous thrombo-embolism
- measurement of FDPs, used in the diagnosis of DIC.

Coagulation defects

Inherited coagulation defects

Only von Willebrand disease is common enough to be described here.

Von Willebrand disease

Von Willebrand factor (vWF) is a large protein released by endothelium that plays an important role in platelet adhesion and aggregation; it is also necessary as a carrier for factor VIII in plasma. Von Willebrand disease is by far the commonest inherited disorder of coagulation and a variety of types have now been described. These differ in whether vWF is present in reduced quantity (type I, type III) or is functionally defective (type II, subtypes A, B, M, N). The commonest (type I) is inherited as an autosomal dominant trait. Typically, there is a lifelong history of mild-to-moderate bleeding, usually from mucosal surfaces, but patients may not be aware that they have a bleeding disorder until they undergo surgery or have an accident, when bleeding may be excessive.

Diagnosis and classification of von Willebrand disease is not always easy, because results of laboratory investigations often vary day-to-day. Classically, patients have a prolonged bleeding time and APTT, but both may be normal. Generally, quantitative abnormalities are detected by measuring plasma von Willebrand antigen, and functional defects by measuring plasma vWF level. Treatment depends upon the situation and the type of von Willebrand disease but may involve tranexamic acid (an inhibitor of fibrinolysis), desmopressin (a synthetic analogue of antidiuretic hormone (arginine vasopressin; p. 305), which causes release of vWF from endothelial stores), vWF concentrate or, occasionally (type IIB), platelet transfusions.

Acquired coagulation defects

The causes of acquired coagulation disorders are listed under the coagulation tests above. You should remember that any GI disease that affects fat absorption may cause vitamin K deficiency. Hepatocellular dysfunction impairs coagulation factor synthesis to such an extent that the PT is a very sensitive test of hepatocellular failure. Clinical implications of this are considered under liver disease (p. 139).

The effects of warfarin and heparin are discussed in the next section and 'consumption coagulopathy' is discussed under DIC (p. 285). Vitamin K is given parenterally to treat malabsorption and to reverse the action of warfarin. It may also improve clotting factor synthesis in mild liver disease. Otherwise, the treatment for coagulation factor deficiencies is infusion of cryoprecipitate or concentrates of specific factors.

Anticoagulation and fibrinolytic therapy

Anticoagulation and fibrinolytic therapies are primarily used in cardiovascular disease including venous thrombo-embolism. Anticoagulation is considered here and fibrinolysis under acute myocardial infarction (p. 17).

Heparin

Unfractioned heparin consists of natural polysaccharides of various molecular weights, which have an almost immediate anticoagulant effect. It markedly potentiates the action of antithrombin III and inhibits serine proteases such as activated factor X (Xa). It has to be given parenterally and either by continuous infusion or as several injections per day because it has a short half-life. It is indicated whenever an immediate anticoagulant effect is required. It may also be used to prevent thrombosis (usually venous). Unfractionated heparin has now been superseded by the newer low molecular weight heparin (LMWH) preparations. These compounds act mainly by inhibition of factor Xa and have a much more predictable effect for a standard dose in different patients. This enables treatment to be given by once or twice daily subcutaneous injections, often without the need for laboratory monitoring. It also allows outpatient treatment of venous thrombo-embolism in selected patients. Warfarin can be introduced while the patient is on heparin, but, in treatment of venous thrombo-embolism, heparin should be continued until warfarinisation is adequate and for at least 5 days. Heparin-induced thrombocytopenia (HIT) is a serious side-effect which can lead to life-threatening thrombosis. More prolonged treatment (as in pregnancy) can cause osteoporosis. Great care should be taken when administering LMWH to patients with renal dysfunction as the drug can accumulate.

Warfarin

Warfarin and other coumarins are used for long-term anticoagulation. They take about 48 hours to become effective, governed by the half-lives of the vitamin K-dependent factors. Warfarin is strongly protein-bound. Anything that affects this binding will affect sensitivity to it. Liver function and levels of the vitamin K-dependent factors also affect sensitivity to warfarin to such an extent that patients may be 'autoanticoagulated'. For this reason, you must always check the PT before starting therapy. Warfarin is given as loading doses over 3 days and a maintenance dose adjusted to prolong the PT (reported as the INR; p. 282) by a factor of 1.5–4 (depending upon the indication). The effect of warfarin is unpredictable in alcoholism and liver disease. Important drug interactions are:

- potentiation of warfarin by displacement from protein binding, e.g. salicylates, sulphonamides
- potentiation of warfarin by inhibiting warfarin metabolism, e.g. metronidazole, amiodarone, cimetidine, isoniazid
- potentiation of the effect of warfarin on the liver, e.g. tetracycline
- reduced effect of warfarin by inducing warfarin metabolism, e.g. phenobarbital, carbamazepine, rifampicin.

Indications for anticoagulation

There are a number of indications for anticoagulation therapy:

- short-term prophylaxis (usually heparin)
  - prolonged recumbency
  - immobilisation, e.g. traction
  - severe heart failure
  - malignant pelvic disease or impediment to venous flow
  - perioperatively, especially after major lower limb orthopaedic surgery
  - in pregnancy in women at high risk of venous thrombo-embolism
  - in air travel (>6 hours) in individuals at high risk of venous thrombo-embolism
- acute (usually heparin)
  - venous thrombo-embolism: deep venous thrombosis, pulmonary embolism
  - arterial disease: peripheral arterial thrombosis or embolism, cardiac mural thrombo-embolism, unstable angina
- chronic (usually warfarin)
  - continued treatment of acute indications
  - prophylactically in cardiac dysrhythmia (e.g. atrial fibrillation, especially if associated with mitral stenosis), poor cardiac function (cardiomyopathy), prosthetic heart valve or vascular prosthesis, after full-thickness anterior myocardial infarct.

Contraindications to anticoagulation

There are both absolute and relative contraindications to anticoagulation therapy:

- absolute
  - cerebral haemorrhage
  - GI, urinary tract or other haemorrhage
  - active peptic ulceration
- relative
  - liver disease
  - alcoholism
  - likely poor compliance
  - concomitant drug therapy likely to cause instability.

Side-effects of anticoagulation

Even if the contraindications listed above are observed, over-anticoagulation may occur and directly cause haemorrhage from the mucosae, into the skin or into the tissues (e.g. cerebral haemorrhage). Warfarin can be reversed within a few hours by giving i.v. vitamin K or immediately by infusion of fresh frozen plasma or clotting factor concentrate. Unfractionated heparin action will wear off after about 4 hours but can be reversed rapidly by i.v. protamine. LMWH acts for 24 hours (longer with renal dysfunction) and is less predictably reversed by protamine.

Sometimes, a decision has to be taken to give anticoagulation therapy to a patient at risk of haemorrhage because the risk of not providing anticoagulation is deemed to be greater than the risk of giving it. Your responsibilities as a prescriber are to:

- vet *all* patients' suitability for anticoagulation in terms of compliance and understanding
- screen for underlying diseases which may complicate treatment
- advise patients about the risks and benefits of treatment and the need to abstain from alcohol and drugs (including over-the-counter drugs) which may complicate anticoagulation
- ensure adequate monitoring of the INR.

Thrombophilic states

Thrombophilic states may be inherited or acquired.

Inherited thrombophilia

The most common cause of inherited thrombophilia is a point mutation in the gene encoding factor V (factor V Leiden), which causes resistance to activated protein C and shifts the delicate balance of the coagulation system towards thrombosis. Antithrombin III (ATIII) deficiency is an autosomal dominant condition that is incompatible with life in its homozygous form. The prevalence of heterozygosity is about 1 per 2000. Protein C and protein S deficiency are similarly inherited but are less common. A prothrombotic variant of the prothrombin gene is also well documented.

Acquired thrombophilia

Antiphospholipid syndrome is an uncommon autoimmune disorder in which an autoantibody triggers coagulation. It may be associated with lupus (lupus anticoagulant which inhibits coagulation in the laboratory) and can cause recurrent fetal loss in young women. Anticardiolipin antibodies are often present. Lesser degrees of thrombophilia occur in any illness that increases fibrinogen levels, in pregnancy and in women taking the oral contraceptive (which is particularly prone to cause thrombosis in women with the factor V Leiden mutation). Malignant diseases frequently lead to a severe prothrombotic state. Nephrotic syndrome also predisposes to thrombosis because of urinary loss of ATIII.

Clinical presentation

Inherited thrombophilia presents with thrombosis at an early age, recurrent thrombosis, thrombosis at unusual sites (e.g. mesenteric vein) and/or a positive family history. The thromboses are usually venous.

Screening for thrombophilia

The following are indications to screen a patient for thrombophilia:

- venous thrombo-embolism in a young person (aged < 40 years)
- recurrent venous thrombosis
- family history of venous thrombo-embolism
- recurrent fetal loss
- venous thrombosis at unusual sites.

Investigations

You should check a full blood count to exclude polycythaemia (p. 273) and thrombocytosis (p. 281): measure plasma fibrinogen and the PT and APTT. Other investigations include anticardiolipin antibodies. A thrombophilia screen usually measures ATIII, activated protein C, protein C and protein S, with genetic testing for factor V Leiden and prothrombin gene variant. It should not be performed at the time of an acute event or when the patient is anticoagulated.

Management

Significant thrombophilia requires anticoagulation to cover high-risk situations (e.g. pregnancy, surgery) and, sometimes on a life-long basis.

6.6 Disseminated intravascular coagulation

Learning objectives

You should:
- know the causes of DIC
- understand its clinical effects and treatment.

Case Study

A middle-aged woman in intensive care with severe sepsis develops DIC. Her platelet count falls to 50×10^9/l. Her PT is prolonged and her FDPs are raised. She becomes anaemic and there are fragmented red cells on her blood film. She develops radiological signs of acute respiratory distress syndrome and her gas exchange worsens.

Pathophysiology

DIC describes widespread activation of the coagulation pathways secondary to a severe illness. There is intravascular fibrin deposition, which may cause microvascular occlusion. Clotting factors and platelets are consumed and may become so depleted that the patient bleeds. Fibrin in the microvasculature may cause mechanical damage to the red cells (microangiopathic haemolysis) leading to haemolytic anaemia, with schistocytes (fragmented cells, p. 266) on the blood film.

Causes

DIC can occur as a result of a number of underlying causes:

- severe sepsis (p. 410)
- incompatible blood transfusion (p. 272)
- trauma
  — particularly crush injury
- systemic diseases
  — disseminated malignancy
  — acute pancreatitis
  — acute promyelocytic leukaemia

- obstetric situations
  — retained fetal products
  — antepartum haemorrhage
  — amniotic fluid embolism.

These factors all have in common the systemic release of toxins which trigger coagulation.

Clinical effects

The dominant clinical features are usually those of the underlying illness. Often a fall in the platelet count is the first sign that the patient is developing DIC. The accompanying features of DIC can be worked out if you think system by system of the effects of small vessel occlusion:

- CNS: impaired consciousness, fits, focal neurological signs
- lungs: acute respiratory distress syndrome
- kidneys: acute renal failure
- gut: bowel infarction
- skin: ischaemic ulceration, digital gangrene.

In addition, there may be haemorrhage into any or all of these tissues. Petechial skin haemorrhages, purpura and bleeding from the mucosae may develop.

Investigations

The investigations follow directly from the pathophysiology. The diagnostic features of DIC are:

- thrombocytopenia ($<100 \times 10^9$ cells/l)
- prolonged PT and APTT
- raised FDPs and D-dimer
- reduced plasma fibrinogen
- signs of microangiopathic haemolytic anaemia (p. 271).

Management and natural history

The development of DIC is a bad prognostic sign in a disease that often already has a bad prognosis. The main aim of treatment is to control the underlying disease; without that, treating the DIC is unlikely to be of value. The treatment of DIC consists of replacing the coagulation factors (as fresh frozen plasma or cryoprecipitate) and platelets.

This narrative has described severe, fulminating DIC. Low-grade DIC may develop in association with malignant disease, vasculitis and other illnesses. Again, treatment is aimed at the underlying disease, and prognosis is determined by the disease itself more than the DIC.

Other related diseases

Detailed knowledge of the haemolytic uraemic syndrome, thrombotic thrombocytopenic purpura and other such rare diseases is not 'core'. You should simply be aware that the pathophysiological processes of consumption coagulopathy and microangiopathic haemolysis can occur in settings other than classical DIC.

Six

Self-assessment: questions

Multiple choice questions

Any or all of each set of five statements may be true or false. Choose your answers and see the reasoning behind the correct answer on page 291.

1. In lymphoma:
   a. If a newly presenting patient has generalised lymphadenopathy, the diagnosis is more likely to be non-Hodgkin's lymphoma than Hodgkin's disease
   b. Early stages of Hodgkin's disease can be cured by radiotherapy alone
   c. Lymphocyte predominance is a favourable histological sign in Hodgkin's disease
   d. Pain in lymph nodes after alcohol is very typical of non-Hodgkin's lymphoma
   e. Bone marrow transplantation has greatly improved the prognosis of low-grade non-Hodgkin's lymphoma

2. The following statements are true:
   a. A neutrophil count of only 0.8×10^9 cells/l is a major risk for infection
   b. A neutrophil count in a febrile patient of 25×10^9 cells/l mostly reflects the production of new neutrophils from the bone marrow
   c. In a patient with less than 0.1×10^9 cells/l neutrophils and a fever, treatment with antibiotics should await the results of blood culture
   d. Neutropenia is common in AIDS
   e. Neutropenia can be caused by carbimazole therapy

Single best answer multiple choice questions

For each numbered question, only one of the options lettered a–e is correct.

1. A 36-year-old man on renal dialysis has the following laboratory results:

Haemoglobin	83 g/l
Mean cell volume	78 fl
Ferritin	200 µg/l

   What is the most likely cause of his anaemia?
   a. Leucoerythroblastic anaemia
   b. Hereditary spherocytosis
   c. Folate deficiency
   d. Iron deficiency
   e. Anaemia of chronic disease

2. Select the single best of the following statements regarding the treatment of thrombocytopenia:
   a. Corticosteroids are given to prevent haemorrhage, whatever the cause
   b. Corticosteroids are routinely given in idiopathic thrombocytopenia
   c. The aim of platelet transfusions is to normalise the platelet count
   d. A platelet count below 10×10^9/l is an indication for platelet transfusion
   e. In severe thrombocytopenia, platelet transfusions have to be repeated up to once a week

3. A woman who has had a life-threatening episode of venous thrombo-embolism during pregnancy is advised to take low molecular weight heparin for the remainder of the pregnancy. Which of the following statements do you most strongly agree with?
   a. Prolonged heparin treatment in this situation may cause thrombocytopenia
   b. Heparin is inappropriate therapy because it is more likely to harm the fetus than warfarin
   c. An important potential side-effect of prolonged heparin therapy is osteomalacia
   d. The dose of heparin should be adjusted according to the prothrombin time
   e. Low molecular weight heparin has to be given four times daily to achieve a stable therapeutic effect

Extended matched questions

EMQ 1

Theme: Haematological diagnoses
Options
1. Hodgkin's disease
2. Acute lymphoblastic leukaemia
3. Myelofibrosis
4. Chronic granulocytic (myeloid) leukaemia
5. von Willebrand's disease
6. Iron deficiency anaemia
7. Thalassaemia trait
8. Anaemia of chronic disease
9. Hereditary spherocytosis
10. Acute myeloid leukaemia
11. Pernicious anaemia
12. Non-Hodgkin's lymphoma
13. Multiple myeloma

For each of the following patients, select the most likely final diagnosis given the clinical feature(s) (more than one may be correct). Each item can be used once, more than once or not at all.

A. An anaemic elderly patient with a palpable spleen has a 'dry tap' on attempted bone marrow aspiration.

B. A 35-year-old woman with weight loss, fever and pruritus has masses of large lymph nodes only in the neck and axillae.

C. A 53-year-old man has an increased count of neutrophil leucocytes showing the 'Philadelphia chromosome'.

D. An otherwise healthy woman with menorrhagia and mild anaemia has a reduced mean red cell volume.

E. An elderly patient with acute renal failure has severe hypercalcaemia.

EMQ 2
Theme: Drug treatments
Options
1. Unfractionated heparin
2. Dipyridamole
3. Reteplase
4. Sinthrome (acenocoumanol/nicoumalone)
5. Aspirin
6. Warfarin adjusted to achieve an INR ≥2
7. Intravenous streptokinase
8. Low molecular weight heparin
9. Intranasal epoprostenol (prostacyclin)

For each of the following patients not currently on any of the drugs on the list above, select the most appropriate drug (more than one may be correct). Each item can be used once, more than once or not at all.

A. A 65-year-old woman with repeated carotid transient ischaemic attacks (TIAs) who has a <70% stenosis of the internal carotid artery and intimal plaque seen on carotid Doppler.

B. A 40-year-old man newly admitted with an acute pulmonary embolism 14 days after fracturing his femur.

C. A 59-year-old patient admitted to the coronary care unit with unstable angina on no treatment.

D. A 72-year-old man with atrial fibrillation and a small stroke, which resolved completely within 5 days, whose echocardiogram shows left atrial thrombus.

E. An 88-year-old man with early dementia and in atrial fibrillation who is to be discharged to live alone, having been admitted after a fall.

EMQ 3
Theme: Anaemia
Options
1. Iron deficiency anaemia
2. Vitamin B_{12} deficiency
3. Folate deficiency
4. Aplastic anaemia
5. Anaemia of chronic disease
6. Leucoerythroblastic anaemia
7. Hereditary spherocytosis
8. Sickle cell disease
9. Thalassaemia
10. Glucose-6-phosphate dehydrogenase deficiency
11. Autoimmune haemolytic anaemia
12. Microangiopathic haemolytic anaemia
13. Hypersplenism

For each of the following anaemic patients, select the most likely diagnosis (more than one may be correct). Each item can be used once, more than once or not at all.

A. A patient with disseminated cancer whose blood film contains immature red and white blood cells.

B. An alcoholic patient with macrocytic anaemia living rough.

C. A Cypriot patient with microcytic anaemia and a raised serum ferritin.

D. An acutely ill patient with disseminated intravascular coagulation.

E. A patient with known polycythaemia vera whose red cells are microcytic.

Objective structured clinical examination (OSCE) stations
OSCE 1
This is a 5-minute station with a normal volunteer on a couch.

Examiner: This 35-year-old man has been found to have a mediastinal mass and lymphoma is suspected. Please examine him.

After you have examined him:

Examiner: What features of any lymph nodes found on examination would help your differential diagnosis?

OSCE 2
A 5-minute finals viva-style OSCE station.

Examiner: Please interpret this blood count from a 70-year-old man:

Haemoglobin	63 g/l
Platelets	15×10^9/l
White blood cell count	1.3×10^9/l

a. What complications might you expect in such a patient?
b. How would you prevent them?

OSCE 3
A 10-minute station with a blood count result.

Examiner: The blood count result that I am about to show you was found incidentally in a 62-year-old man admitted with a chest infection. Please comment on it and offer one or more diagnoses.

Haemoglobin	112 g/l
Mean cell volume	85 fl
White blood cell count	38.0×10^9/l
Neutrophils	3.5×10^9/l
Lymphocytes	34.0×10^9/l
Eosinophils	0.2×10^9/l
Monocytes	0.2×10^9/l
Basophils	0.1×10^9/l
Platelets	97×10^9/l

After you have commented:

Examiner:

a. What findings might you expect on examination?
b. How do you think the chest infection might be related to this blood count?
c. How would you manage him?

Case history questions

Case history 1

Your consultant is concerned that a 73-year-old man in atrial fibrillation is at risk of stroke and asks you to anticoagulate him. You are aware that the patient is vaguely confused and the nursing staff on the ward have received a telephone call from a neighbour stating that he has become increasingly reclusive. He has often been noted to be unsteady on his feet and has once been found lying in the road. At visiting time you have a chance to meet his wife to discuss the plan to use anticoagulation therapy and to give further information.

1. Suggest two important questions which you should ask.
2. Name two haematological investigations which it would be appropriate to perform.
3. Name two possible contraindications to anticoagulation in this case.
4. If a decision were made to proceed with anticoagulation, describe two pieces of advice that you would give to the patient and his wife.

Case history 2

You are called on a Sunday to see a 63-year-old man with non-Hodgkin's lymphoma and a fever of 38.6°C. He is in reverse barrier nursing because his total white cell count is 0.2×10^9/l and his platelets are 15×10^9/l despite daily platelet transfusions. He received intensive chemotherapy (fludarabine) 15 days previously and has been leucopenic for 7 days. You put on your gown, mask and gloves to examine the patient and find that he has no symptoms except those of the fever, mild headache, sweating and an uncomfortable feeling around his bottom.

1. Which of the following actions would be appropriate?
   a. Order a chest X-ray
   b. Take a blood culture
   c. Do a blood count
   d. Do a digital rectal examination
   e. Start him on oral amoxicillin

The senior nurse on the ward encourages you to start him on the 'usual' antibiotics (tazocin and gentamicin). His fever is still elevated 6 hours later despite antibiotics and he looks more toxic. The consultant suggests that you add metronidazole to his regimen. Four days later you are also on call and are asked to see him again. He has had fever up to 38.3°C for 4 days despite tazocin, gentamicin, metronidazole and 2 days of vancomycin. He now has a dry cough, in addition to a painful bottom.

2. What actions should you now take?
   a. Look at his white cell and platelet counts from that morning
   b. Arrange for transfer to an intensive care unit (ITU)
   c. Examine him again carefully
   d. Treat him for a possible fungal infection
   e. Do blood cultures, including a fungal blood culture

On examination, you find crackles at the left base that do not clear on coughing and a black and red perianal area about 2 cm across with surrounding erythema.

3. Should you?
   a. Speak to his consultant at home
   b. Arrange a chest X-ray
   c. Arrange an induced sputum
   d. Call the physiotherapist in
   e. Arrange for a special mattress to help his developing pressure sore

4. Give a differential diagnosis and your thoughts on management.

Key features questions

1. A previously well 19-year-old woman has become very lethargic and has been feverish at times. She has no headache and her conscious level is not impaired. She is pale and has a petechial rash over her lower legs. She has no lymphadenopathy and her liver and spleen are impalpable. Her blood count shows the following:

Haemoglobin	72 g/l
Platelets	15×10^9/l
White cell count	23×10^9/l
Blood film	Leucocytosis; blast cells seen

Which would be the two most important aspects of a more detailed physical examination?

a. Test for Kernig's sign

b. Test carefully for signs of a paraparesis

c. Examine the fundi with an ophthalmoscope

d. Examine carefully for signs of a peripheral neuropathy

e. Perform bedside tests of cognitive function

f. Measure visual acuity

g. Test for an afferent pupil defect

h. Examine her mouth and throat with a torch and spatula

i. Examine the perineum

j. Examine the conjunctivae

k. Examine the neck for signs of an enlarged thyroid gland

l. Auscultate carefully for heart murmurs

m. Auscultate carefully for wheezes

n. Examine the abdomen for signs of an enlarged bladder

o. Measure her temperature

p. Measure peak flow

2. A 40-year-old woman who was warfarinised 5 years ago for a deep venous thrombosis will be flying from London to Sydney. In the past, she has also had an episode of upper gastrointestinal bleeding whilst being treated with diclofenac for reactive arthritis.

Select the most appropriate course of action:

a. Use no specific thromboprophylaxis

b. Wear compression stockings but do not use drug therapy

c. Take aspirin

d. Take clopidogrel

e. Take aspirin and clopidogrel

f. Take low molecular weight heparin

g. Take warfarin

Data interpretation questions

1. Suggest a cause for the findings described in Table 65 for each of six patients.

Table 65 Data obtained for six patients

	A	B	C	D	E	F
Haemoglobin (g/l)	42	78	185	91	87	84
Mean cell volume (fl)	123	69	96	85	80	86
White cell count (×10⁹/l)	2.3	13.6	15.3	8.7	63.0	1.7
Platelets (×10⁹/l)	60	200	600	180	140	48

2. A 22-year-old patient is admitted to hospital 48 hours after a paracetamol overdose, complaining of haematuria. The prothrombin time is 60 sec (control 18 sec). What is the likely diagnosis?

3. A 70-year-old man is referred to hospital because he is anaemic (haemoglobin 82 g/l, mean cell volume 90 fl, platelets 150 × 10⁹ cells/l, ESR 130 mm/hr. Name a possible haematological diagnosis. What biochemical tests should be performed?

Picture questions

1. This skull radiograph (Fig. 71) was taken from a 73-year-old patient who presented in acute renal failure.

   a. What abnormality do you see?

   b. How could the skull radiograph be relevant to the renal failure? Be as precise as you can.

   c. Name one rapid biochemical test which might establish a link.

   d. What would be your immediate management?

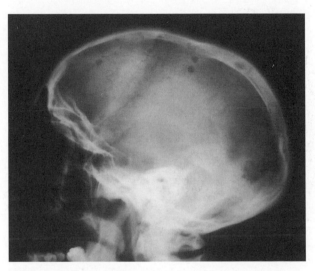

Fig. 71 A skull radiograph of a patient in acute renal failure.

2. A previously fit 28-year-old woman has lost weight.
    She has night sweats and pruritus, and has noticed
    pain in the cervical region after drinking alcohol.
    Her GP arranges a chest radiograph which is
    thought to show hilar enlargement. Figure 72 shows
    thoracic CT scans before (A) and after (B) an
    intravenous contrast agent.

    a. What abnormality is shown?
    b. Suggest, in order of likelihood, a differential
        diagnosis.

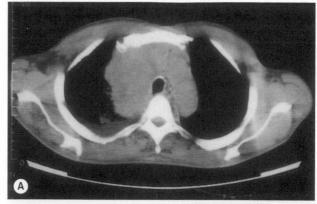

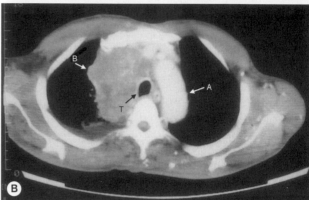

Fig. 72 Thoracic CT scans. **A** Before injection of an intravenous
contrast agent. **B** After. T, trachea; A, aortic arch; B, left brachiocephalic
vein.

Self-assessment: answers

Multiple choice answers

1. a. **True**. In Hodgkin's disease, the lymphadenopathy is often confined to a single site, most commonly the neck, at presentation.

   b. **True**.

   c. **True**.

   d. **False**. Alcohol-related pain is typical of Hodgkin's disease.

   e. **False**. There is no evidence for this in clinical trials to date.

2. a. **False**. A minor risk. It is when the count falls below 0.5×10^9 cells/l and particularly 0.1×10^9 cells/l that the risk becomes major.

   b. **False**. Mostly neutrophil release from the marginating pool. The left shift (or band forms) is the proportion of new neutrophils from the marrow.

   c. **False**. Immediate intravenous broad-spectrum antibiotics are indicated.

   d. **True**. Especially caused by the drugs zidovudine and ganciclovir.

   e. **True**. Neutropenia occurs in 1:10 000 patients treated with carbimazole for thyrotoxicosis.

Single best answer multiple choice answers

1. **e is correct**. The patient is anaemic with mild microcytosis. There are no hints that he might have a haemoglobinopathy. The differential diagnosis is between iron deficiency anaemia and anaemia of chronic disease. The normal serum ferritin indicates the latter.

2. **d is correct**. Corticosteroids are given in selected cases of idiopathic thrombocytopenia and some other haematological diseases, but by no means routinely even to patients with idiopathic thrombocytopenic purpura. Platelet transfusions cannot be expected to normalise the platelet count and, even if they do, the effect is transient. Platelet transfusions have to be given daily in severe thrombocytopenia.

3. **a is correct**. Heparin is less likely to harm the fetus than warfarin. Heparin causes osteoporosis, not osteomalacia. Usually, low molecular weight heparin is not monitored at all, though there is a case for doing so in pregnancy; however, the prothrombin time would not be the appropriate test. One important reason for using low molecular weight rather than unfractionated heparin is that it does not have to be given four times daily; it is given once daily.

Extended matched answers

EMQ 1

A. **3.** The dry tap suggests myelofibrosis and splenomegaly is characteristic.

B. **1.** This patient has 'B' symptoms and pathological lymphadenopathy; the fact that it is in adjacent areas (on only one side of the diaphragm) suggests Hodgkin's disease.

C. **4.** The Philadelphia chromosome is pathognomonic of chronic granulocytic leukaemia.

D. **6.** Either thalassaemia trait or chronic disease could also give a microcytic anaemia, but the clinical details strongly favour iron deficiency.

E. **13.** Of course, there are many causes of renal failure, but the heading makes it clear that you should be making a haematological diagnosis; myeloma is the haematological disease most closely associated with renal failure.

EMQ 2

A. **5.** TIAs are caused by platelet emboli so aspirin is the treatment of choice.

B. **8.** Fibrinolytic therapy is of no proven value, and may cause him to bleed into the fracture site. He will certainly need to take warfarin but must be treated with heparin first. Clinical trials consistently show low molecular weight heparin to be superior to unfractionated heparin so that should be your choice.

C. **8, 5.** Either aspirin or heparin would be correct, but low molecular weight heparin is the better answer.

D. **6 or 4.** Unlike carotid TIAs, arterial thrombo-embolism from cardiac clot should be treated with warfarin (or Sinthrome, although it is less commonly used). Depending on your perception of the danger of recurrence, you might give heparin, but medium- to long-term warfarin is the mainstay of preventing recurrence.

E. **5.** Warfarin is indicated for preventing cerebral embolism in atrial fibrillation unless there are contraindications. Age, falls and concern about this patient's ability to care for himself are relative contraindications. Depending on likely compliance, you might prescribe aspirin.

EMQ 3

A. **6.** The presence of immature cells in peripheral blood indicates marrow replacement with tumour.

B. **3.** Folate deficiency due to poor nutrition.

C. **9.**

D. **12.** Physical damage to red cells caused by strands of fibrin in the circulation causing haemolysis.

E. **1.**

Responses to OSCE stations

OSCE 1

Do not waffle on about 'taking a history' because your instruction is clear and do not attempt to perform a 'general' physical examination. You must use your knowledge to focus the examination on checking:

- all possible sites of lymphadenopathy: the epitrochlear region of the elbow, neck, axillae and groins
- the abdomen for para-aortic nodes (by deep palpation), hepatomegaly and splenomegaly
- the conjunctivae for anaemia.

It is reasonable to examine the chest if you have time, but make less of a play of this than the parts of the examination listed above because chest examination may well be normal, and these other features will be much more informative, whether negative or positive.

The character and distribution of the nodes are both important; see page 264.

OSCE 2

At this stage of your training, you might reasonably be expected — as in this case — to interpret a blood count without being given normal ranges. On request, the examiner could provide you with that information, but you would lose points if you needed to ask for it. The patient is pancytopenic — in other words, each of the three cell types is greatly reduced.

a. This patient's anaemia may precipitate symptoms of coronary, cerebrovascular or peripheral vascular ischaemia and may cause heart failure. His thrombocytopenia may cause purpura, bruising and — in servere cases — mucosal or GI bleeding or cerebral haemorrhage. His neutropenia may cause mouth ulceration, perineal infection and susceptibility to opportunistic infection.

b. Anaemia is treated with blood transfusions. Thrombocytopenia is treated with platelet transfusions if the patient is severely thrombocytopenic and at risk of haemorrhage. Granulocyte transfusions are relatively ineffective and so the treatment of neutropenia is prophylaxis against infection and aggressive treatment of the earliest signs of it.

OSCE 3

This report shows a mild normochromic, normocyitc anaemia. The total white count is raised by a very marked lymphocytosis. The platelet count is reduced. The neutrophil count is relatively low for someone with a chest infection. The likely diagnosis is chronic lymphocytic leukaemia.

a. On examination, mild lymphadenopathy, possibly with splenomegaly, might be expected.

b. It is possible that the chest infection has been caused by a mild immunoparesis.

c. His management will include bone marrow aspiration to confirm the diagnosis, antibiotic prophylaxis after discharge, chemotherapy if required to treat any progression in the anaemia and thrombocytopenia, and long-term follow-up.

Case history answers

Case history 1

1. Whilst anticoagulation is indicated to prevent cerebral embolism in patients with atrial fibrillation, you must not initiate it unless you are sure it will be safe. Age, in itself, is not a contraindication, but there are aspects of the history which suggest there are other contraindications. There are strong hints that he may be abusing alcohol. The confusion is worrying because someone who is having falls and becomes confused could have a subdural haematoma, which is an absolute contraindication to anticoagulation. You should ask about:
   - his alcohol intake
   - dyspepsia or history of blood loss
   - his likelihood of taking tablets and attending for anticoagulant monitoring reliably.

2. You should measure his prothrombin time *before starting anticoagulants*; autoanticoagulation is common and would affect your choice of loading dose. It would also increase your anxiety about the possibility of alcohol abuse (prolonging the PT by causing hepatocellular damage). You should also check the haemoglobin concentration; anaemia would be a relative contraindication to anticoagulation or should, at least, be investigated before anticoagulation.

3. These might include:
   - alcohol abuse
   - dementia (if it would interfere with compliance)
   - difficulty attending for anticoagulant monitoring
   - inability of wife or carer to supervise treatment
   - history of GI bleeding or anaemia
   - history of cerebral haemorrhage
   - concomitant drug therapy affecting the stability of warfarin levels
   - falls.

4. Advice would include:
   - Avoid alcohol.
   - Avoid non-steroidal analgesics and aspirin.
   - Report any excessive or unusual bleeding immediately.
   - Attend regularly for anticoagulant monitoring.
   You should give the patient and his wife an information sheet about anticoagulants, listing drugs to be avoided.

Case history 2

1. a. **True**. This is always appropriate in febrile neutropenia, even in the absence of chest signs or symptoms.
   b. **True**. Very important.
   c. **False**. Unnecessary if done that morning, which it will have been to see whether platelet transfusions were required.
   d. **False**. You must inspect his anal area as he has a symptom there, but a formal rectal examination is not appropriate as it may cause bacteraemia.

e. **False**. Not appropriate; i.v. therapy required with broader coverage.

2. a. **True**.

b. **False**. He is not that ill and you would take him out of protective isolation. In fact, even if he were so ill and requiring ventilation, neutropenic leukaemic patients do so badly in ITU that it is used rarely.

c. **True**. Always true in this group of patients. Especially mouth, chest, skin and rectal area (p. 275).

d. **True**. Candidaemia or invasive aspergillosis is now more likely. This group of patients with persistent fever during neutropenia have a 30% mortality, mostly as a result of fungal infection.

e. **True**. It is always worth repeating blood cultures, even though he is on antibiotics, as these patients develop breakthrough bacteraemia.

3. a. **True**. Now you have a complex problem with two possible sites of infection.

b. **True**. If one was not done that day. A CT scan of his chest is a much better investigation and should be done within the next 24 hours.

c. **False**. Not useful in febrile neutropenia (unlike AIDS), although *Pneumocystis* pneumonia is a diagnostic possibility because fludarabine therapy 'paralyses' T cells.

d. **False**. As the cough is not productive, of no benefit.

e. **False**. His lesion is almost certainly not a pressure sore but a developing infection called icthyma gangrenosum (*Pseudomonas aeruginosa*).

4. He probably has two focal infections: one in his lungs and the other perirectally. The perirectal infection is likely to be caused by *Pseudomonas aeruginosa*, other bacteria including anaerobes, *Aspergillus* or mucormycosis. His lung disease may be caused by any of these or other bacteria or possibly *Pneumocystis*. He needs large doses of antifungals (amphotericin), a CT scan of the lung, which is helpful diagnostically, bronchoscopy, with lavage, to obtain material for microscopy and culture, and a biopsy of his rectal lesion, all as soon as possible.

Key features answers

1. **o and i or h are correct.** She very probably has acute myeloblastic leukaemia. She has a history of fever. She may be infected now and may need antibiotics. To help decide, you must measure her temperature. The perineum is a classical site for unsuspected infection and must be inspected carefully. It is also good practice to examine for treatable oral infection. Whilst the other items might be features of any thorough examination, they are less immediately relevant, particularly the items that have nothing to do with infection.

2. **f is correct.** Someone who has had one venous thrombosis is at increased risk of having another one. She is facing a long-haul flight, which is a risk factor. Antiplatelet agents such as aspirin and clopidogrel would be less effective than heparin or warfarin. Warfarin has a slow onset and has to be monitored. Low molecular weight heparin does not need to be monitored and can be self-administered. It would be an appropriate choice in this case.

Data interpretation answers

1. *Patient A* This is a fairly typical picture of megaloblastic anaemia caused by vitamin B_{12} or folate deficiency with severe macrocytosis, leucopenia and thrombocytopenia; hypersegmented neutrophils on the blood film would confirm the diagnosis, as would bone marrow aspiration, although this is not done as a routine. Haematinics should be measured.

Patient B This is a moderately severe microcytic anaemia. (The differential diagnosis is given on p. 271.) Iron deficiency is the most likely cause. The leucocytosis may be caused by infection or inflammation but could signify acute or subacute blood loss, a possible cause for the iron deficiency.

Patient C There is erythrocytosis, thrombocytosis and leucocytosis, suggestive of polycythaemia vera. The red cell mass is likely to be increased and splenomegaly may be present.

Patient D There is a normocytic anaemia with normal white cell and platelet counts. This would be typical of the anaemia of chronic disease (e.g. renal failure) but could also be caused by a mixed deficiency. This would be suggested by an increased red cell distribution width (RDW) and a 'dimorphic' blood film. You should examine and investigate the patient for an underlying disease.

Patient E There is a normochromic anaemia with mild thrombocytopenia, but the striking abnormality is the marked leucocytosis; this is typical of a chronic leukaemia. A differential white cell count and blood film would be crucial.

Patient F This shows moderate pancytopenia and could be seen in a patient with acute leukaemia, hypoplastic anaemia or after chemotherapy (see p. 269 for a fuller list of causes).

2. Prolongation of the prothrombin time may be caused by warfarin, consumption of clotting factors as in DIC, vitamin K deficiency or deficiency of the vitamin K-dependent clotting factors owing to liver disease. About 48 hours after a massive paracetamol overdose is when hepatocellular damage becomes apparent, and the prothrombin time is quite a sensitive test for this. The likely diagnosis is acute hepatocellular necrosis caused by paracetamol.

3. An extremely high ESR is usually caused by multiple myeloma, giant cell arteritis or chronic/severe infection/inflammation. This patient also has a moderate normochromic anaemia. Multiple

myeloma is a likely diagnosis. Renal failure and hypercalcaemia are common in myeloma. You should measure plasma urea, creatinine and calcium. The definitive diagnosis is made by plasma and urine immunoelectrophoresis, bone marrow examination and skeletal survey.

Picture answers

1. a. Figure 71 shows multiple 'punched-out' lesions, in keeping with multiple myeloma or another cause of osteolytic metastases.

   b. Hypercalcaemia is a common cause of acute renal failure in multiple myeloma. Volume depletion is an important and reversible effect of hypercalcaemia. 'Myeloma kidney' may cause renal failure without hypercalcaemia. This is because of tubular damage by the paraprotein, secondary hyperuricaemia, amyloidosis and infection.

   c. With the history given, you should immediately measure serum calcium. You should also arrange serum and urine immunoelectrophoresis to identify a paraprotein but that is not an emergency investigation.

   d. You should assess the patient's volume status, using a central venous pressure line if necessary, and give saline to increase urinary calcium excretion. Corticosteroid and/or bisphosphonate therapy may be needed as second-line treatment for hypercalcaemia.

2. a. There is a large soft tissue attenuation mass within the mediastinum abutting the trachea and aortic arch and compressing the superior vena cava (which cannot be seen). This is almost certainly a large lymph node mass.

   b. Although you are not told that she has cervical lymphadenopathy, the scenario makes it very likely that she is describing alcohol-related lymph node pain, which is very specific to Hodgkin's disease. The combination with mediastinal lymphadenopathy makes the diagnosis of Hodgkin's by far the most likely. Other causes of a mediastinal soft tissue mass include non-Hodgkin's lymphoma (not associated with alcohol-related pain) or sarcoidosis (the second most likely possibility in this case). Unlikely causes are tuberculosis, retrosternal thyroid (unlikely), thymic tumour, dermoid or lung cancer nodes (especially small cell).

Endocrinology and metabolism

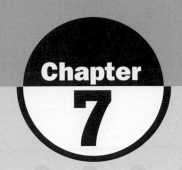

7.1 Background

Learning objectives

You need to:

- know the range of common endocrine diseases
- understand the relationship between the pathological processes of autoimmunity, neoplasia and failure of feedback regulation and those diseases
- understand how biochemical testing and imaging are used to diagnose endocrine disease.

Case Study

A woman in her twenties develops amenorrhoea. The consultant explains to the medical student that dynamic tests are not needed to tell her ovarian failure is primary because her gonadotrophins are very high.

Endocrinology may seem a large and disjointed subject because there are many glands, each with its own diseases and symptomatology. There are, however, some unifying principles of pathology, investigation and management which make learning easier. Remember that glands malfunction in three ways:

- by enlarging
- by becoming overactive
- by becoming underactive.

Sometimes, enlargement is combined with underactivity or overactivity. The pituitary gland has a central, con-trolling function. Remember that there are six anterior pituitary hormones and one posterior pituitary hormone, which control the endocrine 'axes' described in Figure 73. The main endocrine diseases are shown in Table 66.

Pathology

Endocrine underactivity is usually autoimmune (e.g. hypoparathyroidism, hypothyroidism, Addison's disease, type 1 diabetes mellitus (type 1 DM)). The exception is hypopituitarism, which is usually caused by a tumour. Endocrine overactivity usually results from a tumour (e.g. acromegaly, hyperprolactinaemia, Cushing's and Conn's syndromes, phaeochromocytoma, hyperparathyroidism and insulinoma). The exception is hyperthyroidism which is often (but not always) autoimmune. Most endocrino-logically active tumours are benign, because malignant tumours behave in a primitive way and grow at the expense of hormone synthesis. That does not apply to ectopic hormone production; some extremely malignant tumours that are not derived from an endocrine gland synthesise hormones, e.g. adrenocorticotrophic hormone (ACTH), antidiuretic hormone (ADH) and parathyroid hormone (PTH)-related peptide (p. 361) from small cell carcinoma of the bronchus.

Investigations

There are three main types of investigation:

- measurement of hormone concentrations or responses
- imaging
- autoantibody measurement.

Biochemistry

There are two types of biochemical test: static and dynamic. Static tests are single tests measuring blood hormone levels at one point in time. Dynamic tests measure how that hormone level responds to a stimulus. Static tests are used first and may be sufficient. For example, demonstrat-ing that the serum cortisol is unmeasurably low in a patient with a large pituitary tumour and clinically obvious hypo-pituitarism is diagnostic of hypoadrenalism. Some static tests (e.g. thyroid-stimulating hormone (TSH) measure-ment) are now so sensitive that they have made dynamic tests redundant. Dynamic tests are more sensitive but

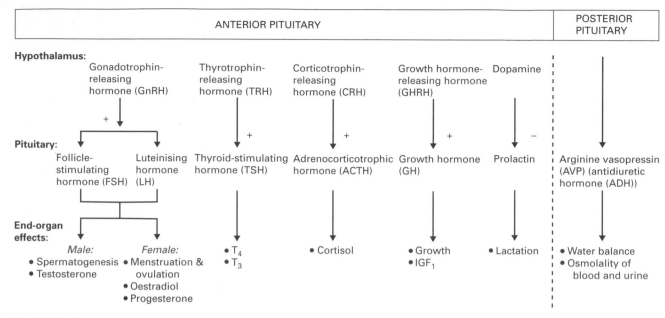

Fig. 73 Hypothalamic and pituitary hormones and their effects. IGF, insulin-like growth factor; T_3, triidothyronine; T_4, thyroxine.

Table 66 A scheme for revising endocrine diseases

	Overactivity	Underactivity	Enlargement
Thyroid	Hyperthyroidism	Hypothyroidism	Thyroid nodule/goitre
Pituitary	Acromegaly, hyperprolactinaemia	Hypopituitarism, diabetes insipidus	Pituitary tumour
Adrenal			
HPA axis	Cushing's syndrome	Hypoadrenalism (including Addison's disease)	
RAA axis	Conn's syndrome		
Medulla	Phaeochromocytoma		
Parathyroid	Hyperparathyroidism*	Hypoparathyroidism*	
Pancreas	Insulinoma	Diabetes mellitus	

HPA, hypothalamo–pituitary–adrenal; RAA, renin–angiotensin–aldosterone.
*See Chapter 8.

more complex and expensive. If there was doubt that the patient described above was hypoadrenal, he would be challenged by ACTH stimulation or insulin hypoglycaemia to see if he could produce cortisol under stress. Dynamic tests have a simple underlying principle:

- If you suspect that a gland is overactive, try to suppress its function.
- If you suspect that it is underactive, stimulate it.

Imaging

Ultrasound, computed tomography (CT) and magnetic resonance (MR) imaging are the most sensitive methods of finding and delineating mass lesions and showing their texture. Radionuclide scanning is generally less sensitive but can show that tissue is endocrinologically active and can find lesions that cannot be found in any other way (e.g. metastases of thyroid cancer located by labelled iodine scanning or use of labelled somatostatin analogue to locate an endocrinologically active tumour).

Immunology

Immunology plays a limited part, usually secondary to clinical diagnosis and biochemistry. For example, high titres of adrenal or thyroid microsomal antibodies support clinical and biochemical diagnoses of autoimmune Addison's disease and Hashimoto's thyroiditis, respectively. They can also predict that a patient is at risk of developing them.

Management

Overactive glands can be treated surgically, with a drug that reduces hormone synthesis or by radiotherapy. If a gland is underactive, the treatment is to replace the missing hormone or give a synthetic analogue.

The efficacy of treatment can be monitored in three ways:

- the end-organ effects (health and wellbeing)
- plasma level of the replaced hormone
- levels of a trophic hormone; for example, measurement of TSH to check the adequacy of thyroid replacement therapy (p. 300).

This chapter will go through diseases, gland by gland, and consider their pathology, clinical presentation, investigations, management and prognosis.

7.2 Thyroid disease

Learning objectives

You should . . .
- know the main clinical features and investigation of thyroid disease
- understand how to approach the patient with 'a lump in the thyroid'
- know how to treat over- and under-production of thyroid hormones
- know how to deal with thyroid swelling.

Case Study

A 30-year-old woman has a flu-like illness, during which her throat and the front of her neck become sore. Over the next 3 weeks, she becomes trembly, tearful and anxious. Her muscles ache and she feels generally lousy. She is found to be mildly thyrotoxic. She has a radioiodine uptake scan, which shows greatly reduced uptake over the thyroid gland. She is told that antithyroid treatment is unhelpful in people like her with subacute thyroiditis and given propranolol. She is warned that her thyroid may swing from being overactive to underactive, but it should all settle down eventually.

Normal thyroid function

The synthesis of thyroid hormone (thyroxine (T_4) and triiodothyronine (T_3)) is controlled by a sequence of hormonal signals:

- thyrotrophin-releasing hormone (TRH) secreted by the hypothalamus into the hypophysial portal system
- thyroid-stimulating hormone (TSH) secreted by the pituitary into the systemic circulation
- feedback inhibition exerted by thyroid hormones on the pituitary and hypothalamus.

Thyroxine and triiodothyronine are largely protein-bound. Thyroxine is converted to triiodothyronine by deiodination in the thyroid and peripheral tissues. The level of thyroid hormone determines tissue metabolic activity.

Hyperthyroidism

Hyperthyroidism is a better term than thyrotoxicosis because overproduction of thyroid hormone is the funda-

mental abnormality and the clinical expression (toxicosis) of the disease is secondary to it and remarkably variable.

Pathology

The common causes of hyperthyroidism are Graves' disease and toxic nodular goitre.

Graves' disease This is also known as diffuse toxic goitre and is the classical cause of hyperthyroidism. It is caused by antibodies formed within the thyroid that bind to TSH receptors on follicular cells and stimulate thyroid hormone synthesis and secretion; other autoantibodies promote thyroid growth and eye disease (see below). It is possible to have ophthalmic signs of Graves' disease without hyperthyroidism and vice versa, presumably because there are different antibodies in different individuals.

Toxic nodular goitre This term describes autonomous solitary or multinodular goitres that are probably not autoimmune in origin; they are not associated with autoimmune skin and eye signs and tend to present in older patients. They are investigated and managed in much the same way as Graves' disease and will be described with it.

Uncommon causes of hyperthyroidism include:

- subacute thyroiditis (p. 302)
- Hashimoto's thyroiditis (p. 300)
- amiodarone therapy
- iodine-induced (e.g. after imaging with iodine — containing contrast medium).

Extremely rarely, hyperthyroidism can be caused by a TSH-secreting pituitary tumour, but this is the exception to the general rule that hyperthyroidism is a primary disease of the thyroid.

Graves' disease is at least five times as common in women as men; it may present at any age but is most common between 40 and 60. Toxic nodular goitre is also more common in women but usually presents in later life.

Clinical presentation

An excess of thyroid hormone increases cell metabolism and sensitises the tissues to catecholamines; hence the similarity between hyperthyroidism and the adrenergically mediated symptoms and signs of anxiety. The classical staring eyes and lid lag of hyperthyroidism are caused by adrenergic stimulation of levator palpebrae superioris. Hyperthyroid patients present with the symptoms listed in Figure 74 or with abnormal thyroid function tests found coincidentally. Elderly patients may present with atrial fibrillation or heart failure. The symptoms and signs are of:

- hyperthyroidism and its complications
- the goitre, if present (p. 301)
- other autoimmune features, notably eye disease.

Thyroid-associated ophthalmopathy

Any hyperthyroid patient may have sore, gritty eyes, lid retraction, lid lag and a staring appearance. Only those with Graves' disease develop the more severe inflammatory changes of thyroid-associated ophthalmopathy

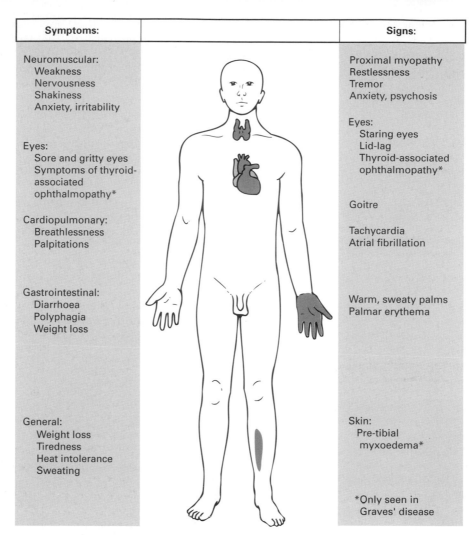

Symptoms:		Signs:

Neuromuscular:
  Weakness
  Nervousness
  Shakiness
  Anxiety, irritability
		Proximal myopathy
		Restlessness
		Tremor
		Anxiety, psychosis

Eyes:
  Sore and gritty eyes
  Symptoms of thyroid-
  associated
  ophthalmopathy*
		Eyes:
		  Staring eyes
		  Lid-lag
		  Thyroid-associated
		  ophthalmopathy*

Cardiopulmonary:
  Breathlessness
  Palpitations
		Goitre
		
		Tachycardia
		Atrial fibrillation

Gastrointestinal:
  Diarrhoea
  Polyphagia
  Weight loss
		Warm, sweaty palms
		Palmar erythema

General:
  Weight loss
  Tiredness
  Heat intolerance
  Sweating
		Skin:
		  Pre-tibial
		  myxoedema*
		
		*Only seen in
		  Graves' disease

Fig. 74 Symptoms and signs of hyperthyroidism.

which include enlargement and (later) fibrosis of ocular muscles.

The symptoms are watering eyes, photophobia, retro-orbital pain, double vision and (in a few cases) visual loss. Patients are very self-conscious of their abnormal appearance. They have proptosis, which may be asymmetrical, and conjunctival and periorbital oedema. They may develop corneal ulceration and/or diplopia. Reduced visual acuity is an indication for urgent action. Physical examination should include measurement of visual acuity, fields and fundoscopy. CT scan is indicated, particularly if the disease is asymmetrical, to demonstrate the swollen eye muscles and exclude a retro-orbital tumour.

Treatment is with artificial tears, sunglasses and diuretics for severe oedema. Raising the head of the bed at night helps to reduce periorbital oedema. In severe cases, the treatment is high-dose steroids, azathioprine, surgical decompression and/or radiotherapy.

Investigations

Investigation of hyperthyroidism has been greatly simplified by the sensitive and reliable assays now available. In most cases, both total thyroxine and triiodothyronine are raised. Occasionally only triiodothyronine is raised (T_3 toxicosis). Measurement of total thyroxine can be misleading because increased thyroid-binding globulin (as in patients who are pregnant or on the contraceptive pill) gives a raised total thyroxine, suggesting hyperthyroidism, when the 'free' (unbound) fraction of thyroxine is in reality normal. Many laboratories measure free thyroxine routinely to avoid this catch.

Measurement of TSH gives extra information because:

- thyroid autonomy causes feedback suppression of TSH; serum TSH may be low before the thyroid hormones are measurably increased, making it a very sensitive test for hyperthyroidism
- serum TSH will be normal if total thyroxine is artificially raised by an increased level of thyroid-binding globulin (see previous paragraph)
- it will detect the very rare cases in which thyrotoxicosis is caused by increased pituitary TSH secretion.

Table 67 summarises some common abnormalities of thyroid function tests.

Table 67 Typical thyroid function test results in a range of diseases

	Thyroxine		Triiodothyronine	TSH
	Total	Free		
Primary hypothyroidism	↓	↓	↓	↑
Secondary hypothyroidism	↓	↓	↓	↔ or ↓
'Euthyroid sick' syndrome	↔ or ↓	↔ or ↓	↓	↔ or ↓
Hyperthyroidism	↑	↑	↑	↓
T_3 toxicosis	↔ or ↓	↔ or ↓	↑	↓
Raised TBG (e.g. pregnancy, contraceptive pill)	↑	↔	↔ or ↑	↔

TBG, thyroid-binding globulin.
↓ fall; ↑, increase; ↔ no change from normal.

Neither immunology nor imaging has any major part in the routine investigation of hyperthyroidism because measurement of the thyroid-stimulating immunoglobulins of Graves' disease is not routinely available and the exact nature of the goitre rarely influences management. The only exception is the solitary toxic nodule, which can be diagnosed by an isotope scan in a patient with hyperthyroidism and a clinically obvious solitary nodule.

Management

Antithyroid drugs

Most patients are treated with antithyroid drugs first and later with **ablative treatment**, usually radioiodine but sometimes surgery. Antithyroid drugs (carbimazole and propylthiouracil) work by preventing iodine-trapping and suppressing antithyroid autoimmunity. Their main side-effect is neutropenia, which is not dose-related and usually occurs in the first 8 weeks of treatment. Rashes, nausea and cholestatic jaundice are other side-effects. Graves' disease may remit and is more likely to do so after treatment with antithyroid drugs, so it is common practice to give drug treatment for a period and then withdraw it. The alternatives are to start a moderately large dose and taper it once hyperthyroidism is controlled ('titration' regimen) or continue a full dose and add levothyroxine (the drug form of thyroxine) when euthyroid ('block–replace' regimen). Block–replace therapy must not be used in pregnant women, as the fetus may become hypothyroid. The drug is continued for about 1 year, although the optimum duration is controversial. The long-term results are disappointing, since only one-half of patients remit and, of those who do, one-half relapse. Causes of hyperthyroidism other than Graves' disease do not usually remit. Long-term antithyroid drug therapy is a treatment option that may occasionally be used: for example, in elderly patients who refuse radioiodine or do not respond to it.

Beta-blockade Since many thyrotoxic symptoms (particularly tremor and palpitations) are adrenergic, beta-blockers give very rapid and effective symptom relief at the start of treatment. In some cases, they may be used as sole therapy: for example, in mild, transient hyperthyroidism postpartum, in subacute thyroiditis, and when antithyroid drugs are contraindicated.

Radioiodine

Radioiodine treatment is non-invasive and relatively free of immediate side-effects, although it can precipitate a hyperthyroid crisis in a patient with uncontrolled hyperthyroidism. It is slow to act, taking up to 3 months to have its effect. For that reason, radioiodine therapy that produces an acceptable rate of euthyroidism (e.g. 95% cured within 12 months of treatment) carries a 50% likelihood of hypothyroidism within 12 months and a 90% or higher lifetime risk. If a first dose of radioiodine fails to control hyperthyroidism — for example, in a patient with multinodular goiter — it can be given more than once. Radioiodine is absolutely contraindicated in children, nursing mothers and women likely to become pregnant within 4 months because of the risks of thyroid cancer, transmission in breast milk and congenital malformations, respectively. Men, also, should be advised not to stop contraception within 4 months. It can produce thyroiditis-like side-effects acutely and slightly increases the (small) risk of cancer or lymphoma of the thyroid.

Surgery

Surgery is indicated for a small number of patients, including those who have large goitres or respond poorly to other modalities of treatment. Surgery may be complicated by recurrent laryngeal nerve palsy, permanent hypoparathyroidism and hypothyroidism. Patients whose thyrotoxicosis is inadequately controlled beforehand with potassium iodide may have a thyroid crisis during surgery. A small number of patients are uncontrolled by surgery and late relapse of hyperthyroidism may also occur. There is a trend for fewer patients to be treated with surgery.

Whichever form of ablative therapy is chosen, it is usual to pretreat all but the mildest cases with antithyroid drugs and/or beta-blockers for rapid symptom relief and to prevent hyperthyroid crisis. All successfully treated patients, whichever treatment they have received, need annual thyroid function tests for the rest of their lives to detect late hypothyroidism or relapse.

Prognosis

Hyperthyroidism can usually be cured without serious sequelae. Many patients, particularly those who have received radioiodine, eventually become hypothyroid. The most severe acute effects are hyperthyroid crises, psychoses and cardiac dysrhythmias. Atrial fibrillation is a particularly important complication because it may cause embolic stroke. Patients with hyperthyroidism and atrial fibrillation should be given anticoagulation therapy unless there are strong contraindications. They should be considered for cardioversion once they are euthyroid. Every patient with atrial fibrillation should have thyroid function tests to exclude hyperthyroidism.

Hypothyroidism

Pathology

Hypothyroidism is *commonly* primary or secondary to radiotherapy or surgery, and *uncommonly* secondary to pituitary tumours.

Primary hypothyroidism is now almost always autoimmune in developed countries, although iodine deficiency used to be the most common cause. The most common diagnosis is **primary atrophic hypothyroidism** and so the majority of hypothyroid patients have no palpable goitre; **Hashimoto's thyroiditis**, a more florid autoimmune disease with a firm rubbery goitre, lymphocytic infiltration and high-titre thyroid autoantibodies, is less common. Rarely, patients with Hashimoto's thyroiditis may go through a short phase of hyperthyroidism (hashitoxicosis). Hashimoto's disease is 10 times more common in women than men and usually presents in middle age. **Previous ablative therapy** for hyperthyroidism is another common cause of hypothyroidism. Less common causes include viral thyroiditis and amiodarone or lithium treatment. Hypothyroidism is not a presenting feature of thyroid cancer.

Clinical presentation

Figure 75 summarises the specific clinical features of hypothyroidism. The condition may also cause non-specific symptoms. Thyroid function tests are cheap, reliable and often performed, so many cases of hypothyroidism are found almost by chance. A particularly high yield is in women with gynaecological complaints, because menorrhagia and infertility can be caused by hypothyroidism. Hypothyroidism rarely *presents* with obesity (p. 314), although patients often admit to weight gain.

Investigations

Like hyperthyroidism, hypothyroidism is easily diagnosed from the serum thyroxine and TSH concentrations (Table 67). Patients with *primary* hypothyroidism have a low serum thyroxine with a compensatory increase in TSH. Deficiency of thyroid-binding globulin causes a low serum thyroxine without a raised TSH. *Secondary* (pituitary) hypothyroidism should be suspected if the patient is truly hypothyroid (low free thyroxine concentration, p. 298) with no compensatory increase in serum TSH. Measurement of serum triiodothyronine adds nothing and is actually unhelpful because it can be reduced by non-specific intercurrent illness (low T3 syndrome or 'euthyroid sick syndrome').

Imaging the thyroid is not indicated in uncomplicated primary hypothyroidism, even if accompanied by a diffuse goitre. Rarely, pressure symptoms or a suspicious-feeling nodule justify aspiration cytology and/or ultrasound scanning (p. 302). If a patient has stridor or other evidence of tracheal compression, a radiograph of the thoracic inlet and CT scan of the neck are indicated.

Management

Thyroxine deficiency is treated by replacement with levothyroxine. Unless hypothyroidism has come on suddenly (as after surgery), a small dose is started and increased at 2–4-weekly intervals. It has a long half-life and is given once daily. The serum thyroxine and TSH concentrations often normalise before patients feel back to normal; consequently the response to treatment must be monitored both clinically and biochemically.

The longer the history and more severe the symptoms, the more cautiously levothyroxine should be given because hypothyroidism causes hypercholesterolaemia and coronary artery disease. Speeding up metabolism with injudicious doses of levothyroxine can cause myocardial infarction and death. Even if levothyroxine is started in a small dose, angina may be precipitated or worsened; however, that is not a reason to stop treatment because untreated hypothyroidism leaves patients feeling unwell and a persistently high serum cholesterol causes progression of coronary artery disease. By analogy with other lipid-lowering treatments, levothyroxine replacement may be expected to cause long-term regression of coronary atherosclerosis.

A combination of triiodothyronine and levothyroxine therapy can be given to patients whose wellbeing is not fully restored by levothyroxine alone, although the research evidence of benefit is somewhat controversial.

Prognosis

Hypothyroidism, left untreated, is a risk factor for ischaemic heart disease. If diagnosed and treated early, life expectancy is good.

Myxoedema coma

This is a rare medical emergency caused by severe hypothyroidism, usually in elderly people. It presents with coma and, usually, hypothermia. It is fatal in over 50% of patients despite treatment, which consists of:

- intensive nursing care
- nasogastric suction
- cautious fluid therapy
- passive rewarming
- corticosteroid therapy
- i.v. triiodothyronine (liothyronine)
- treatment of underlying infection
- oral levothyroxine.

If there is reason to suspect the myxoedema coma is secondary to hypopituitarism, or there is other reason to

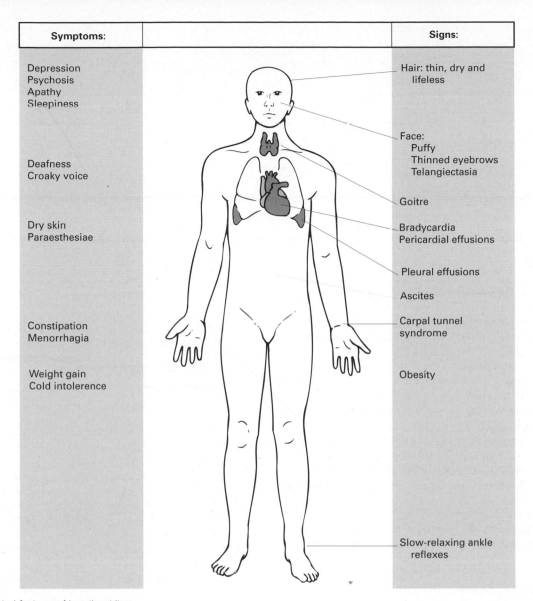

Symptoms:			Signs:
Depression Psychosis Apathy Sleepiness			Hair: thin, dry and lifeless

			Face:
			   Puffy
			   Thinned eyebrows
			   Telangiectasia

Deafness Croaky voice			Goitre
			Bradycardia Pericardial effusions
Dry skin Paraesthesiae			Pleural effusions
			Ascites
Constipation Menorrhagia			Carpal tunnel syndrome
Weight gain Cold intolerence			Obesity
			Slow-relaxing ankle reflexes

Fig. 75 Clinical features of hypothyroidism.

believe the patient is hypoadrenal, cortisol replacement must be given for several days before giving thyroid hormone. Otherwise, increasing metabolism with thyroid hormone can precipitate a hypoadrenal crisis.

Goitre

Thyroid swelling matters because it may be:

- unsightly
- a cause of pressure symptoms
- accompanied by hypothyroidism or hyperthyroidism
- caused by a tumour (in up to 10% of patients).

The clinical approach is determined by:

- The context: thyroid enlargement in patients with hypothyroidism, hyperthyroidism, pregnancy or puberty rarely needs investigation.
- Feel: diffuse goitres are rarely malignant.

- History: onset in childhood, a rapid onset at any age, or a history of previous thyroid radiation is suggestive of malignancy.
- Local policy: some clinicians perform fine needle aspiration cytology on all goitres.

Even benign thyroid enlargement may need surgery for cosmetic reasons, for comfort or to control hyperthyroidism. If the goitre extends retrosternally, surgery may be needed for pressure symptoms. In most cases, the aim is to exclude or treat malignancy. Table 68 shows causes of thyroid enlargement.

Pathology of thyroid tumours

Thyroid tumours are typically unifocal and solid. Apart from toxic adenomas, they are non-functioning ('cold') on isotope scanning.

Papillary carcinoma This constitutes about 60% of thyroid cancers and is the most differentiated and least

Table 68 Causes of thyroid enlargement

	Hypothyroid	Euthyroid	Hyperthyroid
Diffuse	Iodine deficiency Hashimoto's thyroiditis	Simple goitre Pregnancy Puberty	Graves' disease
	Subacute thyroiditis (tender)	Subacute thyroiditis (tender)	Subacute thyroiditis (tender)
Nodular/asymmetrical		Thyroid cyst	
		Adenoma	Adenoma
		Nodular goitre	Nodular goitre
		Carcinoma: papillary, follicular, medullary, anaplastic	
		Lymphoma	
		Metastasis	

aggressive of the malignant tumours. It may present in children.

Follicular carcinoma Follicular carcinoma (20%) is less differentiated and more likely to metastasise (typically to lung or bone).

Medullary carcinoma This form (5%) may arise as a lone abnormality or as part of the syndrome of **multiple endocrine neoplasia**; it is relatively slow-growing but prone to recur and spread locally. Its biochemical hallmark is calcitonin secretion.

Anaplastic carcinoma Anaplastic carcinoma (10%) affects elderly people and is extremely locally invasive.

Lymphomas (<5%) These may arise in longstanding autoimmune goitres.

Investigations and management

The investigation and treatment of thyroid swelling is summarised in Figure 76. Relevant investigations are:

- fine needle aspiration cytology
- thyroid ultrasound
- surgical biopsy.

Isotope scintigraphy is only useful to demonstrate that a solitary solid nodule is functional and, therefore, not likely to be malignant. Aspiration cytology can diagnose or give an index of suspicion of malignancy. Ultrasound can demonstrate that a lesion is cystic, multinodular, solid and/or invasive. It can also be used to guide a biopsy needle. The definitive investigation/treatment is surgical removal of a nodule or partial or total thyroidectomy.

Papillary and follicular carcinomas are treated by total thyroidectomy with high-dose radioactive iodine for metastases. Anaplastic carcinoma is so invasive that it is untreatable. Lymphoma is treated with chemotherapy.

Thyroiditis

A number of conditions can present as subacute thyroiditis, which is characterised by:

- pain in some patients
- swelling
- thyroid dysfunction in some patients.

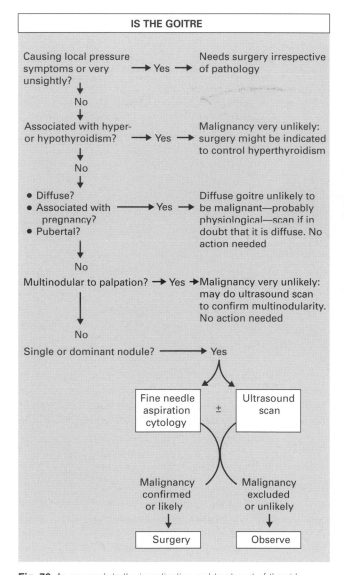

Fig. 76 An approach to the investigation and treatment of thyroid enlargement.

Commoner syndromes include:

- postpartum thyroiditis
- Hashimoto's thyroiditis
- subacute (de Quervain's or viral) thyroiditis.

Very uncommon forms of thyroiditis are acute suppurative thyroiditis and Riedel's (invasive fibrous) thyroiditis.

Hashimoto's disease

Hashimoto's disease may present with classical thyroiditis but far more often presents with painless goitre and thyroid dysfunction.

Subacute thyroiditis

Subacute thyroiditis is a distinctive syndrome that, though less common than Hashimoto's disease, is prevalent enough to be important, because it can be treated if recognised. It causes rapid, painful thyroid enlargement, sore throat with dysphagia, systemic malaise and myalgia. The gland is enlarged and tender. There is fever and a high erythrocyte sedimentation rate (ESR). Thyroid function progresses over days or weeks from euthyroidism to hyperthyroidism, then hypothyroidism before spontaneously returning to normal. The aetiology is thought to be a viral infection with release of stored thyroid hormone, causing hyperthyroidism, and impaired synthesis, causing hypothyroidism. The gland shows absent uptake on an isotope scan. The condition resolves spontaneously with time but a short course of high-dose prednisolone rapidly relieves systemic symptoms and speeds recovery.

7.3 Pituitary disease

Learning objectives

You should . . .
- know the significance of the anatomical location of the pituitary and its role in directly and indirectly controlling many vital processes
- know the clinical features, investigations and treatment of pituitary over- and underactivity.

Case Study

A 55-year-old man takes early retirement because he can no longer cope with the pace of work. Despite finishing work, he continues to get bad headaches. His optometrist finds a bitemporal hemianopia and refers him to the eye clinic. An MR scan shows a tumour greater than 1 cm in diameter extending upwards from the pituitary fossa and compressing the optic chiasm. Blood tests show low testosterone and cortisol levels but he is not hypothyroid. He is treated with hydrocortisone and referred for trans-sphenoidal pituitary surgery.

Normal anatomy and physiology

The pituitary is located in the pituitary fossa, bounded by the anterior and posterior clinoid processes, diaphragma sellae and (laterally) cavernous sinuses. A narrow plate of bone separates the pituitary fossa from the sphenoid sinus, which is accessible to the surgeon.

The pituitary gland is connected to the hypothalamus by the pituitary stalk. It is composed of the anterior pituitary, which synthesises and secretes the anterior pituitary hormones (Fig. 73), and the posterior pituitary, an extension of neurones of the hypothalamus, which secretes antidiuretic hormone (ADH; arginine vasopressin). ADH diffuses down these neurones but is not synthesised in the posterior pituitary; therefore, pituitary enlargement does not necessarily cause ADH deficiency.

Secretion of all the anterior pituitary hormones except prolactin is stimulated by hypothalamic trophic hormones. Prolactin secretion is under the *inhibitory* control of hypothalamic dopamine. These controlling hormones reach the anterior pituitary through the blood vessels of the hypophysial portal system. Signalling by hormones is a complex process and some of its intricacies have a bearing on clinical practice. For example, gonadotrophin-releasing hormone (GnRH) is secreted by the hypothalamus in a pulsatile fashion. Pulsatile GnRH infusion stimulates gonadotrophin secretion and can be used as a treatment for infertility, whereas non-pulsatile GnRH therapy down-regulates the GnRH receptors and actually inhibits gonadotrophin secretion. Long-acting GnRH analogues can be used, for example, to treat 'precocious puberty' or carcinoma of the prostate.

Pituitary tumours

Pathology

The significance of the anatomical location of the pituitary in the development of symptoms from pituitary tumours is shown in Figure 77. At postmortem, up to one-third of pituitary glands contain microscopic or macroscopic

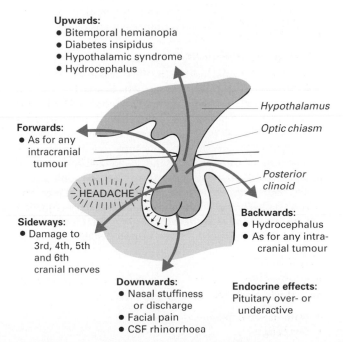

Upwards:
- Bitemporal hemianopia
- Diabetes insipidus
- Hypothalamic syndrome
- Hydrocephalus

Hypothalamus

Optic chiasm

Forwards:
- As for any intracranial tumour

Posterior clinoid

HEADACHE

Sideways:
- Damage to 3rd, 4th, 5th and 6th cranial nerves

Backwards:
- Hydrocephalus
- As for any intra-cranial tumour

Downwards:
- Nasal stuffiness or discharge
- Facial pain
- CSF rhinorrhoea

Endocrine effects:
Pituitary over- or underactive

Fig. 77 How expanding pituitary tumours cause symptoms.

Seven

adenomas. They are known about in life only if they grow large enough to compress adjacent structures (e.g. the optic chiasm) or overproduce a hormone which causes symptoms. Most do neither. Even tiny tumours can cause serious disease if they are secretory (e.g. Cushing's disease). Hyperprolactinaemia is the most common pituitary overactivity, usually presenting in women during their menstrual years. Most such women have **micro-adenomas** (<1 cm diameter). Pituitary tumours can secrete any anterior pituitary hormone and sometimes several, but prolactin, growth hormone (GH) and ACTH are the most clinically important. Tumours need to be over 1 cm in diameter (i.e. **macroadenomas**) to present with 'mass effects'. Most pituitary tumours are benign, but the pituitary fossa is so small and so close to important structures that relatively modest expansion can cause serious damage. They can expand in any direction (Fig. 77):

- **upwards:** towards the optic chiasm, hypothalamus and third ventricle
- **sideways:** into the cavernous sinus, compressing the cranial nerves in its walls
- **downwards:** into the base of skull, sphenoid sinus and nasopharynx
- **forwards:** large/invasive tumours into the anterior cranial fossa
- **backwards:** large/invasive tumours into the middle and posterior fossae.

Secondary tumours can deposit in or near the pituitary fossa and several types of primary intracranial tumour can affect the pituitary and its hypothalamic connections. Of these, craniopharyngioma is the most important; its embryonic origin from Rathke's pouch places it in the suprasellar cistern. The commonest presentations of such a tumour are visual impairment, hypothalamic dysfunction, hypopituitarism and (in children) disorders of growth and puberty. Granulomas, cysts and tuberculomas are rare pathologies that can cause pituitary expansion.

Clinical presentation

Headache and visual loss are the most common symptoms of an expanding pituitary tumour. The headache is frontal or retro-orbital. As the tumour expands upwards and comes into contact with the optic chiasm, it first causes superior temporal field loss, then complete bitemporal hemianopia, progressing to concentric visual field loss and blindness. Central fields and visual acuity are sometimes affected relatively early. There may be some asymmetry, but both fields are usually affected. Later, the optic discs become pale and atrophic. Optic nerve function can be saved by early decompression; established optic atrophy is irreversible. Other symptoms are shown in Figure 77.

Investigations

Investigation includes assessment of:

- optic nerve damage
  — perimetry
  — visual acuity

- endocrine status, testing for
  — hypopituitarism
  — overactivity (prolactin and GH in particular)
- the tumour mass
  — high-resolution MR scan (CT is second-best here)
  — MR angiography, sometimes needed to exclude an aneurysm mimicking a tumour.

Management and prognosis

There are three types of treatment:

- medical
- surgery
- radiotherapy.

If the optic nerves are compromised by a large pituitary tumour, urgent action is needed. Two classes of drug — dopaminergic agonists (bromocriptine, cabergoline and quinagolide) and a somatostatin analogue (octreotide) — can shrink some types of pituitary tumour. Dopaminergic agonists are highly effective for prolactinomas and may also shrink GH-secreting tumours. Octreotide is mainly used for GH-secreting tumours. In practice:

1. Your first step when presented with a large pituitary tumour is to measure serum prolactin.
2. If it is high (>2000 mU/l), the first-line treatment is to give an oral dopaminergic agonist, which acts so rapidly that it can be used for a 'medical' optic nerve decompression without the need for surgery.
3. In all other patients, urgent decompressive neuro-surgery is needed.

If visual acuity and fields are normal, there is less urgency, and medical therapy, surgery and radiotherapy are tailored to the individual patient. Dopaminergic agonists are so effective for prolactin-secreting tumours that there is little place for surgery in the management of prolactinoma. Surgery is the best choice for other secretory *micro*adenomas because the surgeon can directly inspect the gland, remove the tumour and cure the endocrine disease, often without causing hypopituitarism. It may also be indicated to debulk *macro*adenomas (see previous paragraph). Radiotherapy is slow to act and likely to damage residual normal pituitary function, so it is reserved for tumours of any size when drugs and/or surgery have failed to control overactivity or there is a residual large tumour mass. The advent of high-quality non-invasive imaging, less invasive neurosurgical techniques and effective medical therapies means that most patients, even with large pituitary tumours, have a good prognosis. This is highly specialised medicine, not for the generalist.

Hypopituitarism and diabetes insipidus

Hypopituitarism may present out of the blue or develop in a patient with known pituitary disease following surgery or radiotherapy. Transient diabetes insipidus and hypopituitarism are common immediately after pituitary surgery and may resolve within days or weeks. If they last longer than 1 month, they are likely to be permanent. In contrast, radiotherapy causes hypopituitarism months or years later. In patients with hypopituitarism as their first presentation of pituitary disease, MR scanning has revolutionised management. Together with a careful clinical history, it can usually narrow the diagnosis down to just one cause. Common causes are:

- pituitary and hypothalamic tumours
  — primary: intra- and extrasellar
  — secondary
- iatrogenic
  — surgery
  — radiotherapy
- idiopathic hypopituitarism, including the empty sella syndrome.

Rare causes include:

- cysts, granulomas
- autoimmune: lymphocytic hypophysitis
- vascular: Sheehan's syndrome.

Since ADH is secreted by hypothalamic neurones, diabetes insipidus is a symptom of hypothalamic damage. It may occur without anterior pituitary underactivity and vice versa. Extensive damage is needed to cause simultaneous anterior and posterior pituitary underactivity.

Clinical presentation

Anterior pituitary underactivity

The symptoms and signs of anterior pituitary underactivity are determined by which hormones are deficient. Prolactin differs from the others in that it is under the *inhibitory* control of hypothalamic dopamine. Hypoprolactinaemia rarely occurs and is clinically unimportant when it does. The other anterior pituitary hormones are under *stimulatory* hypothalamic control. With progressive anterior pituitary dysfunction, they are usually lost in the order:

1. GH
2. gonadotrophins
3. ACTH
4. TSH.

GH deficiency causes growth failure in children and lethargy, impaired wellbeing, altered body composition, dyslipidaemia and osteoporosis in adults. Gonadotrophin deficiency (like hyperprolactinaemia, p. 306) causes amenorrhoea/infertility in women and impotence/infertility in men. ACTH deficiency causes hypoadrenalism (p. 308) and TSH deficiency causes hypothyroidism.

The hypoadrenalism of hypopituitarism differs from primary adrenal failure in that the patient does not become pigmented and is not aldosterone-deficient.

The hypothyroidism of pituitary disease differs from primary hypothyroidism in that it rarely causes weight gain because of accompanying hypoadrenalism.

The patient with panhypopituitarism is pale, hypotensive, impotent, weak and lethargic. Advanced disease may present with collapse, hyponatraemic fits (as a result of cortisol and thyroxine deficiency) or symptoms of an underlying tumour. A tumour that oversecretes one hormone (typically prolactin or GH) may cause deficiency

of the others, although tumours presenting with hypopituitarism are more often than not non-functioning.

Diabetes insipidus

The symptoms of diabetes insipidus are overwhelming thirst, polyuria (often over 4 litres/day), frequency and nocturia. Patients have to get up and drink during the night. One patient was known to fantasise about drinking whole swimming pools before he received treatment. The diagnosis is obvious if those symptoms develop suddenly after neurosurgery or a head injury but may be unrecognised if they develop slowly and spontaneously.

Investigations

Anterior pituitary underactivity

Hypopituitarism is confirmed by 'static' and 'dynamic' tests (p. 304). Examples of helpful static tests are:

- hypothyroidism without a compensatory rise in TSH, strong presumptive evidence of pituitary or hypothalamic underactivity
- hypogonadotrophic hypogonadism
- lack of appropriately high gonadotrophins in postmenopausal women.

Cortisol, GH and ACTH have short half-lives and their plasma levels are very variable in health, so random measurements are of limited value. GH and ACTH deficiency can be diagnosed by measuring the cortisol and GH responses to insulin-induced hypoglycaemia. This is unpleasant, potentially dangerous and contraindicated in

- elderly people (age > 70 years)
- patients with histories of ischaemic heart disease or epilepsy
- patients who appear profoundly hypopituitary.

However, insulin stress testing remains the gold standard test today. If it is performed on a patient with suspected hypopituitarism, the dose of insulin should be kept small (0.1 U/kg) to avoid dangerous hypoglycaemia. A short Synacthen test is now widely used to detect long-standing (> 3 months) secondary hypoadrenalism. An arginine stimulation test may be used to assess GH reserve.

Diabetes insipidus

The diagnosis of diabetes insipidus is obvious if a patient develops polyuria after pituitary surgery or a head injury (provided he or she is not clearing an iatrogenic fluid load). Treatment is with desmopressin, a synthetic ADH analogue.

If diabetes insipidus develops insidiously and/or the diagnosis is uncertain, a 'water deprivation test' is performed. The patient is given nothing to drink for 8 hours and then has an injection of desmopressin. Urine volume, urine osmolality and plasma osmolality are measured. The test distinguishes between:

- Normal: urine volume falls, urine osmolality rises and plasma osmolality remains normal.
- Diabetes insipidus: there is no fall in urine volume, no rise in urine osmolality, plasma osmolality rises and the patient loses weight.

Patients with **nephrogenic diabetes insipidus** have no response to injected desmopressin because their kidneys are insensitive to it. Patients with **cranial diabetes insipidus** respond as normal (see above) to desmopressin.

Management and prognosis

Cortisol and thyroxine are replaced as described under hypoadrenalism (p. 308) and hypothyroidism (p. 300). GH is of proven value in children with short stature and is increasingly being given to GH-deficient adults. Gonadotrophin deficiency is treated by sex steroid replacement and diabetes insipidus by intranasal or oral desmopressin. Patients newly presenting with panhypopituitarism should receive corticosteroids for at least a week before thyroxine is started because increasing the metabolic rate can precipitate a hypoadrenal crisis. Sex steroid therapy can safely be deferred (but must not be forgotten). If diabetes insipidus is proven, it should be treated without delay because starting corticosteroids will exacerbate diabetes insipidus in a patient with panhypopituitarism.

The most serious risk to the hypopituitary patient is a hypoadrenal crisis because of either non-compliance or inadequate therapy, particularly during intercurrent illness (p. 308). Any vomiting/ill patient with hypopituitarism must receive parenteral hydrocortisone. They should wear an alert bracelet and carry a steroid card to advise others of their need for steroid replacement when ill. Even with adequate replacement treatment, there is an increased risk of cardiovascular disease in hypopituitary patients.

Pituitary overactivity

Hyperprolactinaemia

Hyperprolactinaemia most commonly presents as galactorrhoea, menstrual disturbance and/or infertility in a young woman and is usually caused by a **microadenoma** (tumour < 1 cm) or **lactotroph hyperplasia** (no tumour seen on scan). In men, hyperprolactinaemia causes impotence/infertility. Male reproductive function is less sensitive to hyperprolactinaemia so men usually present later in life with larger tumours. **Macroprolactinomas** can present at any age and are the second most common pituitary macroadenoma (after non-functioning tumours). Particularly in elderly people, there may be no symptoms directly related to the hyperprolactinaemia. There are many causes of hyperprolactinaemia. Primary hyperprolactinaemia is caused by a pituitary tumour or lactotroph hyperplasia. **Secondary causes** include:

- mass lesions preventing inhibitory control of prolactin secretion: intra- or suprasellar tumours or granulomas
- drugs: metoclopramide, phenothiazines, antidepressants, histamine H_2 antagonists
- endocrine: primary hypothyroidism, polycystic ovarian syndrome
- systemic disease: renal failure
- chest wall/breast stimulation or disease
- fitting.

Physiological causes include:

- pregnancy
- breast-feeding
- stress, anxiety
- sleep.

Secondary hyperprolactinaemia is most commonly a chance biochemical finding but it can cause the same symptoms and signs as idiopathic hyperprolactinaemia. Once secondary causes have been excluded, investigation consists of MR scanning and pituitary function testing. Treatment is with dopaminergic agonists (chiefly cabergoline), which are very successful at relieving galactorrhoea, menstrual disturbance and infertility and reducing tumour size. The place of surgery and radiotherapy has been discussed earlier (p. 304).

Acromegaly and gigantism
Pathology

GH oversecretion is the second most common pituitary overactivity and almost invariably results from a pituitary adenoma, usually large enough to expand the pituitary fossa and often to extend outside it. A minority of GH-secreting tumours also secrete prolactin. Extremely rarely, acromegaly may be caused by a tumour secreting GHRH ectopically. There are two distinct presentations:

- Most often, GH excess presents in middle or later life as acromegaly.
- Rarely, GH excess before epiphyseal fusion presents with the syndrome of gigantism.

The mass effects, investigation and treatment of macroadenomas have been covered earlier (p. 304).

Clinical presentation and investigations

Figure 78 shows the symptoms and signs of acromegaly other than those caused by tumour expansion and accompanying hypopituitarism or hyperprolactinaemia. Enlargement of the hands and feet is the classical symptom. Most patients admit to the symptom and there are few other causes in adults. However, that is rarely how the diagnosis is made. It is usually a chance observation by a doctor.

GH excess is confirmed by glucose tolerance testing (GTT). In normal people, serum GH suppresses to unmeasurable levels after oral glucose whereas it is not suppressed and may actually rise in acromegaly/gigantism. Serum prolactin must always be measured and pituitary function tests performed to exclude hypopituitarism. In almost every patient, MR scanning will demonstrate a pituitary adenoma, usually a macroadenoma.

Management and prognosis

Surgery is the first-line treatment for most patients with acromegaly. Trans-sphenoidal surgery can cure 80% of microadenomas with little morbidity; however, it is less effective for macroadenomas. A dopaminergic agonist (cabergoline) can suppress GH secretion and alleviate symptoms but is rarely curative. A somatostatin analogue such as octreotide is much more effective but:

- is extremely expensive
- has to be given by injection

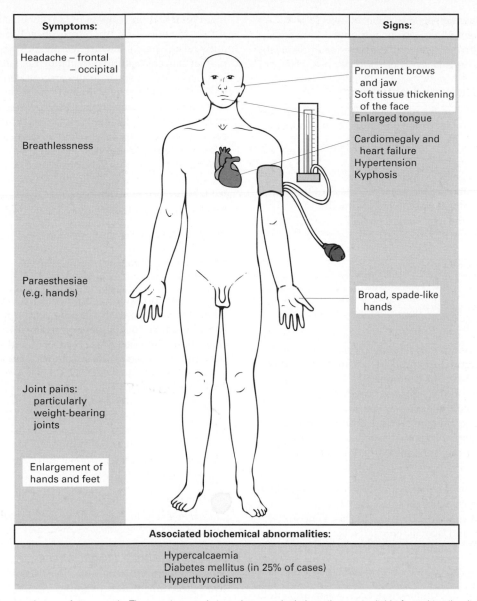

Symptoms:		Signs:
Headache – frontal – occipital		Prominent brows and jaw Soft tissue thickening of the face Enlarged tongue
Breathlessness		Cardiomegaly and heart failure Hypertension Kyphosis
Paraesthesiae (e.g. hands)		Broad, spade-like hands
Joint pains: particularly weight-bearing joints		
Enlargement of hands and feet		

Associated biochemical abnormalities:

Hypercalcaemia
Diabetes mellitus (in 25% of cases)
Hyperthyroidism

Fig. 78 The symptoms and signs of acromegaly. The symptoms and signs shown unshaded are the most reliable for making the diagnosis.

- has many side-effects, including gall stone formation owing to stasis of bile.

Radiotherapy is also effective but is slow to act; it is indicated for patients not cured by surgery. Pegvisomant, a GH receptor antagonist, is a novel treatment for acromegaly that has not responded to conventional treatments. Because it does not suppress GH (indeed, it has the opposite effect) there is concern about its long-term effect on tumour size, which must be monitored by serial MR scans.

Acromegaly causes unpleasant symptoms, major morbidity from joint, heart and respiratory disease and increased mortality from cardiorespiratory and malignant disease (particularly carcinoma of the colon); consequently there are strong arguments for treating it aggressively. Colonoscopic surveillance has been advocated.

7.4 Adrenal disease

Learning objectives

You should . . .
- understand the roles of the adrenal medulla and cortex
- know the main clinical features, investigation and management of adrenal over- and underactivity.

Case Study

A woman in her seventies has been on steroids for asthma for years. Although her asthma is now well controlled with inhalers, she has not been able to come off prednisolone. On holiday, she gets a stomach upset.

She is given an antiemetic but just gets worse. A nurse staying in the same hotel insists she goes to hospital. She is given intravenous hydrocortisone for Addisonian crisis and told she is lucky to be alive.

Normal anatomy and physiology

The two adrenal glands are situated at the upper poles of the kidneys. There are three main adrenal hormones:

- cortisol (cortex), controlled by the hypothalamo–pituitary–adrenal axis
- aldosterone (cortex), controlled by the renin–angiotensin–aldosterone system
- adrenaline (epinephrine) (from the medulla) controlled by the hypothalamus and the sympathetic nervous system.

Hypoadrenalism

The clinical effects of hypoadrenalism are caused by glucocorticoid and mineralocorticoid deficiency. Adrenaline (epinephrine) deficiency does not cause disease. Adrenal cortical underactivity may be:

- primary, i.e. because of disease in the adrenal itself, in which case both glucocorticoid and mineralocorticoid secretion are likely to be impaired
- secondary to pituitary disease, in which case mineralocorticoid secretion is unimpaired
- secondary to prolonged corticosteroid therapy and suppression of the hypothalamo–pituitary–adrenal axis, in which case mineralocorticoid secretion is unimpaired.

The main clinical situation described here is primary hypoadrenalism or **Addison's disease**. Iatrogenic hypoadrenalism is the cause you are most likely to encounter (or have to prevent) and is considered later. Isolated hypoaldosteronism is a rare condition not discussed in this chapter.

Pathology

Over 80% of cases of primary hypoadrenalism are autoimmune, caused by a lymphocytic adrenalitis and associated (in about half the patients) with measurable adrenal antibodies in plasma. Other causes are:

- Infectious
  - tuberculosis is an important cause in developing countries, now rare in developed countries
  - acquired immunodeficiency syndrome (AIDS), cytomegalovirus and histoplasmosis
  - the Waterhouse–Friedrichsen syndrome, adrenal haemorrhage complicating meningococcal septicaemia.
- Tumour: tumours often metastasise to the adrenals but hypoadrenalism is uncommon because both glands would have to be destroyed.

Clinical presentation

The symptoms of hypoadrenalism are non-specific and include weight loss, lethargy, weakness, nausea and abdominal pain. Both glucocorticoid and mineralocorticoid deficiency cause hypotension, particularly on stand-

ing. Pigmentation (caused by a compensatory increase in ACTH secretion and, therefore, absent in *secondary* hypoadrenalism) affects the nipples, recent scars, face and neck, palmar skin creases and buccal mucosa. Patients with incipient hypoadrenalism are often precipitated into 'hypoadrenal crisis' by intercurrent illness because the failing adrenals cannot mount an appropriate response. Treatment with rifampicin, which induces hepatic enzymes and increases cortisol metabolism, can have the same effect. The clinical picture of hypoadrenal crisis is collapse and vomiting with characteristic changes in electrolytes (see below).

Investigations

The biochemical signs of hypoadrenalism are:

- hyponatraemia
- hyperkalaemia
- a raised urea concentration
- mild acidosis.

Random cortisol measurements are unreliable because what appears 'normal' may be inappropriately low for someone who is 'ill'; however, a markedly low cortisol concentration with raised ACTH in an ill patient is diagnostic. All patients should have the following investigations.

Synacthen test

This tests the ability of the adrenals to increase cortisol secretion in response to (synthetic) ACTH stimulation. The short synacthen test measures the response over 30 minutes. If there is no response, ACTH can be given for 24 hours to exclude temporary adrenal suppression (long Synacthen test).

Abdominal CT or MR scan

This will exclude tuberculous calcification and adrenal tumours.

Adrenal antibody measurement

This is a pointer to autoimmune Addison's disease if positive but is unhelpful if negative.

Renin and aldosterone levels

These test the integrity of the renin–angiotensin–aldosterone axis.

Management

The treatment of adrenal crisis is saline repletion and intravenous hydrocortisone. You should look for evidence of underlying infection and treat it. Maintenance treatment is with oral hydrocortisone. Most, but not all, patients are also mineralocorticoid-deficient and need oral fludrocortisone. Patients with tuberculous hypoadrenalism should receive antituberculous chemotherapy. *All patients should be taught to increase their steroid doses during intercurrent illness and advised to carry a security disc or steroid card at all times. They must receive parenteral steroid if they are vomiting or seriously ill.*

Iatrogenic adrenal suppression

Corticosteroid therapy suppresses the hypothalamo–pituitary–adrenal axis. When it is stopped, there may be a delay before the axis recovers. After prolonged suppression, it may never do so. If corticosteroids are withdrawn from an individual whose axis is permanently suppressed, or withdrawn too quickly from an individual who has the potential to recover, hypoadrenalism results. It may also result if patients do not increase their steroid dose during intercurrent illness. You should follow the rules below:

- Remember the risk of adrenal suppression in any patient who has had corticosteroid therapy for longer than 3 weeks.
- Reduce steroid doses slowly in patients who have had prolonged therapy and warn them of the risk and symptoms of hypoadrenalism.
- Teach all patients to increase 'maintenance' steroid doses during intercurrent illness and report symptoms of hypoadrenalism immediately.

Withdrawal of steroids in patients who have received them long-term can be difficult and requires expert supervision. Synacthen testing is of no value in this situation.

Congenital adrenal hyperplasia

A number of inherited adrenal enzyme defects affect cortisol and/or aldosterone biosynthesis. The commonest is 21-hydroxylase deficiency, which is inherited as an autosomal recessive trait. The homeostatic response to cortisol deficiency is increased ACTH secretion. This cannot overcome the enzyme deficiency but does increase androgen synthesis. There may also be mineralocorticoid deficiency; consequently 21-hydroxylase deficiency often presents in the first week of life with salt-losing crises. It causes virilisation of female infants and can cause precocious puberty in males. Treatment is with glucocorticoid and mineralocorticoid replacement, as for Addison's disease. Congenital adrenal hyperplasia can also present with hirsutism in adult women. Serum 17-hydroxyprogesterone concentration (the steroid 'upstream' of the enzyme block) is the definitive investigation. In infants, the basal level is grossly abnormal. When the disease presents in adulthood, the abnormality is more subtle but 17-hydroxyprogesterone rises exces-sively, and cortisol rises subnomally, after ACTH (Synacthen) stimulation.

Cushing's syndrome

Pathology

Cushing's syndrome has the following characteristics:

- Two-thirds of cases are caused by pituitary disease, usually microadenomas.
- The remainder of cases split roughly equally between adrenal tumours (usually benign) and ectopic ACTH secretion, usually from carcinoid tumours.
- Prolonged corticosteroid therapy can cause a similar clinical picture, but the aetiology is obvious.
- Alcohol abuse can give a similar clinical picture: 'alcohol-induced pseudo-Cushing's'.
- Obesity and depression can produce changes in cortisol metabolism which are almost indistinguishable from Cushing's.

Clinical presentation

The clinical features of Cushing's syndrome are given in Figure 79. The diagnosis is often made late and depends on an observant clinician spotting the facial appearance and body habitus in a non-specifically unwell, hypertensive and/or diabetic person. Around 95% of patients with Cushing's have the triad of hypertension, proximal myopathy and skin changes. It is impossible to distinguish between Cushing's caused by a pituitary adenoma, an adrenal tumour or carcinoid ectopic ACTH secretion on clinical grounds. Ectopic ACTH secretion from *malignant* tumours (see Respiratory disease, p. 81) usually presents quite differently because the patients are very ill, wasted and heavily pigmented.

Investigations

The diagnosis of Cushing's syndrome is made by demonstrating increased plasma or urinary cortisol levels. There is loss of the normal circadian rhythm of plasma cortisol (lowest at midnight) and it remains inappropriately high after dexamethasone; this glucocorticoid is used here because, unlike hydrocortisone, it does not cross-react with cortisol in the laboratory assay.

Having demonstrated unsuppressible hypercortisolism, the next step is to measure plasma ACTH. If this is suppressed, the presumptive diagnosis is an adrenal adenoma, which can be confirmed by abdominal CT or MR scanning.

If ACTH is unsuppressed, the patient may have either an ectopic or a pituitary source of ACTH. MR scanning of the pituitary may show an adenoma and MR or CT scan of the thorax may show an occult carcinoid tumour.

Further investigation of 'high ACTH Cushing's' depends on determining the anatomical source and on the physiological principle that feedback responsiveness will only be retained for pituitary Cushing's syndrome — the secretory function of ectopic tumours is autonomous. Consequently a high dose of dexamethasone will suppress cortisol secretion only in the former. Localisation is achieved by bilateral simultaneous inferior petrosal sinus sampling with corticotrophin-releasing hormone (CRH) stimulation. This involves placing catheters in the veins draining both sides of the pituitary and stimulating ACTH secretion with CRH. Although complex to perform, it is the best way to distinguish pituitary from ectopic Cushing's syndrome. In pituitary Cushing's, ACTH levels are higher in pituitary venous efferent than peripheral blood and rise further after CRH injection because the hypothalamo–pituitary axis remains responsive. In Cushing's syndrome secondary to an ectopic tumour, pituitary ACTH secetion is suppressed and unresponsive to CRH stimulation and the ectopic tumour does not respond.

Management

Adrenal adenomectomy is the definitive treatment for adrenal Cushing's. Likewise, tumours secreting ectopic ACTH should be excised if possible. Selective adenomectomy is the first-line treatment for pituitary Cushing's. Whatever the cause, patients need to be prepared for surgery with a drug such as metyrapone, mitotane, aminoglutethimide or ketoconazole, which blocks cortisol

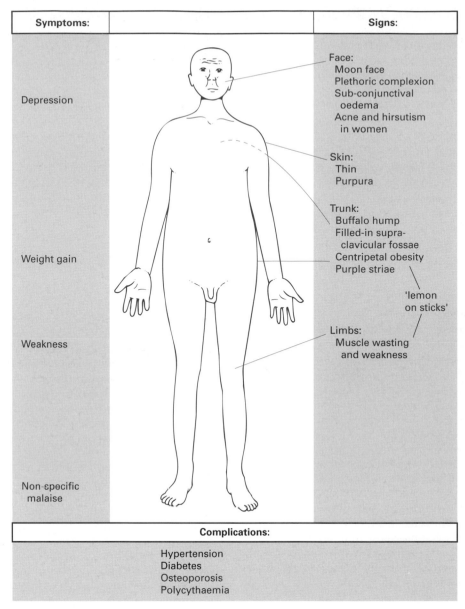

Symptoms:		Signs:

Depression

Weight gain

Weakness

Non-specific malaise

Face:
Moon face
Plethoric complexion
Sub-conjunctival
oedema
Acne and hirsutism
in women

Skin:
Thin
Purpura

Trunk:
Buffalo hump
Filled-in supra-
clavicular fossae
Centripetal obesity
Purple striae

'lemon
on sticks'

Limbs:
Muscle wasting
and weakness

Complications:

Hypertension
Diabetes
Osteoporosis
Polycythaemia

Fig. 79 The clinical features of Cushing's syndrome.

biosynthesis. If pituitary surgery for ACTH-dependent Cushing's fails to cure the patient, bilateral adrenalectomy is an option but it carries a risk of late pituitary tumour expansion and optic nerve compression (Nelson's syndrome). Radiotherapy is indicated for pituitary tumours that have not been cured by neurosurgery.

Prognosis

Cushing's is a disabling disease that often causes irreversible physical and psychological morbidity before it is diagnosed and may respond poorly to treatment. Pituitary microsurgery has improved the prognosis but is not always successful and tumours may recur.

Hyperaldosteronism

Secondary hyperaldosteronism, caused by reduced effective arterial volume/reduced renal perfusion, is a homeo-

static response that causes saline retention in heart failure and hypoalbuminaemic states (p. 196).

Primary hyperaldosteronism (**Conn's syndrome**) is a rare disorder that:

- presents with hypokalaemia and characteristically mild-to-moderate (occasionally severe) hypertension
- may be caused by a discrete adrenal adenoma or bilateral hyperplasia of the zona glomerulosa
- accounts for fewer than 1% of cases of hypertension.

Patients with Conn's syndrome may have symptoms of hypokalaemia (muscle weakness, cramps, polyuria) but are usually asymptomatic. The disease can be screened for by measuring plasma electrolytes in all hypertensive patients before they start treatments which affect potassium (diuretics, angiotensin-converting enzyme (ACE) inhibitors, etc.). The disease should be suspected in hypertensive patients with those features:

1. <40 years old
2. hypokalaemic hypertension
3. resistance for drug therapy.

or who have a family history of multiple endocrine neoplasia or Conn's syndrome. The diagnosis is confirmed by measuring renin and aldosterone after overnight recumbency and again after 4 hours in the upright posture:

- Patients with adrenal adenomas have suppressed renin and a raised serum aldosterone concentration which does not change with posture.
- Those with bilateral hyperplasia also have hyporeninaemic hyperaldosteronism but plasma aldosterone rises with posture.

Adrenal adenomas can be demonstrated by CT, MR or ultrasound. Bilateral hyperplasia can be confirmed by catheterising the renal veins and demonstrating that aldosterone levels are similar on both sides.

All forms of hyperaldosteronism can be treated with spironolactone, although not all patients can tolerate the high doses required. Adrenal adenomas are treated surgically. Whilst hypokalaemia can be expected to resolve, hypertension does so in <50% of patients.

Phaeochromocytoma

Phaeochromocytoma is the one disease of the adrenal medulla. Like Conn's syndrome, it is a cause of secondary hypertension but it is even rarer than Conn's. It is an important disease to recognise because it causes florid and potentially fatal hypertensive crises. The diagnosis is often made postmortem, patients dying of haemorrhagic stroke or cardiovascular complications. It is usually caused by a solitary adrenal adenoma but there are exceptions, which lead to the nickname 'the 10% tumour':

- 10% are bilateral
- 10% malignant
- 10% extra-adrenal.

The tumours usually secrete noradrenaline (norepinephrine). Symptoms are classically paroxysmal, the commonest being the triad of:

- headache
- sweating
- palpitations.

Nervousness, panic attacks and flushing may also occur. Hypertension can be paroxysmal or sustained. Patients may be hypotensive between paroxysms and on standing. This hypotension results from two homeostatic responses: downregulation of catecholamine receptors and plasma volume contraction. The diagnosis is made:

- first and foremost by thinking of it
- by measuring urinary or plasma catecholamines in patients with suggestive symptoms, severe or labile hypertension or a positive family history.

Once a biochemical diagnosis is made, the adrenals are imaged by MR rather than CT because the appearance of phaeochromocytoma on T_1-weighted images is quite characteristic. In addition, radionuclide scanning with a labelled precursor of catecholamine synthesis can demonstrate hormone synthesis in the tumour.

Treatment is first with i.v. then with oral alpha-blockers (phentolamine and phenoxybenzamine, respectively). Intravenous fluids should be given to stabilise blood pressure once alpha-blockade has been instituted. Beta-blockers are often added later. A period of stabilisation on antihypertensive therapy precedes surgery.

7.5 Hypogonadism

Learning objectives

You should . . .
- know the main causes and clinical features of hypogonadism.

Case Study

An elderly widower is taken aback when his specialist suggests he should have testosterone treatment. When it is explained to him that testosterone can improve wellbeing and prevent osteoporosis, as well as restore erectile function, he agrees to give it a try.

Hypogonadism may be primary (i.e. caused by ovarian/testicular failure) or secondary to disease of the hypothalamus or pituitary. The commonest form of primary hypogonadism, the menopause, is covered in gynaecology text books so this section will concentrate on male hypogonadism, although the same general principles can be applied to females.

In primary hypogonadism the sex steroid levels are low, and the gonadotrophins are high (hypergonadotrophic hypogonadism), whereas in secondary hypogonadism the gonadotrophins are low (hypogonadotrophic hypogonadism).

Sex steroid secretion is vulnerable to hypothalamo–pituitary disease because, as described on p. 304, the gonadotrophins are among the first hormones to be affected by pituitary disease. They are also affected by hyperprolactinaemia, which suppresses them.

Male impotence and infertility are rarely caused by hypogonadism but the latter should be suspected if the patient has:

- loss of drive and libido
- reduced beard growth
- erectile failure
- anorgasmia
- a reduced volume of ejaculate
- reduced testicular volumes.

The diagnosis is made by measuring testosterone, luteinising hormone, follicle-stimulating hormone and prolactin; a full list of causes is given in Box 19.

Box 19: Causes of hypogonadism

Hypogonadotrophic causes
- Hypopituitarism (p. 304)
- Hyperprolactinaemia
- Hypothalamic tumours
- Kallmann's syndrome

Hypergonadotrophic causes
- Testicular injury
- Klinefelter's syndrome

Hypogonadotrophic or hypergonadotrophic cause
- Haemochromatosis

Hyperprolactinaemia is treated with a dopaminergic agonist (p. 306). Otherwise, treatment is by testosterone replacement therapy, which can be given:

- orally
- by monthly injection
- as a 6-monthly subcutaneous implant
- transdermally by a skin patch on the trunk
- by 3-monthly depot injection
- by application of a gel to non-hairy skin
- by a buccal gel.

Untreated hypogonadism predisposes to osteoporosis and may cause non-specific lethargy and weakness, so testosterone treatment should be offered even to patients who do not wish to be sexually active. Induction of spermatogenesis requires gonadotrophin injection or infusion therapy.

7.6 Hyperlipidaemia

Learning objectives

You should:
- understand the common hyperlipidaemias and their relationship to cardiovascular disease
- be familiar with the *current* consensus guidelines for starting treatment
- be aware of the management options.

Case Study

An alcoholic man presents to accident and emergency with abdominal pain. When you take blood, you notice that his plasma is milky. You see in his electronic record that his plasma triglyceride level on a previous hospital admission was 68 mmol/l, over 30 times the upper limit of normal for fasting trigycerides (0.3–2.0 mmol/l). A plasma amylase of 3500 IU/l clinches the diagnosis of acute pancreatitis.

Hyperlipidaemia can seem a very confusing subject. This discussion follows a simple, pragmatic approach, emphasising key points. These are:

- Hyperlipidaemia is an important public health problem because it increases the risk of cardiovascular disease.
- Severe hyperlipidaemia may, in addition, cause skin lesions and pancreatitis.
- Hyperlipidaemia may be secondary to systemic disease or primary (genetic).
- Treatment is first with diet and second with one of a limited range of drugs.

You should be familiar with current consensus guidelines used to decide when to start treatment. They change too rapidly for any textbook to remain up-to-date.

Investigations

To diagnose hyperlipidaemia and assess cardiovascular risk, you need to measure:

- serum total cholesterol
- high-density lipoprotein (HDL) cholesterol
- low-density lipoprotein (LDL) cholesterol
- triglyceride.

Ideally, lipids should be measured after a 12-hour fast (necessary for triglycerides but not cholesterol). LDL cholesterol increases cardiovascular risk. HDL (involved in cholesterol disposal) reduces it. The result should be interpreted in the light of the patient's age and gender and the presence or absence of cardiovascular risk factors and disease. Lipids should not be measured between 24 hours and 3 months after a severe illness (e.g. myocardial infarct), which will make them artificially high. Table 69 summarises the main primary and secondary types of hyperlipidaemia.

Lipids and coronary risk

Hypercholesterolaemia is one of the three main factors, together with smoking and hypertension (the 'unholy trinity'), that predispose to cardiovascular disease. Serum cholesterol accounts for as much as two-thirds of the variance in cardiovascular risk between different populations. There is no such thing as a *normal* cholesterol because cardiovascular risk rises progressively with increasing serum cholesterol, particularly above 6.5 mmol/l. Presence of more than one major risk factor increases cardiovascular risk multiplicatively. Triglycerides are a weaker risk factor for coronary artery disease but can cause acute pancreatitis in high concentration (>20 mmol/l). There is an inverse relationship between triglyceride and HDL cholesterol concentrations and it is controversial how far this accounts for the apparent protective effect of HDL.

Clinical presentation

Symptoms and signs

Hyperlipidaemia is usually detected by screening. Hypercholesterolaemia may cause:

- corneal arcus: a white ring at the junction of cornea and sclera
- xanthelasma: subcutaneous cholesterol deposits at the inner margins of the eyelid
- xanthoma: thickening of tendons.

Table 69 Types of hyperlipidaemia

Type	Cholesterol	Triglycerides	Prevalence
Primary (genetic)			
Polygenic hypercholesterolaemia	↑		++++
Familial hypercholesterolaemia			
Heterozygous	↑		++
Homozygous	↑↑		Rare
Familial combined hyperlipidaemia	↑	↑	+++
Familial hypertriglyceridaemia		↑	+
Remnant hyperlipoproteinaemia	↑↑	↑↑	+
Hyperchylomicronaemia		↑↑	Rare
Secondary to systemic disease			
Obesity	↑	↑	
Hypothyroidism	↑		
Nephrotic syndrome	↑	(↑)	
Liver disease	↑		
Diabetes		↑	
Alcohol abuse		↑	

↑, increased.

Hypertriglyceridaemia can cause:

- eruptive xanthoma: subcutaneous deposits of triglyceride
- lipaemia retinalis: milky appearance of the retinal vessels on ophthalmoscopy.

Specific syndromes

Primary hypercholesterolaemia is usually inherited in a simple polygenic pattern. Heterozygous autosomal dominant familial hypercholesterolaemia is less common and causes moderate hypercholesterolaemia. Homozygous familial hypercholesterolaemia causes extremely severe hypercholesterolaemia, which is usually fatal in early adult life. Hypercholesterolaemia may be secondary to hypothyroidism, obstructive jaundice or nephrotic syndrome.

Hypertriglyceridaemia may be caused by obesity, alcoholism, uncontrolled diabetes or the uncommon condition of familial hypertriglyceridaemia. Familial combined hyperlipidaemia is dominantly inherited and may produce different patterns of hyperlipidaemia in different family members.

Management

Who and when to treat

There are two underpinning points.

1. The decision to treat depends on the patient's absolute risk of having a cardiovascular event. Reducing plasma total cholesterol by 0.6 mmol/l with a statin can be expected to reduce risk by 25% over 5 years. For people with a 50% risk of a heart attack, eight would have to be treated (seven ineffectively) to prevent one of them having a heart

attack. If the risk were only 10%, 40 would have to be treated (39 ineffectively) to prevent one, clearly less of a bargain!

2. More than just lipids determine absolute risk: specifically, whether the patient already has cardiovascular disease, smokes, is hypertensive and is at high risk because of diabetes or a positive family history of cardiovascular disease.

So, plasma lipids are never interpreted in isolation. Tables and computer programes are widely available to calculate risk.

Both in deciding who to treat and whether their treatment has been effective, just remember two simple threshold values: total cholesterol ≥4 mmol/l and LDL cholesterol ≥2 mmol/l. The two are broadly correlated so a patient who exceeds one is likely to exceed the other.

Broadly, there are three categories of individuals for treatment:

1. people who have established cardiovascular disease
2. people who do not have established cardiovascular disease but have a 10-year risk ≥30%
3. people who do not have cardiovascular disease but do have a condition known to be associated with cardiovascular disease (e.g. chronic kidney disease) and a 10-year risk ≥15%.

Since hypercholesterolaemia as an isolated problem is asymptomatic, the question is who should be screened to detect it. It follows logically from the above that any patient who is at increased risk by virtue of smoking, hypertension or a positive family history of cardiovascular disease should be screened.

How to treat

Diet and exercise Every patient should be advised to restrict calories to normalise their body weight, reduce their intake of saturated fat and take regular aerobic exercise. These measures, alone, will bring cholesterol below threshold in only a minority.

Lipid-lowering therapy A statin (e.g. simvastatin, pravastatin) is the first-line drug treatment. It should be started at the dose used in the major treatment trials (e.g. simvastatin 20 mg daily, pravastatin 40 mg daily) and adjusted according to the lipid response. Fibrates (bezafibrate, fenofibrate, gemfibrozil) lower triglycerides as well as cholesterol and may be considered as first-line treatment in patients with combined hyperlipidaemia: for instance, in diabetes. Newer statins (atorvastatin, rosuvastatin) are more potent at lowering cholesterol and may be considered first-line drugs. Statins and fibrates can be combined. Treatment is successful if total and LDL cholesterol are lowered below threshold values. An alternative criterion of success is a >30% lowering of cholesterol.

Ezetimibe, a cholesterol esterase inhibitor, reduces the absorption of cholesterol across the intestinal wall and is used as an adjunct to statins or where statins are not tolerated. Bile acid sequestrants (colestyramine and colestipol), taken as oral resins, are relatively effective at lowering cholesterol but very unpalatable. Nicotinic acid and derivatives (acipimox) lower triglycerides but are poorly tolerated. A slow-release preparation of nicotinic acid (Niaspan) is better tolerated and raises HDL as well as lowering triglycerides. These drugs are usually only given by specialists in lipid disease.

Treatment of other cardiovascular risk factors It follows logically from the multifactorial nature of cardiovascular risk and the additive effects of different risk factors that no single risk factor should be treated in isolation. All patients should be given lifestyle and dietary advice; those who smoke should be supported in stopping it (including regular consultation and nicotine replacement therapy or bupropion), and blood pressure should be effectively treated. Cardioprotective drugs such as aspirin, beta-blockers and ACE inhibitors are often indicated. The aim is not just to improve the plasma cholesterol measurement but to take a broad, effective and continuing approach to cardiovascular risk.

7.7 Obesity

Learning objectives

You should:
- be aware of the health hazards associated with obesity
- understand the management of obesity and how to counsel patients

Case Study

A woman in her twenties with congenital adrenal hyperplasia has a body mass index of 35 because she has needed so much hydrocortisone to suppress her adrenals. After bariatric surgery, she loses 4 stone in weight and forms the first serious sexual relationship of her life.

Obesity is an epidemic disease in developed countries, contributing to vascular disease, diabetes, hypertension, arthritis, shortened life expectancy and many other major public health problems. It is a common lay belief that obesity is caused by 'something wrong with the glands'. Do not fall into the trap of thinking that obesity is an 'endocrine disease'. Obese patients may deposit their food more readily into their fat stores than non-obese people but they also eat more and exercise less. There are few organic causes of obesity, and patients with those diseases do not usually present with obesity. Those organic causes include:

- hypothyroidism
- Cushing's syndrome
- hypothalamic tumours causing polyphagia
- insulin or sulphonylurea treatment of diabetes
- insulinoma.

Some of these causes are common and obvious; others are exquisitely rare. Investigation of obese patients for endocrine disease is generally unrewarding. It is important to convince patients that there is not something wrong with their glands rather than entrench their belief by investigating them fruitlessly.

The first-line management of obesity is sympathetic dietary advice, emotional support, exercise and counselling to encourage and support behaviour change. Weight loss is indicated in patients with a body mass index (BMI) over 30 kg/m^2, or over 28 kg/m^2 with other risk factors. Drug treatment can be useful in conjunction with diet and exercise. Orlistat, which blocks intestinal fat breakdown, is licensed to be used for 2 years in patients who have already succeeded in losing 2.5 kg over 4 weeks of dietary effort. Its usefulness is limited by steatorrhoea and flatulence. Sibutramine is an appetite suppressant, whose side-effects include hypertension and tachycardia. Bariatric surgery (gastroplasty) is an effective treatment for morbid obesity, or obesity in association with a disease like diabetes or severe hyperlipidaemia.

7.8 Diabetes mellitus and spontaneous hypoglycaemia

Learning objectives

You should:
- know the main types of diabetes and understand their causes and the rationale for their treatment
- be able to describe the management of the common metabolic emergencies of diabetes (hypo- and hyperglycaemia)
- understand what is meant by 'diabetic tissue complications' and know their features and management.

Case Study

A student nurse in her early twenties develops type 1 diabetes. With insulin aspart before each meal and detemir at bedtime, she achieves a haemoglobin A1c of 6.8% and is able to take vigorous exercise and avert hypoglycaemia by regular glucose monitoring and attention to what she eats. She is not eligible for an insulin infusion pump 'on the NHS' because her control is so good. Perhaps she is still in the 'honeymoon period' but, if she can sustain this level of control, her risk of complications is greatly reduced.

Diabetes

Diabetes mellitus is the most common endocrine disease. It is caused by insulin deficiency and/or insulin resistance, the relative contributions of which vary between different types of diabetes. The net effect is hyperglycaemia. The metabolic disturbance ranges from an asymptomatic biochemical abnormality to a fatal metabolic emergency. Over months or years, diabetes causes tissue damage, seen clinically as diabetic complications. Diabetes:

- shortens life expectancy by up to one-third
- increases the risk of ischaemic heart disease threefold
- increases the risk of amputations 15-fold; it is responsible for nearly half of lower limb amputations
- is the most common cause of blindness in middle age
- is responsible for one in ten cases of renal failure and is the most common single cause of dialysis/transplantation.

Much of this morbidity is preventable by well-structured medical care, with an emphasis on good control of blood glucose and other risk factors (blood pressure, smoking, cholesterol), and detection of complications at an early stage. Diabetic patients have to take responsibility for much of their own care and need good education and support. You will inevitably care for diabetic patients early in your career because over 5% of UK hospital bed-days are associated with diabetes.

Carbohydrate metabolism

Normal metabolism

Think of insulin as a 'storage hormone', which is secreted by the pancreatic β cell when blood glucose rises after a carbohydrate meal. Insulin causes:

- increased glucose uptake in many tissues by activation of glucose transporter molecules
- increased glycolysis
- decreased gluconeogenesis
- storage of glucose in liver and muscle as glycogen.

Insulin also affects protein and fat metabolism:

- Protein synthesis is stimulated and protein breakdown inhibited.
- Fat is deposited in adipose tissue.
- Ketogenesis is reduced.

Insulin is formed by cleavage of a connecting peptide (C-peptide) from the precursor proinsulin. C-peptide can be measured as a marker of endogenous insulin secretion. Glucagon, adrenaline (epinephrine), cortisol and GH have opposite metabolic effects and can be thought of as 'anti-insulin hormones'.

During starvation, insulin levels fall and increased levels of the anti-insulin hormones maintain blood glucose by glycogenolysis, and gluconeogenesis from the substrates alanine, lactate and glycerol.

Reduced insulin action also causes release of amino acids from protein, and glycerol and fatty acids from adipose tissue. Free fatty acids are metabolised to the ketones acetoacetate, β-hydroxybutyrate and acetone, which can be used as a fuel.

In health, continuous variation in the rate of insulin secretion maintains plasma glucose within narrow limits. The brain, in particular, has a high demand for glucose and is absolutely reliant on an adequate blood glucose level. Even a modest fall to a glucose concentration of 3 mmol/l provokes adrenaline (epinephrine) secretion and impairs cognitive function. Profound hypoglycaemia (<2 mmol/l) causes coma and, ultimately, permanent neurological damage or death.

Abnormal carbohydrate metabolism

Diabetes is caused by absolute or relative insulin deficiency from one or more of:

- β cell failure
- tissue resistance to insulin caused by a receptor or postreceptor defect
- excess of one or more anti-insulin hormones.

The earliest abnormality is an increased blood glucose after ingesting carbohydrate. The **glucose tolerance test** (GTT) — in which blood glucose is measured before and 2 hours after 75 g oral glucose — is a sensitive test for impaired insulin secretion/action. At this early stage, the feedback loop between glucose and insulin is able to maintain a normal fasting blood glucose but, with worsened insulin action, fasting hyperglycaemia (≥7 mmol/l) develops. This is the biochemical hallmark of diabetes. Symptoms do not develop until there is quite marked fasting hyperglycaemia. With severe insulin deficiency, excessive ketone body formation and acidosis develop, as well as severe hyperglycaemia (diabetic ketoacidosis). Impaired glucose tolerance, type 2 diabetes mellitus (type 2 DM) and type 1 diabetes mellitus (type 1 DM) represent three points on a spectrum of insulin deficiency.

Hypoglycaemia is caused by:

- excessive insulin given to treat diabetes
- excessive insulin secretion from an insulin-secreting pancreatic tumour or from sulphonylurea therapy (see below)
- underproduction of the anti-insulin hormones: for example, in hypoadrenalism or hypopituitarism
- starvation or liver disease, in which the glycogen stores are depleted and/or gluconeogenesis fails.

Glycation and other metabolic effects of hyperglycaemia

Glucose attaches to proteins throughout the body by the process of glycation. This is not dependent on enzymes and occurs in proportion to blood glucose levels averaged over the life of the protein. Glycation is important because:

- it damages tissues and is one of the processes causing diabetic complications
- measuring its degree gives a time-averaged measure of hyperglycaemia.

Haemoglobin is a readily accessible protein with a long half-life. Glycation alters the electrophoretic mobility of haemoglobin A. This glycated form of haemoglobin A is termed haemoglobin A_{1c} (HbA_{1c}). The percentage of haemoglobin A in this glycated form (usually <6%) is a measure of blood glucose control and a predictor of diabetic complications. Fructosamine is a measure of the degree of glycation of plasma proteins. It is a less precise and less stable measure of glycaemic control than HbA_{1c}.

Diabetic patients have many other metabolic abnormalities that predispose to vascular disease including hyperlipidaemia, increased fibrinogen levels, increased blood viscosity and high insulin levels.

Epidemiology

Diabetes affects 2% of Caucasians, up to a quarter of whom are insulin-dependent. Its prevalence rises to 10% in elderly people and is 3–4 times higher in Asians than Caucasians in the UK. Some non-UK populations have prevalences as high as 50% (e.g. Pima Indians in the USA).

Types of diabetes

In temperate countries there are two main types of diabetes (Table 70): types 1 and 2. Internationally, 'tropical diabetes' is another important type which may be insulin-treated or non-insulin-treated. It is not discussed here.

The stereotypes in Table 70 are far from absolute. Patients with type 2 DM may present in young adult life; those with type 1 may present in old age. That is why the terms maturity-onset and juvenile-onset diabetes have been abandoned. There is another problem in that about 10% of patients with type 2 DM per year after diagnosis become uncontrollable with tablets and progress to insulin treatment without becoming ketosis-prone. Such patients are best described as having insulin-treated type 2 DM.

Causes

Type 1 DM is caused by autoimmunity against the β cells of the pancreas, which eventually destroys them com-

pletely and causes absolute insulin deficiency. It is thought that this process may be triggered by a viral infection or some other environmental insult. It can be halted by immunotherapy (for example, with ciclosporin) but over 90% of β cells are destroyed by the time a patient presents with type 1 DM, so immunotherapy gives no lasting benefit. Type 2 DM is less well understood; insulin is still produced but the response to an increase in plasma glucose is 'too little and too late', probably because the capacity of the β cells to recognise and respond to hyperglycaemia is impaired. Likewise, the responsiveness of insulin's target tissues is impaired. Type 2 DM is, therefore, an effect of both insulin deficiency and insulin resistance: **relative insulin deficiency**. Since neither the feedback loop between plasma glucose and the β cell nor the capacity to secrete insulin is lost completely, hyperglycaemia is not usually as severe as in type 1 DM and ketosis does not occur. Why patients with type 2 DM progress to insulin treatment is unexplained by this mechanism; a leading theory is that deposits of amyloid in the islets of Langerhans are somehow associated with progressive dysfunction of the β cells, a process quite distinct from the lymphocytic inflammation which destroys the islets in type 1 DM.

Primary and secondary diabetes

Diabetes can be caused by any process that interferes with the production or action of insulin. Type 1 and type 2 DM, as described above, could be termed *primary* or idiopathic diabetes. There are many causes of *secondary* diabetes, which can be insulin-dependent or non-insulin-dependent, depending on the degree of insulin deficiency. Secondary diabetes may be accompanied or unaccompanied by pancreatic exocrine deficiency. Causes can be categorised by the underlying mechanism.

Failure of insulin secretion Common causes are:

- pancreatitis, pancreatectomy
- pancreatic carcinoma
- alcohol abuse
- drugs: beta-blockers, thiazides (including diazoxide).

Rare causes include haemochromatosis.
Insulin resistance Common causes are:

- steroid therapy
- gross obesity.

Table 70 Characteristics of the two main types of diabetes mellitus*

	Type 1	Type 2
Age of onset	Younger: peak incidence in late teenage years	Older: incidence increases progressively with age
Weight	Lean	Obese
Onset	More abrupt	May be very insidious
Treatment	Absolute dependence on insulin therapy	Treatable initially with diet alone or tablets
Ketosis	Develops if insulin not given	Not ketosis-prone

*These stereotypes are not absolute.

Rare causes include:

- endocrine diseases: Cushing's disease, acromegaly, thyrotoxicosis, phaeochromocytoma.

Associated with congenital syndromes These are all rare and the causes unknown. They are not discussed here.

Gestational diabetes This is a special case, which will be considered below (p. 323).

Clinical presentation

Symptoms

Mild-to-moderate hyperglycaemia can be asymptomatic or can cause any or all of these symptoms:

- thirst, polyuria and polydipsia
- blurred vision
- balanitis in men and pruritus vulvae in women
- lethargy and somnolence
- weight loss and weakness
- anorexia and nausea
- recurrent skin infections.

Severe hyperglycaemia causes:

- severe thirst
- drowsiness or coma
- vomiting.

Ketosis causes:

- nausea, vomiting
- breathlessness.

It is important to think of the ways in which diabetes may present. There are four main ways.

1. Classically, type 1 DM presents with a short history (days or weeks) of severe symptoms, sometimes culminating in ketoacidosis.
2. Type 2 DM can also cause severe hyperglycaemic symptoms but more typically presents with less severe symptoms over a longer time (months or even years).
3. Even quite severe hyperglycaemia may cause no symptoms at all and type 2 DM is commonly diagnosed by screening (e.g. well-person checks, insurance or employment medicals). Even if found by chance, diabetes must be taken seriously because asymptomatic hyperglycaemia can cause complications (see below).
4. Finally, diabetes may present with its complications:
   — infections, e.g. staphylococcal skin infections, foot ulcers, candidiasis
   — visual impairment caused by cataract or retinopathy
   — arterial disease, e.g. myocardial infarction, peripheral vascular disease
   — neuropathy, e.g. mononeuritis multiplex or polyneuropathy
   — renal failure.

Investigations

You can infer that patients have diabetes if they have glycosuria, but different people 'spill' glucose into the urine at different levels of blood glucose (renal threshold). If anything, urine glucose testing is over-sensitive so it is used to screen for, but cannot be used to diagnose, diabetes.

- If a patient is symptomatic, a single plasma glucose measurement that is raised according to the diagnostic criteria below confirms the diagnosis.
- If asymptomatic, two abnormal blood glucose concentrations are needed to exclude laboratory error or other spurious causes; the appropriate investigation is the *fasting* blood glucose, because random measurements are influenced by the timing and size of the most recent meal.
- A GTT is needed occasionally: for example, in an asymptomatic patient with borderline fasting or random blood glucose values.

The GTT can define a second category of abnormality in which fasting blood glucose is normal but there is an abnormally high level after oral glucose: **impaired glucose tolerance**. Such patients do not have diabetes and are not at risk of its microvascular complications but are at increased risk of coronary heart disease. The GTT has recently been shown to be a better predictor of morbidity than the fasting glucose concentration; as a result, the GTT is more widely used after a period of being 'out of fashion'.

Diagnostic criteria for diabetes

The World Health Organization revised its criteria in 2000, the main change being a reduction in the fasting glucose level diagnostic of diabetes from 7.8 to 7.0 mmol/l. In a patient with suggestive symptoms (e.g. thirst, polyuria, weight loss), the diagnosis can be made on:

- a random venous plasma glucose concentration ≥11.1 mmol/l, *or*
- a fasting plasma glucose concentration ≥7.0 mmol/l (whole blood 6.1 mmol/l), *or*
- a plasma glucose concentration ≥11.1 mmol/l 2 hours after 75 g anhydrous glucose in an oral GTT.

The same criteria are applied to patients who are asymptomatic, but an abnormal plasma glucose concentration must be found on two occasions on different days. Two other categories of abnormality are recognised:

- impaired glucose tolerance (IGT), a stage of impaired glucose regulation (fasting plasma glucose <7.0 mmol/l and oral GTT 2-hour value ≥7.8 but <11.1 mmol/l)
- impaired fasting glycaemia (IFG), introduced to classify individuals who have fasting glucose values above the normal range but below those diagnostic of diabetes (fasting plasma glucose >6.1 but <7.0 mmol/l).

Management

The principles of treatment follow directly from the pathophysiology. Type 1 can only be treated by insulin replacement. Type 2 is treated by lessening insulin resistance and/or boosting or supplementing insulin secretion.

Diet

Diet is central to the management of all types of diabetes. Patients with type 2 DM are usually obese and their insulin resistance can be improved by weight loss. Many can be treated by diet alone. For those on tablets or insulin, diet is an essential adjunct. The aim of the diet is to:

- optimise glycaemic control
- combat hyperlipidaemia and minimise the risk of vascular disease
- minimise the risk of hypoglycaemia if on tablets or insulin.

For all types of diabetes, the approach is similar:

- Restrict calories if overweight.
- Take starchy and high-fibre foods in preference to simple sugars to prevent violent swings in blood glucose.
- Take frequent and small meals and snacks to match the sluggish insulin response from the diseased pancreas and/or the slow absorption of injected insulin.
- Limit total fat intake and encourage mono- and polyunsaturates in preference to animal fat to aid weight loss and reduce plasma lipids.

Patients with diabetic nephropathy are sometimes recommended a reduced-protein diet.

Tablets

Oral treatment is indicated in type 2 DM if diet fails to achieve satisfactory glycaemic control. There are five types:

1. *biguanides*: metformin, which works by reducing hepatic gluconeogenesis
2. *sulphonylureas*: tolbutamide, chlorpropamide, glibenclamide, glipizide, gliclazide, glimepiride, gliquidone, which work by increasing insulin secretion
3. α-*glucosidase inhibitors*: acarbose, which works by inhibiting intestinal brush border saccharidases and delaying glucose absorption
4. *glitazones (thiazolidinediones)*: rosiglitazone or pioglitazone, which increase the sensitivity of muscle and fat to insulin
5. *meglitinides*: repaglinide, natiglinide, which enhance meal-related insulin secretion.

Metformin does not increase insulin secretion and, therefore, does not cause weight gain. Since many patients with type 2 DM are obese, this makes it the treatment of choice for those who cannot be controlled with diet alone. It is as effective as sulphonylureas but causes intolerable side-effects (nausea, anorexia and diarrhoea) in up to 20% of patients. It can cause lactic acidosis, a fatal metabolic complication, in patients with severe heart failure, liver disease and renal failure and is, therefore, contraindicated in those conditions. The glitazones constitute a second class of insulin sensitisers. They can be given in conjunction with metformin or sulphonylurea. Unlike metformin they cause weight gain.

Although sulphonylureas cause weight gain by increasing insulin secretion, they are effective, well tolerated and widely used. Hypoglycaemia is their main complication. Patients over 70, particularly if they live alone, should not be given long-acting sulphonylureas like glibenclamide and chlorpropamide, which can cause profound, prolonged and potentially fatal hypoglycaemia. Meglitinides, although chemically different, have a similar effect to sulphonylureas.

Acarbose is used as first-line or adjunctive treatment for type 2 DM. It has proved effective in some clinical trials but its practical usefulness is limited by flatulence and diarrhoea.

Metformin, the glitazones, sulphonylureas and acarbose (and, indeed, insulin) all have different modes of action and can be used for type 2 DM in combination, though the combination of glitazones and insulin can cause heart failure.

Insulin

Insulin is indicated in patients who present with classical type 1 DM or who, having originally presented with type 2 DM, become ketosis-prone or hyperglycaemic despite sulphonylureas. The mystique that surrounds insulins is largely unjustified and can be dispelled if they are thought of generically rather than by trade name. Insulin preparations differ in their:

- species of origin: beef, pork or human
- length of action: ultrashort (lispro or insulin aspart), short (soluble), medium/long (isophane, lente), long (ultralente, glargine, detemir).

Almost all patients can be controlled with ultrashort/short and medium/long in various combinations.

The advent of insulin analogues has revolutionised insulin therapy, although therapy with human (and even animal) insulin is likely to be common for some time yet. Treatment with a long-acting analogue insulin (detemir or glargine) is the foundation of most contemporary insulin regimens. In many patients with type 1 DM, this is supplemented with ultrashort insulin (lispro or aspart) each time the patient eats, typically three times per day. In patients with type 2 DM, detemir/glargine may be given alone or combined with metformin. Premixed combinations of short- and long-acting insulin are also used. The choice of regimen depends on the preferences of patients and physicians and, sometimes, trial and error. Pen injectors have almost entirely taken the place of conventional syringes and needles.

Monitoring

Monitoring can be divided broadly into self-monitoring and clinic monitoring:

- Home urine and blood testing are the common forms of self-monitoring.
- Clinic monitoring is by enquiry about hyperglycaemic and hypoglycaemic symptoms, and measurement of weight and glycated haemoglobin.

All patients who are able should at least do home urine tests. A typical recommendation is to do one test per day on 3 days per week and in addition whenever they feel unwell. Home blood glucose testing is usually reserved for those who are younger, using insulin or more inquisitive about their control. How often patients should do blood tests is a matter of individual choice. One test per day at a minimum, varying the time, would be a usual regimen.

Education

Responsibility for controlling diabetes rests primarily with the patient. It may involve complex day-to-day decisions about insulin doses. Education of the patient and ready availability of advice are key aspects of diabetes management. There are a number of common issues.

- Hypoglycaemia. All patients taking sulphonylureas or insulin and their partners must be acquainted with the symptoms and know how to prevent and treat them. The partners of patients with type 1 DM should be provided with glucagon and/or oral glucose gel (p. 324) and taught how to use it.
- Exercise. Advice is needed on how to tailor the regimen to regular or unexpected exercise by taking extra carbohydrate and/or reducing insulin doses.
- Illness. Every patient should be taught never to reduce insulin doses during illness, given instructions on how to manage their diabetes if their tests are high and/or they cannot eat, and advised who to contact if they lose control.
- Shift work and travel across time zones.
- Pregnancy. Every diabetic woman of child-bearing potential must be educated about the need for good control at the time of conception, and about other aspects of pregnancy (p. 323).
- Employment, careers, etc.
- Insurance.
- Complications. In particular, the reasons not to smoke and the need for retinal screening and preventive foot care.

The multidisciplinary diabetes team

Diabetes care is most effectively delivered by a team of doctors, nurses, dietitians, podiatrists and other professionals working closely together. In particular, diabetes specialist nurses are key members of this multidisciplinary team, available to educate and advise students and doctors in training as well as diabetic patients.

Complications of diabetes

The effects of diabetes include:

- tissue complications
- pregnancy-related complications
- metabolic complications (hypoglycaemia and hyperglycaemia)
- psychosocial complications (a major cause of morbidity, which will not be further considered here)
- increased susceptibility to infections.

Tissue complications

These are largely caused by vascular disease:

- *Macrovascular* (large vessel) complications include cardiovascular disease, peripheral vascular disease and stroke; these are more prevalent in diabetes but not specific to it.

- *Microvascular* complications include retinopathy, nephropathy and neuropathy; they are specific to diabetes.

Macrovascular complications and hypertension

Figure 80 lists the manifestations and causes of macrovascular disease. The important point to remember is that diabetes is a potent risk factor for all types of large vessel disease, which may present at younger ages and is diffuse, affecting smaller as well as larger arteries. Apart from the surgical difficulties posed by diffuse disease, there is nothing special about the management of arterial disease in diabetes.

Hypertension Hypertension and diabetes are linked in a number of ways:

- Hypertension is so common in patients with type 2 DM that it is thought the two diseases have a pathophysiological link, either genetic or acquired in utero or in early life. Many hypertensive patients with type 2 DM are also hyperlipidaemic and hyperinsulinaemic. This cluster of factors is potently atherogenic and is termed the metabolic syndrome.
- The treatment of hypertension with beta-blockers may precipitate type 2 DM by impairing insulin secretion and causing insulin resistance.
- Hypertension increases the risk of both microvascular and macrovascular disease in diabetics.
- Patients with nephropathy may be caught in a vicious circle of rising blood pressure and worsening renal function, which can be broken by antihypertensive therapy.

The prevalence of hypertension is not increased in uncomplicated type 1 DM, unless nephropathy has developed, but the prevalence is greatly increased in type 2 DM. The clinical presentation and investigation of hypertension are as described on page 41. There are some specific points about its treatment in diabetes:

- Diabetic patients should be regarded as high-risk hypertensives.
- Hypertension should be treated aggressively in patients with nephropathy; unless there is evidence of renal artery stenosis (p. 187) or a possibility of pregnancy, use ACE inhibitors.
- ACE inhibitors or angiotensin receptor antagonists are the first-line treatment in many situations, particularly for patients with heart failure or left ventricular dysfunction.
- Beta-blockers and calcium antagonists are indicated, usually with an ACE inhibitor, in patients with myocardial infarction or angina.
- Beta-blockers worsen glucose tolerance and hyperlipidaemia. Their role as first-line antihypertensives in type 2 DM is debated.

Prevention of macrovascular disease This consists of primary prevention, the early identification and correction of risk factors, and secondary prevention, the management of established disease. All patients should have as good glycaemic control as possible, although this has not yet been *proven* to prevent macrovascular disease. All risk

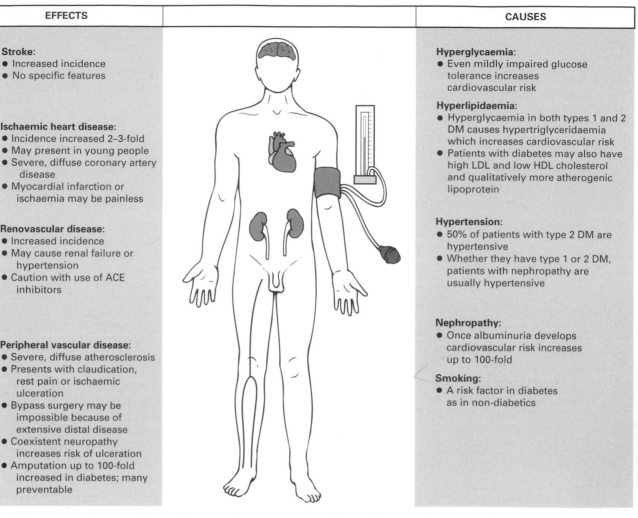

EFFECTS		CAUSES

Stroke:
- Increased incidence
- No specific features

Ischaemic heart disease:
- Incidence increased 2–3-fold
- May present in young people
- Severe, diffuse coronary artery disease
- Myocardial infarction or ischaemia may be painless

Renovascular disease:
- Increased incidence
- May cause renal failure or hypertension
- Caution with use of ACE inhibitors

Peripheral vascular disease:
- Severe, diffuse atherosclerosis
- Presents with claudication, rest pain or ischaemic ulceration
- Bypass surgery may be impossible because of extensive distal disease
- Coexistent neuropathy increases risk of ulceration
- Amputation up to 100-fold increased in diabetes; many preventable

Hyperglycaemia:
- Even mildly impaired glucose tolerance increases cardiovascular risk

Hyperlipidaemia:
- Hyperglycaemia in both types 1 and 2 DM causes hypertriglyceridaemia which increases cardiovascular risk
- Patients with diabetes may also have high LDL and low HDL cholesterol and qualitatively more atherogenic lipoprotein

Hypertension:
- 50% of patients with type 2 DM are hypertensive
- Whether they have type 1 or 2 DM, patients with nephropathy are usually hypertensive

Nephropathy:
- Once albuminuria develops cardiovascular risk increases up to 100-fold

Smoking:
- A risk factor in diabetes as in non-diabetics

Fig. 80 Macrovascular disease in diabetes. ACE, angiotensin-converting enzyme; LDL and HDL, low- and high-density lipoproteins respectively.

factors, including hypertension, should be treated because their effects are additive:

- Hyperlipidaemia is common in diabetes and should be treated aggressively (p. 312).
- Smoking is even more dangerous than in the general population.
- Blood pressure should be monitored regularly and treated early (see above).

Patients who already have macrovascular disease have a very high risk of disease progression and mortality, so secondary prevention should be even more strenuous than primary prevention. There is compelling evidence that ACE inhibitors and angiotensin receptor antagonists are beneficial and may have effects beyond lowering blood pressure in diabetic patients at increased cardiovascular risk. These topics are also covered under hyperlipidaemia (p. 312), hypertension (p. 41) and ischaemic heart disease (p. 11).

Microvascular complications

Retinopathy Diabetes is the single most common cause of blindness in middle age and a cause of visual loss at all ages. Retinopathy may be present when diabetes is diagnosed, particularly in old people, and becomes increasingly prevalent with longer durations of diabetes. Clinical features are summarised in Figure 81. Diabetic retinopathy results from occlusion and leakage of retinal capillaries. There are two causes of visual loss:

- **Maculopathy** is loss of visual acuity caused by background retinopathy involving the fovea.
- **Proliferative retinopathy** is the formation of new blood vessels or fibrous tissue on the surface of the retina in response to retinal ischaemia; ultimately, those vessels bleed and/or the fibrous tissue related to them contracts.

Blindness is caused by progressive macular damage, bleeding from new vessels, contraction of fibrous tissue leading to retinal detachment and 'rubeotic glaucoma' (obstruction of the filtration angle in the anterior chamber by new vessels).

Retinopathy can be prevented in both type 1 and type 2 DM by excellent glycaemic control. Once maculopathy or proliferative retinopathy has developed, visual loss can usually be prevented by laser photocoagulation. Vision

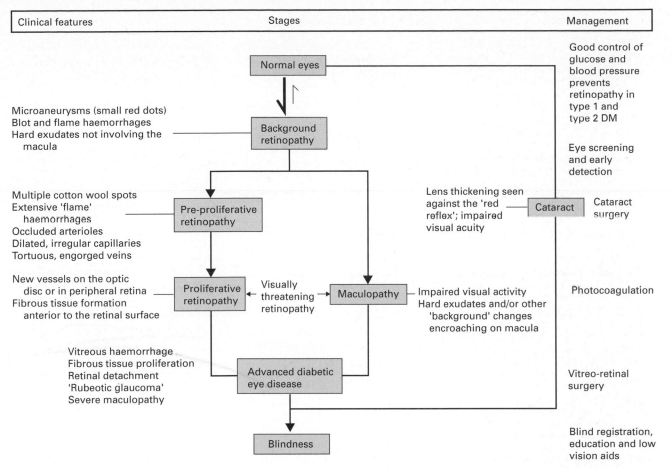

Clinical features	Stages	Management

Normal eyes

Good control of glucose and blood pressure prevents retinopathy in type 1 and type 2 DM

Eye screening and early detection

Microaneurysms (small red dots)
Blot and flame haemorrhages
Hard exudates not involving the macula → **Background retinopathy**

Multiple cotton wool spots
Extensive 'flame' haemorrhages
Occluded arterioles
Dilated, irregular capillaries
Tortuous, engorged veins → **Pre-proliferative retinopathy**

Lens thickening seen against the 'red reflex'; impaired visual acuity — **Cataract** — Cataract surgery

New vessels on the optic disc or in peripheral retina
Fibrous tissue formation anterior to the retinal surface → **Proliferative retinopathy** ← Visually threatening retinopathy → **Maculopathy** — Impaired visual activity Hard exudates and/or other 'background' changes encroaching on macula

Photocoagulation

Vitreous haemorrhage
Fibrous tissue proliferation
Retinal detachment
'Rubeotic glaucoma'
Severe maculopathy → **Advanced diabetic eye disease**

Vitreo-retinal surgery

Blindness

Blind registration, education and low vision aids

Fig. 81 Diabetic eye disease: progression and management.

may be salvaged by vitreo-retinal surgery for advanced proliferative retinopathy. Patients with proliferative retinopathy may have normal visual acuities until their new vessels bleed and patients with maculopathy may not complain of visual loss. If you wait until the patient has symptoms, you will detect diabetic retinopathy too late. It should be detected by regular (at least annual) eye examination consisting of:

- measurement of visual acuity
- retinal examination by an experienced observer through dilated pupils
- retinal photography, the 'gold standard' for retinopathy screening.

Presence of anything more than mild background retinopathy and/or *any* degree of visual impairment are indications for immediate ophthalmic referral.

Cataracts and glaucoma These are not microvascular complications but are mentioned here because they are part of 'diabetic eye disease'.

Cataracts These are more prevalent in diabetes and present at younger ages, but their clinical features are little different from cataracts in non-diabetics. The association is so strong that all patients with cataracts should be screened for diabetes. Treatment is by lens extraction. Many old people go blind needlessly because their diabetic cataracts are not treated.

Glaucoma Various types of glaucoma are more common in diabetes and can cause visual loss.

Nephropathy Diabetes is one of the most common causes of chronic renal failure. Up to one-third of patients with type 1 DM and 10% with type 2 DM develop it. Once nephropathy is established, it is likely to progress to renal failure. Also, it increases the risk of ischaemic heart disease up to 100-fold. The stages are illustrated in Figure 82.

Nephropathy can be prevented by good control. Proteinuria is the first sign and is virtually diagnostic of nephropathy if the patient has retinopathy (signifying microvascular disease elsewhere in the body) and no other cause for proteinuria (such as a urinary tract infection). Occasionally, a renal biopsy is needed to distinguish diabetic nephropathy from other causes of proteinuria. Once nephropathy is established, ACE inhibitors and angiotensin receptor antagonists reduce proteinuria and delay progression. Moderate dietary protein restriction may confer some additional benefit. Many patients with nephropathy die of ischaemic heart disease, so all cardiovascular risk factors (smoking and hyperlipidaemia as well as hypertension) should be treated and aspirin given. Diabetic patients with end-stage renal failure are treated by dialysis or transplantation.

Neuropathy Neuropathy is caused by small vessel disease within the nerves and a direct metabolic effect of

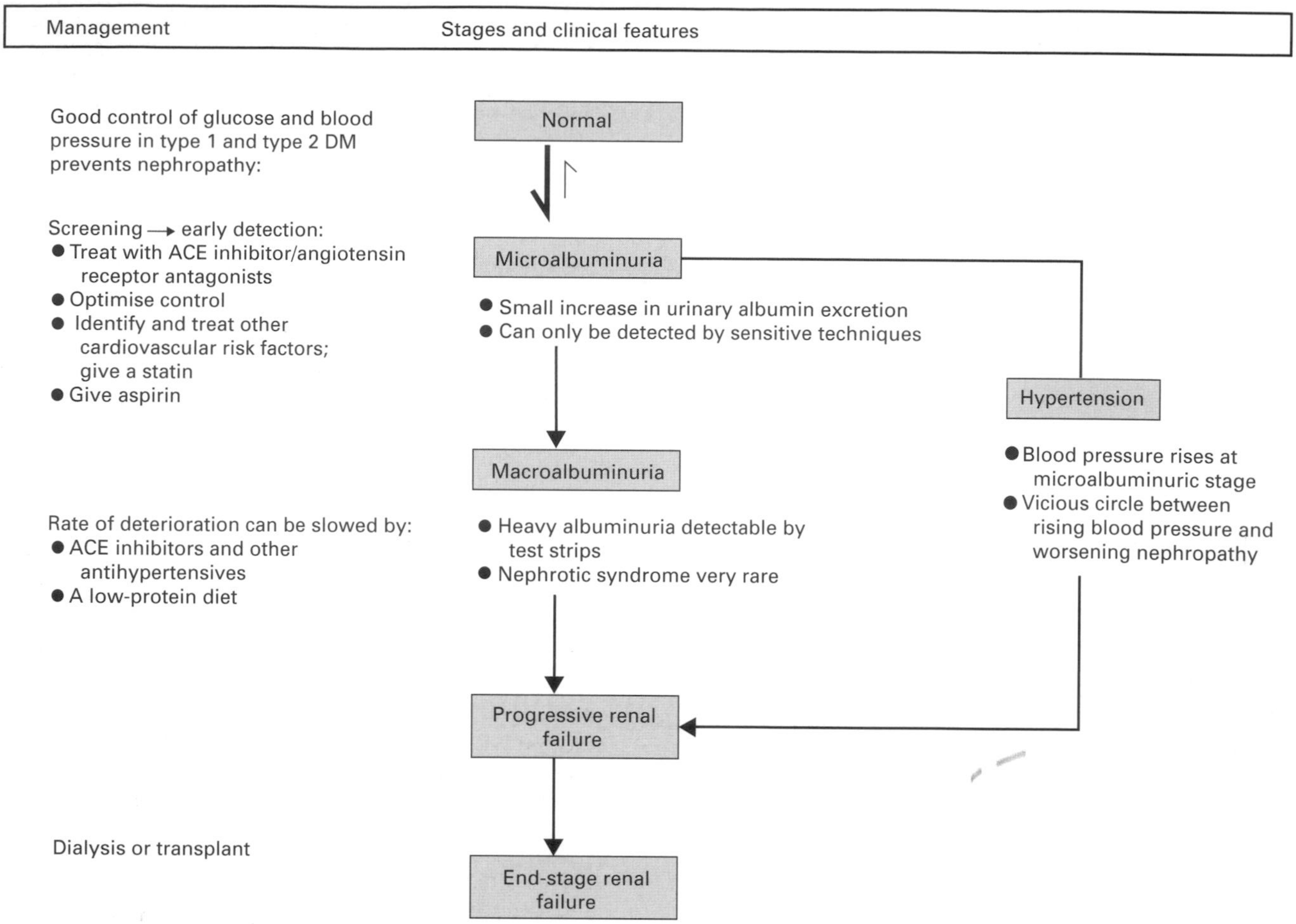

Management	Stages and clinical features

Good control of glucose and blood pressure in type 1 and type 2 DM prevents nephropathy:

```
                              Normal
```

Screening → early detection:
- Treat with ACE inhibitor/angiotensin receptor antagonists
- Optimise control
- Identify and treat other cardiovascular risk factors; give a statin
- Give aspirin

```
                          Microalbuminuria
```

- Small increase in urinary albumin excretion
- Can only be detected by sensitive techniques

```
                                                    Hypertension
```

- Blood pressure rises at microalbuminuric stage
- Vicious circle between rising blood pressure and worsening nephropathy

```
                          Macroalbuminuria
```

Rate of deterioration can be slowed by:
- ACE inhibitors and other antihypertensives
- A low-protein diet

- Heavy albuminuria detectable by test strips
- Nephrotic syndrome very rare

```
                       Progressive renal
                            failure
```

Dialysis or transplant

```
                        End-stage renal
                            failure
```

Fig. 82 Stages of nephropathy; ACE angiotensin-converting enzyme.

diabetes on them. Clinical presentations are summarised in Figure 83 and include:

- motor and sensory polyneuropathy in a 'glove and stocking' distribution, affecting the legs more than the arms
- mononeuritis multiplex, causing sudden dysfunction of peripheral nerves or nerve roots, typically painful and resolving spontaneously over time; typical examples include cranial mononeuropathy causing isolated oculomotor palsies, radiculopathy (diabetic amyotrophy) or peripheral nerve lesions (peroneal mononeuropathy causing foot drop)
- autonomic neuropathy, including excessive upper body sweating, postural hypotension, atonia of the bladder, gastropathy (episodic vomiting), bowel involvement (episodic nocturnal diarrhoea) and erectile impotence.

Diabetic foot disease This may be caused by neuropathy, peripheral vascular disease (see above) or both. Neuropathy is usually painless but can sometimes cause deep 'toothache' or burning superficial leg pain, often worse at night. There is loss of pinprick and vibration sense. Motor involvement causes 'clawing' of the toes and callus formation or ulceration under the metatarsal heads. Every patient should have:

- an annual foot examination
- education about the risks of foot disease and how to prevent it
- access to preventive chiropody
- appropriate footwear.

Ulceration This results from:

- accidental damage owing to insensitivity
- foot deformity caused by motor neuropathy
- autonomic neuropathy, which causes loss of sweating, dry skin and fissuring
- impaired resistance to infection
- disordered neurogenic control of the distal circulation.

Ulceration requires immediate expert attention and, often, hospital admission. It is treated with chiropody, rest, debridement and antibiotics. Amputation is needed for severe infection, osteomyelitis or chronic, disabling ulceration. These problems often result from late presentation or inadequate care. Painful neuropathy is treated with a tricyclic antidepressant (amitriptyline), gabapentin or pregabalin, and capsaicin cream.

Erectile dysfunction

Its prevalence is increased in diabetes, because of neuropathy, vascular disease and psychosocial factors. Once

Stages of nephropathy

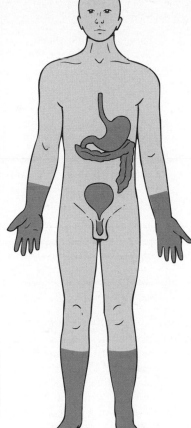

Mononeuropathies:
Cranial: e.g.
3rd nerve palsy
Plexopathies,
radiculopathics
Peripheral nerve lesions

Autonomic neuropathy:
Excessive, inappropriate
upper body sweating
Gastropathy: episodes
of vomiting
Bowel disease:
alternating constipation
and nocturnal diarrhoea
Bladder dysfunction
Erectile dysfunction
Postural hypotension

Peripheral neuropathy:
Sensory loss
Pain
Small muscle wasting
Clawed feet
Foot ulceration

Fig. 83 Clinical presentation of diabetic neuropathy.

hypogonadism (p. 311) is excluded, a phosphodiesterase inhibitor (sildenafil or tadalafil) is the first-line treatment, though these are contraindicated in patients taking nitrates for ischaemic heart disease. Intraurethral or intracaverno-sal alprostadil has been used much less often since phosphodiesterase inhibitors have been available.

Diabetes and pregnancy

Established diabetes is the most common medical disorder complicating pregnancy in the UK, occurring in about 4 of 1000 pregnancies. This is because many patients with type 1 DM are of childbearing age and type 2 DM is becoming increasingly common in young women. In addition, pregnancy can precipitate transient or permanent diabetes (see below).

Complications

Several decades ago, diabetes was usually lethal to the fetus and sometimes to the mother too. With good control *throughout pregnancy*, the outlook is now almost as good in diabetic as non-diabetic women.

Glucose crosses the placenta. Hyperglycaemia is terato-genic in early pregnancy and stimulates excessive fetal insulin secretion as pregnancy progresses. Complications are associated with poor glycaemic control.

In early pregnancy Major congenital malformations are 2–3 times more common than in non-diabetic women and include neural tube and cardiovascular defects; the main risk factor for them is poor glycaemic control *at the time of conception*.

In later pregnancy Complications include:

- intrauterine death, hydramnios and pre-eclampsia
- fetal macrosomia (large-for-dates)
- neonatal complications, including hyaline membrane disease and hypoglycaemia.

Other complications Nephropathy and retinopathy may deteriorate during pregnancy and must be monitored carefully. Women with these complications have a worse fetal outcome.

Management

There are three stages, all requiring good glycaemic control: at conception, during pregnancy and during labour.

At conception All diabetic women who are 'at risk' of pregnancy should be informed of the increased risk of congenital malformations if they become pregnant when poorly controlled. Some hospitals run prepregnancy clinics to counsel, give contraceptive advice, optimise control and advise on the timing of pregnancy.

During pregnancy Blood glucose levels and HbA_{1c} should be kept as close to normal as possible. Insulin doses have to be increased as pregnancy progresses because the hormones of pregnancy cause insulin resistance. Women who are treated with twice-daily insulin outside pregnancy are often treated with four injections per day. Dietary advice is reinforced. Blood glucose needs to be measured several times each day. Tight control increases the risk of hypoglycaemia, so the patient's partner should be instructed in the use of glucagon or oral glucose gel (p. 324). Hypoglycaemia, though unpleasant to the mother, is not known to be harmful to the fetus. Patients are seen every 2–4 weeks, ideally in a joint diabetic/ antenatal clinic. If good control is achieved and pregnancy progresses well, the aim is a spontaneous vaginal delivery at term.

During labour As during surgery (p. 325), blood glucose is kept within normal limits by constant infusion of glucose and insulin. A patient with diet-treated diabetes can be managed without insulin, provided their blood glucose is monitored closely and remains normal.

Type 2 DM is becoming increasingly common in women of reproductive age. Oral hypoglycaemic therapy is con-traindicated in pregnancy, so they are switched from tablets to insulin before any planned pregnancy.

Gestational diabetes

Just as pregnancy hormones increase insulin requirements in women with established diabetes by causing insulin resistance, they can actually precipitate diabetes, usually in the third trimester. This is termed gestational diabetes if it remits after delivery. Type 1 DM and type 2 DM can also first present during pregnancy. Women at risk of gestational diabetes are those with a history of

- large-for-dates babies
- previous gestational diabetes
- diabetes in the family.

Gestational diabetes increases the risk of macrosomia and perinatal complications. It is usually asymptomatic and diagnosed by measuring random blood glucose levels backed up by GTT. It is treated with a sugar-free diet and, in many cases, insulin. Good glycaemic control has been shown to improve the fetal outcome. Within 10 years of delivery, 50% of women with gestational diabetes have developed permanent diabetes, usually type 2 DM.

Metabolic complications

Hypoglycaemia

Hypoglycaemia in diabetes only occurs in patients on insulin or sulphonylureas. Sulphonylurea-induced hypoglycaemia is usually the result of over-aggressive treatment and should, therefore, be an infrequent occurrence. Hypoglycaemia in those using insulin, however, can occur despite the best care because:

- insulin is absorbed erratically from injection sites
- sensitivity to it varies with the patient's emotional state, menstruation, drugs and many other factors
- variations in exercise and eating habits also affect glucose metabolism.

Hypoglycaemia is disruptive to the patient and their family and friends but rarely has lasting sequelae unless it causes injury. The incidence of severe hypoglycaemia can be reduced by good education, regular home blood glucose monitoring and regular eating habits. Patients are particularly vulnerable to it if, as may occur with long-standing diabetes, the early warning symptoms are lost (hypoglycaemia unawareness). This is particularly likely to occur in those with the best glycaemic control because frequent, low blood glucose levels desensitise the hypothalamus to hypoglycaemia. Sulphonylurea-induced hypoglycaemia can be prevented by starting on small doses of drugs and not increasing them too quickly. Long-acting sulphonylureas (glibenclamide, chlorpropamide) should not be used in patients over the age of 70 because they can cause fatal hypoglycaemia.

Whatever the cause, the symptoms of hypoglycaemia include:

- **the adrenergic, anti-insulin response:** sweating, shaking, pallor, anxiety, headache
- **neuroglycopenia:** loss of concentration, personality change, drowsiness and coma.

It is loss of the adrenergic response that causes patients to go into coma without warning.

Except in patients with hypoglycaemia unawareness, the adrenergic symptoms come first. Mild hypoglycaemia is treated by taking extra carbohydrate. All patients on insulin should be encouraged to carry glucose tablets at all times, particularly when driving. Severe hypoglycaemia is best treated with a glucose gel rubbed on to the gums, or intramuscular glucagon, which can be given by relatives, friends or ambulance personnel and acts within 10 minutes. Intravenous glucose is harder to give and damaging to veins. Emergency treatment of hypoglycaemia is described in the box below.

> **Clinical Box:** Emergency treatment: management of hypoglycaemia
>
> - Diagnosed by typical symptoms in a known diabetic
> - May be confirmed by finger-prick testing (plasma glucose <3 mmol/l)
> - If able to cooperate, treat with oral glucose
> - More severe hypoglycaemia can be treated with proprietary glucose solution or glucose gel squirted or smeared in the mouth
> - If comatose or uncooperative, give glucagon 1 mg i.m.
> - If still unresponsive after 15 minutes, give 25 g glucose (50 ml, 50%) i.v.
> - Feed as soon as conscious
> - Consider how to prevent recurrence

Spontaneous hypoglycaemia — not treatment induced — is discussed below.

Severe hyperglycaemia/ketoacidosis

Although often described as two distinct conditions, there are more similarities than differences between diabetic ketoacidosis (DKA) and the diabetic hyperosmolar non-ketotic state (HONKS). Ketoacidosis occurs in patients with type 1 DM or those with type 2 DM who have unusually high levels of anti-insulin hormones caused by intercurrent illness, such as myocardial infarction or severe infection. HONKS develops slowly in type 2 DM patients (with some residual insulin secretion) and is characterised by profound depletion of sodium and water. Keto-acidotic patients are also dehydrated because of an uncontrolled osmotic diuresis. The diagnosis and management of DKA and HONKS are similar and described together here.

Causes are divided roughly equally between:

- newly presenting diabetes
- intercurrent illness (particularly bacterial infection)
- mistakes with insulin doses
- no cause identified, sometimes a result of deliberate manipulation or underdosing.

Clinical presentation Features include vomiting, hyperglycaemic symptoms, unexplained unconsciousness or the symptoms of a precipitating illness. Hyperglycaemic symptoms come on over hours or days, compared with the symptoms of hypoglycaemia, which come on over minutes. There are signs of volume depletion unless the illness is complicated by cardiac or renal failure. If the patient is ketoacidotic, there is deep, sighing respiration and a smell of acetone on the breath.

Management Your priorities are to:

- confirm the diagnosis
- search for and treat any precipitating cause
- assess hydration and give fluid
- give insulin
- monitor the biochemistry (particularly plasma potassium) and clinical signs.

Immediate clinical assessment Take a quick history, examine carefully for signs of a precipitating illness and assess hydration (p. 195). The emergency treatment of DKA/HONKS is given in the box below.

Immediate investigations Measure glucose, urea, electrolytes and bicarbonate; record an ECG, culture blood and urine and arrange a chest X-ray.

Immediate management Set up a drip, give saline and start an insulin infusion or hourly intramuscular insulin injections. If central venous pressure is uncertain, a central venous pressure line may be inserted and fluid replacement adjusted to maintain a pressure of approximately 10 cmH$_2$O.

Fluid therapy Initial resuscitation is with isotonic saline. If the patient is hypernatraemic, some of the fluid should be hypotonic saline. Potassium is given, even if the plasma level is high initially, because insulin lowers it by driving it into cells. Patients with profound acidosis complicated by shock or cardiac dysrhythmias may be given sodium bicarbonate, but this will cause an even greater potassium shift into cells and can precipitate severe hypokalaemia. Once plasma glucose is at or below 15 mmol/l, the infusion is changed to 5% dextrose.

General care Patients who are comatose and cannot protect their airways should have a nasogastric tube to prevent vomiting and aspiration and, if necessary, an airway. Severely ill and/or oliguric patients should have a urinary catheter. Antibiotics are given if there is evidence of infection or the patient is severely ill; such patients should be treated in an intensive care unit.

Clinical Box: Emergency treatment: management of ketoacidosis/hyperosmolar coma

- Put up a drip
- If comatose, protect the airway; consider nasogastric tube and urinary catheter
- Establish the diagnosis: measure glucose, venous bicarbonate and urine or plasma ketones
- Quick history and examination. What has caused it?
- Assess hydration: give saline (see text)
- Start insulin infusion (e.g. soluble insulin 6 units/hour)
- Urgent ECG, chest X-ray, blood and urine cultures
- Give potassium (see text) from the second bottle of fluid onwards
- Observe state of hydration, urine output and conscious level repeatedly
- Monitor plasma glucose and potassium repeatedly
- Infuse 5% dextrose when plasma glucose reaches 15 mmol/l

Monitoring Careful and repeated observation of the conscious level and state of hydration is essential. Plasma glucose and electrolytes should be measured 1–2-hourly initially and less frequently thereafter. Once the i.v. fluid

is changed to dextrose, bedside glucose monitoring can be used to adjust the insulin infusion rate.

Prevention of recurrence Severe hyperglycaemia carries a mortality up to 50% in old people and can be lethal at any age so it is important to search for causes. A common preventable cause of ketoacidosis is to reduce the insulin dose misguidedly during intercurrent illness. All diabetic patients should be advised against this when they are first started on insulin.

Surgery and special situations

In hospital, managing diabetes perioperatively or during intercurrent illness is the skill most commonly required of non-specialists. The subject is too complex to be discussed in detail. However, the general principles are:

- Insulin rather than oral hypoglycaemic drugs should be used to control hyperglycaemia in all acute situations.
- If a patient is fasting or too ill to eat, a constant infusion of insulin (given through a syringe pump or added to isotonic dextrose and potassium) is the best approach.
- Unless the volume of i.v. fluid has to be minimised because of heart failure, it is always best to infuse dextrose simultaneously with insulin to achieve stable glycaemic control; potassium should be added to the infusion.
- Patients who are well enough to eat can usually be managed with subcutaneous insulin given four times daily before meals and before bed; doses need to be reviewed regularly and adjusted according to four-times daily glucose measurements.
- In less acute situations, twice-daily insulin or sulphonylureas can be used.

Spontaneous hypoglycaemia

Hypoglycaemia is defined by the triad of:

- a plasma glucose <2.5 mmol/l *and*
- typical symptoms *and*
- relief of the symptoms by carbohydrate.

Patients who are not diabetic and not on insulin or sulphonylureas may become spontaneously hypoglycaemic through:

- excessive secretion of insulin from the β cells
- other insulin-like hormones (sometimes secreted by mesenchymal tumours)
- antibodies with insulin-like activity.

Hypoglycaemia may also result from:

- excessive sensitivity to insulin, as in hypoadrenalism
- surreptitious abuse of insulin or sulphonylureas.

The classical cause of spontaneous hypoglycaemia is an insulinoma: a rare, usually benign, pancreatic tumour. Table 71 gives a more complete list of causes of spontaneous hypoglycaemia, all of which are rare.

Suspected hypoglycaemia must be confirmed biochemically; blood taken at the time of hypoglycaemia is crucial in determining the cause. Your tasks are to:

Table 71 Causes of spontaneous hypoglycaemia

Cause	Biochemical profile
Excessive insulin	
Insulinoma	High insulin, high C-peptide
Benign	
Malignant	
Sulphonylurea abuse	High insulin, high C-peptide
Insulin abuse	High insulin, low C-peptide
Excessive sensitivity to insulin	Low insulin, low C-peptide
Hormone deficiency	
Hypoadrenalism	
Hypothyroidism	
Hypopituitarism	
Impaired gluconeogenesis	
Liver disease	
Alcoholism	
Other insulin-like factors	Low insulin, low C-peptide
Hormones	
Antibodies with agonist activity	

- recognise hypoglycaemia when it presents with confusion, coma or a fit; a bedside glucose test gives you a working diagnosis
- recognise that it is spontaneous, i.e. the patient is not known to be on treatment for diabetes
- measure blood glucose on a fluoride sample (yellow tube) to confirm the diagnosis of hypoglycaemia
- obtain blood at the time of hypoglycaemia for insulin, C-peptide and other measurements
- treat the hypoglycaemia.

Insulinomas are located by CT scanning, angiography and preoperative ultrasound. Removal of the tumour can be curative. Diazoxide can be used as a medical treatment in patients who are not fit for surgery.

Self-assessment: questions

Any or all of each set of five statements may be true or false. Choose your answers and see the reasoning behind the correct answer on pages 335–336.

Multiple choice questions

1. Epidemiology of diabetes:
   a. Asian people in the UK have a more than twofold increased prevalence of diabetes
   b. The incidence of diabetes peaks at the age of 60
   c. If you are going to develop type 1 DM, you will do so by the age of 30
   d. The prevalence of type 1 and 2 DM is increasing in the UK
   e. There are more insulin-treated people in the UK over the age of 30 than below it

2. In hypoglycaemia:
   a. Insulin-dependent patients may recover from hypoglycaemic coma without treatment
   b. Sweating and shaking are always late symptoms of insulin-induced hypoglycaemia
   c. Insulin-dependent patients may lose their warning symptoms of hypoglycaemia after many years of diabetes
   d. Metformin is responsible for as many cases of hypoglycaemia as sulphonylureas
   e. The symptoms characteristically come on over hours rather than minutes

3. Diabetic retinopathy:
   a. Characteristically causes arterio-venous nipping
   b. Should be referred to an ophthalmologist only if the patient has visual symptoms
   c. Inevitably causes blindness
   d. May cause cotton wool spots (soft exudates)
   e. Is more likely to cause blindness in type 1 than in type 2 DM

4. Instituting intensive insulin treatment aiming to normalise glycated haemoglobin in type 1 diabetes mellitus:
   a. Increases the risk of severe hypoglycaemia
   b. Reduces the incidence of diabetic retinopathy
   c. Reduces the incidence of diabetic nephropathy
   d. Increases mortality
   e. Is more hazardous if the patient does not do regular home blood glucose monitoring

5. Regarding hypertension in diabetes:
   a. It is more prevalent in type 1 than in type 2
   b. Its treatment slows the deterioration of nephropathy in type 1 DM
   c. Thiazide diuretics should not be used in diabetes

   d. Beta-blockers may increase the risk of severe hypoglycaemia in insulin-treated patients
   e. It increases the risk of stroke in diabetes

6. Diabetic pregnancy:
   a. Insulin-dependent women should be advised not to contemplate pregnancy
   b. Diabetes increases the risk of neural tube defects
   c. Poor glycaemic control at conception increases the risk of congenital malformations
   d. There is a less than 10% chance that an episode of ketoacidosis will cause intrauterine death
   e. Sulphonylureas are the treatment of choice for gestational diabetes

7. Which of the following are true?
   a. Most tumours causing overactivity or underactivity of endocrine glands are malignant
   b. Surgery can cure many diseases of endocrine overactivity
   c. Autoimmunity is a common cause of endocrine underactivity
   d. The best way to tell if an endocrine gland is overactive is to stimulate it and test how it responds
   e. Most endocrine diseases can be managed without radionuclide imaging

8. The following are true of hypothyroidism:
   a. Thyroid cancer sometimes (>20% of patients) causes hypothyroidism
   b. It may be caused by pituitary tumours
   c. Most cases are autoimmune
   d. Ultrasound scanning is usually indicated
   e. It predisposes to ischaemic heart disease

9. Thyroid nodules:
   a. Are best investigated by isotope scanning followed by surgery
   b. Are usually (>50%) malignant
   c. May be associated with hyperthyroidism
   d. Can safely be ignored if they present in children
   e. Can be investigated by aspiration cytology

10. In pituitary tumours:
    a. Surgery is the treatment of choice for patients with hyperprolactinaemia
    b. The usual early visual field defect of chiasmal compression is superior temporal hemianopia
    c. Diabetes insipidus suggests hypothalamic dysfunction
    d. Optic atrophy may be an effect of pituitary tumours
    e. Radiotherapy may cause hypopituitarism up to 10 years later

327

11. Acromegaly:
    a. Has no effect on life expectancy
    b. Often causes headaches
    c. Can be cured by surgery
    d. Can be treated medically if surgery is impossible or unsuccessful
    e. Is associated with an increased risk of malignant disease

Single best answer multiple choice questions

For each numbered question, only ONE of the options lettered a–e is correct.

1. A 24 year-old woman with previously good health has lost weight over the preceding 2 months but has noticed no other abnormal symptoms. Her thyroid function tests are:

Total thyroxine	248 (normal 50–150 nmol/l)
Triiodothyronine	5.3 (normal 1.9–2.9 nmol/l)
Thyroid-stimulating hormone	<0.01 (normal 0.02–5.0 mU/l)

   She has moved in with her boyfriend recently and is having unprotected intercourse. You find a diffuse non-tender goiter, which she had not noticed until you point it out to her. She has mild proptosis of the left eye. Which would be the best single first-line treatment?
    a. A beta-blocker
    b. Radioiodine
    c. Subtotal thyroidectomy
    d. Carbimazole
    e. Lugol's iodine

2. A previously healthy 63-year-old man is found at a health check to have a plasma cholesterol of 8.9 mmol/l. His thyroid function tests are:

Total thyroxine	<10 (Normal 50–150 nmol/l)
Thyroid-stimulating hormone	<100 (Normal 0.02–5.0 mU/l)

   Which would be the best single first-line treatment?
    a. Thyroxine
    b. Simvastatin
    c. Atorvastatin
    d. Triiodothyronine
    e. Ezetimibe

3. In a patient with type 1 DM, which of the following statements is true?
    a. Because they have type 1 rather than type 2 DM, their risk of ischaemic heart disease is no higher than if they did not have diabetes at all
    b. The presence of microalbuminuria signifies increased cardiovascular risk
    c. The presence of sensory neuropathy signifies reduced cardiovascular risk
    d. Excellent glycaemic control increases rather than reduces cardiovascular risk
    e. The lifetime risk of renal failure requiring dialysis or a transplant exceeds 50%

4. An alcoholic man in his forties develops diabetes secondary to chronic pancreatitis. Which of the following statements is true?
    a. His risk of diabetic retinopathy is more than twice as high as in a person with primary diabetes
    b. His risk of experiencing hypoglycaemia is half that of a person with primary diabetes
    c. His risk of developing peripheral sensory neuropathy is one-quarter that of a person with primary diabetes
    d. His risk of diabetic retinopathy is approximately the same as a person with primary diabetes of the same duration and severity
    e. He is less likely to respond to a sulphonylurea than a patient with type 2 DM with diabetes of equivalent severity

5. When an obese patient with type 2 DM is no longer controlled on oral hypoglycaemic therapy and has to start insulin, the most suitable regimen would be:
    a. Once-daily long-acting insulin with metformin
    b. Once-daily long-acting insulin with rosiglitazone
    c. An ultrashort-acting analogue insulin four times daily
    d. Three times daily long-acting analogue insulin
    e. Once-daily long-acting analogue and three times daily short-acting analogue insulin

Extended matched questions

EMQ 1

Theme: Treatment options
Options
1. Acarbose
2. Insulin detemir (long-acting)
3. Metformin
4. Glibenclamide
5. Rosiglitazone
6. Gliclazide
7. Twice-daily medium/long-acting insulin
8. Metformin and once-daily long-acting insulin
9. Repaglinide
10. Three times daily ultrashort/short-acting and night-time medium/long-acting insulin

For each of the following outpatients, select the best treatment (more than one may be correct). Each item can be used once, more than once or not at all.

A. An 80-year-old diet-treated woman with a body mass index of 22, who is losing weight and has an HbA$_{1c}$ (glycated haemoglobin) of 11% (ideal <7.0%).

B. A well-motivated patient with type 1 diabetes on twice-daily isophane insulin who is found to be 8 weeks pregnant.

C. A 63-year-old obese man on maximum dose gliclazide, metformin and rosiglitazone with an HbA$_{1c}$ of 11.5%.

D. A 52-year-old obese woman who was diagnosed diabetic 3 months ago and is symptomatically hyperglycaemic on diet alone.

E. A 20-year-old university student newly presenting with type 1 diabetes.

EMQ 2

Theme: Investigation/treatment options
Options
1. Fine needle aspiration cytology
2. A therapy dose of radioiodine
3. Propranolol
4. Thyroid lobectomy
5. ^{131}Iodine uptake measurement
6. Carbimazole
7. Lugol's iodine (potassium iodide)
8. Levothyroxine
9. Propylthiouracil
10. Triiodothyronine (liothyronine sodium)
11. Subtotal thyroidectomy
12. Total thyroidectomy followed by radioiodine therapy

For each of the following patients, select the investigation or treatment listed above that would be the first line of management (more than one may be correct). Each item can be used once, more than once or not at all.

A. A 32-year-old woman with a pituitary tumour, treated with hydrocortisone, who has been found to have a low serum thyroxine and a low thyroid-stimulating hormone.

B. A 60-year-old man with mild hyperthyroidism on no treatment admitted for thyroid surgery in 6 days' time.

C. A 24-week pregnant woman on full-dose propylthiouracil with uncontrolled hyperthyroidism.

D. A 50-year-old woman on atenolol for hypertension who, after an influenza-like illness with a sore throat, has an extremely tender thyroid and is shaky and sweaty.

E. A 35-year-old man who, on palpation, has a solitary nodule in the right lobe of the thyroid and is euthyroid.

EMQ 3

Theme: Cushing's syndrome
Options
1. Normal
2. Alcohol-induced pseudo-Cushing's
3. Obesity
4. Depression
5. Adrenal suppression due to prolonged glucocorticoid treatment
6. Cushingoid state due to glucocorticoid anti-inflammatory therapy
7. Cushingoid state due to excessive glucocorticoid replacement therapy
8. Type 2 diabetes
9. Metabolic syndrome
10. Type 4 hyperlipidaemia
11. Cushing's syndrome of uncertain cause
12. Adrenal Cushing's
13. Cushing's syndrome that could be pituitary or ectopic in origin
14. Pituitary Cushing's
15. Cushing's syndrome due to ectopic adrenocorticotrophic hormone (ACTH) from a carcinoid tumour
16. Cushing's syndrome due to ectopic ACTH from small cell carcinoma of the bronchus

For each of the following situations, select a diagnosis (more than one may be correct). Each item can be used once, more than once or not at all.

A. A long-term asthmatic patient on inhaled steroids who develops thin skin and easy bruising. Her 9 a.m. cortisol is <50 nmol/l.

B. A patient with weight gain, hypertension, hyperglycaemia and osteoporosis who does not drink alcohol, and whose 24-hour urinary free cortisol excretion and 9 a.m. plasma cortisol do not suppress by 50% or more after 48 hours on dexamethasone 2 mg 6-hourly (high-dose dexamethasone).

C. Patient B who, after further investigation, has a high 9 a.m. ACTH level tested on more than one occasion.

D. A patient with proven Cushing's; blood taken from his petrosal sinus soon after being given intravenous corticotrophin-releasing hormone shows a rise in ACTH.

E. A teetotal patient with thirst, polyuria and a fasting blood glucose >7 mmol/l who has a strong family history of ischaemic heart disease, is hypertensive, has combined hyperlipidaemia and has central obesity. Her raised 24-hour urine free cortisol excretion suppresses after dexamethasone 0.5 mg 6-hourly (low-dose dexamethasone).

EMQ 4

Theme: Treatment of diabetes

Options

1. Change to a once-daily long-acting insulin regimen
2. Change to a twice-daily medium/long-acting insulin regimen
3. Change to a four times daily 'basal bolus' regimen
4. Increase the dose of long-acting insulin
5. Reduce the dose of long-acting insulin
6. Reduce the dose of short-acting insulin before breakfast
7. Reduce the dose of short-acting insulin before the midday meal
8. Reduce the dose of short-acting insulin before the evening meal
9. Add metformin to the insulin regimen
10. Reduce the proportion of dietary calories taken as carbohydrate
11. Reduce the proportion of dietary calories taken as protein
12. Have a larger breakfast
13. Have a larger midday meal
14. Have a larger evening meal
15. Have a mid-morning snack
16. Have a mid-afternoon snack
17. Have a snack before bed

For each of the following people with unsatisfactory glycaemic control, select an action (more than one may be correct). Each item can be used once, more than once or not at all.

A. A 24-year-old pregnant woman with type 2 DM on twice-daily medium-acting insulin who has poor glycaemic control and is motivated to improve it.

B. An obese middle-aged woman with type 2 DM on once-daily long-acting insulin who has a high haemoglobin A_{1c} and is gaining weight.

C. A patient with type 1 DM on a basal bolus regimen who takes three meals per day without snacks and is repeatedly having nocturnal hypoglycaemic fits.

D. A patient with type 1 DM on a basal bolus regimen who has an excellent haemoglobin A_{1c} but is trying to lose weight and is prone to mid-morning hypoglycaemia.

Objective structured clinical examination (OSCE) stations

OSCE 1

This is a 5-minute station with a normal volunteer on a couch.

Examiner: Please show me how you would screen this person for diabetic foot disease

Examiner: You find hard skin under the ball of the foot; what significance does that have?

OSCE 2

A 5-minute viva-style OSCE station.

Examiner: You are a general practitioner. A patient with Addison's disease, who normally takes hydrocortisone 10 mg at breakfast, 5 mg at lunch, and 5 mg at teatime, is due to fly off on a business trip in 24 hours. He comes to the emergency surgery because he has a heavy cold and is feeling nauseated and light-headed. His blood pressure is 102/60 mmHg, with 20 mm systolic postural drop. You advise him not to travel but he insists that he will. What actions should you take?

OSCE 3

A 10-minute viva-style OSCE station.

Examiner: A 23-year-old woman with type 1 DM since the age of 10 has attended clinics infrequently. She has recently married and attends clinic at her husband's insistence. Please look at these data and comment on them:

Blood pressure, averaged over three measurements at weekly intervals 162/94 mmHg
24-hour urine protein excretion 2 g
Haemoglobin A_{1c} 11% (recommended <6.5%)
Pregnancy test Negative

a. Please tell me three things you would look for when you examine her.
b. What diagnosis and action should be considered as a result of her urinary protein excretion?
c. Apart from discussing her current treatment regimen, what else should she be counselled about?

OSCE 4

A 10-minute finals OSCE in which the candidate is required to give telephone advice to an actor.

At the other end of the line is the husband of a 48-year-old insulin-dependent patient who has caught a heavy cold. His wife is normally well controlled on a twice-daily medium-acting insulin regimen. It is teatime and she is due for her injection. She is not sure that she can face a cooked meal. Her fingerprick blood glucose level is 9 mmol/l. He requests advice.

Case history questions

Case history 1

A 68-year-old diabetic man who has been on gliclazide and furosemide for 5 years presents breathless, vomiting and collapsed 12 hours after an episode of precordial chest pain. His blood glucose stick test is unrecordably high.

1. Which of the following are true?
   a. Intravenous fluid should be given before the patient is examined or any investigations are done

b. The fact that he has diabetes and has had chest pain makes a diagnosis of myocardial infarction unlikely

c. An ECG should be done soon after presentation

d. If he is able to take tablets, his hyperglycaemia should be controlled with gliclazide

His ECG confirms acute myocardial infarction and his biochemistry shows him to be in ketoacidosis with a serum potassium of 3 mmol/l.

2. Which of the following are true?

a. His relatives should be told that he is critically ill and may not survive

b. Acidosis should be corrected with bicarbonate as a priority

c. He may eventually return to tablet therapy

d. Insulin should not be given without a dextrose infusion

Case history 2

A 78-year-old patient has had type 2 DM for 1 year and is being treated with glipizide. She is very thin and continuing to lose weight. She has become incontinent.

1. Suggest how these problems may be linked and what investigations you would do.

Case history 3

You are an officer in accident and emergency. At 10 p.m., a young man with type 1 DM is brought in by the police having been found wandering and confused. He is pale and sweating and has a finger-prick glucose <2 mmol/l. He is aggressive and agitated.

1. How would you manage him?

Once he has recovered, you want to know the cause.

2. Name four points you would enquire about.

You cannot identify a cause for his attack. His diabetes is normally well controlled. He is fully recovered and ready to go home.

3. Suggest one action that you should take.

Case history 4

A 48-year-old woman presents with irritability, restlessness and poor energy. She has a palpable goitre. Plasma thyroxine is 200 nmol/l (normal up to 150) and triiodothyronine 3.4 nmol/l (normal up to 2.9).

1. What other biochemical abnormality would confirm your suspected diagnosis of hyperthyroidism?

The diagnosis of hyperthyroidism is confirmed biochemically.

2. What investigations would be useful in elucidating the pathology of the condition?

A diagnosis of solitary toxic nodule is made.

3. How might the patient be treated?

Key features questions

1. An 85-year-old woman is admitted to an elderly care ward because she is 'not coping at home'. In the past, she managed to live independently despite quite severe angina, for which she was reluctant to take treatment. Over several years, she has become increasingly withdrawn and confused. Responding to the concern of her family, her general practitioner visited her a week ago and took blood tests which showed:

Total thyroxine	<20 (normal 50–150 nmol/l)
Thyroid-stimulating hormone	>100 (normal 0.02–5.0 mU/l)
Total cholesterol	15 mmol/l
Creatinine	130 μmol/l

Over the few days before admission, she has taken to her bed. She does not complain of chest pain. The nursing staff find it hard to persuade her to take very much by mouth. Her pulse is 48 beats/min, sinus rhythm; temperature is 34.5°C. Her jugular venous pulse cannot be seen, even when she is lying flat. Plasma glucose is 7.6 mmol/l.

Select the most important elements of her immediate management:

a. Passive rewarming

b. A hot bath

c. Intensive nursing care

d. Intravenous 0.9% saline

e. Intravenous 5% dextrose

f. Intravenous 4.2% sodium bicarbonate

g. Gliclazide

h. Insulin

i. Simvastatin

j. Atorvastatin

k. Intravenous hydrocortisone

l. Oral prednisolone

m. Intravenous triiodothyronine

n. Oral levothyroxine

o. Atenolol

p. Amlodipine

q. Ramipril

r. Intravenous nitrate

2. A 72-year-old man had a subtotal thyroidectomy for hyperthyroidism 8 years ago. The histology showed a multinodular goiter. For the first 7 years, blood tests were repeatedly normal. He feels well, but a routine blood test shows the following abnormality:

Total thyroxine	120 (normal 50–150 nmol/l)
Triiodothyronine	3.1 (normal 0.9–2.4 nmol/l)
Thyroid-stimulating hormone	<0.02 (normal 0.02–5.0 mU/l)

The abnormality is confirmed on repeat testing 1 month later. The most appropriate course of action would be to:

a. Explain that minor abnormalities of thyroid function are common in this situation and not necessarily significant
b. Perform a thyrotrophin-releasing hormone test
c. Refer for repeat thyroid surgery
d. Repeat in 3 months
e. Recommend carbimazole therapy

3. A 35-year-old diabetic man complains of erectile dysfunction. His serum testosterone, luteinising hormone and follicle-stimulating hormone are low. His serum prolactin is very high.

3.1 The most likely explanation for this scenario is that:
   a. He has typical diabetic erectile dysfunction
   b. Diabetes has caused hypothalamic failure
   c. Diabetes has caused hypopituitarism
   d. He has coincidental hypopituitarism
   e. His primary disorder is hyperprolactinaemia

3.2 The most appropriate immediate course of action would be to:
   a. Prescribe testosterone
   b. Request a pituitary MR scan
   c. Prescribe cabergoline
   d. Perform a luteinising hormone-releasing hormone (gonadotrophin-releasing hormone) test
   e. Take a detailed drug history

4. You are flattered that a well-known middle-aged male TV chat show host comes to see you as a patient at your very exclusive and well-resourced private hospital. He looks 'cuddly' on the screen, but in real life he is really quite fat. However, that is not his only problem. He has mild exertional angina, for which a cardiologist plans to stent him. He smokes five cigars per day and drinks 21 units of alcohol per week. He has a family history of diabetes and ischaemic heart disease, and his plasma glucose 2 hours after an oral 75 g glucose load is 12.3 mmol/l. His fasting triglyceride level is 4 mmol/l though his plasma cholesterol is only 4.5 mmol/l. His blood pressure is 135/94 mmHg. He has normal renal function and no proteinuria. He is on no treatment at all.

He is rather taken aback by the number of health problems that have been identified. Which of the following treatments would it be appropriate to recommend over his first month under your care?

a. Acarbose
b. Metformin
c. Gliclazide
d. Rosiglitazone
e. Insulin
f. High complex carbohydrate, low-fat diet
g. Behaviour change therapy from a nutritionist
h. Orlistat
i. Sibutramine
j. Bariatric surgery
k. Written information about the health risks of smoking
l. Nicotine replacement therapy
m. A consultation with a smoking cessation adviser
n. Written information about the health effects of drinking alcohol
o. Statin therapy
p. Bendroflumethiazide
q. Furosemide
r. Lisinopril
s. Atenolol
t. Amlodipine

5. An able-bodied 80-year-old lady who has been admitted with pneumonia is nearly ready to go home. In accident and emergency, her random blood glucose was 16 mmol/l. She was started on a variable-rate intravenous insulin infusion, which was stopped when she became hypoglycaemic. Now, 5 days later, her pre-meal blood tests are running at 6 mmol/l. She has not had insulin for 5 days, and is not on an oral hypoglycaemic.

What action would you take at the time of discharge with regard to her glycaemic control?

a. Recommend a sugar-free diet
b. Recommend a low-carbohydrate diet
c. Start metformin
d. Start gliclazide
e. Start rosiglitazone
f. Start insulin
g. Start home urine testing
h. Start finger-prick blood glucose testing
i. Measure her haemoglobin A_{1c}
j. Arrange review by the primary care team within 4 weeks
k. Arrange a glucose tolerance test 1 month after discharge
l. Discharge her without follow-up

Data interpretation questions

1. In an oral glucose tolerance test with 75 g glucose, the venous whole blood glucose values for three patients were as shown in Table 72. How would you interpret the results?

Table 72 Venous whole blood glucose values (mmol/l)

	Fasting	2 hours after glucose
Patient A	5	8
Patient B	8	12
Patient C	3	4

2. A 45-year-old who has had type 1 DM for 20 years presents with swollen hands and feet. Biochemical results are as shown below. How do you interpret these findings?

Plasma urea 24 mmol/l

Creatinine 250 mmol/l

Albumin 24 g/l

24-hour urine protein excretion 15 g

3. A 60-year-old man with type 2 DM of 5 years' duration is taking no regular treatment and has the following results:

HbA_{1c} 9.5% (normal up to 6.2%)

Total cholesterol 6 mmol/l (Table 2, p. 6)

Triglycerides 6 mmol/l

a. Comment on the results.

b. What other information would help to interpret these results?

c. How would you treat him?

4. A young woman with no history of diabetes is brought to accident and emergency, having had a fit. Her previous health has been good but she has gained weight over the last year. Her finger-prick glucose is <2 mmol/l. Laboratory glucose is 1.1 mmol/l. Her serum insulin and C-peptide are both found to be high. What is the differential diagnosis?

5. Interpret the three sets of thyroid function test results given in Table 73.

6. In a water deprivation test, a patient is not allowed to drink for 8 hours and the hourly urine volume, plasma and urine osmolalities are measured hourly. Intramuscular desmopressin (ADH analogue) is then given and the measurements are continued for 2 hours more, during which time the patient is allowed to drink. Interpret the three sets of results given in Table 74.

Table 73 Thyroid function test for three patients

	Total thyroxine (nmol/l)	Total triiodothyronine (nmol/l)	Thyroid-stimulating hormone (mU/l)
Patient A	48	–	2.4
Patient B	210	5.3	<0.1
Patient C	30	–	>50
Normal range	50–150	1.9–2.9	0.5–5.0

Table 74 The results of a water deprivation test

	Measurement	After 8 hours of water deprivation	2 hours after desmopressin
Expected results	Serum osmolality (mosmol/kg)	≤295	≤295
	Urine osmolality (mosmol/kg)	>750	>750
Patient A	Serum osmolality (mosmol/kg)	302	298
	Urine osmolality (mosmol/kg)	180	800
	1-hour urine volume (ml)	100	0
Patient B	Serum osmolality (mosmol/kg)	294	293
	Urine osmolality (mosmol/kg)	820	900
	1-hour urine volume (ml)	15	10
Patient C	Serum osmolality (mosmol/kg)	298	300
	Urine osmolality (mosmol/kg)	200	200
	1-hour urine volume (ml)	80	85

Picture questions

1. Figure 84 is the coronal magnetic resonance image of the pituitary region in a young woman complaining of amenorrhoea, infertility and galactorrhoea. The pituitary gland is in the midline immediately above the sphenoid sinus, which shows black. To the left of the midline is an oval lesion.

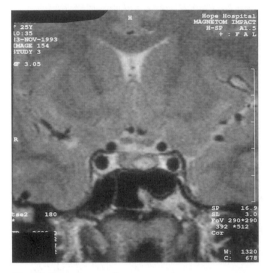

Fig. 84 Coronal magnetic resonance image.

    a. What is this lesion likely to be?

    b. How would you confirm the diagnosis?

    c. How would you treat her?

2. A 65-year-old cigarette smoker is admitted to hospital so weak that he cannot stand. He complains of cough and a painful right upper arm. He has lost 2 stone in weight over the last 3 months. He is pigmented. His serum potassium is 1.8 mmol/l.

    a. Figure 85A shows his thoracic computed tomographic (CT) scan. What abnormality does it show?

    b. Figure 85B shows his right humerus. Describe the abnormality shown.

    c. Suggest a diagnosis and give your reasons.

    d. Assuming the diagnosis was confirmed, how would you treat him?

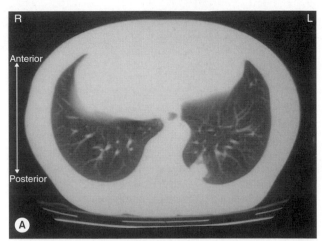

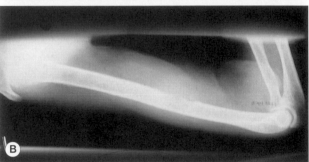

Fig. 85 Images for picture question 2. **A** CT scan of the thorax. **B** Radiograph of the right humerus.

3. Figure 86 is a radiograph of the foot of a 58-year-old man with type 2 diabetes mellitus. He has a painless discharging ulcer under the forefoot.

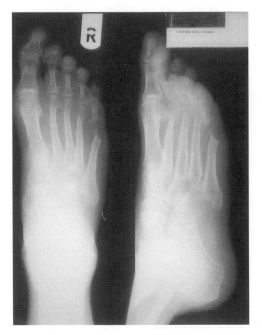

Fig. 86 Radiograph of a man with type 2 diabetes mellitus.

    a. What abnormality is shown?

    b. What is the likely diagnosis?

    c. How should it be treated?

Self-assessment: answers

Multiple choice answers

1. a. **True.**
   b. **False.** It increases progressively with age and there is no peak.
   c. **False.** Type 1 can present at any age.
   d. **True.** Both are becoming more prevalent.
   e. **True.** Many patients with type 2 (which is much commoner than type 1) need insulin and type 1 itself may present after the age of 30. Almost all of those who present before age 30 survive well into middle age.

2. a. **True.** The anti-insulin hormones can bring the patient round and the insulin which caused the coma can 'wear off'.
   b. **False.** They are early warning symptoms for many patients.
   c. **True.** About 50% of patients who have had type 1 DM for 20 years or more develop 'hypoglycaemia unawareness'.
   d. **False.** Metformin does not cause hypoglycaemia.
   e. **False.** Hypoglycaemic symptoms typically come on over minutes rather than hours.

3. a. **False.** This is a sign of hypertensive retinopathy.
   b. **False.** Ophthalmic referral for laser photocoagulation is often made in asymptomatic patients with visually threatening retinopathy seen on ophthalmoscopy but without symptoms.
   c. **False.** Provided it is detected early, even visually threatening retinopathy should not cause blindness.
   d. **True.** These may also occur in hypertension and other ischaemic retinopathies.
   e. **False.** It may cause visual loss in patients with all types of diabetes. It is wrong to think of type 2 DM as 'mild diabetes'; its complications can be anything but 'mild'.

4. a. **True.**
   b. **True.**
   c. **True.**
   d. **False.**
   e. **True.**

5. a. **False.** Hypertension is associated with type 2 more strongly than with type 1 DM.
   b. **True.**
   c. **False.** There is no absolute contraindication to their use, particularly in type 1 and if used in low dose.
   d. **True.** This is true primarily of non-cardioselective beta-blockers.
   e. **True.**

6. a. **False.** Type 1 DM is rarely a contraindication to pregnancy.
   b. **True.** Neural tube defects are 2–3 times more common.
   c. **True.** Hyperglycaemia is teratogenic in early pregnancy; major congenital malformations are 2–3 times more common.
   d. **False.** Ketoacidosis carries a high risk of intrauterine death.
   e. **False.** If the patient is significantly hyperglycaemic on a sugar-free diet, insulin is given.

7. a. **False.** Most are benign.
   b. **True.** Apart from hyperthyroidism, which is usually treated with drugs or radioiodine, and hyperprolactinaemia, which is treated with dopaminergic agonists, surgery is the most likely treatment to cure endocrine overactivity.
   c. **True.**
   d. **False.** Suppression tests are used to confirm overactivity.
   e. **True.** Radionuclide scans are used occasionally to locate elusive tumours or to demonstrate overactivity but are less often useful than ultrasound, MR or CT.

8. a. **False.** Thyroid cancer would have to destroy the entire gland to cause hypothyroidism and this rarely occurs.
   b. **True.** Pituitary tumours cause secondary hypothyroidism.
   c. **True.**
   d. **False.** Imaging is rarely required in hypothyroidism.
   e. **True.** Hypothyroidism causes hypercholesterolaemia, which predisposes to ischaemic heart disease.

9. a. **False.** Isotope scans are often unhelpful. Fine needle aspiration cytology and isotope scanning usually make surgery unnecessary.
   b. **False.** 10% or fewer are malignant.
   c. **True.** 'Toxic nodular goitre'.
   d. **False.** Nodules in children should be taken seriously as they may be malignant.
   e. **True.**

10. a. **False.** Hyperprolactinaemia, even if the patient has a large pituitary tumour, is best treated medically.
    b. **True.**
    c. **True.** Pituitary tumours usually do not cause diabetes insipidus unless there is hypothalamic involvement or the patient has had surgery.

d. **True.** Optic atrophy is a late effect of optic nerve compression.

e. **True.** Radiotherapy is slow-acting and can have an effect decades later.

11. a. **False.** Acromegaly reduces life expectancy significantly.

b. **True.** Headache is common and hard to treat effectively.

c. **True.** The cure rate for smaller tumours (≤1 cm) is approximately 80%.

d. **True.** Dopaminergic agonists, octreotide and pegvisomant are effective.

e. **True.** Also cardiorespiratory disease.

Single best answer multiple choice answers

1. **d is correct.** You would only use a beta-blocker as sole treatment if she had mild short-lived hyperthyroidism, as in subacute thyroiditis. The fact that her goitre is asymptomatic and the length of history make subacute thyroiditis very unlikely. Radioiodine is contraindicated both by her eye disease and the possibility of pregnancy. Surgery could be considered as primary treatment, but she would have to be pretreated with iodine. Iodine alone would only control her hyperthyroidism in the very short term. The presence of eye disease, a diffuse goitre and hyperthyroidism makes Graves' disease the most likely diagnosis. Given all the other circumstances, treatment with an antithyroid drug is the best answer.

2. **a is correct.** This is hypercholesterolaemia secondary to hypothyroidism. The treatment is to correct the primary cause. Thyroxine therapy is likely to improve his wellbeing (even if he is unaware there is anything wrong with him). It will also bring down his plasma cholesterol. If it does not normalise, that could be an argument for statin treatment, but it would not be first-line.

3. **b is correct.** Diabetes, whatever the type, increases cardiovascular risk, and the presence of any complication signifies further increased cardiovascular risk. Excellent glycaemic control slightly reduces cardiovascular risk. The lifetime risk of a patient with type 1 DM requiring renal replacement treatment is much lower than 50%.

4. **d is correct.** In the respects covered by this question, secondary diabetes behaves very similarly to primary diabetes. Its severity (i.e. how hyperglycaemic patients become and whether or not they are prone to ketosis) depends on how much pancreatic damage they have sustained. They are no more prone to retinopathy. Their risk of hypoglycaemia is similar, unless they continue to abuse alcohol, in which case it will be higher. From the diabetes viewpoint, their risk of sensory neuropathy is no different, through alcohol abuse itself causes sensory neuropathy. There is no reason

why they should respond to a sulphonylurea better or worse than a patient with primary diabetes.

5. **a is correct.** The combination of insulin and glitazone is relatively contraindicated because it can cause heart failure. Any patient given four times daily ultrashort-acting analogue insulin will have very unstable control because the insulin effect will wear off between doses. Long-acting analogue insulin has such as long half-life that it is unnecessary (and burdensome to the patient) to give it three times daily. A four times daily 'basal bolus' regimen would be appropriate for a motivated patient with type 1 DM, but unlikely to achieve better glycaemic control than long-acting insulin with metformin, more likely to cause hypoglycaemia and more likely to cause weight gain.

Extended matched answers

EMQ 1

A. **6.** She is insulin-deficient and needs a treatment that will boost insulin supply, e.g. gliclazide. Insulin would be an alternative, though it is usual to try a sulphonylurea first. Glibenclamide is contraindicated by her age, and metformin and rosiglitazone are not first-line therapy in a thin person.

B. **10.** She is likely to comply with a demanding regimen; most diabetologists would use insulin four times daily.

C. **8.** He plainly needs insulin. Clinical trials have shown the combination of metformin and night-time insulin to achieve at least as good glycaemic control with less weight gain and hypoglycaemia than twice-daily insulin.

D. **3.** Metformin is the first-line treatment in obese type 2 diabetes uncontrolled by diet alone. Glitazones are currently recommended as second-line treatment in obese patients.

E. **7 or 10.** Depending on the patient's psychological state and level of motivation it would be appropriate to start them an either a twice-daily or four times daily regimen.

EMQ 2

A. **8.** She has (secondary) hypothyroidism and should be treated with levothyroxine.

B. **7.** Potassium iodide will both reduce the vascularity of the gland and control his hyperthyroidism; some surgeons have advocated using just a beta-blocker in preparation for surgery, so that would also be an acceptable answer.

C. **11.** Carbimazole will be no better, and radioiodine cannot be given in pregnancy so the treatment is subtotal thyroidectomy.

D. **5.** This is classical subacute thyroiditis. She is already taking atenolol; beta-blockers are the only treatment of any value in the hyperthyroid phase of thyroiditis, so the correct answer is a measurement of ^{131}I uptake. Absent uptake will confirm the diagnosis. The patient may need a short course of steroid therapy.

E. **1.** Fine needle aspiration cytology is the first-line investigation; in some centres, it is done under ultrasound control.

EMQ 3

A. **5 and 6.** The thin skin and easy bruising tell you she is Cushingoid. The low 9 a.m. cortisol level tells you she has adrenal suppression; the inhaled glucocorticoid is not detected by the cortisol assay, so she appears to have a low level of glucocorticoid in her blood, but actually she has a high level. Her inhaled glucocorticoid is anti-inflammatory, not replacement therapy.

B. **11** is the only safe option; the patient certainly seems to have Cushing's, but it could be adrenal, pituitary or ectopic.

C. **13.** The patient has 'high ACTH Cushing's', which could be pituitary or ectopic, but we do not yet have sufficient information to decide which.

D. **14.** This is the definitive evidence of Cushing's disease. The rise in ACTH shows that the feedback loop is still intact, which is characteristic of Cushing's disease.

E. **3, 8 and 9** are all true, though the examiner might only give full marks for metabolic syndrome, because that is clearly what this patient has. The raised basal 24-hour urine free cortisol is due to obesity, as shown by the fact that it suppresses after low-dose dexamethasone.

EMQ 4

A. **3.** She requires 'intensive therapy', which means a basal bolus regimen. You have not been given any information that would lead you to change her diet or alter the dose.

B. **9.** Whilst diet might help, none of the dietary options that you have been offered is appropriate. Metformin, on the other hand, is proven effective in this situation.

C. **5 and 17.** You want to take quite urgent action to prevent further fits. A patient who does not have a snack before bed has a very long gap during which long-acting insulin can make them hypoglycaemic. You can improve the situation by recommending a pre-bed snack; it would be quite appropriate to reduce the dose of long-acting insulin as well, irrespective of what time of the day it was taken.

D. **6.** The choice is between increasing the size of the patient's breakfast, recommending a mid-morning snack, or reducing the dose of insulin at breakfast. Reducing the insulin dose is the only one of those that would not counteract her efforts to lose weight. Depending on the patient's blood glucose profile, 5 might also be appropriate.

Responses to OSCE stations

OSCE 1

Your examination should exclude active foot ulceration and identify neuropathy, peripheral vascular disease and any other risk factors for it. The way the instruction has been phrased suggests you are not expected to ask about symptoms, though you may wish to check that with the examiner.

Screening for diabetic foot disease

- **Look at the foot**, including under the heel and between the toes, for ulceration or skin changes such as hairlessness, injury or signs of previous surgery.
- **Examine for neuropathy**
  - Loss of vibration sense and ankle jerks is sensitive for neuropathy, though it ceases to be specific in patients over 70.
  - Loss of the ability to feel a 10 g nylon monofilament or pain to a sterile point is specific for neuropathy.
  - Temperature and light touch sensation are lost variably in patients with neuropathy.
- **Examine for peripheral vascular disease.** Feel the dorsalis pedis, posterior tibial and popliteal pulses in both feet; record them as present or absent ('weak' is too subjective to be reliable); loss of both pulses in a foot or a more proximal pulse is diagnostic of peripheral vascular disease.

Significance of hard skin

- *Cause*: must be assumed to be from excessive pressure, caused by imbalance of the foot muscles and/or sensory loss.
- *Consequences*: can lead to pressure ulceration, because the hard skin acts like a pebble under the insensitive foot.
- *Treatment*: needs podiatric care to pare off the hard skin, and probably special shoes to relieve the pressure point; should be kept under podiatric follow-up.

OSCE 2

He is probably in early Addisonian crisis. He needs not just his normal dose of hydrocortisone but an increased dose, and yet his nausea may prevent him from taking any by mouth. You should give him hydrocortisone 50–100 mg parenterally (either intravenously or intramuscularly) at once. An overnight hospital admission may render him fit enough to travel. In hospital, parenteral hydrocortisone should be continued, and he should be given intravenous 0.9% saline to correct his probable hypovolaemia. Assuming his nausea improves, he should double his oral hydrocortisone to 20 mg at breakfast, 10 mg at lunch, and 10 mg at teatime until he is fully recovered. He should be given an ampoule of parenteral hydrocortisone and shown how to self-inject. He should be advised to report to a hospital immediately if his symptoms recur. He should carry a steroid card in case he is admitted to hospital in a state of collapse, or is not able to communicate his problem to non-English-speaking staff. It is noteworthy that he is not taking mineralocorticoid replacement. Whilst about 50%

of Addisonian patients do not need mineralocorticoid, the decision should be reviewed since he has become Addisonian. A raised plasma renin, when he has recovered, would indicate that he is mineralocorticoid-deficient.

OSCE 3

a. The following should form part of the examination:
- Examine fundi through dilated pupils.
- Test for peripheral neuropathy (light touch, pinprick, cold metal and vibration sense).
- Test for peripheral vascular disease.
- Examine for foot ulceration.
- Examine for left ventricular hypertrophy/failure.

b. She probably has diabetic nephropathy as the cause of her proteinuria; the diagnosis is even more likely if she also has severe retinopathy. She needs antihypertensive therapy. An ACE inhibitor or angiotensin receptor antagonist is most beneficial to the kidneys but she should not have an ACE inhibitor if she is contemplating pregnancy.

c. She should be counselled about pregnancy including:
- the risks to the fetus if she becomes pregnant while poorly controlled
- the risk that her diabetic nephropathy will worsen during pregnancy
- the increased fetal loss in diabetic women with nephropathy
- the dangers of fetal malformations associated with ACE inhibitors.

OSCE 4

She should:

- test her urine for ketones
- take her normal evening insulin dose; *she should not reduce it*
- take whatever carbohydrate calories she can up to her normal
  amount as milk, biscuits or glucose tablets/drink
- test her urine for ketones and blood glucose before bed
- ensure that she is admitted directly to hospital if she starts vomiting or develops uncontrolled hyperglycaemia or ketosis.

It is very tempting to suggest that she should reduce or omit her insulin because she and her husband may be afraid that she will become hypoglycaemic. However, intercurrent illness will make her insensitive to insulin, so there is a far greater risk of hyperglycaemia/ketosis than of hypoglycaemia, and hypoglycaemia is a far less serious complication. Advising her to reduce or omit her insulin would be a dangerously incorrect answer.

Case history answers

Case history 1

1. a. **False.** Since it sounds as though he has had a myocardial infarct; he may be in heart failure, in which case i.v. fluid would be contraindicated. Assessment of his fluid status must be done first.

   b. **False.** Diabetes may cause painless myocardial infarction but painful infarction is more common.

   c. **True.** An ECG is needed urgently.

   d. **False.** Tablet treatment of diabetes has no place in the management of acutely ill patients.

2. a. **True.** Diabetic ketoacidosis at his age has a mortality of >25% and myocardial infarction has an equally high mortality in diabetic patients. The two together are a serious combination.

   b. **False.** There is a high risk of heart failure and sodium-containing fluids must be given cautiously. In addition, correcting his acidosis with bicarbonate will further lower serum potassium (by shifting potassium into cells) and could cause cardiac arrest.

   c. **True.** Diabetic ketoacidosis can be precipitated by intercurrent illness, and patients can sometimes return to tablets when they have recovered.

   d. **False.** Insulin is given without a glucose infusion during the initial management of diabetic ketoacidosis. If there is a risk of fluid overload (as in a patient with acute myocardial infarction), it may be safer to give insulin without infusing glucose even when hyperglycaemia has been controlled, although more stable control is achieved if both are infused together.

Case history 2

1. She may have:
- type 1 or insulin-requiring type 2 diabetes which has not been recognised and is causing weight loss and osmotic diuresis
- carcinoma of the pancreas causing diabetes and weight loss
- urinary tract infection, possibly causing hyperglycaemia
- thyrotoxicosis, which exacerbates diabetes and causes weight loss.

Other possibilities include dementia, depression or other psychiatric or social problems. Other organic diseases include tuberculosis, occult neoplasia, renal failure, hypercalcaemia. Investigations that could be done include:

- fasting or random glucose
- HbA_{1c}
- testing urine for ketones
- thyroid function tests
- renal, hepatic function and calcium
- chest X-ray
- urine culture
- abdominal ultrasound scan.

Case history 3

1. Try to persuade him to take carbohydrate, e.g. glucose tablets or drink. If this is unsuccessful, he should be given an oral glucose gel or intramuscular glucagon. Avoid i.v. 50% dextrose if possible because it is difficult to give to an agitated patient and may permanently thrombose veins.

2. Enquire about:
   - whether he has eaten normally
   - whether he has drunk alcohol (note the time of his admission)
   - whether he has taken different insulin doses from normal
   - his physical activity before the hypoglycaemic attack
   - previous history of hypoglycaemia
   - whether he does or does not experience hypoglycaemic warning symptoms.

3. Notify his normal carers, e.g. general practitioner or diabetes centre. On the evidence given here, there is no reason to adjust his insulin doses and you should feel no obligation to do so. A hypoglycaemic attack may be a 'one-off'.

Case history 4

1. Serum thyroid-stimulating hormone. This is likely to be suppressed.

2. If the goitre is diffuse, no other investigation is indicated. If it seems clinically to be nodular, isotope scanning may be of value to identify a solitary toxic nodule.

3. First, her thyrotoxicosis should be controlled with antithyroid drugs. Surgical removal of the toxic nodule will be curative. Alternatively the patient may be treated with radioiodine.

Key features answers

1. **a, c, d and k are correct.** She has very severe hypothyroidism against a background of ischaemic heart disease. Indeed, she is close to or actually in myxoedema coma. Although she does not have symptoms of angina, her reduced metabolism may be masking it. She needs passive rewarming and intensive nursing care. Active rewarming could cause complete circulatory collapse and death. She is hypovolaemic and in renal failure, so she needs intravenous saline. Mild hypoglycaemia is common in hypothermia; it can simply be monitored. Her severe hypercholesterolaemia is caused by hypothyroidism and will improve spontaneously. She is not well enough to be given non-essential tablets. Steroid therapy is appropriate for suspected myxoedema coma. It is too important to be given by mouth. She is so critically ill that she needs to be resuscitated before considering thyroid hormone therapy. Given her precarious cardiovascular state, intravenous triiodothyronine could be hazardous. It would not

be wrong to give her oral levothyroxine, but it is not an immediate priority.

2. **e is correct.** The biochemical picture is of T3 toxicosis. Whilst the test is not severely abnormal, it is significantly abnormal, and the abnormality has emerged after a period of normality and been confirmed on repeat testing. If the thyrotoxicosis is left untreated, he may develop atrial fibrillation or osteoporosis, or become symptomatic. Option d is not strictly wrong, but the situation is unlikely to be any better 3 months later. Whilst b might have been true some years ago, modern-day TSH assays are so sensitive and specific that it is not necessary. Repeat surgery would not be the treatment of choice in this situation. The alternatives are radioiodine or antithyroid drug therapy. Since radioiodine therapy is not offered, e would be the most appropriate action; however, it is likely he will be referred for radioiodine when his hyperthyroidism is controlled.

3. 3.1. **e is correct.** In the patient with erectile dysfunction due to diabetes, no endocrine abnormality would be expected. So, only d or e should be considered. It is possible that the has coincidental hypopituitarism but hyperprolactinaemia could be the primary disorder, and so that is the correct answer.

   3.2. **e is correct.** Secondary hyperprolactinaemia should always be excluded before any further action. In this case, it turns out that the patient is taking high-dose metoclopramide for vomiting caused by diabetic autonomic neuropathy. Metoclopramide causes hyperprolactinaemia. Before doing any of the other things listed, it would be sensible to see if he could be taken off metoclopramide, and whether his problem improved.

4. **b, f, g, o, p and t are correct.** It would be reasonable, depending on his preference, to prescribe metformin early, or to start with a diet and see how his blood glucose settled. Successful dietary treatment will help his diabetes, blood pressure, angina and hypertriglyceridaemia. Since he is apparently wealthy and your clinic is well resourced, intensive nutritional therapy might be very beneficial. Statin therapy is indicated, irrespective of his 'normal' plasma cholesterol, because he has ischaemic heart disease. Because his cardiovascular risk is so high, antihypertensive treatment is indicated. Following the A, B, C, D approach, a thiazide diuretic or calcium antagonist would be a reasonable first-line antihypertensive.

5. **a, g or h, j and k are correct.** It may be that the hyperglycaemia was induced by her pneumonia and that she is not truly diabetic. However, diabetes is common in old people and the pneumonia may have brought to light an important diagnosis. The bedside tests before discharge have not given you a firm answer one way or the other. It is advisable for people with diabetes to reduce the amount of sugar they eat, but starchy and high-fibre foods are

entirely appropriate, so b is wrong. There is no indication to start treatment. It would be sensible for her to learn to test her diabetes; blood testing is not strictly incorrect, but is perhaps unnecessarily complex in this situation. It would be entirely appropriate for her to be reviewed by the primary care team. If she is willing and local resources permit, a glucose tolerance test when she is fully over the illness will give a more definitive diagnosis.

Data interpretation answers

1. Patient A. Impaired glucose tolerance.

   Patient B. Diabetes

   Patient C. Normal.

2. The patient has nephrotic syndrome (oedema, albuminuria and hypoalbuminaemia) and renal failure (raised urea and creatinine). Diabetic nephropathy is the likely cause but there is insufficient information here to make that diagnosis.

3. a. Glycaemic control is poor and he is hypertriglyceridaemic, probably because of his poor control but possibly also because of obesity and/or alcohol excess.

   b. His body mass index.

   c. His hyperglycaemia and hypertriglyceridaemia need to be controlled by diet and lipid-lowering (statin) therapy.

4. She is not known to be diabetic; she has 'hyperinsulinaemic hypoglycaemia'. The insulin could be endogenous (from her own pancreas) or injected. C-peptide is released when endogenous proinsulin is processed to insulin so the fact that it is high tells you that her insulin excess is endogenous. She probably has an insulinoma. People with insulinomas often gain weight as she has done. Sulphonylurea abuse causes oversecretion of insulin so that should also be considered.

5. Patient A. Secondary hypothyroidism. Serum TSH should rise as thyroxine falls. If it does not, the patient should be investigated for hypothalamic or pituitary disease.

   Patient B. Thyrotoxicosis.
   Patient C. Primary hypothyroidism, with an appropriate rise in TSH.

6. Patient A. The patient has a high plasma osmolality and continues to pass dilute urine; this is diagnostic of diabetes insipidus. There is a good response to desmopressin so the diagnosis is cranial diabetes insipidus.

Patient B. Normal.

Patient C. This patient differs from patient A because there is no response to desmopressin; the diagnosis is nephrogenic diabetes insipidus.

Picture answers

1. a. A prolactin-secreting pituitary tumour.

   b. Measure serum prolactin; there is no need to do a stimulation or suppression test. A raised serum prolactin with this history and radiological appearance would confirm the diagnosis of prolactinoma.

   c. She should be treated medically, with cabergoline, quinagolide or bromocriptine. The tumour does not extend outside the pituitary fossa and is not causing mass effects. Even if it were, the treatment would be medical rather than surgical in the first instance because dopaminergic agonists can relieve symptoms, restore fertility and shrink even large tumours.

2. a. Figure 85A is of a small mass lesion lying in the posterior left lower lobe (magnified images of the mediastinum after contrast).

   b. There is a lucency on the medial side of the humerus. This lytic lesion extends through the cortex into the medulla.

   c. He has a nodular lesion on the thoracic CT scan and a lytic bone lesion elsewhere. He is a smoker with a cough. He probably has a malignant lung tumour with distant metastases. The muscle weakness is probably caused by his severe hypokalaemia. The picture is strongly suggestive of ectopic ACTH secretion from a malignant tumour.

   d. First, he should receive potassium supplements and analgesics. If the diagnosis of small cell carcinoma is confirmed, you should consider chemotherapy. Local radiotherapy may help to relieve the pain in his arm. If he has ectopic ACTH secretion (confirmed by measuring his serum cortisol and ACTH), you may improve his symptoms by giving a treatment to suppress cortisol secretion. Metyrapone is rapidly effective and usually the first choice.

3. a. There is loss of the right fifth metatarsal head.

   b. Osteomyelitis secondary to a penetrating, neuropathic foot ulcer.

   c. Surgical exploration, removal of necrotic bone, prolonged bed rest and antibiotic treatment.

Musculoskeletal disease

8.1 Clinical aspects

Learning objectives

You should be able to:

- formulate a differential diagnosis based on the history and examination findings together with the results of investigations; this must take into account the pattern of joint and other organ involvement
- discuss the key investigations for particular diseases and why these are important, and be able to interpret them
- discuss the principles of management
- demonstrate a working knowledge of the main classes of drug used in rheumatological disorders, know the broad indications for their use and know the potential harm.

Case Study

Sam has been troubled with back pain for most of his life and now, having reached the age of 59 years, he feels that he has learned to live with it. However, in these last few weeks, things seemed to have changed. The pain seems to be present all the time and is getting steadily worse. He cannot remember when it came on; he just noticed it one day. Generally he feels awful and his wife says that he has lost weight. It also worried him when his GP examined him and found a particular tender spot.

Normal anatomy and physiology

You need to know the basic structure and working of a joint in order to follow what happens when a joint becomes inflamed and/or damaged. A synovial joint consists of two articular surfaces, enclosed by a fibrous capsule lined with synovium. The space between the articular cartilages is filled with synovial fluid acting as a lubricant. Surrounding the joints are tendon insertions on bone (**entheses**), muscles, ligaments and bursae. Any of these may be affected by an inflammatory process.

The **articular** surface is covered by avascular hyaline cartilage. The **synovium** is a specialised vascular membrane whose main function is to produce synovial fluid. The cells can be divided into two types: synovial macrophages, which are phagocytic, and synovial fibroblasts, which are secretory. The fluid is derived from plasma and has a high concentration of hyaluronic acid giving a high viscosity. Joint sensation and pain come from the capsule, periosteum and ligaments.

Common symptoms and signs

You should think of symptoms and signs in terms of:

- joints
- bone
- muscles and their connections
- systemic features
- whether the problem is acute or chronic.

The age of the patient is important. Giant cell arteritis (p. 354) is rare before the age of 60 years; osteoarthritis is much more common in elderly people. Rheumatoid arthritis can affect adults of any age, though the age-specific prevalence increases through life. Systemic lupus erythematosus (SLE) and Reiter's syndrome are more common in younger people.

Joints

Arthritis is characterised by:

- pain
- swelling
- increased local heat
- deformity.

In the absence of any joint inflammation, pain is described as **arthralgia**.

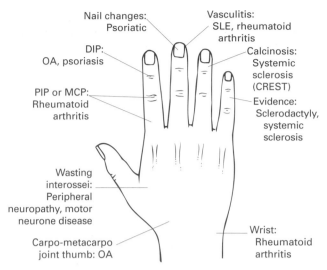

Fig. 87 Involvement of the joints and soft tissues in the hand in various musculoskeletal diseases. CREST, see page 356; DIP, distal interphalangeal; PIP, proximal interphalangeal; MCP, metacarpophalangeal; OA, osteoarthritis; SLE, systemic lupus erythematosus.

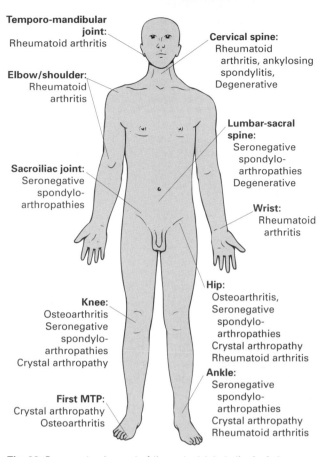

Fig. 88 Common involvement of the major joints in the body in musculoskeletal disease. MTP, metatarsophalangeal.

Swelling is common in arthritis and may be identified from either the history or the examination. It may be caused by:

- synovial thickening
- joint effusion
- bony overgrowth.

Furthermore the pattern of joint involvement must be noted when talking to the patient and during your examination. Is it monoarticular (e.g. gout), oligoarticular (less than five joints, e.g. reactive arthritis) or polyarticular (five or more, e.g. rheumatoid arthritis)? Is the arthropathy symmetrical (e.g. rheumatoid arthritis) or asymmetrical (e.g. psoriatic)? Does it involve small joints (hands (Fig. 87) wrists, feet) or large joints and/or the spine (Fig. 88)? Is there evidence of an active arthritis, with local heat, effusion and synovial thickening? How is the range of movement affected?

A combination of this information will frequently point to the diagnosis. For example, if the patient is a middle-aged woman with a symmetrical polyarthritis affecting the proximal interphalangeal (PIP) joints and metacarpophalangeal (MCP) joints with marked synovial involvement and systemic disturbance, then she has an inflammatory arthropathy, probably rheumatoid arthritis. In contrast, an elderly woman with a slowly progressive problem involving the right hip with pain on exercise, short-lived stiffness after resting and marked limitation of movement, particularly rotation, probably has osteoarthritis.

Back pain

Back pain is a very common symptom. As with many diagnostic problems, a rewarding approach is to consider a number of options and target the questions accordingly, gradually homing in on a probable cause. Above all, does the pain represent a serious underlying problem such as infection or malignancy ('red flag' symptoms or 'sinister' back-pain)? Clues may be recent onset, unremitting severe pain with marked localised tenderness and associated symptoms such as weight loss and fever.

Examples of diseases causing back pain are:

- an inflammatory arthropathy such as ankylosing spondylitis, which may be differentiated by the age of the patient, pattern of joints affected, effect of exercise, rest and systemic features
- osteoporosis, which is seen in older people and may present with increasing kyphosis, loss of height and episodes of severe pain resulting from vertebral collapse
- intervertebral disc prolapse, in which the onset of pain is sudden with marked muscle spasm and radiation of pain if there is radicular involvement. Neurological symptoms and signs may be present.

By means of exclusion, the residual diagnosis may be non-specific back pain. It is necessary to decide at which point to stop: after taking a history and performing an examination, or following a few basic tests or, in a small number of cases, more complex investigations. In reaching a diagnosis of non-specific back pain, the important points are that you have considered other possible causes and reassured the patient.

Bone

In bone, the common symptoms and signs are pain/tenderness and deformity.

Bone pain is often deep and poorly localised. It may be very severe and unremitting, particularly if caused by malignancy. The history of the pain will be a clear pointer to its cause. If the patient is an elderly female and the pain was sudden in onset, is localised in the middle of the lower back and then has gradually improved over several days/weeks, this points to osteoporotic collapse.

The other symptom (and sign) is deformity. If localised, it may imply a fracture or a malignant process. If the whole bone is involved in an older patient, Paget's disease may be suspected. Rarely, it may be caused by osteomalacia.

Muscle

Patients often complain of fatigue, but unless this is accompanied by a clear onset and other symptoms, it is often very difficult to make a specific diagnosis. If the patient has a pattern of increasing weakness during repetitive exercise, myasthenia gravis can be considered (p. 244). Proximal weakness might suggest a myositis (especially with pain/tenderness), sometimes as part of a generalised connective tissue disease. The major effects of proximal weakness are related to activities such as climbing stairs or getting up out of a chair.

Stiffness of muscles or joints is a very important symptom and patients need to be asked directly about this. Common causes are:

- osteoarthritis
- rheumatoid arthritis
- polymyalgia rheumatica.

In osteoarthritis, the stiffness is usually shortlived and improves within about 15–30 minutes, even after prolonged resting. In contrast, stiffness in the morning or following inactivity is a dominant and disabling feature of an inflammatory process such as rheumatoid arthritis or polymyalgia rheumatica. **Morning stiffness** may take a few hours to disappear and improvement in the duration of stiffness is a clear sign of improvement.

Systemic features

In your assessment, it is very important to enquire about systemic disturbance. Connective tissue disease cannot be regarded as confined to joints. For example, rheumatoid arthritis is a systemic disease not only affecting joints. Patients feel generally unwell and may lose weight, as well as having specific problems such as breathlessness (lung involvement) or a peripheral nerve lesion.

Other symptoms

Within the history, there are a number of other features that should be sought as they may provide a key to the diagnosis. Acute gout is *uncommon* in women, but rheumatoid arthritis and SLE are more common. Repeated stress and minor trauma on joints, such as in professional sport, may cause osteoarthritis in later life. A recent viral illness or episode of diarrhoea may have been triggers for arthritis.

In the family, there may be a history of rheumatoid arthritis (and other autoimmune disease), psoriasis or ankylosing spondylitis (with HLA-B27).

In addition to the symptoms, it is very important that particular attention is paid to the effect the disease/problem is having on the patient's lifestyle. You have to be able to describe the patient's disability as well as document the examination findings. You should also go through the drug history carefully, noting which drugs have been taken and for how long, the patient's response and any side-effects.

Investigations

Haematology

A full blood count is mandatory in musculoskeletal disease. **Anaemia of chronic disease** is seen in many of these (p. 270). In the inflammatory arthritides, anaemia is common and broadly reflects disease activity. The level of haemoglobin may fall to around 90 g/l and the anaemia characteristically has a normochromic normocytic pattern. The serum iron is normal and total iron-binding capacity reduced, reflecting impaired iron utilisation. Serum ferritin is difficult to interpret as it is an acute-phase reactant and will be elevated in any inflammatory process. Low values do suggest iron deficiency. High values are likely to indicate anaemia of chronic disease. A result in the 'normal range' is less helpful. In some patients, there may be iron deficiency secondary to blood loss from the gastrointestinal (GI) tract (peptic ulcer: non-steroidal anti-inflammatory drugs (NSAIDs)). If the mean cell volume (MCV) is low, you should investigate for a cause. Red cell aplasia or haemolysis rarely occurs in SLE.

A **leucocytosis** may be seen in a number of different diseases, including gout and bacterial infection. Remember that corticosteroid therapy commonly causes a granulocytosis. A high white cell count is sometimes seen in polyarteritis nodosa.

A low white cell count can occur. In active SLE, **lymphopenia** is characteristic. **Felty's syndrome** is seen in rheumatoid arthritis where hypersplenism (splenomegaly with associated lymphadenopathy) causes granulocytopenia. **Thrombocytosis** is seen in patients with active rheumatoid arthritis, whereas thrombocytopenia is observed in SLE.

In addition, you should consider the effects of drugs. Not only may cytotoxic agents such as azathioprine cause bone marrow depression, but others, including NSAIDs, can cause haematological problems such as an iron deficiency anaemia.

Measures of inflammation

Erythrocyte sedimentation rate (ESR) The ESR is a nonspecific marker for an inflammatory process and, like **plasma viscosity** (PV), reflects changes in fibrinogen and other globulins. Unlike PV, the ESR is influenced by age, gender (normal values, Table 1, p. 5) and haematocrit, with reduced values in erythrocytosis and higher values in anaemia. It can be used to monitor disease activity.

C-reactive protein (CRP) This is one of a family of acute-phase proteins, others being fibrinogen, haptoglobin, caeruloplasmin, ferritin and α_1-antitrypsin. They increase in concentration in active inflammatory joint disease. Like ESR, the C-reactive protein is used to monitor response to treatment.

Eight

Biochemistry

The key biochemical abnormalities are disturbances in renal function, particularly in SLE and the vasculitides. Rheumatoid arthritis may cause renal amyloidosis (chronic inflammation leads to amyloid deposition, causing renal impairment and nephrotic syndrome) and many of the drugs used in treatment can affect renal function. In addition to serum urea, creatinine and urinalysis, measurement of 24-hour protein excretion and creatinine clearance may be indicated.

In any patient with suspected crystal arthropathy, you must measure serum urate. A low value makes the diagnosis of gout unlikely, but a raised value does not necessarily confirm the diagnosis (joint aspiration is needed to do so).

Immunology

The diagnosis of most autoimmune diseases can be supported with an antibody test (Table 75). This does not mean that the antibody causes the damage (epiphenomena). There are two major immunopathological processes involved in autoimmunity:

- direct antibody attack with complement activation and/or cellular attack, e.g. Goodpasture's syndrome, myasthenia gravis, thyroiditis and organ-specific autoimmune diseases
- formation of immune complexes (type III hypersensitivity) (Table 76).

There is a relatively strong genetic component to the development of autoimmune diseases. In all of them, T cell involvement appears to be critical. Continous exposure to the inciting antigen (exogenous or endogenous) is probably important for perpetuating the disease.

Autoimmune diseases vary from highly specific single organ diseases (as in male infertility, thyroiditis or pemphigus vulgaris) to multisystem disease. As a general rule, the greater the specificity of the antibody for an organ or tissue, the more the autoimmune disease is confined to a single site. Antibodies to cellular targets present in many cell types, such as cardiolipin or antinuclear antibody, lead to multisystem disease.

For more detailed explanation of abnormalities of the immune system, see Chapter 9.

Table 75 Useful autoantibody tests

Antibody	Interpretation
Nuclear and nucleic acid antigens	
Antinuclear antibodies (ANA)	High titre: systemic lupus erythematosus (SLE)
Double-stranded DNA	Highly specific for SLE (high titre) some correlation with disease activity
Ro and La	SLE, Sjögren's syndrome
Jo-1	Fibrosing alveolitis, polymyositis
Ribonucleoprotein	Connective tissue disease overlap syndromes
Centromere	Limited cutaneous systemic sclerosis and CREST
Scl-70	Systemic sclerosis, diffuse pattern (20%)
Phospholipids	
Cardiolipin	Antiphospholipid syndrome
Mitochondria	
Antimitochondrial antibodies	Primary biliary cirrhosis
Neutrophils	
Cytoplasmic antineutrophil cytoplasm antibodies (ANCA)	Generalised Wegener's granulomatosis
Perinuclear ANCA	Microscopic polyarteritis, idiopathic glomerulonephritis, Churg–Strauss syndrome
Circulating proteins	
Rheumatoid factor (RF: Fc portion of IgG)	Low titre: normal, connective tissue disease, rheumatoid arthritis
	High titre: rheumatoid arthritis and extra-articular disease (70%)
Structure-specific antibodies	
Basement membrane	Goodpasture's syndrome
Acetylcholine receptors	Myasthenia gravis, Eaton–Lambert syndrome
Cell (organ)-specific antibodies	
Adrenal cortex	Addison's disease
Thyroid antibodies	Thyroiditis
Intrinsic factor, gastric parietal cells	Pernicious anaemia
Skin	Pemphigus and pemphigoid
Red cells, specific blood group antigens	Haemolytic anaemia
Platelets	Idiopathic thrombocytopenic purpura
Islet cell antibodies	Diabetes mellitus
Spermatozoa	Male infertility

Table 76 Examples of diseases linked to immune complex deposition

	Sites of deposition of immune complex and inflammatory processes						
	Brain	Kidney	Vessels	Joints	Skin	Lungs	Muscle
Systemic lupus erythematosus (SLE)	+	+	+	+	+	+	
Rheumatoid arthritis			+	+			
Vasculitis			+		+		
Polyarteritis nodosa		+	+				+
Cryoglobulinaemia		+	+	+	+		

Rheumatoid factors

Rheumatoid factors (RF) are autoantibodies which are directed against the Fc fragment of IgG. They are predominantly IgM. Seropositivity is defined as agglutination in the latex test at a serum dilution of 1 : 20 (1 : 32 in the sheep cell agglutination test: SCAT). RFs can be found in the normal population (increasing with age), a whole range of other connective tissue diseases (e.g. Sjögren's syndrome, SLE, polyarteritis nodosa, systemic sclerosis), chronic infections and other immunological disorders (e.g. sarcoidosis). You must *not* interpret the presence of RF as diagnostic of rheumatoid arthritis. Similarly, in some patients with rheumatoid arthritis the test may be negative. However, strong seropositivity (high dilutions) is associated with rheumatoid arthritis and predicts a worse outcome and extra-articular disease. Overall approximately 20% of patients with rheumatoid arthritis remain negative for RF.

Antinuclear antibodies

As with RFs, there are a wide range of conditions in which antinuclear antibodies (ANA) are found. Antibodies against *double*-stranded DNA (in high titres) are highly specific for SLE (the only exception is autoimmune hepatitis), whereas antibodies against *single*-stranded DNA are a feature of drug-induced SLE. Antibodies against *extractable nuclear antigen* are characteristic of connective tissue overlap syndromes (p. 356).

Complement

A detailed explanation of complement function is given on page 381. Low serum levels of C3 or C4 (or total haemolytic complement) are found in SLE. Particularly low concentrations are found in **lupus nephritis**, because of consumption of complement. Serial measurements can help in monitoring disease activity and response to treatment.

Imaging

Other than requesting plain radiographs of affected joints, you should order radiographs of the hands and feet, since diagnostic features may be present despite the *absence* of symptoms and signs. The common features seen with specific conditions are given in the separate sections. In certain instances, other imaging may be useful, including computed tomographic (CT) and magnetic resonance (MR) scan and arthrography.

CT and MR imaging is being used increasingly in the evaluation of musculoskeletal disease. Close to bone (e.g. spinal column), CT suffers from interference, but MR gives clear images of all the soft tissues. In trauma (including sports injury), MR allows visualization of small amounts of damage to ligaments, muscles and tendons as well as microfractures and meniscal tears.

In degenerative or inflammatory conditions, MR can be used to assess the joint surface and surrounding tissues. Similarly, it is used in the diagnosis of osteomyelitis and bone tumours (where CT scanning is also used).

MR is the preferred imaging modality in spinal disease including trauma, disc degeneration and herniation. In rheumatoid arthritis, MR can delineate the inflammation and destruction of the cartilage, bone and ligaments with associated instability, subluxation and damage to the spinal cord.

Bone scanning

Bone scans can be useful in the assessment of acute and chronic osteomyelitis and metastatic disease of bone. Patients receive a small dose of labelled technetium linked to phosphate and the whole skeleton is imaged after 2–4 hours. Increased uptake is sometimes seen in healing fractures or arthritis.

Joint aspiration (arthrocentesis)

The two key diagnoses that *require* joint aspiration are:

- crystal arthropathy
- septic arthritis.

The aspirate is divided into three portions for:

- white cell count and differential
- Gram stain and culture
- polarised light microscopy for crystals.

Table 77 gives details of the findings in different diseases.

Management

With any disease, you should have a broader view of management than simply drug therapy. All patients need to have three things discussed with them:

- What is it? Explanation and discussion of the disease process.

Table 77 Synovial fluid abnormalities with different joint disorders

	Appearance	White cells	Culture	Crystals (polarising light)
Normal	Clear viscous	<200	Sterile	None
Rheumatoid arthritis	Yellow, very low viscosity, may be turbid	Very high (5000–50 000)	Sterile	None
Osteoarthritis	Viscosity preserved	High (<2000)	Sterile	Small (<5%), pyrophosphate
Crystal arthritis	Clear, reduced viscosity	Very high (50 000–100 000)	Sterile	Negatively birefringent: urate – gout Weakly positive birefringent: pyrophosphate – pseudogout
Septic arthritis	Turbid, reduced viscosity	Extremely high (>50 000)	Positive (may be on Gram stain)	None

- What will happen? Explanation of natural history, investigations prognosis for morbidity (including disability) and any threat to life.
- What can be done? Discussion of treatment options, monitoring and recommendations.

Management is aimed at the person, not just the disease. Consequently, the major end-points are survival, disability (p. 211) and handicap (p. 211). You need to know when and how to involve the allied health professions (including physiotherapists and occupational therapists). Other medical disciplines may need to be consulted and surgery may be required. A doctor in training may only see the patient for a short time, but that person's relation-ship with the multi-professional team is likely to extend over a number of years.

Common drugs

Non-steroidal anti-inflammatory drugs

The NSAIDs are important in the management of inflammation. There is a whole range of drugs available; you need to know their common properties. The prime action is to block the **cyclo-oxygenase** (COX) pathway, producing various inflammatory mediators (prostaglandins). One potential consequence of blockade is an overactivity of the **lipo-oxygenase** pathway, with increase in leucotrienes. As the leucotrienes include powerful bronchoconstrictors, the disturbance in balance between the two systems can produce bronchoconstriction. In aspirin-induced asthma, there is a hypersensitivity reaction over and above this mechanism.

Another consequence of COX blockade is a reduction of **intrarenal** generation of prostaglandins. This can have deleterious affects on intrarenal vascular control, causing a deterioration in renal function and hyperkalaemia.

The third, and most important, problem associated with the use of NSAIDs is an increased risk of the complications of peptic ulcers. Numerous epidemiological studies have shown a clear relationship between NSAIDs and perforation, bleeding and risk of death, particularly in older people. The use of rectal preparations, prodrugs or enteric-coated drugs does *not* protect against gastric damage.

Of the currently available non-selective NSAIDs (see below for COX-2 drugs), **ibuprofen** appears safest, with diclofenac and naproxen being relatively safe despite stronger anti-inflammatory action. The mechanism of gastric mucosal damage is linked, like the renal changes, to alteration in prostaglandin production. **Misoprostol**, which is a prostaglandin analogue, helps to prevent damage to the mucosa (p. 124), as do the proton pump inhibitors (e.g. omeprazole).

Drugs (e.g. celecoxib, rofecoxib) that specifically act by blocking the COX-2 isoenzyme were developed in an attempt to avoid the gastric damage linked to COX-1 blockade (the non-selective NSAIDs such as ibuprofen inhibit both isoenzymes). After initial enthusiasm and widespread prescription of the COX-2 inhibitors, these drugs have come under close scrutiny. There is evidence for an increased risk of cardiac events (e.g. myocardial infarct) with their prescription and this may be a class effect rather than linked to a particular drug (e.g. rofecoxib). Similarly, there appears to be an increased risk of upper gastrointestinal problems (e.g. haematemesis, peptic ulcer). For both see COX-2 inhibitors and the non-selective NSAIDs, the prescription of ulcer healing drugs (e.g. proton pump inhibitors — omeprazole) reduces the risk of gastrointestinal problems and should be co-prescribed in high-risk patients (e.g. also on steroids or previous history of peptic ulceration).

There are other problems with NSAIDs: for example, fluid retention and resistance to treatment for heart failure or hypertension (particularly indometacin). Individual drugs have their own spectrum of side-effects.

The main recommended use of NSAIDs is in inflammation. They can bring marked relief in inflammatory arthropathies, including osteoarthritis if there is an inflammatory component. However, most patients do *not* have any active inflammation. NSAIDs do *not* influence the underlying disease process. The principle should always be to initiate treatment with ibuprofen in moderate doses. Only if there is no relief at high doses of ibuprofen, should you change to one of the more potent drugs (such as diclofenac or naproxen). It is better to be familiar with two or three drugs, getting to know these well.

There are other situations in which NSAIDs are of benefit:

- bone pain from metastatic disease
- renal and biliary colic (**diclofenac sodium** is as effective as narcotic analgesics).

Simple analgesics

The use of simple analgesics in musculoskeletal disease is often not fully exploited. They are the drugs of choice in osteoarthritis. The order of potency is paracetamol, codeine, dihydrocodeine and morphine. Patients should always be on the full dose of the least potent drug before moving on to the next one. Compound preparations are frequently used and you need to be aware of their constituents and dose. All narcotic analgesics cause constipation and a laxative should be prescribed as a preventative measure.

Corticosteroids

Corticosteroids are effective in suppressing inflammatory disease activity. However, corticosteroids have many long-term adverse effects, including osteoporosis, cataracts, skin atrophy, susceptibility to infection and adrenal suppression. It is still not clear whether oral corticosteroids improve the outcome in rheumatoid disease. When used as intra-articular therapy, repeated injection of the same joint may very rarely result in joint destruction but it does have a place in treating flares of rheumatoid arthritis.

Surgery

The two aims of surgery are **prophylactic**, to prevent further damage, and **reconstructive**, to restore function and stability. Procedures include synovectomy, tendon reconstruction, arthroplasty and arthrodesis. Surgery has an important role in the management of musculoskeletal disease.

8.2 Infection

Learning objectives

You should be able to:

- recognise the clinical features and initiate appropriate investigations of an acutely inflamed joint
- discuss the common organisms causing septic arthritis and appropriate initial investigation and management
- describe how both acute and chronic osteomyelitis present clinically, which investigations are useful and the management strategies.

Case Study

A 16-year-old presents with acute back pain of 3 days' duration. He has low-grade fever, a normal white cell count and a CRP of 120 mg/l. There is no injury history. He reports recent cuts related to 'mucking about on his bike'. Plain X-rays of his back are normal. He requires morphine to control the pain.

Septic arthritis

Septic arthritis is an infection (usually bacterial) of one or more joints. Bacteria invade the synovial membrane and fluid and the inflammatory response (especially neutrophils) leads to cartilage and joint destruction. It is a medical emergency and the immediate, appropriate management of septic arthritis is critically important to the preservation of function of the joint over the long term, as the infecting organisms and the neutrophil response will lead to substantial damage to cartilage in 1–2 days. As part of your management, you should always exclude other causes of an acutely inflamed joint (such as gout or an inflammatory arthritis). Around 250–300 cases occur annually in the UK.

Clinical presentation

The primary symptoms of septic arthritis are:

- fever
- acute joint pain (not always in the elderly)
- acute joint swelling.

In your initial evaluation of the patient, you should establish whether the problem is a monoarthritis, oligoarthritis or polyarthritis. Monoarthritis is caused particularly by *Staphylococcus aureus*, β-haemolytic streptococci and *Mycobacterium tuberculosis*. The first two commonly present more acutely than the last. Previously damaged joints are at greater risk of infections.

Oligoarthritis or polyarthritis has a wider aetiology, including *Neisseria gonorrhoeae*, postinfectious or reactive arthritis, rheumatic fever (p. 420), erythrovirus or rubella infection (p. 419) or Lyme borreliosis (p. 421).

Investigations

The key investigation is joint aspiration. You may be able to aspirate fluid from the knee relatively easily, but most other joints require specialist help, particularly small joints such as the elbow or sternoclavicular joint. If the area of inflammation is large and fluid has collected above or directly over a smaller joint, then direct aspiration is appropriate. If, on aspiration of the joint, the fluid is obviously turbid, then the joint should be aspirated to dryness as this is an important part of the management regardless of the organism. The fluid should be examined for total cell count, for differential white cell count and by Gram stain and culture (see Table 77).

It is important to try to do the aspiration before antibiotics are started, although these should not be delayed for very long while you wait for appropriate expertise.

The white cell count is usually raised. A blood culture should be done. Serology for erythrovirus, rubella and Lyme borreliosis and antistreptolysin O (ASO) titre for rheumatic fever are appropriate for an oligo- or polyarthritis, as may be RF and other autoimmune antibody tests.

Management

The principles of management are:

- appropriate i.v. antibiotics (e.g. flucloxacillin 2 g every 6 hours for *Staph. aureus*)

- repeated aspiration of joints (at least once a day) or arthroscopy and joint washout to prevent cartilage destruction
- complete rest of the affected joint, particularly if weight-bearing, until there is substantial improvement
- pain relief.

In some patients, septic arthritis is a manifestation of disseminated or systemic infection. This is particularly true of staphylococcal septic arthritis if there has been no injury. You should seek other sites of infection (e.g. endocarditis) and treat appropriately. Septic arthritis may also be the presentation of SLE, sarcoidosis and a number of other rare diseases. Expert advice should be sought if there are other clinical features suggesting a generalised disease.

Osteomyelitis (osteitis)

Osteomyelitis is infection of bone. It may be acute or chronic. The presentation and management of acute and chronic osteomyelitis are substantially different.

Acute osteomyelitis

Acute osteomyelitis occurs following a bacteraemic episode usually with *Staph. aureus*, but occasionally with Gram-positive, Gram-negative (e.g. *Salmonella*) or anaerobic bacteria. The most common site is the vertebral column, but no bone in the body is exempt.

Clinical presentation

The patient almost always has fever and localised pain. Sometimes patients are very ill when bacteraemia develops and do not complain of pain. Often the osteomyelitis presents days or weeks after the episode of bacteraemia that precipitated it. In other slightly less acute cases, complaints such as back pain caused by acute osteomyelitis are shrugged off by patients and doctors. There are two features that will help you:

- The pain is persistent.
- Usually palpation over the affected area is painful.

Investigations

There may be a raised white cell count and the ESR or CRP is almost always extremely high. Blood cultures are often positive for *Staph. aureus*. Plain radiographs are normal for at least the first 10 days of infection and may then show lucency and bone destruction. Bone scan and white cell scans show abnormalities earlier than radiographs.

Management

The principles of management are:

- Establish the extent of infection by radiology and isotope scanning of the affected site.
- Ascertain the microbiological cause using direct needle puncture under radiographic control.
- Give i.v. antibiotic therapy with large antibiotic doses as concentrations in bone tend to be low, after needle aspiration.
- Immobilise the area, particularly if a critical part of the vertebral column is involved or there is evidence of epidural compression.

- Organise review by an orthopaedic surgeon of the need for surgery; if there is extensive involvement or localised abscess formation impinging on important structures such as the spinal cord, then surgery is often mandatory.

Chronic osteomyelitis

Chronic osteomyelitis presents with symptoms over months or years. Typical forms of infection include:

- tuberculous osteomyelitis
- osteomyelitis of the metatarsals or other bones in the feet in diabetic patients with chronic foot ulcers
- chronic discharging sinus overlying a prior fracture or injury involving foreign bodies (e.g. shrapnel)
- fracture site with infected metalwork within it
- chronic vertebral osteomyelitis caused by fungi (such as *Aspergillus* or *Coccidioides* spp.), which is often initially mistaken for bony metastases
- osteomyelitis of the head or neck related to chronic sinus or ear infections.

Clinical presentation

The clinical presentation falls into two groups: those with chronic pain or deformity (such as patients with tuberculous osteomyelitis who develop Pott's disease of the spine) and patients with a chronically discharging sinus overlying an area of osteomyelitis. Unlike in acute osteomyelitis, where plain radiographs are often normal, in chronic osteomyelitis the plain radiographs are almost always abnormal. The primary exception is diabetic foot osteomyelitis, in which the area of involvement is often small. White cell scans or bone scans also show areas of infection. Most patients do not have a raised white cell count, although they usually have a raised ESR and CRP.

Management

The principles of management are:

- Determine the cause by needle biopsy or surgery *before* antibiotics are given; submit cultures for aerobic, anaerobic, mycobacterial and fungal culture.
- If bacterial in origin, organise complete debridement and removal of all dead bone (sequestrum), metalwork, foreign bodies, etc.
- Give high-dose i.v. antibiotic therapy for at least 3 weeks, followed by long-term oral antibiotic therapy.
- If caused by *Mycobacterium tuberculosis* or fungi, medical therapy is used initially unless the deformity is so extensive or dangerous that surgery is required.

The prognosis of chronic osteomyelitis is poor, partly because of the underlying disease and partly because of the chronicity and difficulty in removing all dead infected bone. Exceptions include tuberculous osteomyelitis, which has a good outlook, although it takes weeks or even months for pain and symptoms to improve. You will find chronic osteomyelitis to be a major therapeutic challenge and accurate determination of the cause together with susceptibility testing is critical to a good outcome.

8.3 Arthropathies

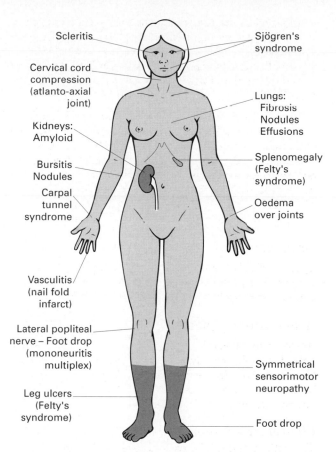

Fig. 89 Systemic manifestations of rheumatoid **arthritis**.

Learning objectives

You should be able to:

- describe the systemic manifestations of rheumatoid arthritis and its management and prognosis
- set out the differences between the seronegative spondyloarthropathies and seropositive rheumatoid arthritis
- discuss the range of conditions within the seronegative spondyloarthropathies and the similarities and differences between them.

Case Study

Meera has had rheumatoid arthritis for about a year. She was very keen to stay off tablets as long as possible and concentrate on diet and lifestyle, but things have got worse. She is finding it difficult to use her hands because of pain, and walking has also become troublesome because of painful feet. She is not keen on taking any anti-inflammatory drugs because of the recent publicity, but wants to talk to you about her options.

Rheumatoid arthritis

Rheumatoid arthritis is the most common disorder of the connective tissues and is characterised by:

- a symmetrical chronic polyarthritis that often results in joint damage
- disease affecting many body systems (Fig. 89)
- the presence of RF in most patients.

Epidemiology

Rheumatoid arthritis has prevalence of around 2–3% and a male to female ratio of 1 : 3. The onset is most commonly between the ages of 30 and 60 years. Within families, approximately 10% have a first-degree relative affected and there may be a 12–15% concordance in identical twins. A strong association exists between the disease and HLA-DR4 with a 6–12-fold increase in risk. Most recently there has been interest in the 'shared epitopes' of certain HLA-DR4 and HLA-DR1 subtypes.

Pathology and pathogenesis

The cause of rheumatoid arthritis is unknown, but there is strong evidence of disordered immunity. RFs (particularly IgG) play a part in forming immune complexes, which are found in the circulation and within the synovium. These can activate the complement cascade, generating inflammatory and chemotactic factors (p. 379).

The vascularity of the synovium increases, and the membrane thickens and becomes oedematous with infiltration by T lymphocytes, plasma cells and macrophages. Within the synovial fluid there are large numbers of granulocytes. A chronic inflammatory **pannus** is formed in the synovium, which encroaches from the joint margins leading to cartilage and joint destruction.

Changes are also found in other tissues. Rheumatoid nodules, which are pathognomonic, show *palisading* macrophages (histiocytes) around a central zone of hyaline necrosis.

Clinical presentation

Rheumatoid arthritis usually comes on insidiously over a few months, though in a minority there is an acute onset with marked systemic disturbance. In some patients, an episodic arthralgia may have been present for months/years (**palindromic rheumatism**).

Joints

Characteristically, the joint involvement is symmetrical and affects the small joints of the hands (PIPs, MCPs, wrists) and feet. In a smaller proportion, the large weight-bearing joints are affected first. The natural history is usually involvement of increasing numbers of joints. The main symptoms are joint pain and swelling together with marked morning stiffness. In the early inflammatory phase, there may be tenderness and swelling over a greater area than simply the joints. As the disease progresses, permanent joint damage occurs, with bone and cartilage damage as well as rupture of tendons resulting in joint subluxation and dislocation. In the hands this produces typical changes (Fig. 90).

Small joints: hands and feet Rheumatoid arthritis characteristically affects the small peripheral joints. The wrists, MCPs and PIPs show swelling, increased warmth

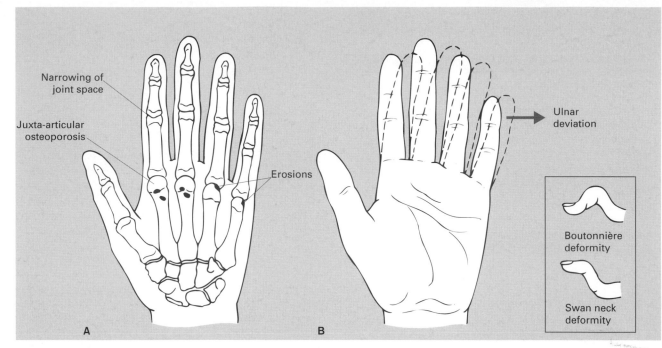

Fig. 90 Schematic representation of changes in rheumatoid arthritis. **A** Radiographic changes. **B** Hand deformities.

and tenderness. Disease activity over years leads to limitation of movement, wrist subluxation, ulnar styloid resorption, ulnar deviation of the fingers and swan neck and boutonnière deformity of the fingers (Fig. 90); most of these are caused by tendon displacement or damage. Wasting of the interossei muscles may be apparent. In the feet, there is tenderness over the metatarsal heads and eventually subluxation. The patients may complain that it feels as though they are walking on pebbles.

Large joints The knees may be warm and swollen because of effusions, synovial thickening or, in the later stages, bony overgrowth. A varus or a valgus deformity may result. Quadriceps wasting is often prominent and the joint may be unstable owing to damage to the cruciate and lateral ligaments. The ankles, elbows, shoulders and hips may be involved.

Other joints Rheumatoid arthritis may affect the temporomandibular joint, giving pain on mastication. Damage to the atlanto-axial joint may cause odontoid peg destruction and instability. Symptoms include:

- pain radiating to the occiput (C1, C2 dermatomes): most common
- paraesthesia, sensory loss
- sudden deterioration in hand function
- abnormal gait
- urinary retention or incontinence.

If the patient requires intubation for a general anaesthetic, care has to be taken not to flex the neck excessively as this increases atlanto-axial subluxation. The lower cervical vertebra can be involved, again with cord problems. Management initially involves stabilisation using a *firm* collar and a neurosurgical opinion.

Periarticular involvement Rheumatoid nodules are associated with high titres of RF and are found over the extensor surfaces of the elbows, pressure points and, sometimes, along tendons. They are usually not fixed and are not painful, though they can sometimes ulcerate. They are pathognomonic for the disease.

Tenosynovitis and bursitis These are common. The latter involves the olecranon and the prepatellar, subacromial and trochanteric bursae.

Systemic involvement

You must think of rheumatoid arthritis as a systemic disease not only affecting joints. This is why it is sometimes termed rheumatoid *disease* (see Fig. 89). Patients feel unwell when the disease is active; they lose weight and are anaemic. They are also more susceptible to infection, especially if treated with corticosteroids.

Pulmonary involvement Rheumatoid arthritis frequently affects the lung and pleura. Effusions occur and can mimic empyema. Pulmonary nodules may be difficult to differentiate from other causes (p. 84). They may predate the arthropathy and are associated with aggressive disease and high titres of RF. Pulmonary fibrosis occurs, particularly affecting the lower zones and causing a restrictive defect.

Nervous system A sensorimotor neuropathy may develop, with predominantly sensory disturbance. A vasculitis can affect individual nerves causing a mononeuritis (multiplex). Common nerves affected are the median, ulnar, lateral popliteal, tibial and oculomotor. There may be *entrapment* neuropathies in which nerves are compressed by the swelling and tissue thickening around joints. The ulnar, median, lateral popliteal and tibial nerves are the usual ones affected. The most common entrapment is carpal tunnel syndrome (p. 242). Disease involvement of the **cervical spine** with cord and root signs has been discussed.

Vascular involvement Vasculitis is one of the hallmarks of aggressive disease with high RF titres. It can affect all sizes of vessel:

- small end-arteries: nailfold and small areas of skin infarction
- large arteries (rarely affected): stroke, mesenteric ischaemia or limb ischaemia
- medium (and small calibre) arteries: mononeuritis multiplex (through involvement of the vasa nervorum) and patchy muscle ischaemia.

The renal vasculature is *spared*.

Eye Main ocular complications are:

- Sjögren's syndrome
- uveitis and scleritis.

Primary Sjögren's syndrome is a combination of kerato-conjunctivitis sicca (dry eyes) and xerostomia (dry mouth). The salivary and lacrimal glands are infiltrated with lymphocytes. The syndrome is seen in association with other connective tissue diseases (e.g. SLE). Diagnosis is by **Schirmer's test** for impaired tear secretion, or a lip salivary gland biopsy. Dry eyes are helped by artificial tears.

Other complications Rheumatoid arthritis can affect most body systems. The **kidney** may be affected by:

- amyloidosis (severe disease): nephrotic syndrome and renal impairment
- the drugs used (see above).

Lymphadenopathy is occasionally seen but is more common in juvenile arthritis. Splenomegaly can lead to hypersplenism and granulocytopenia (**Felty's syndrome**). There is also an association with leg ulceration (vasculitis). Often a pericarditis occurs with a small effusion.

Investigations

The investigation of a symmetrical inflammatory polyarthritis has been described (p. 343). Additional considerations are monitoring of disease activity and drug therapy. Disease activity is measured using a composite of different indices: clinical assessment, ESR, CRP and full blood count.

Radiological assessment must always be carried out, including radiographs of the hands and feet. The typical features are shown in Figure 90. **Erosions** occur and are associated with high RF titres. An important consideration is the change in radiographic appearances over time.

Management and prognosis

The management of musculoskeletal disease has been outlined. The emphasis in the management of rheumatoid disease is now the early use of disease-modifying antirheumatic drugs (DMARDs) such as sulfasalazine or methotrexate. The evidence is that these have improved the outcome with retardation or prevention of disease progression (joint destruction and subsequent loss of function). The prognosis is variable, with only around 1 in 10 patients becoming severely disabled. A worse prognosis is predicted by:

- male gender
- HLA-DR4
- insidious onset
- systemic disease
- high antibody titre
- early appearance of erosions.

Potential DMARDs

Early treatment with chloroquine, methotrexate or sulfasalazine over time may modify the underlying disease. Initiation of therapy and monitoring of response and side-effects are best done within a specialised unit.

Chloroquine Chloroquine and hydroxychloroquine are antimalarial drugs that coincidently suppress disease activity in rheumatoid arthritis. The main toxicity occurs in the retina, with deteriorating visual acuity.

Gold Gold therapy (either by injection or orally) takes 2–3 months to have any impact on disease activity. At least one-third of patients develop side-effects, many of which are serious. These include rashes, thrombocytopenia, leucopenia, aplastic anaemia and glomerulonephritis (nephrotic syndrome). Consequently, it is necessary to monitor the patient's full blood count and renal function (particularly for proteinuria). The use of gold is gradually being phased out.

Sulfasalazine, 5-aminosalicylic acid Sulfasalazine is a compound of sulfapyridine and 5-aminosalicylic acid. These are usually well tolerated, with a low incidence of serious adverse effects. Main problems are with GI upset and depression. A reversible oligospermia also occurs.

Leflunomide This is proven to slow radiographic progression and joint damage. The mechanism of action is not fully understood but may relate to inhibition of tyrosine kinase. As with other DMARDs, it takes several weeks to be fully effective. The main side-effects are on the liver, and hair loss (alopecia) also occurs. It should not be given in pregnancy.

Immunosuppressives Methotrexate is now commonly used early in rheumatoid disease, particularly in those with bad prognostic indicators (RF positive, high ESR) or if sulfasalazine is ineffective or not tolerated. Methotrexate has greater efficacy and most patients can tolerate it long-term. It may cause intrahepatic fibrosis and a pneumonitis. Because of bone marrow suppression, monitoring of the blood count is necessary.

Ciclosporin This was first introduced to prevent transplant rejection. It interferes with T cell functioning by inhibiting interleukin-2. The main side-effects are on the kidney.

Biologic agents

Biologic therapies, targeting cytokines, are being increasingly used for active rheumatoid arthritis unresponsive to other therapies. Those antagonising the action of tumour necrosing factor alpha (TNF-α) are currently most commonly used. Examples include etanercept (protein binds to TNF-α) and infliximab (monoclonal antibody against TNF-α). Biologic therapies should be not be used in pregnancy. Side-effects include increased susceptibility to infection and also demyelination. More recently, an interleukin-1 receptor antagonist (anakinra) has been introduced.

Eight

Seronegative spondyloarthropathies

The seronegative spondyloarthropathies are a group of conditions that share several common features:

- *absence* of RF in the serum
- a peripheral arthritis which is usually *asymmetrical*
- sacroiliitis
- extra-articular manifestations
- association with HLA-B27.

The term *spondyl* is derived from the Greek *spondylos* (vertebra). Radiological examination may show asymmetric bony ankylosis (fusion) and marginal periostitis. The main histopathological abnormalities are at insertion of tendons and ligaments (**enthesopathy**) rather than in the synovium.

There is a strong familial tendency. Almost all patients with ankylosing spondylitis are positive for the **HLA-B27** histocompatibility antigen. Approximately half of patients with psoriatic arthropathy are also positive for HLA-B27.

The cause of the seronegative spondyloarthropathies is unclear apart from the association with HLA-B27.

Psoriatic arthropathy

Many of your patients will have psoriasis (usually it is incidental to the reason for which they are consulting) and about 1 in 10 of these will have an arthropathy. The skin disease often predates the arthropathy by many years. There is no close correlation between the severity of the skin problem and the joint disease; the exception is the association between nail psoriasis and arthritis of the DIP.

The arthritis may take different forms:

- a symmetrical polyarthritis (relatively common)
- an asymmetrical oligoarthritis affecting the hands and feet and sometimes larger joints
- spondylitis with evidence of sacroiliitis (one-third)
- nail and DIP disease together
- arthritis mutilans with severe deformity of the fingers and hands.

The treatment is similar to that of rheumatoid arthritis and the prognosis is *better*.

Ankylosing spondylitis

Ankylosing spondylitis is approximately 2–3 times more common in men; in women it tends to be mild and can be missed. In most patients, the disease will have started in young adulthood and around 95% of patients are HLA-B27 positive.

The most important pathological changes are seen in enthesis rather than synovium. The joints of the spine are affected with damage to the discs and ligament attachments. Eventually ankylosis occurs with calcification of intervertebral ligaments and annulus fibrosus.

Clinical presentation

Most patients present with back pain and may be systemically unwell. The pain is worse after rest, may wake the patient during the night and is usually associated with marked morning stiffness. Unlike other arthropathies, symptoms *improve* with exercise.

On examination, you will commonly find that the lumbar lordosis is lost and that there is sacroiliac tenderness. Costochondral joint involvement leading to decreased chest expansion is an important sign. In late, severe cases, there is a typical posture with marked kyphosis, stiff pelvis and limited back movement, making the diagnosis easy.

Other large joints are involved, particularly lower limb, in approximately 20–30% of patients. Tenderness at the insertions of tendons (enthesopathy) is common.

There are extra-articular manifestations:

- constitutional upset
- upper lobe fibrosis: restrictive pulmonary function
- aortic incompetence and conduction problems
- iritis
- amyloidosis (renal impairment, peripheral neuropathy)
- cauda equina syndrome.

Investigations

Investigations fall into several groups:

- haematology: raised ESR in active disease, anaemia (normochromic, normocytic)
- biochemistry: renal impairment, features of nephrotic syndrome (amyloidosis)
- radiology: sacroiliitis, characteristic syndesmophytes (calcification around the intervertebral disc) giving a **bamboo spine** and **squaring** of the vertebra
- tissue typing: HLA-B27.

Management

The treatment plan is continued activity. All patients will need the help of a physiotherapist for an exercise programme (this is the most important aspect of management), together with NSAIDs (p. 346). Long periods of bed rest are *avoided* as much as possible.

Prognosis

For most patients, the outlook is good, with severe progressive disease in only a small minority.

Reactive arthritis

Reactive arthritis is defined as a non-specific arthritis strongly linked to a recognised episode of infection with no viable microorganisms in the affected joint.

Reactive arthritis may follow a lower genital tract or bowel infection. The dysenteric form is associated with *Shigella flexneri*, *Yersinia enterocolitica* and *Salmonella typhimurium*. *Chlamydia trachomatis* is often the responsible organism in genital tract infection.

Reiter's syndrome is part of the spectrum of reactive arthritis and is associated with urethritis, cervicitis or both.

Clinical presentation

Most urogenital cases occur in young men; the postdysenteric syndrome has an equal sex incidence. Often the first element to appear is urethritis. There are superficial ulcers that coalesce as a **circinate balanitis** of the glans penis. The skin manifestation on the palms of the hands and soles of the feet looks identical to pustular psoriasis and is called keratoderma blenorrhagica. Commonly a **sterile conjunctivitis** occurs, and occasionally a severe anterior uveitis. Cardiac complications include heart block, aortic valve disease and pericarditis.

The arthritis ranges from mild synovitis to a chronic progressive arthropathy. It is usually asymmetrical in the fingers and toes, with some large joint involvement. The problem usually lasts for a few months.

Investigations

The ESR is elevated when the disease is active and there may be juxta-articular osteoporosis and, characteristically, **periostitis. Plantar spurs** occur in about one-third of patients and may be painful. Spondylitis may develop together with sacroiliitis.

Management

Most patients are treated with NSAIDs. Eye disease should be managed by an ophthalmologist; treatment includes corticosteroid drops.

Enteropathic arthropathy

Enteropathic arthropathy is defined as an arthritis associated with inflammatory bowel disease. Both sacroiliitis and synovitis (affecting weight-bearing joints) occur.

With ulcerative colitis, the arthritis tends to occur at times of flares of the bowel disease and in patients with severe involvement. A pan-colectomy cures the arthropathy. Similarly, in Crohn's disease, the synovitis correlates with disease activity.

The back can be involved with typical changes of ankylosing spondylitis. This may predate the bowel disease and does not follow the disease activity.

8.4 Systemic lupus erythematosus

Learning objectives

You should be able to:

- use your knowledge of SLE as a multisystem disorder with an autoimmune basis and, from this, be able to predict its manifestations
- investigate a person with possible SLE and be able to interpret the results
- discuss the principles of management.

Case Study

Janet has been a frequent attender at her doctor's with different symptoms such as mouth ulcers, headaches, pains in her joints and some rashes, but then it all changed when she developed widespread joint swelling and a generalised rash. After seeing a number of doctors, she was relieved when she was finally told the diagnosis and had an explanation for all her symptoms. Now, her main concern is with the side-effects of the various tablets she is taking and what will happen to her bones, eyes and kidneys.

Epidemiology and immunopathogenesis

SLE can affect virtually any organ, but skin, joints, kidneys and brain are most often involved. It affects women 10 times more often than men and there is likely to be a hormonal (probably oestrogenic) component to the pathogenesis. It is more common in the Afro-Caribbean population. Within families, there is a higher than expected incidence and a significant concordance between identical twins.

Patients with the disease undoubtedly have a disordered immune response. There is activation of B lymphocytes, leading to hyperglobulinaemia, impaired T cell regulation of the immune response and production of autoantibodies. Immune complexes are formed and deposited widely, particularly in the blood vessels (vasculitis) and kidney (glomerulonephritis). The formation of immune complexes leads to consumption of complement. Pathologically, SLE is characterised by widespread vasculitis and deposition of fibrinoid.

Clinical presentation

The onset of SLE is usually in those between 20 and 40 years of age. The criteria used for the diagnosis and classification of SLE are the presence of any four of the following together or separately in time:

- malar rash
- discoid rash
- photosensitivity
- oral ulcers
- arthritis
- pleurisy or pericarditis
- renal disease
  — cellular casts
  — proteinuria >0.5 g in 24 hours
- seizures or organic psychosis without other cause
- blood dyscrasia
  — haemolytic anaemia
  — leucopenia
  — lymphopenia
  — thrombocytopenia
- raised ANA titre
- immunological features, e.g. raised double-stranded DNA antibody titre.

Classical initial presentations of SLE include the following:

- joint pain without arthritis but with positive ANA
- butterfly rash over the bridge of the nose with or without other features of photosensitivity
- pleurisy with other features to suggest a multisystem disease
- haematological abnormalities.

Your assessment of the patient with possible SLE depends to some extent upon the presentation. All patients require a thorough physical examination, including individual joint assessment. Consideration of other associated diseases such as Sjögren's syndrome and antiphospholipid antibody syndrome is important.

Investigations

Investigations should include ANA and double-stranded DNA antibodies, complement levels with assessment of renal function and haematology. Measurement of CRP can help to distinguish between active disease (normal) and infection (high).

Management

Once the diagnosis is established, the patient should be referred to physicians who specialise in SLE. The patient will need lifelong supervision. As the disease waxes and wanes over time, the intensity of support varies. There should be regular assessments of renal function. General treatment measures include:

- rest when the disease is active
- low-fat diet in patients with hyperlipidaemia
- protection from photosensitivity with sun-block creams
- NSAIDs for symptoms.

Management of the more serious complications includes use of corticosteroids, azathioprine and cyclophospha-mide for accelerating renal disease. Chloroquine (or hydroxychloroquine) is the mainstay of treatment for skin or joint disease; the main drug complication is ocular toxicity. Renal and cerebral disease are the major determinants of outcome. Without these, the disease is usually relatively mild and has a good long-term outcome.

8.5 Vasculitides

● ●

Learning objectives

You should be able to:
- distinguish the overlapping conditions involving vasculitis
- discuss the management approaches involved in the varying vasculitides.

Case Study

Two months ago, Lawrence felt extremely fit for his 71 years, but then it seemed to change overnight. He just does not feel well, his appetite has gone, he aches and it takes a couple of hours to get going in the morning. His general practitioner has taken a blood test and has said that he needs to start steroids immediately, but Lawrence has been on the Internet and wonders whether he needs a biopsy first because he has heard a lot about steroids.

In many connective tissue diseases, vasculitis occurs and can have serious consequences in terms of morbidity and mortality. There is also a range of conditions in which vasculitis is the major feature. The simplest classification is to think of the calibre of the vessel affected:

- large, e.g. temporal arteritis
- medium, e.g. polyarteritis nodosa
- small, e.g. SLE.

Temporal arteritis and polymyalgia rheumatica

It is very important for you to recognise these overlapping clinical problems because:

- temporal arteritis poses a major threat to vision and is easily treated with corticosteroids
- polymyalgia rheumatica is debilitating and easily treated with corticosteroids.

They are diseases of later life, so be very wary of making the diagnosis in a person aged under 60 years; look for other causes of their symptoms. Histopathological examination in temporal arteritis shows a vasculitis with giant cells ('giant cell arteritis'); characteristically the inflammatory process 'skips' certain sections of an affected artery whilst damaging others.

In temporal arteritis, it is the arteries of the scalp and the ophthalmic artery that are predominantly affected, though occasionally it can cause a stroke through intracranial involvement, particularly of the vertebro-basilar system.

In polymyalgia rheumatica, pathological findings are variable and may be mild or absent. Changes of vasculitis in the muscle bed may be found. There are no typical changes in the muscle.

Temporal arteritis

Headache and scalp tenderness are the dominant features. The headache is usually severe and the patient will say that it is unlike any previous ones (p. 211). Sometimes the first manifestation is monocular blindness (p. 213), which is often permanent. In a few, vision may be impaired temporarily. The patient will often complain of general malaise. Some patients complain of pain on chewing or talking (jaw claudication). On examination, you may find tender temporal arteries, which may be thickened and non-pulsatile. You should make full visual assessment (e.g. visual fields, acuity, ophthalmoscopy, eye movement).

Polymyalgia rheumatica

It is easy to miss this diagnosis because the features are non-specific. Patients complain of general ill-health, with anorexia, weight loss and fatigue. The cardinal feature is *morning stiffness*. It is important to ask specifically about the symptoms of temporal arteritis.

Diagnosis

The diagnosis is based on the clinical features supported by a high ESR, plasma viscosity or CRP, indicating a general inflammatory process. You should consider a temporal artery biopsy using the following criteria:

- It is most useful in temporal arteritis (but one-third are negative), much less so in polymyalgia rheumatica.
- When diagnosis is in doubt.
- Do not delay treatment in patients with a high probability of having the condition
- The yield is greatest when performed within 24 hours of starting treatment (after a week only 10% of biopsies are positive)

- A negative result does not exclude the diagnosis
- A positive result may help if the diagnosis is questioned later (lack of response to treatment or complications of treatment).

Management

Treatment is the immediate administration of corticosteroids. In temporal arteritis, this should be 60 mg prednisolone and the patient should obtain symptomatic relief within 24–48 hours. In polymyalgia rheumatica, a lower dose (10–20 mg) is used and improvement may take 1–2 weeks but is usually quicker. The disease activity is monitored by the patient's wellbeing and changes in the ESR (or plasma viscosity). The dose of steroids is gradually reduced over weeks or months to the lowest maintenance dose that keeps the disease in remission; ideally this should be less than 10 mg prednisolone to prevent long-term side-effects. Corticosteroids *suppress* but do not cure the condition; the natural history is for the arteritis to burn itself out over 2 or more years. Bone protective agents (e.g. bisphosphonates) should be given to reduce osteoporosis (particularly if the patient is over 65 years).

Polyarteritis nodosa

Polyarteritis nodosa is characterised by a patchy vasculitis of medium and large vessels, with fibrinoid necrosis and small aneurysm formation. It is more common in males and usually starts in middle age. In the UK, <10% of the patients are hepatitis surface antigen-positive but in the USA the proportion rises to 50%.

Clinical presentation

The symptoms and signs depend on the vessels affected, but most patients present with non-specific malaise and weight loss. Abdominal pain caused by bowel ischaemia is common. Involvement of the renal vasculature leads to renal failure and malignant hypertension. Elsewhere, brain and limb ischaemia develops. As with all the vasculitides affecting the vasa nervorum, mononeuritis multiplex can occur.

Investigations

The ESR may be raised and there may be a polymorphonuclear leucocytosis. Arteriography of the renal or GI vasculature will demonstrate the microaneurysms. A firm diagnosis may be established by biopsy.

Management

Treatment is with corticosteroids and cyclophosphamide, which has transformed the prognosis to a 10-year survival of 80%. Untreated, the outlook is bleak with death commonly from renal failure. Treatment can usually be tapered and stopped within 12–18 months.

Small vessel vasculitis

Many connective tissue diseases have a small vessel vasculitis. **Henoch–Schönlein purpura** and mixed cryoglobulinaemia (globulins which may cause agglutination below a certain temperature) have, as a major feature, a small vessel vasculitis. In the skin, this causes a purpura which is *palpable* (cf. thrombocytopenia). Features of mixed cryoglobulinaemia are abdominal pain, haematuria, polyarthritis and a mononeuritis. Cases are often self-limiting.

Vasculitis with granulomas

In **Wegener's granulomatosis**, there is a vasculitis with granulomas affecting the respiratory tract (p. 95), nasopharynx and the kidneys. It often presents with a bloody nasal discharge and haemoptysis. Renal failure supervenes. A chest radiograph shows multiple ill-defined nodules that may cavitate. Untreated, most patients will die within 12 months; the use of cyclophosphamide has dramatically altered this.

A variant of the above is Churg–Strauss syndrome, with asthma, pulmonary infiltrates and a very high eosinophil count.

8.6 Systemic sclerosis

> ### Learning objectives
>
> You should be able to:
> - describe the clinical features of systemic sclerosis.

> ### Case Study
>
> Amanda has been troubled for a few months with heartburn. Apart from this and not liking the cold weather because it affects her hands, she has been well, though she will confess to being embarrassed by the 'broken blood vessels' on her face and also that her skin has become 'blotchy' with some white patches.

Systemic sclerosis is a rare condition that is more common in females and has an onset between the third and fifth decades. It is characterised by connective tissue fibrosis. It is often called scleroderma because of the skin involvement, but the preferred term is systemic sclerosis because it is a multisystem disease with variable organ involvement.

Pathology

The cause of the condition is unknown. The histopathological sequence is inflammation, followed by fibrosis and atrophy. As well as the connective tissue changes, there is concentric proliferation and thickening of the intima within the vascular bed. Morphoea is a condition in which the changes are seen only in a patch of skin.

Clinical presentation

Raynaud's phenomenon often predates the other changes and is present in almost all patients with established disease. In the skin, the disease develops with painless oedema, which is followed by thickening of the fingers, hands and face; sometimes it is more widespread. As atrophy develops, the face becomes 'pinched', with a beaked nose, small mouth (microstomia) and widespread telangiectasia. There is also pigmentation and vitiligo. Subcutaneous calcification occurs in nodules, particularly around the fingertips, and these may ulcerate.

The second most common system affected is the GI tract. In the oesophagus, there is decreased/absent peristalsis with dilatation. Patients may be asymptomatic or may have marked dysphagia and heartburn. In the small bowel, stasis and dilatation occur with bacterial overgrowth and malabsorption.

In the musculoskeletal system, there are flexion and spindling deformities of the fingers. Other problems are myositis and myocardial fibrosis (conduction defects and arrhythmias). The lungs may show fibrosis and honeycombing leading to a restrictive defect. Sjögren's syndrome may be present. Progressive renal failure and malignant hypertension are due to an obliterative endarteritis. More deaths in systemic sclerosis are due to lung and heart disease than renal disease because of the aggressive management of hypetension.

Investigations

A positive speckled or nucleolar ANA is present in the majority of patients and RF is found in up to one-third. A minority have a normochromic normocytic anaemia with a raised ESR. Careful monitoring of the blood pressure and renal function is required. Radiographs show deposits of calcium and erosion of the tufts of the distal phalanges. A barium swallow will show oesophageal involvement and a barium meal and follow-through may demonstrate dilatation and flocculation.

Management

No treatment alters the prognosis except for angiotensin-converting enzyme (ACE) inhibitors in accelerated hypertension, which do preserve renal function. Symptomatic treatment for various features may help:

- antibiotics for blind loop syndrome
- electrically heated gloves for Raynaud's phenomenon
- epoprostenol (prostacyclin) infusion for digital ischaemic episodes.

Limited cutaneous systemic sclerosis (CREST) syndrome

A variant of systemic sclerosis has been described by the acronym CREST (calcinosis, raynaud's, esophagitis, sclerodactyly and telangiectasia). Anticentromere antibodies are specific to this condition (now termed **limited cutaneous systemic sclerosis**). It runs a more benign early course than the diffuse type because of the absence of renal involvement, but the patients are still subject to pulmonary hypertension, cardiac lesions, GI involvement and digital ischaemia.

Connective tissue overlap syndromes

These were previously called mixed connective tissue disease but have been renamed because of the overlap between the features of systemic sclerosis, SLE and myositis.

Dermatomyositis and polymyositis

These are covered on page 245.

Raynaud's phenomenon

Raynaud's phenomenon is characterised by:

- episodic colour change of fingers (toes less common) in response to cold
- the colour changes, which are white (ischaemia) then blue (stasis) then red (reactive hyperaemia).

Raynaud's phenomenon is common, affecting about 5% of the population. Over 90% of sufferers are female. It can be associated with connective tissue disease but this is uncommon (<5%). The associations are with:

- systemic sclerosis (most common)
- SLE, Sjögren's syndrome, myositis
- rheumatoid arthritis (least common).

The likelihood of an association with a connective tissue disease is increased if the condition starts for the first time in middle life. Similarly, the presence of ANA is helpful in predicting the probability of underlying disease.

8.7 Crystal arthropathies

Learning objectives

You should be able to:

- describe how gout and pseudogout commonly present
- describe the metabolism of uric acid and how abnormalities lead to gout
- set out the principles of acute treatment and long-term management.

Case Study

Alex is in agony because of pain, swelling and tenderness in his right big toe and ankle. He feels unwell and his wife measured his temperature and found it to be 38°C. He has never had anything like this before and the only thing that has changed is that his general practitioner has told him that he has high blood pressure and has started him on a tablet to bring it down and also a junior aspirin.

Gout

Uric acid is produced by the breakdown of purine bases. The enzyme responsible is xanthine oxidase, which metabolises xanthine. The main pathway for uric acid excretion is in the kidney with filtration at the glomerulus. The uric acid is then reabsorbed in the proximal tubule and subsequently excreted in the distal tubule. *Low-dose* aspirin blocks this distal secretion and causes hyperuricaemia; *high-dose* aspirin blocks proximal reabsorption and, as this is of greater magnitude, the net effect is urate excretion.

Classical gout with monoarthritis affecting the big toe is seen predominantly in men. The first attack is severe, but subsequent attacks are less severe and involve joints other than the big toe. There may be systemic disturbance, including pyrexia. Gout is very uncommon in premeno-

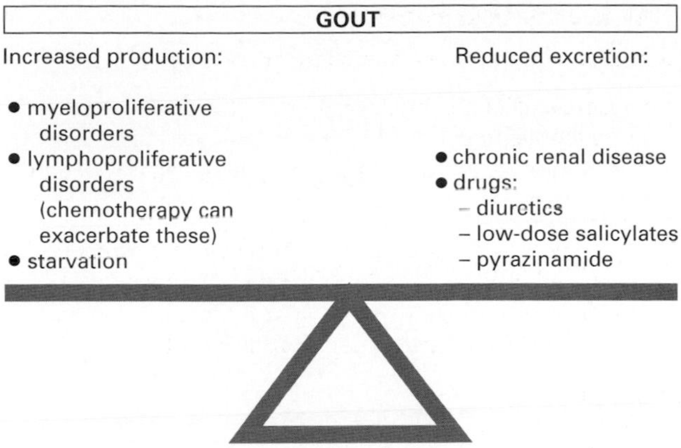

GOUT

Increased production:	Reduced excretion:
• myeloproliferative disorders	
• lymphoproliferative disorders (chemotherapy can exacerbate these)	• chronic renal disease
	• drugs:
	– diuretics
	– low-dose salicylates
• starvation	– pyrazinamide

Fig. 91 Factors affecting the balance between production and excretion of uric acid.

pausal females; in older women it may cause a chronic polyarthritis.

The underlying problem is excess urate production, which cannot be excreted by the kidney. The urate is deposited as crystals in the joints and also in the tissues as **tophi**. The diagnosis is made by identification of urate crystals by polarising microscopy. Asymptomatic hyperuricaemia is not usually treated. Gout can occur secondary to some other process and factors affecting the balance between production and excretion are illustrated in Figure 91.

Management

Management involves:

• identifying any cause, such as drugs or excess alcohol intake most cases will be idiopathic
• treating the acute attack with an NSAID such as diclofenac; occasionally colchicine is used
• unless there is a definite precipitating factor which can be removed, starting *prophylactic* treatment.

Prophylaxis is usually with **allopurinol**, which acts by blocking the enzyme xanthine oxidase. Xanthine is much more water-soluble and can be excreted by the kidneys. You must remember to continue NSAID treatment for a few months because allopurinol treatment allows mobilisation of the urate that was deposited in the tissues and this may precipitate a further attack of gout.

Extremely rapid rises of urate (e.g. in the treatment of leukaemia) can precipitate renal failure, not gout. Consequently, leukaemic patients require allopurinol prophylaxis.

Pseudogout

Pseudogout is predominantly a disease of older people and is often associated with osteoarthritis. Like gout, it is a crystal arthropathy, but it tends to occur in the knees and ankles. The patients often present with a monoarthritis. A radiograph may show a line of calcification within the joint space and examination of the joint aspirate under a polarising microscope will show the crystals of pyrophosphate (Table 77). The principles of management are:

• rest of the joint
• analgesics, particularly NSAIDS, for the inflammatory component
• intra-articular injection of steroids.

8.8 Osteoarthritis and soft tissue rheumatism

Learning objectives

You should be able to:
• diagnose osteoarthritis, distinguish it from rheumatoid arthritis and establish whether it is primary or secondary
• outline the principles of management.

Case Study

Laura feels her knees have all but given up. She knows that she is overweight (BMI 32 kg/m²), but the pain when she walks even 50 m is bad. The diclofenac seems to help, but her general practitioner is not happy about her staying on this even with another tablet 'to protect her stomach'. He has referred her to an orthopaedic consultant to see what her options are.

Osteoarthritis

Some texts use the terms osteo*arthrosis* to mean signs and symptoms of joint damage without a marked inflammatory component and osteo*arthritis* to indicate the presence of inflammation. This can be a difficult distinction (cf. diverticulosis and diverticulitis). You should be aware of why the terms are used and stick to one of them (prefer osteoarthritis).

Osteoarthritis is the most common arthropathy in the UK. The prevalence rises with age, affecting the great majority of patients over the age of 75 years. Most cases are *primary*: that is, no cause can be found; however, you should always ask yourself whether one can be identified, in which case the problem is *secondary* osteoarthritis.

Primary osteoarthritis has a strong familial tendency and is associated with increasing age and obesity.

Pathogenesis and pathology

The cause of osteoarthritis is not known. It is a metabolically active condition that shows a variable balance between anabolic and catabolic processes. At different times, there is increased activity in all the joint tissues. The primary problem seems to be either mechanical damage to cartilage or a biochemical abnormality of the cartilage itself. The chondrocyte releases enzymes, which can degrade collagen and proteoglycans. Crystals released into the synovial fluid initiate and perpetuate inflammation. With repair comes remodelling, producing the characteristic osteophyte.

The list of conditions associated with secondary osteoarthritis is long but can be categorised into:

- mechanical joint damage: occupational, inflammatory arthritis, neuropathic joints, congenital dysplasia, fracture through the joints
- abnormal cartilage: pyrophosphate arthropathy, haemochromatosis.

The joint shows **fibrillation** of the superficial cartilage layer with deeper **fissures**. With advanced disease there is complete cartilage loss and **eburnation** ('polishing') of bone. The synovium is infiltrated with mononuclear cells and the subchondral bone is thickened and may contain cysts.

Clinical presentation

The joints most often affected are the knees and hips. Particularly in **primary generalised osteoarthritis**, the small joints of the hands are involved. **Heberden's nodes** occur in the DIPs (which can be hot and painful when they first arise) and **Bouchard's nodes** in the PIPs. The carpometacarpal joint of the thumb is commonly damaged with *squaring* of the hand at the base of thumb. The apophyseal joints in the cervical and lumbar spine may be involved. Rarely affected, unless there is pre-existing joint abnormality, are the elbows, shoulders and ankles.

The characteristic features of osteoarthritis are:

- pain that is worse in the evenings and is aggravated by use
- stiffness following rest, lasting for only 15–30 minutes, unlike that caused by inflammatory arthritis
- reduced mobility
- disability as the disease progresses.

On examination, the joint is swollen either through bony overgrowth or an effusion. There is limitation of movement, crepitus, deformity and instability.

One important complication, associated with any chronic arthropathy, is the formation of a **Baker's cyst** in the knee. This consists of a degenerative outpouching of the synovium, which can be palpated in the popliteal fossa. It can rupture, allowing tracking of synovial fluid into soleus and gastrocnemius muscles. The fluid sets up an inflammatory response, the signs of which closely mimic those of a deep vein thrombosis. The use of anticoagulants makes the situation worse. It can be diagnosed by ultrasound or an arthrogram.

Investigations and management

There are no haematological or biochemical abnormalities in primary osteoarthritis. The radiological features are shown in Figure 92.

The mainstay of drug therapy is simple analgesia (p. 346). The use of NSAIDs should be limited, particularly in elderly people, because of potential gastrotoxicity. NSAIDs do have a place in those patients with either an acute or a chronic inflammatory component.

Physiotherapists can help by giving guidance on muscle-strengthening exercises (e.g. quadriceps), local therapy (e.g. heat), provision of walking aids and rehabilitation after surgery.

For many patients with severe disability and pain, surgery has been a major advance. Joint replacement of the

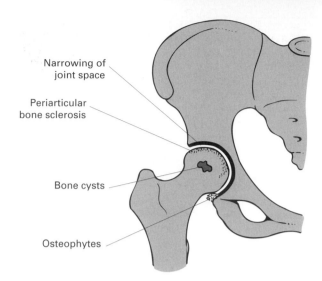

Fig. 92 Schematic representation of radiographic changes in osteoarthritis.

Labels: Narrowing of joint space; Periarticular bone sclerosis; Bone cysts; Osteophytes

hip is extremely successful and replacement of other joints — for example, the knee — gives good results. Other options are arthrodesis and osteotomy.

Fibromyalgia (fibrositis)

Fibromyalgia is a very common condition seen in general practice and rheumatology clinics. The patient has chronic musculoskeletal pain that is poorly localised. Other features include tiredness, headaches and association with irritable bowel syndrome. It is much more common in women. All investigations are normal and just serve to exclude other more serious causes. The management includes reassurance and treatment with antidepressants if a mood disorder is present. Low-dose tricyclic antidepressants can also improve the sleep pattern.

Frozen shoulder (capsulitis)

Patients present with marked unilateral shoulder pain, restriction of movement and tenderness on examination. Over several months, the pain subsides, but the movements become more restricted. Treatment is with analgesics and mobilising exercises as the pain subsides. The whole cycle with recovery (at least in part) takes 1–2 years.

8.9 Calcium metabolism and metabolic bone disease

Learning objectives

You must:

- understand calcium metabolism in terms of its control mechanisms (principally parathyroid hormone (PTH) and vitamin D) and intestinal and renal calcium and phosphate handling
- understand bone formation and resorption in relation to the bone matrix, the 'remodelling unit' of osteoblast and osteoclast and the process of mineralisation

- be able to interpret serum calcium, phosphate and alkaline phosphatase and related parameters (urea, creatinine and albumin)
- understand the causes and management of hypercalcaemia and hypocalcaemia
- understand the causes, clinical presentations and prevention of osteoporosis
- know about some other disorders of bone including Paget's disease.

Case Study

A middle-aged Yemeni woman who always wears traditional dress has many complex symptoms but non-specific pain in her bones and joints has become an increasingly dominant complaint. Her serum calcium is 1.9 mmol/l and phosphate 0.5 mmol/l. Six weeks after starting alfacalcidol, her pain is much improved and she is getting out of the house more.

Calcium and phosphate are measured routinely on multiple channel analysers and abnormalities are not rare so you must be ready to interpret and respond to them from the start of your career. Hypercalcaemia and hypocalcaemia are important — if infrequent — medical emergencies. Amongst bone diseases, osteoporosis is a major and potentially preventable cause of debility in old age. Metabolic bone disease is *par excellence* a topic in which command of simple anatomical and physiological principles makes learning easy.

This section will combine a problem-orientated (hypo- and hypercalcaemia) and disease-orientated approach to metabolic bone disease. Table 78 shows the relationships between them.

Functional anatomy of bone

Bone is composed of a collagen matrix (osteoid) impregnated with calcium phosphate (hydroxyapatite crystals). It has a dense cortex and a less dense medulla composed of trabecular bone. Long bones have a central marrow cavity. Bone is vascular and contains:

Table 78 Bone diseases related to serum calcium

	Serum calcium		
	Low	High	Normal
Parathyroid			
Hyperparathyroidism		*	
Hypoparathyroidism	*		
Vitamin D			
Vitamin D excess		*	
Osteomalacia/rickets	*		
Malignant hypercalcaemia		*	
Renal bone disease	*	*	*
Osteoporosis			*
Paget's disease			*

- osteoblasts that form the osteoid and initiate the process of crystallisation
- osteoclasts: multinucleate cells that erode and resorb mineralised bone.

It is important to conceive of bone as a dynamic structure in a constant state of turnover, adapting to injury and mechanical stress. About 10% of its mass is remodelled each year. Remodelling units consist of osteoclasts and osteoblasts, and move slowly through bone, completing remodelling in about 100 days. Alkaline phosphatase is an enzyme secreted by the osteoblasts that indicates the activity of remodelling units.

Calcium and phosphate metabolism

Calcium comprises 1.5% of body weight and 99% of it is within the skeleton. A small fraction of skeletal calcium is in a rapidly exchangeable pool, but the majority can only be released by increased osteoclast activity. In blood, calcium is about 50% albumin-bound (and biologically inactive). Most unbound calcium consists of free calcium ions ('ionised') and this is the biologically active fraction, essential to blood coagulation and nerve and muscle function. An important practical point is that a low plasma albumin reduces the total calcium concentration reported by the biochemistry laboratory without any change in the ionised fraction, and vice versa. Moreover, the ionised fraction (which cannot easily be measured) increases with acidosis and falls with alkalosis. That is why hyperventilation causes hypocalcaemic tetany without any change in total plasma calcium.

Calcium is actively absorbed from the gut under the control of vitamin D. There is obligatory reabsorption of calcium in the proximal renal tubule and variable reabsorption in the distal tubule controlled by parathyroid hormone (PTH).

Like calcium, most phosphate is in a skeletal pool. It is absorbed from the gut in direct proportion to dietary intake and reabsorbed from the glomerular filtrate in the proximal tubule, a process inhibited by PTH. Apart from the hormonal control mechanism described below, there is a direct relationship between plasma calcium and phosphate concentrations because calcium phosphate comes out of solution once the product of their concentrations exceeds a critical value.

Vitamin D and parathyroid hormone

The vitamin D/parathyroid interrelated hormone systems control calcium absorption and excretion and influence the balance between bone deposition and resorption. There are two sources of 'parent' vitamin D:

- the skin, where it is formed in response to sunlight
- intestinal absorption.

Vitamin D undergoes two hydroxylation steps (25-hydroxylation in the liver and 1-hydroxylation in the kidneys) to become the biologically active 1,25-dihydroxy-cholecalciferol (calcitriol). Active vitamin D increases intestinal calcium absorption.

PTH is secreted by the parathyroid glands in direct response to changes in plasma calcium and phosphate and is under negative feedback control from 1,25-dihydroxy-cholecalciferol. Its effects are to increase plasma calcium and lower phosphate by:

- increasing osteoclast activity
- increasing 1-hydroxylation of vitamin D
- increasing renal calcium reabsorption
- reducing renal phosphate reabsorption.

The actions of vitamin D and PTH are intimately interrelated and conjointly regulate serum calcium and phosphate within tight limits.

Other hormones and the skeleton

Calcitonin

It is secreted by the parafollicular cells of the thyroid in response to hypercalcaemia and reduces bone resorption. It does not have a major physiological role, as illustrated by the fact that diseases of calcitonin deficiency and excess do not disrupt calcium metabolism; however, pharmacological doses can be used to reduce bone remodelling in Paget's disease and net bone resorption in malignant hypercalcaemia.

Glucocorticoids

They reduce calcium and phosphate absorption (an important therapeutic effect in vitamin D excess) and inhibit net bone formation the basis for steroid-induced osteoporosis.

Thyroid hormones

They reduce bone mineral density and can cause osteoporosis in hyperthyroidism.

Sex steroids

They increase bone formation over resorption by a direct effect on osteoblasts.

PTH-related peptide (PTH-rp)

This hormone is produced by some malignant tumours. It is chemically related to native PTH and causes malignant hypercalcaemia (see below) but is not detected by PTH assays.

Clinical presentation

Symptoms and signs can be caused by:

- hypocalcaemia
- hypercalcaemia
- bone pain, deformity and/or fractures.

Hypocalcaemia

Clinical manifestations result from irritability and dysfunction of nerves and muscles and include:

- paraesthesiae in the hands and around the mouth
- weakness
- spasms of skeletal muscles (tetany); laryngeal stridor and asphyxia in severe cases
- mental confusion and fits.

Signs can be precipitated by:

- tapping the facial nerve over the parotid gland; a positive response is twitching of the ipsilateral facial muscles (Chvostek's sign)

- occluding the brachial artery by inflating a sphygmomanometer above systolic pressure for 3 minutes; a positive response is carpal spasm (Trousseau's sign).

These signs are, at best, a stop-gap and cannot substitute for measuring plasma calcium.

Hypercalcaemia

The symptoms and signs are vague and non-specific but hypercalcaemia is common so you must have a high index of suspicion; measure serum calcium if there is anything to suggest the diagnosis. The signs affect a range of systems.

Renal

These are caused by hypercalcaemia-induced insensitivity to ADH (nephrogenic diabetes insipidus):

- thirst, polyuria, nocturia
- symptoms and signs of volume depletion
- symptoms of renal stones/nephrocalcinosis.

Intestinal

- Nausea and vomiting
- Constipation
- Dyspeptic abdominal pain
- Symptoms and signs of pancreatitis (acute pancreatitis is a sign of **severe** hypercalcaemia).

Neurological

- Lassitude
- Mood disturbance, particularly depression
- Confusion: sign of severe hypercalcaemia
- Drowsiness: sign of severe hypercalcaemia.

Ocular

There is corneal calcification: a visible band at the medial and lateral corneo-scleral junction. Corneal calcification, like renal stones, is evidence of longstanding hypercalcaemia. It is asymptomatic and best seen with a slit lamp.

Cardiovascular

Hypertension is a sign of hypercalcaemia.

Investigations

It follows from the basic physiology of calcium metabolism that you should measure calcium, phosphate and alkaline phosphatase as a triad. Alkaline phosphatase is raised if there is increased bone remodelling but may be normal in patients with abnormal serum calcium and phosphate (e.g. hyperparathyroidism without significant bone disease) and abnormal in patients with normal calcium and phosphate (Paget's disease and malignant bone destruction). The interpretation of calcium and phosphate is considered under the individual diseases. Once an abnormality of plasma calcium or phosphate has been established, these additional tests may be informative:

- 24-hour urinary calcium and phosphate excretion
- renal function (urea and creatinine)
- PTH and 25-hydroxyvitamin D
- urinary cyclic AMP, an index of PTH activity

- urinary hydroxyproline excretion (best measured as the hydroxyproline:creatinine ratio in an early morning urine sample), an index of bone remodelling.

Radiological investigations

Radiological investigations include:

- plain radiology, which is not sensitive for early disease but may show specific abnormalities in Paget's disease, hyperparathyroidism, osteomalacia/rickets, renal bone disease, malignancy and osteoporosis
- densitometry (by photon absorptiometry or quantitative CT), which is much more sensitive than plain radiology for a reduced bone mass
- radionuclide scanning, which is sensitive to increased bone remodelling, showing areas of increased vascularity as 'hot spots'
- CT and MR, used to investigate bone and joint structure in detail.

Bone biopsy

This provides detailed morphological information but is needed in only a small number of patients.

Hypercalcaemia

In its clinical presentations, hypercalcaemia ranges from a mild and asymptomatic biochemical abnormality to a medical emergency. The 'big two' causes are hyperparathyroidism and malignant hypercalcaemia. Vitamin D excess is less common but important to remember because it is steroid-responsive. Immobilisation can worsen all causes of hypercalcaemia by increasing bone resorption. The causes you are most likely to encounter are shown bold in this list:

- hyperparathyroidism
  — **primary**
  — tertiary
- malignancy
  — **solid tumours**: breast, bronchus, thyroid, kidney, prostate
  — **haematological**: myeloma, leukaemias
- vitamin D excess
  — excess intake, e.g. excessive consumption of vitamin tablets or cod liver oil
  — excess formation: granulomatous diseases including sarcoidosis and tuberculosis, glucocorticoid deficiency, lymphoma.

Hyperparathyroidism

Hypercalcaemia results from increased delivery of calcium into the extracellular pool, which is reinforced, in hyperparathyroid states, by increased renal reabsorption. As serum calcium rises, total urinary calcium excretion increases (though fractional excretion may not). Thus, hypercalcaemia can remain mild so long as glomerular filtration and flow are maintained and the patient experiences thirst and responds to it by drinking. Unfortunately, more severe hypercalcaemia causes anorexia, vomiting and drowsiness which, in the face of continued polyuria, lead to volume depletion and, ultimately, renal hypofiltration. When this occurs, the escape route for calcium is blocked and severe hypercalcaemia occurs (e.g. serum calcium >3.5 mmol/l). The immediate management of severe hypercalcaemia follows from this:

- You should first assess blood volume and renal function; volume depletion and renal impairment (very high urea, high creatinine (low estimated GFR)) are usually seen in severe hypercalcaemia.
- If the patient is volume-depleted, give i.v. saline, aiming for a urine output >4 litres daily; furosemide may help, once volume has been replaced, to increase calcium excretion.

Management is then directed at establishing the cause and achieving a cure. Appropriate steps include:

- careful history and physical examination for evidence of neoplasia, parathyroid disease, vitamin D excess, sarcoidosis, etc.
- measurement of PTH and 25-hydroxycholecalciferol
- steroid suppression test.

The definitive treatment depends upon the final diagnosis but emergency treatment with bisphosphonates (see below) should always be considered if rehydration fails to control hypercalcaemia.

Primary hyperparathyroidism

Primary hyperparathyroidism has a prevalence of 1 in 1000, making it one of the commoner endocrine diseases. Around 80% of cases are caused by a parathyroid adenoma and 5% by multiple adenomas. The remaining 15% are caused by diffuse parathyroid hyperplasia and (least commonly) carcinoma. Rarely, hyperparathyroidism is part of the syndrome of multiple endocrine neoplasia. The prevalence of hyperparathyroidism increases with age. Modes of presentation in decreasing order of frequency are:

- a chance biochemical finding
- thirst, polyuria or abdominal symptoms
- symptoms of bone disease, including pain, fractures and deformity
- renal stones
- hypercalcaemic crisis, particularly after periods of immobilisation
- hypertension.

The parathyroid glands are rarely palpable.
Investigations The diagnostic features are:

- a raised serum calcium
- a low phosphate
- a raised or 'inappropriately normal' serum PTH
- hypercalciuria; urinary calcium excretion must always be checked to exclude 'familial benign hypercalcaemia' caused by reduced calcium excretion, distinguishable from primary hyperparathyroidism by not having a raised fractional calcium excretion and being unresponsive to parathyroidectomy.

Subperiosteal resorption of the phalanges is the commonest radiological sign; localised areas of bone resorption with fibrosis ('osteitis fibrosa et cystica') may also be seen on plain radiographs of the long bones and ribs. Plain radiographs and bone densitometry may show generalised osteopenia. Ultrasound, CT, MR and radionuclide (sestamibi) scanning and venous catheterisation studies can be used to localise parathyroid adenomas, but exploration by an experienced surgeon is the most sensitive technique. Many clinicians proceed directly to surgery once the biochemical diagnosis has been made.

Management Surgery is the only effective treatment and is indicated for:

- more severe hypercalcaemia; calcium ≥2.8 mmol/l
- symptoms
- complications, including renal stones, osteoporosis, pancreatitis and renal failure.

If surgery fails, treatment with a bisphosphonate may be needed to control hypercalcaemia. The availability of better imaging modalities and minimally invasive surgery is making it increasingly appropriate to operate on asymptomatic hypercalcaemia and/or older people to prevent long-term complications.

Malignant hypercalcaemia

There are four mechanisms by which malignant diseases cause hypercalcaemia:

- direct destruction of bone
- secretion of osteoclast-activating cytokines (as in multiple myeloma)
- secretion of PTH-rp (p. 361)
- overproduction of 1,25-dihydroxycholecalciferol (as may occur in lymphomas).

Malignant disease can cause extremely severe hypercalcaemia. This usually signifies widespread bone involvement. It has an aggressive course and patients may develop severe hypercalcaemia very rapidly because they are already anorexic as an effect of their underlying disease and get into a vicious circle of volume depletion and worsening hypercalcaemia. It has an extremely poor prognosis.

Investigations

Consider the possibility of malignancy, including myeloma, and arrange the following in every case of severe hypercalcaemia:

- haemoglobin and ESR
- liver function tests
- plain radiographs of the chest and pelvis
- plasma protein and urine electrophoresis to exclude myeloma.

A radionuclide bone scan may detect malignant deposits not seen on plain radiology.

Management

The importance of volume replacement has been considered above. Remember that severely hypercalcaemic patients may develop acute renal failure because of volume depletion or myeloma kidney, so the neck veins and urine output must be carefully observed. Corticosteroids can lower calcium in myeloma and some other haematological malignancies but are otherwise ineffective. If these measures fail, the treatment is a parenteral bisphosphonate, such as pamidronate or clodronate, which prevents bone resorption by coating hydroxyapatite crystals. This can normalise serum calcium within a few days.

States of vitamin D excess

Vitamin D excess causes hypercalcaemia by increasing intestinal calcium absorption. Vitamin D intoxication is uncommon, although it may occur inadvertently in the treatment of renal bone disease or hypocalcaemia. Uncommon, but important, is the synthesis of 1,25-dihydroxycholecalciferol in the granulomas of sarcoidosis (p. 94) and tuberculosis, in which case the diagnosis may be made from a chest radiograph. Glucocorticoids antagonise the effect of vitamin D on calcium absorption so a trial of glucocorticoids can control hypercalcaemia and confirm the diagnosis.

Hypocalcaemia

Hypoparathyroidism is the main cause of severe hypocalcaemia because intact parathyroid glands can restore serum calcium to near normal in most other diseases. The causes of hypocalcaemia include:

- hypoparathyroidism
  — surgical
  — autoimmune
- resistance to PTH (pseudohypoparathyroidism)
- vitamin D deficiency (see osteomalacia/rickets)
- renal failure (see renal bone disease, p. 184)
- binding of calcium (usually obvious from the clinical context)
  — acute pancreatitis
  — massive blood transfusion.

Clinical presentation

As in hypercalcaemia, the presentation of hypocalcaemia ranges from an asymptomatic biochemical finding to a life-threatening emergency (symptomatic with a serum calcium <1.8 mmol/l). Management is summarised in the box.

Clinical Box: Emergency treatment: management of severe hypocalcaemia

1. Establish venous access and quickly take blood for:
   - Calcium, phosphate, alkaline phosphatase, PTH
   - Urea and creatinine

2. Give i.v. 10% calcium gluconate, 10 ml over 10 minutes

3. Call for senior help

4. Give repeated doses or a slow infusion of calcium gluconate according to symptomatic response

---

Hypoparathyroidism

Hypoparathyroidism is most often a result of surgery for thyroid, parathyroid or pharyngeal disease and may present as a postoperative emergency. Less common is idiopathic hypoparathyroidism which:

- may be familial or sporadic
- is caused by autoimmunity

- is associated with other organ-specific autoimmune diseases such as Addison's disease and hypothyroidism
- may be associated with chronic mucocutaneous candidiasis and malabsorption syndrome.

With prolonged hypoparathyroidism, whatever its cause, calcification may be seen in the basal ganglia on a plain skull radiograph or CT scan. The biochemical signs of hypoparathyroidism are:

- hypocalcaemia
- a raised serum phosphate
- low serum PTH.

If PTH is unexpectedly high, the patient has pseudohypoparathyroidism (tissue PTH insensitivity).

Management

PTH, though now available as a therapeutic agent, is not used for hypoparathyroidism and treatment is with a combination of oral calcium and a vitamin D metabolite or analogue (calcitriol 1,25-dihydroxycholecalciferol) or alfacalcidol (1α-hydroxycholecalciferol) to increase its absorption.

Osteomalacia

The syndrome of vitamin D deficiency is termed rickets if it occurs in children and osteomalacia once growth has ceased. Failure of calcium absorption is compensated for by increased PTH secretion ('secondary hyperparathyroidism'), which reduces the bone mineral content and leaves osteoid unmineralised. The biochemical signs are:

- a low-normal or (uncommonly) low serum calcium
- a low phosphate, because of the phosphaturic effect of PTH.

Note that this low phosphate distinguishes rickets/ osteomalacia from hypoparathyroidism. Alkaline phosphatase may be normal or raised if there is parathyroid bone disease. The serum 25-hydroxycholecalciferol level is low.

Osteomalacia is rarely caused by pure dietary deficiency, because vitamin D synthesis in skin can compensate; however, chronically ill or old people may lack sunlight exposure and an adequate diet and become vitamin D-deficient. Asian people may have the same risk factors, compounded by a diet high in phytates (chapati), which bind calcium in the gut. Other causes include:

- malabsorption syndrome, reducing the absorption of fat-soluble vitamin D
- renal disease, in which there is impaired 1-hydroxylation of vitamin D
- liver disease, with impaired 25-hydroxylation of vitamin D
- anticonvulsant therapy, in which there is impaired 25-hydroxylation and tissue vitamin D resistance.

Clinical presentation

Adults with osteomalacia experience bone pain and may have weakness and a waddling gait. Radiological signs are:

- osteopenia
- Looser zones: localised areas of decalcification on the concave surfaces of bones, particularly the femur and pelvis
- biconcave deformity of vertebrae.

Management

Osteomalacia is treated with calcium and vitamin D supplements.

Renal bone disease (renal osteodystrophy)

This is covered in Chapter 4 (p. 184).

Osteoporosis

Bone mass is determined by the relative activities of osteoblasts and osteoclasts. During growth, bone formation exceeds resorption. In the fourth decade, age-related bone loss begins. A reduced bone mass, predisposing to fractures after relatively mild trauma, is termed osteoporosis. Unlike osteomalacia, the mass of osteoid is reduced, although the bone that is present is normally mineralised. Trabecular bone is lost more than cortical bone, so fractures occur at sites composed mostly of trabecular bone.

Epidemiology and causes

Loss of bone mass is a feature of ageing. An individual is predisposed to osteoporosis by having a low peak bone mass, a rapid rate of loss thereafter or advanced age. Having reached a level of bone mass that predisposes to fractures, only a small further reduction greatly increases the fracture risk. Women differ from men in undergoing an abrupt and severe reduction in sex steroid secretion at the menopause, which accelerates their rate of bone loss. As a result, they are more prone to osteoporosis. Osteoporosis is a major socioeconomic problem. One in two women and one in six men will sustain a fracture related to osteoporosis by age 90. These fractures may cause permanent disability. Mortality is increased over the months after an osteoporotic fracture.

Osteoporosis may present at several stages of life:

- associated with the rapid loss of bone mass after the menopause
- associated with progressive bone loss into old age
- 'idiopathic' osteoporosis, caused by premature bone loss, presenting in middle age.

Osteoporosis may be 'primary' or secondary to:

- endocrine/metabolic disease
  — glucocorticoid excess: Cushing's disease, steroid therapy
  — hyperthyroidism
  — hypogonadism
  — growth hormone deficiency (hypopituitarism)
  — hyperparathyroidism
  — diabetes mellitus
  — renal osteodystrophy
- neoplasia: multiple myeloma
- GI disease: malabsorption, gastrectomy, liver disease
- rheumatological disease: rheumatoid arthritis

- other: immobility, substance abuse, malnutrition, any chronic, debilitating disease.

Clinical presentation

Until fractures occur, osteoporosis is asymptomatic. They are as painful as any other fracture. Typical sites are:

- distal radius
- femoral neck
- vertebral bodies.

Patients may lose height and develop increased spinal curvature and a protuberant abdomen.

Investigations

Radiologically, there may be generalised osteopenia, wedge collapse of vertebrae, 'codfish vertebrae' (caused by herniation of the discs into the centre of the vertebral body) and increased spinal curvature. Bone densitometry (p. 361) is used to confirm the diagnosis and estimate fracture risk. Plain radiology and bone scanning can be used to demonstrate fractures. Biochemistry is normal, apart from a raised alkaline phosphatase during fracture healing.

You should suspect secondary osteoporosis in young or middle-aged patients and investigate them for the diseases listed above.

Management

Patients with fractures need adequate analgesia; those with vertebral osteoporosis may have relentless pain. There are various treatments that reduce bone resorption and the risk of future fractures but do nothing for fractures which have already occurred. They include:

- bisphosphonates (alendronate), which are proven to reduce the rate of vertebral fracturing
- a physiological dose of vitamin D with calcium, which may reduce fracture risk and is relatively safe
- Selective oestrogen receptive modulators (e.g. raloxifene) which have an oestrogen-like effect on bone
- PTH (teriparatide).

Patients with osteoporosis should be physically active, take a high-calcium diet and avoid the risk factors listed below. Their response to treatment can be monitored densitometrically.

Prevention

Risk factors for osteoporosis are:

- hypogonadism or an early menopause
- family history of osteoporosis
- substance abuse (alcohol and tobacco)
- inactivity
- corticosteroid therapy and the endocrine diseases listed above.

It is part of general health education to encourage weight-bearing exercise, a high-calcium diet, a moderate alcohol intake and not smoking; this is particularly important in high-risk individuals. High-risk individuals can be selected for preventive therapy by densitometry. The value of densitometric screening of the general population is unproven.

Paget's disease of bone

Paget's disease affects 4% of the population over age 40 years, the prevalence increasing with age. It is more common in men than in women and most prevalent in Anglo-Saxons, particularly in the north-west of England. The primary abnormality is in the osteoclasts, which are enlarged, have more nuclei than normal and resorb bone excessively. This is thought to be the late effect of a virus infection. Osteoblast function is also increased. The bone is formed chaotically, expanded, poorly calcified and unusually vascular. It is soft and prone to deformity and fractures. Paget's disease affects the tibia, femur, vertebrae, pelvis and skull.

Clinical presentation

Increased osteoblast activity causes an increased plasma alkaline phosphatase and a characteristic radiographic appearance (see below). The disease is usually asymptomatic and found by chance radiographically or by measurement of alkaline phosphatase. It may, however, cause symptoms which can be disabling:

- pain, caused by bone expansion, deformity and fractures
- warmth, as a result of increased vascularity
- deformity, causing immobility and secondary osteoarthritis
- nerve root compression, typically deafness because of skull involvement; spinal compression may occur
- osteogenic sarcoma, which may rarely develop.

Investigations

Alkaline phosphatase and the hydroxyproline:creatinine ratio (p. 361) are high, reflecting increased osteoblast and osteoclast activity, respectively. Radionuclide bone scans show areas of increased uptake, caused by increased vascularity. Plain radiographs show:

- thickening of the cortex
- trabecular thickening and sclerosis
- areas of osteolysis
- deformity.

Management

The bisphosphonates bind to hydroxyapatite and increase the resistance of bone to osteoclasts. They are highly effective at relieving pain and can normalise the biochemical markers and prevent progression.

Self-assessment: questions

Any or all of each set of five statements may be true or false. Choose your answers and see the reasoning behind the correct answer on pages 372–373.

Multiple choice questions

1. The following are seen with non-steroidal anti-inflammatory drugs (NSAIDs):
   a. Improvement in renal function
   b. Increase in serum potassium
   c. Increased risk of peptic ulcer complications
   d. Improved long-term prognosis of rheumatoid arthritis
   e. Improvement in coexistent asthma

2. In giant cell arteritis:
   a. The erythrocyte sedimentation rate (ESR) falls with steroid treatment
   b. Radiographs of MCP (metacarpophalangeal) and IP (interphalangeal) joints are normal
   c. The patient often gains weight
   d. Muscle biopsy may be abnormal
   e. Pain may occur during mastication

3. The following are features of systemic lupus erythematosus (SLE):
   a. Raynaud's phenomenon
   b. Mononeuritis multiplex
   c. Thrombocytopenia
   d. Lymphopenia
   e. A very high C-reactive protein

4. Rheumatoid factor is:
   a. An antibody to sheep erythrocytes
   b. Present when rheumatoid nodules are present
   c. Diagnostic of rheumatoid arthritis
   d. Usually of the IgA subtype
   e. Not found in rheumatoid synovial, pleural or pericardial fluid

5. In primary osteoarthritis:
   a. The ESR is normal
   b. Proximal interphalangeal (PIP) joints are not usually affected
   c. Radiographs show characteristic erosions of articular margins
   d. Morning stiffness usually lasts over 1 hour
   e. Carpometacarpal joint of the thumb involvement is a common finding

6. In gout:
   a. Tophi are an early sign
   b. Allopurinol is used to treat the acute attack
   c. Furosemide helps to increase urate excretion
   d. Large joints are not affected
   e. Raised serum urate makes the diagnosis certain

7. Clinical features characteristic of psoriatic polyarthritis include:
   a. Distal interphalangeal (DIP) joint involvement
   b. Asymmetrical small joint involvement
   c. Arthritis mutilans
   d. Sacroiliitis
   e. Temporomandibular joint involvement

8. Ankylosing spondylitis:
   a. Is more common in females
   b. May present as a severe oligoarthritis
   c. Is associated with the histocompatibility antigen HLA-DW3
   d. Is associated with pulmonary fibrosis
   e. Involves the PIP joints

9. The following statements are true of normal synovial fluid:
   a. The fluid is clear and colourless
   b. Calcium pyrophosphate crystals may be found
   c. The viscosity is low
   d. The fibrin content is high
   e. The predominant white cell is the lymphocyte

10. Presenting features of rheumatoid arthritis indicating a poor prognosis include:
    a. Rheumatoid factor in high titre
    b. Systemic features
    c. Rheumatoid nodules
    d. Erosive joint changes
    e. Hand involvement

11. The following are true:
    a. Three inflamed painful joints occurring together makes septic arthritis very unlikely
    b. If *Staphylococcus aureus* is cultured from an inflamed joint, oral flucloxacillin and bed rest are the primary treatments
    c. Viruses do not cause acutely inflamed, swollen joints
    d. Absence of fever rules out septic arthritis
    e. A chronic monoarthritis may be caused by *Mycobacterium tuberculosis*

12. Concerning osteomyelitis:
    a. Debridement of infected bone is essential for cure in chronic bacterial osteomyelitis
    b. It is usually accompanied by a very high ESR
    c. A distinctive feature of chronic osteomyelitis is a discharging sinus
    d. A positive culture from a sinus track is a good indication of the bacterial cause of the chronic osteomyelitis
    e. Usually 2 or 3 weeks' antibiotic therapy is adequate for cure

13. The following autoantibody tests are matched with the relevant diseases:

    a. Antibasement membrane antibodies and Goodpasture's syndrome

    b. Intrinsic factor antibody and pernicious anaemia

    c. Perinuclear antineutrophil cytoplasm antibodies (ANCA) and polyarteritis

    d. Antinuclear antibody and secondary Raynaud's phenomenon

    e. Antimitochondrial antibodies and antiphospholipid syndrome

14. With regard to reactive arthritis:

    a. It may be caused by either *Salmonella* or *Campylobacter* spp.

    b. It is usually chronic and unremitting over 3–4 years

    c. Confidence in the diagnosis rests on growing a bacterium from stool or other sites

    d. NSAIDs are appropriate therapy

    e. Rheumatic fever should be excluded

15. The following are true:

    a. Plasma calcium and phosphate alter independently of one another

    b. Dietary calcium intake is the main determinant of plasma calcium

    c. Plasma alkaline phosphatase is a marker of the activity of osteoblasts

    d. Normal mineralisation of bone depends upon adequate intestinal calcium absorption

    e. Renal failure causes phosphate retention

16. The following are true:

    a. Osteoporosis is among the more common causes of hypercalcaemia

    b. Granulomatous diseases, whatever their aetiology, may cause hypercalcaemia

    c. A characteristic of parathyroid hormone (PTH)-mediated hypercalcaemia is a low serum phosphate

    d. Renal bone disease never causes hypercalcaemia

    e. A haematological malignancy should be considered as a possible diagnosis in a patient presenting with hypercalcaemia

17. The following are true:

    a. Osteoporosis is characterised by deficiency of osteoid and bone mineral

    b. Bone mass peaks at the age of 55 and declines thereafter

    c. Prolonged inactivity causes loss of bone mass

    d. An incidental effect of corticosteroid therapy is to increase bone mass

    e. Hypogonadism only causes osteoporosis in old age

18. The following are true:

    a. Hypocalcaemia may present as epilepsy

    b. Bedside examination is a highly sensitive way of detecting hypocalcaemia

    c. Calcitonin is an effective treatment for recurrent hypocalcaemia

    d. Cerebral calcification may occur in hypoparathyroidism

    e. Patients with hypoparathyroidism are treated with recombinant human PTH

Single best answer multiple choice questions

For each numbered question, only ONE of the options lettered a–e is correct.

1. A 57-year-old woman is seen in the outpatient clinic with a 6-month history of pain and swelling in both wrists and her metacarpophalangeal and proximal interphalangeal joints. On direct questioning, she says that she is taking a couple of hours to get 'her hands going in the morning'. There is no previous history of note. Your examination confirms the swelling of the joints with local increase in temperature. The results of the blood tests you order show:

   Haemoglobin 103 g/l
   Mean cell volume 80 fl
   Erythrocyte sedimentation rate 63 mm/hr
   Antinuclear antibodies and rheumatoid factor Not detected

   What is the most likely diagnosis?

   a. Osteoarthritis

   b. Gout

   c. Systemic lupus erythematosus

   d. Reactive arthritis

   e. Rheumatoid arthritis

2. A 29-year-old man attends his general practitioner because of pain in his left ankle and knee as well as his right elbow. He says that he came back from holiday in Greece about 2 weeks ago and had an 'upset stomach' there with some loose motions. He also has noticed that his eyes have been 'a bit red' for the last couple of days. What is the most likely diagnosis?

   a. Ankylosing spondylitis

   b. Gout

   c. Septic arthritis

   d. Reactive arthritis

   e. Rheumatoid arthritis

3. A 71-year-old woman has been experiencing pain in her hands which has gradually been getting worse over the last 3–4 years. During this time, she has noticed some swelling of her finger joints and moving her thumb can be particularly painful. It takes a few minutes to 'get her hands going' at the start of the day, and the pain tends to be worse by

the end of the day but has been helped by paracetamol. On examination, there is some pain on moving her thumbs and bony swellings at her distal interphalangeal joints. Results of blood texts show:

Haemoglobin 129 g/l
Mean cell volume 80 fl
Erythrocyte sedimentation rate 12 mm/hr
Antinuclear antibodies and rheumatoid factor Not detected

What is the most likely diagnosis?

a. Rheumatoid arthritis
b. Psoriatic arthropathy
c. Pseudogout
d. Osteoarthritis
e. Systemic sclerosis

4. A 32-year-old woman is seen in the rheumatology clinic because of mild pain in her hands and feet, as well as a red rash over her nose and cheeks. This is unsightly and she was also troubled by an itchy red rash when she went on holiday to Spain. Her investigations show:

Haemoglobin: 130 g/l
White cell count: 6.6×10^9/l
Lymphocytes: 1.2×10^9/l
Erythrocyte sedimentation rate: 50 mm/hr
Urinalysis: Negative
Urea and electrolytes, liver function tests: Normal
Rheumatoid factor: Negative
Antinuclear factor: Positive titre 1:320
Pregnancy test: Negative

What would be the best treatment?

a. Ibuprofen
b. Prednisolone
c. Methotrexate
d. Sulfasalazine
e. Hydroxychloroquine.

5. A 54-year-old man presents with a 2-month history of severe pain affecting his hands, feet and knees. He has morning stiffness lasting for up to 2 hours. The symptoms persist despite regular naproxen. On examination there is a symmetrical polyarthritis with some nodules on the extensor surfaces of his arms. Investigations show:

Haemoglobin: 100 g/l
Mean cell volume: 84 fl
Erythrocyte sedimentation rate: 73 mm/hr
Urinalysis: Negative
Urea and electrolytes, liver function tests: Normal
Rheumatoid factor: Positive: 1:640 titre
Antinuclear factor: Negative
Radiographs hands, feet: Normal

What would be the best treatment?

a. Diclofenac sodium
b. Sulfasalazine

c. Prednisolone
d. Colchicine
e. Hydroxychloroquine

Extended matched questions

EMQ 1

Theme: Possible diagnoses in arthropathy
Options
1. Acute septic arthritis
2. Ankylosing spondylitis
3. Enteropathic arthropathy
4. Gout
5. Haemarthrosis
6. Psuedogout
7. Osteoarthitis
8. Psoriatic arthritis
9. Reactive arthritis
10. Rheumatoid arthritis
11. Systemic lupus erythematosus

For patients, A–E, choose the most likely diagnosis.

A. A 61-year-old man is complaining of a painful ankle. In the previous medical history, he started on diuretics for hypertension 2 weeks ago. On examination, his temperature is 37.3°C and he has a painful, hot, swollen left ankle.

B. A 69-year-old woman with a chronic burn-out inflammatory arthropathy has been unwell for 2 days, feeling hot and cold. On examination, her temperature is 38.9°C and her left elbow is swollen, hot and 'boggy'.

C. A 23-year-old man has recently returned from several months of travelling through Asia. In the last month, he has been troubled with severe bloody diarrhoea, but this settled after a couple of weeks. He has not had any previous gastrointestinal problems. On examination, his temperature is 36.7°C and he is generally well. In his locomotor system, he has some evidence of a mild asymmetrical synovitis affecting his feet and knees.

D. A 51-year-old man has had a progressive asymmetrical arthropathy for the past 27 years. On examination, he has a significant degree of joint damage and disruption in his hands, including the proximal and distal interphalangeal joints. He also has discrete erythematous patches that are scaly and widespread over his body.

E. An 83-year-old woman is increasingly troubled with pain on walking. This is particularly noticeable if she sits down for any length of time, but after about 10 minutes she then 'loosens up'. On examination, she is overweight and there is reduction in hip abduction and rotation, particularly on the left side.

EMQ 2

Theme: Drug treatment in arthropathy
Options
1. Azathioprine
2. Codeine phosphate
3. Ibuprofen
4. Joint injection of corticosteroid
5. Infliximab
6. Morphine
7. Oral prednisolone
8. Paracetamol
9. Sulfasalazine
10. Topical diclofenac

For each patient, choose the most beneficial treatment.

A. A 79-year-old man is having a lot of difficulty with pain in his shoulder that is limiting his activities. It has been present for a few months and is not settling. Examination shows limited movement with pain. A plain radiograph confirms degenerative changes.

B. A 64-year-old woman with generalised mild osteoarthritis is troubled by pain during the day. There is no history of morning stiffness or any inflamed joints. On examination, there are changes of osteoarthritis but no evidence of an active arthropathy.

C. A 58-year-old man has a further attack of gout affecting his right big toe. On examination, the first metatarsophalangeal joint is swollen, hot and very tender to touch.

D. A 67-year-old man presents with marked morning stiffness and muscle pain for about 3 months. He feels unwell, but there is no history of headaches or visual disturbance. In your investigations, you find that he has a mild normochromic normocytic anaemia and his ESR is 102 mm/hr. A myeloma screen is negative, as are all the other investigations.

E. A 57-year-old woman presents with a symmetrical inflammatory polyarthritis affecting her hands and feet. Her rheumatoid factor is strongly positive.

EMQ 3

Theme: Raynaud's phenomenon
Options
1. Cryoglobulinaemia
2. Dermatomyositis
3. Ergotamine
4. Hyperthyroidism
5. Occupational injury
6. Rheumatoid arthritis
7. Sjögren's syndrome
8. Systemic lupus erythematosus
9. Systemic sclerosis
10. Thermal injury
11. Thoracic outlet syndrome

The following patients have Raynaud's phenomenon. Please choose the most appropriate underlying diagnosis.

A. A 47-year-old woman presents with 4-month history of food sticking in her mouth, poor taste and her dentures not seeming to fit as well. She also says that her eyes feel quite 'gritty'. On examination, you find that there is a smooth swelling at the angle of the jaw on both sides.

B. A 40-year-old woman is seen in the outpatient department with a 6-month history of aching in her hands and feet with some tightness of the skin of her fingers. She has also become troubled by acid reflux. On examination, there is restriction of movement of the fingers of the hand.

Objective structured clinical examination (OSCE) stations

OSCE 1

This is a structured oral with an examiner for data interpretation in the locomotor system.
Examiner: If I showed you a picture of a patient with arthritis of both hands, what would you think about?

OSCE 2

This is a 5 minute station with an examiner and a real patient, who is seated and has her hands on her lap. It tests your skill at observation and then linking your findings with other possible disease manifestations.

Examiner: Please ask this patient to open her mouth. What do you notice?
Student: She seems to have restricted opening.
Examiner: Very good. Apart from anything to do with her joints or skin, what questions would you like to ask her?
   Now, what specific signs would you like to examine her skin and joints for?

Case history questions

Case history 1

A 28-year-old rugby player presents 2 days after a match in which he was not injured, other than a graze on the left shin, with a painful, swollen, red right knee and a slightly painful left elbow. He has a temperature of 38.6°C.

1. What is your initial differential diagnosis?
2. What further history should you seek?
3. List the four most appropriate immediate investigations.

Case history 2

A 65-year-old man presents to accident and emergency drowsy and vomiting. He has a short history of thirst, polyuria and weight loss and has complained to his wife of backache. He is drowsy and confused. A note from his GP states that a recent biochemical profile showed his serum calcium to be 3.9 mmol/l.

1. Name three other biochemical measurements that you would wish to know without delay.
2. Give two likely causes for the hypercalcaemia.
3. List two forms of treatment for his hypercalcaemia.

Key feature questions

1. A 37-year-old woman who works as a cleaner has been under review at her general practitioner's with low back pain that has been present continuously for about 3 months. She has been off work during this time and feels that returning will exacerbate her pain. The pain does not radiate, it has not worsened and she has not had any problems with weakness or sensory disturbance. It started when she tripped over an uneven pavement. The pain did not start immediately but came on a couple of days later. She has rung a 'no win, no fee' firm of solicitors because of this accident. On examination, there is minimum tenderness over the lower lumbosacral spine but nothing else of note. In the past, she has had bouts of low back pain and also episodes of low mood. She had an acrimonious divorce a couple of years ago and is bringing up her three children (4, 6 and 14 years) alone.

Give four features that indicate her pain is not due to an underlying serious pathology.

2. A 73-year-old woman who has had rheumatoid arthritis for 20 years is seen in the outpatients clinic for a review. Her main complaint is difficulty in using her hands. She has also had pain, particularly in the right arm, that has been waking her up at night and is relieved by hanging the arm out of bed. On examination, she has ulnar deviation, much worse at the right wrist, and also significant swan-neck deformity of her fingers, also on the right. There is wasting of the thenar muscles bilaterally. The hands are generally weak, particularly abduction of the right thumb. There is also some subjective numbness of the index and middle fingers of both hands.

Give three features indicating that her symptoms are not simply due to arthritic changes.

3. A 75-year-old man comes to see you with headaches that have been present for about 6 weeks. He describes the headaches as being very severe and affecting one side. It has also been painful when he has been washing his hair. He has noticed some aching around his jaw when he is eating. About a week ago, he had some flashing lights in his vision in his right eye, but this settled over a few hours.

Give two features that strongly point to temporal arteritis.

4. An 83-year-old woman who lives independently has had type 2 diabetes for 5 years. Over the last 2 months, she has 'gone off her legs'. She has thirst and polyuria and is clinically hypovolaemic. Her laboratory results are as follows:

Calcium	3.6 mmol/l
Phosphate	1.3 mmol/l
Urea	18 mmol/l
Creatinine	130 µmol/l
Potassium	5.6 mmol/l
Alkaline phosphatase	360 IU/l
Haemoglobin A$_{1c}$	7%
Fasting blood glucose	7.2 mmol/l
Haemoglobin	90 g/l
Erythrocyte sedimentation rate	110 mm/hr

a. What is the most likely cause of her thirst and polyuria?
  1. Renal failure
  2. Hyperkalaemia
  3. Hypercalcaemia
  4. Diabetes mellitus
  5. Cranial diabetes insipidus
  6. Psychogenic polydipsia
  7. Anaemia
  8. Raised alkaline phosphatase

b. What is the most likely cause of her presentation?
  1. Sarcoidosis
  2. Tuberculosis
  3. Osteoporosis
  4. Disseminated malignancy
  5. Paget's disease
  6. Hyperparathyroidism

Data interpretation questions

Table 79 gives the biochemical results for six patients. Suggest an interpretation with reasons.

Picture questions

1. Figure 93 shows the hand of a 48-year-old man with rheumatoid disease, which he says causes 'some bruises'.
   a. What is the problem?
   b. What does this mean in terms of the disease?

2. A 65-year-old man has developed a very painful joint (Fig. 94). He has had several attacks in the past affecting different joints; he is supposed to be on treatment to reduce the frequency of the attacks but has not been taking it regularly.
   a. What is the diagnosis?

Table 79 Biochemical results for data interpretation question

	A	B	C	D	E	F
Calcium (mmol/l)	3.5	3.9	2.0	1.2	2.3	2.05
Phosphate (mmol/l)	0.5	2.3	0.6	2.1	0.9	2.5
Alkaline phosphatase (IU/l)	230	190	200	120	280	320
Urea (mmol/l)	10	35	6	5.3	5.1	34
Creatinine (µmol/l)	118	500	100	98	110	480

Reference ranges: as a final-year student you should aim to know the reference ranges for all of these measurements (p. 5).

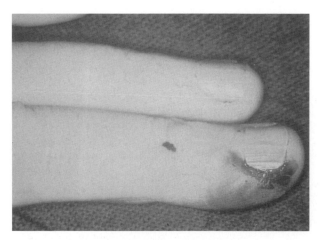

Fig. 93 The hand of a man with rheumatoid disease.

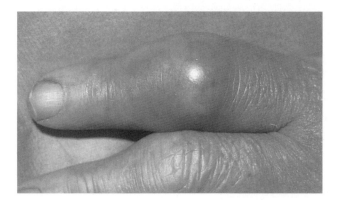

Fig. 94 A painful joint.

b. What treatment should he have been taking?
c. How should you treat this attack?
d. What precipitating factors should you ask about?
e. What preventative treatment should be given?

3. Figure 95 is a computed tomographic (CT) scan of the lower chest on 'bone windows' to demonstrate bone and soft tissue defects. The descending aorta is seen just to the left of centre.

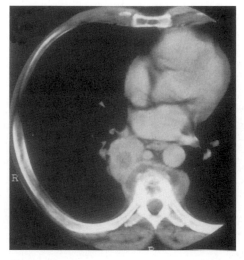

Fig. 95 CT scan of the lower chest on 'bone windows'.

a. Looking at the aorta, what is your estimate of the patient's age?

Just posterior to the aorta is some abnormal 'tissue' in front of the vertebrae with an outpouching slightly to the right of centre adjacent to this abnormal area.

b. What do you think this might be?
c. What is the correct term for this?

Regarding the adjacent vertebra:

d. Is it normal?
e. What would you call this?
f. Give a differential diagnosis.
g. State your plan of investigation, knowing that the spine was not unstable and that there were no focal neurological signs but the patient was in great pain (requiring morphine).

4. Figure 96 is a radiograph of the lower leg of an 80-year-old man who has been admitted to an elderly care ward because of immobility. He complains of pain in the left knee.

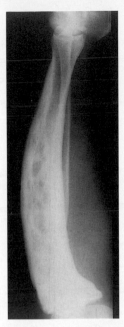

Fig. 96 A radiograph of the lower leg in an elderly man with a painful knee.

a. Describe the abnormalities.
b. What is the diagnosis?
c. What biochemical tests would support the diagnosis?
d. What imaging investigation would you use to assess how extensively his bones are affected?
e. How could you treat him?

Short notes

1. In a patient with a symmetrical polyarthritis, what, apart from enquiring about joint problems, would you want to ask about and why?

2. In a patient suspected of having temporal arteritis, outline your immediate and, presuming the diagnosis is confirmed, long-term management plans.

3. Which investigations should you request in a person with an acute symmetrical polyarthritis? Given that the diagnosis is rheumatoid arthritis, what abnormalities might there be in the investigations that you ordered?

4. Outline how you would approach the management of a patient with rheumatoid arthritis.

5. You are asked to see a 77-year-old woman with known osteoarthritis in accident and emergency. She has been reasonably well but 3 days earlier she noticed some pain in her calf which had progressed. Now her calf is swollen, indurated and tender with increased local warmth. What is the differential diagnosis and what investigations would you request?

6. A 45-year-old patient presents with right wrist drop. He has weakness of dorsiflexion of his left foot and he has also been complaining of some diplopia on looking to the right. Generally, he has not been very well for a few months with some weight loss and abdominal pain. What is the differential diagnosis? What is the basis for this? What investigations would you carry out and why?

7. Write short notes on:

a. The symptoms of hypercalcaemia
b. The factors which predispose to osteoporosis
c. How you would manage a patient with severe hypercalcaemia
d. How you would manage a patient with severe hypocalcaemia

Self-assessment: answers

Multiple choice answers

1. a. **False.** A consequence of cyclo-oxygenase blockade is a reduction in intrarenal generation of prostaglandins, which causes a deterioration in renal function.
   b. **True.** The change in renal function results in hyperkalaemia.
   c. **True.** There is a clear relationship between NSAID use and complications such as perforation, bleeding and death, particularly in old people.
   d. **False.** NSAIDs relieve inflammation; they do not influence disease progression.
   e. **False.** A consequence of NSAID action is increased leucotriene production; leucotrienes are powerful bronchoconstrictors.

2. a. **True.** Disease activity is monitored by measuring ESR, C-reactive protein or plasma viscosity.
   b. **True.** Some patients may have arthralgia but there is no damage to the joints.
   c. **False.** Weight loss is characteristic of polymyalgia rheumatica.
   d. **True.** A muscle biopsy may show patchy vasculitis; however, it is not a useful diagnostic test.
   e. **True.** Pain during mastication is a characteristic feature of temporal arteritis.

3. a. **True.**
   b. **True.**
   c. **True.** This is one of the typical blood-associated dyscrasias.
   d. **True.** As with thrombocytopenia.
   e. **False.** Characteristically the C-reactive protein is normal; if high, then another cause should be sought (e.g. infection).

4. a. **False.** They are directed against the Fc fragment of IgG.
   b. **True.** Nodules are associated with high titres of rheumatoid factor.
   c. **False.** It is not diagnostic of rheumatoid disease (for example, it can occur in endocarditis).
   d. **False.** The antibody is usually of the IgM class against normal IgG (sometimes it is IgG against IgG).
   e. **False.**

5. a. **True.** There are no haematological abnormalities.
   b. **False.** Bouchard's nodes are osteoarthritis of the PIP joints.
   c. **False.** Erosions are typical of rheumatoid disease.
   d. **False.** It should not last longer than 30 minutes.

   e. **True.** This is common, resulting in 'squaring' of the hand.

6. a. **False.** Tophi indicate chronic deposition of urate.
   b. **False.** Use of allopurinol would make an acute attack worse by stimulating the tissue mobilisation of uric acid.
   c. **False.** Furosemide causes urate retention. Bumetanide is better.
   d. **False.** After the big toe, the ankle and knees may be affected.
   e. **False.** Raised serum urate *supports* the diagnosis; you need to demonstrate crystals within the synovial fluid for a definitive diagnosis.

7. a. **True.** There is close correlation between nail psoriasis and DIP involvement.
   b. **True.** The joint involvement is characteristically *asymmetrical*. However, up to 25% of patients have symmetrical joint involvement.
   c. **True.** Joint involvement can be severe: 'mutilans'.
   d. **True.** Sacroiliitis is a key feature of all spondylo-arthropathies.
   e. **False.** Temporomandibular joint involvement is characteristic of *rheumatoid disease*.

8. a. **False.** It is 2–3 times more common in men.
   b. **True.** Commonly affects several joints and often presents with back pain.
   c. **False.** It is associated with HLA-B27.
   d. **True.** It is associated with upper lobe fibrosis and aortic incompetence.
   e. **False.** The hands and feet are not affected.

9. a. **True.** A clear viscous fluid.
   b. **False.** The presence of pyrophosphate crystals is indicative of gout.
   c. **False.** The viscosity is high.
   d. **False.** Fibrin is indicative of disease.
   e. **False.**

10. a. **True.**
    b. **True.** Systemic features are indicative of severe disease.
    c. **True.** Rheumatoid nodules are pathognomonic for the disease and are associated with high levels of rheumatoid factor.
    d. **True.** Erosions, particularly their early appearance, predict a poor prognosis.
    e. **False.**

11. a. **True.** It is less likely to be septic arthritis than a monoarthritis but septic oligoarthritis is quite common. It does rule out tuberculous arthritis, however. If joints are affected sequentially, consider rheumatic fever and Lyme borreliosis

(or reactive arthritis); if together, consider *Neisseria gonorrhoeae*, rubella and erythrovirus.

b. **False.** The keys to successful management and to preserving the joint cartilage are i.v. antibiotic treatment, joint aspiration to dryness and resting of the joint.

c. **False.** Rubella and parvovirus are common causes.

d. **False.** Although it would be unusual in a young, previously well person; it is more common with advancing age.

e. **True.** Not always with an acute presentation.

12. a. **True.** It is often difficult to remove all dead infected bone.

b. **True.** Virtually always and it is a useful marker of response to treatment and relapse.

c. **True.** Although there are other causes of a sinus including actinomycosis, implanted foreign body (such as shrapnel), mycetoma (fungal soft tissue and bony infection of the leg in the tropics).

d. **False.** If *Staph. aureus* is grown, this is helpful, but otherwise there is no relationship at all between bony cultures and sinus cultures.

e. **False.** Usually 3–6 weeks of i.v. therapy followed by 4–12 weeks of oral therapy is necessary and even then this often fails. Longer treatment is necessary for chronic osteomyelitis. It always fails if dead bone or metalwork remains.

13. a. **True.**

b. **True.**

c. **True.**

d. **False.**

e. **False.**

14. a. **True.** It usually occurs 3–12 weeks after the episode of diarrhoea.

b. **False.** It is self-limiting over several weeks or occasionally months.

c. **False.** It is helpful if it can be done if negative does not rule out the diagnosis.

d. **True.**

e. **True.** However, this is usually easy, as the flitting polyarthropathy seen in rheumatic fever is *not* characteristic of reactive arthritis, which usually afflicts large joints and does not 'move around'.

15. a. **False.** They are intimately interrelated.

b. **False.** Plasma calcium is regulated independently of dietary intake.

c. **True.** However, because osteoblasts and osteoclasts are 'coupled' as bone remodelling units, diseases which increase the activity of one will increase the activity of the other, and alkaline phosphatase may increase even in disease which primarily activates osteoclasts (such as metastatic cancer).

d. **True.**

e. **True.** This is one of the main pathophysiological processes in renal bone disease, lowering serum calcium and secondarily 'activating' parathyroid hormone secretion.

16. a. **False.** Osteoporosis rarely causes hypercalcaemia unless the patient is immobile.

b. **True.** Sarcoidosis, tuberculosis, berylliosis and other granulomatous diseases all cause increased vitamin D synthesis in the granulomas.

c. **True.** PTH increases renal phosphate excretion and lowers serum phosphate. The exception to this is renal bone disease in which the parathyroid glands may become autonomous (tertiary hyperparathyroidism) and cause hypercalcaemia with hyperphosphataemia, but this is very much the exception rather than the rule.

d. **False.** See the answer to (c).

e. **True.** Haematological malignancies are a close second to solid tumours as a cause of malignant hypercalcaemia.

17. a. **True.** Osteoporosis is characterised by low bone mass and microarchitectural disruption.

b. **False.** It peaks in early adult life, around age 25.

c. **True.** Weight-bearing exercise protects against bone loss and immobility exacerbates it; this can become a vicious circle for osteoporotic patients immobilised by fractures.

d. **False.** Steroids *reduce* bone mass.

e. **False.** Severe hypogonadism (as in hypopituitarism and some genetic disorders) can cause osteoporosis even in young adult life.

18. a. **True.** Both acute and chronic hypocalcaemia may present with epilepsy.

b. **False.** The bedside tests are insensitive and have been largely superseded by availability of calcium measurements as an emergency.

c. **False.** Calcitonin is used for treating *hyper*calcaemia.

d. **True.** In prolonged disease.

e. **True.** PTH is now available for treatment of hypoparathyroidism.

Single best answer multiple choice answers

1. **e is correct.** The patient has a inflammatory (morning stiffness) symmetrical arthritis affecting the hands and wrists. The blood tests show a normochromic, normocytic anaemia consistent with inflammatory disease. Less than half the patients with early rheumatoid arthritis may have circulating rheumatoid factor. Reactive arthritis is usually asymmetrical and affects large joints as well. There is no trigger in the history.

2. **d is correct.** He has an asymmetrical arthritis affecting large joints, possibly with some iritis. The recent travel and episode of diarrhoea are all consistent with the diagnosis.

3. **d is correct.** The gradual onset, lack of early morning stiffness and pain at the end of the day point to a primary osteoarthritis. Psoriatic arthritis can affect the DIPs, but there are no skin changes and the description is of Heberden's nodes.

4. **e is correct.** The diagnosis is systemic lupus erythematosus with predominantly skin involvement (butterfly rash and photosensitivity). The systemic features are the arthralgia, the lymphopenia and the moderately elevated ESR. The treatment is dependent on the systems affected and to what degree. An NSAID could be used to treat the arthralgia but would not help the skin (which is the patient's main concern). Renal or central nervous system disease will require immunosuppressives.

5. **b is correct.** The patient has developed seropositive rheumatoid arthritis. He needs early treatment with a disease-modifying antirheumatic drug (DMARD) to prevent disease progression.

Extended matched answers

EMQ 1

A. **4.** The main differential diagnosis is between sepsis, gout and pseudogout. The ankle is a common site for the last two conditions and the recent treatment with a diuretic (e.g. furosemide or bendroflumethiazide) points to gout. Urate arthropathy is associated with a temperature and systemic disturbance.

B. **1.** Damaged joints are much more prone to infection. You should consider it in any patient who is non-specifically unwell with a chronic arthritis.

C. **9.** The patient could have an enteropathic arthropathy associated with inflammatory bowel disease. However, the self-limited episode of diarrhoea linked to travelling makes a reactive arthropathy the probable diagnosis.

D. **8.** A progressive mutilating arthritis associated with a scaling, red rash is most likely due to psoriasis. Reiter's syndrome can cause a pustular rash similar to psoriasis over the palms, but there is no history of urethritis. It is very unusual for SLE to cause severe joint damage.

E. **7.** Osteoarthritis at the hip commonly affects abduction and rotation early in the disease. Although the patient stiffens on rest, this is different to the stiffness associated with an inflammatory arthropathy.

EMQ 2

A. **4.** This patient has problems limited to one joint that is causing disability. Initial treatment is with physiotherapy and an exercise regimen. Oral simple analgesics may be prescribed, but he could be helped by a single injection of a local anaesthetic and a long-acting corticosteroid (e.g. triamcinalone) into the joint.

B. **8.** NSAIDs should not be used as a first-line treatment in generalised osteoarthritis with no evidence of joint inflammation. You should start on the first rung of the analgesic ladder with regular paracetamol.

C. **3.** In gout, the joint is intensely inflamed and the pain very severe. You should prescribe regular ibuprofen or another NSAID.

D. **7.** The history, examination and investigations indicate that the most likely diagnosis is polymyalgia rheumatica. He should respond to 10–20 mg/day of prednisolone within 1–2 weeks.

E. **9.** Patients with rheumatoid arthritis will derive benefit from NSAIDs and simple analgesics. However, the most beneficial treatment will be a disease-modifying agent (DMARD) (others being chloroquine, methotrexate, gold and penicillamine). Infliximab would be used for patients not responding to a first-line DMARD.

EMQ 3

Raynaud's disease has no underlying cause. The most frequent association of Raynaud's phenomenon is with systemic sclerosis (where it affects almost all patients). Other associations are with SLE, vibrating tools (occupation), Sjögren's syndrome, previous thermal injury (frostbite) and cryoglobulinaemia. There should be at least two colour changes (white —pallor, blue — cyanosis, red — hyperaemia) to establish the diagnosis and these should be reversible.

A. **7.** Patients with Sjögren's syndrome may complain of dryness of the mouth and eyes (and sometimes skin or vagina) or the problems caused by this. They may have recurrent episodes of parotitis, or the enlarged parotid gland may be found on examination. About 1 in 5 patients will have Raynaud's phenomenon.

B. **9.** The diagnosis of systemic sclerosis can be difficult from the history, as the symptoms can be non-specific and stem from a number of different body systems. The tightness of the skin (often with some induration in the early stages) and the restricted movement on examination point to the diagnosis. On examination, you should also look for:

- skin changes: pigmentation, telangiectasias, tight and shiny skin (or induration), loss of skin folds, calcium deposits, restriction of movement of the hands, small mouth — restricted opening
- other system involvement: GI, respiratory, cardiovascular, neurological and renal (must check BP).

Responses to OSCE stations

OSCE 1

Most likely the examiner would show you a picture, rather than telling you about it. You would then have to describe the abnormalities. Here are some possible scenarios.

Examiner: I agree that it shows a patient with swelling and deformity of the proximal and distal interphalangeal joints. What else would you comment on in the hands?

A crucial point at this stage is the pattern of joint involvement and whether the arthritis is symmetrical. From here, you would want to examine the other joints to check for involvement and confirm the pattern.

Examiner: So you think that the patient has a severe asymmetrical arthritis affecting the hands, and I have told you that there is some involvement of the feet. What do you want to do now?

You would need to examine the other systems: for example, looking for neurological involvement (e.g. mononeuritis). You would also need to examine the skin carefully (psoriasis, vasculitis and subcutaneous nodules — rheumatoid, gout).

Examiner: Here is a picture of the person's trunk. What do you notice?
Student: Given the discrete patches of red scaling skin, I think the most likely cause is psoriasis.
Examiner: What tests do you want to do?

There are no specific tests for psoriatic arthritis — it is a clinical diagnosis. You could discuss:

- plain radiographs of hands and feet (erosions)
- rheumatoid factor and antinuclear factor (ANF) (SLE is an unusual cause of a severe arthritis; mostly it causes arthralgia)
- urate levels (can be severe deforming arthritis)
- full blood count and ESR (normochromic normocytic anaemia — chronic disease).

Suggestions for further practice Many students lack confidence in joint examination. You need to seek out stable patients that you can practise on. In medicine, rheumatology clinics are the obvious source, but these may be oversubscribed by students or held infrequently in your hospital. You should also consider:

- orthopaedic clinics: large, frequent clinics, mostly osteoarthritis, but also some inflammatory arthropathies
- elderly care medicine: outpatients or rehabilitation units (orthogeriatric units); generally very good for patients with lots of physical signs but patients less robust (for long practice sessions!).

OSCE 2

The difficulty in opening the mouth (microstomia) is a strong pointer towards systemic sclerosis and the student has done well to notice this (it is easy to miss unless you specifically consider it). Given that the patient probably has systemic sclerosis, questions could cover:

- general: fatigue, weight loss
- gastrointestinal system: heartburn, bowel disturance (diarrhoea and constipation) and dyspepsia
- respiratory system: breathlessness (fibrosis and pulmonary hypertension)
- cardiovascular system: breathlessness and palpitations (conduction abnormalities)

- ear, nose and throat: dry mouth and eyes (Sjögren's syndrome)
- central nervous system: weakness or numbness (nerve entrapment)
- vascular: Raynaud's phenomenon.

On examination, you need to look for:

- skin induration and tightness
- restricted hand movements
- telangiectasia
- calcinosis
- any pigmentary changes (hyper- or hypopigmentation)
- any loss of parts of digits (vasospasm).

Case history answers

Case history 1

1. The differential diagnosis is:
   - staphylococcal septic arthritis (slightly less likely if two joints)
   - gonococcal arthritis (need sexual history)
   - reactive arthritis (Reiter's syndrome)
   - erythrovirus infection (less likely as knee inflamed).

2. Sexual contact history, urethral discharge and any other current or recent symptoms relevant to erythrovirus or reactive arthritis (e.g. diarrhoea, rash, prodromal illness, etc.).

3. Investigations:
   - joint aspiration for cells and Gram stain and culture (including *Neisseria gonorrhoeae*)
   - blood culture
   - white cell count
   - erythrovirus serology (IgM).

Case history 2

Note the symptoms of hypercalcaemia and bone symptoms (backache). Apply the same principles as under the data interpretation questions below.

1. Phosphate, urea, creatinine, alkaline phosphatase, sodium, potassium and bicarbonate are all needed. In a seriously ill patient, the immediate priority is to measure renal function and electrolytes to guide emergency management; assessment of acid–base status may also be needed if there is renal failure. Phosphate and alkaline phosphatase are needed to explore the differential diagnosis.

2. Malignant disease or hyperparathyroidism is the most likely diagnosis. Other causes are rare.

3. The priority is to assess the patient's state of hydration; he is likely to be volume-depleted. Saline will increase renal perfusion and calcium excretion. If that alone fails to control hypercalcaemia rapidly, a bisphosphonate can be given, even if the diagnosis is not firmly established, because it reduces osteoclastic bone resorption. The remainder of the management plan will be to diagnose and treat the underlying disease.

Key features answers

1. Features include the following:
   - a patient with previous episodes of back pain and considerable personal stress
   - a possible claim for compensation and being off work
   - no radiation of the pain and no neurological features
   - pain not severe and not worsening
   - minimal findings on examination.

   MR scanning or other imaging in this patient is not indicated. If carried out, there may be degenerative or other changes present, but this does not mean that these are the cause of her pain. The best management is a cognitive behavioural approach with an active exercise plan.

2. Features include the following:
   - pain in her arms that is worse at night and helped by a particular posture
   - weakness of abductor pollicis brevis on the right
   - numbness in a nerve distribution.

   Patients with longstanding rheumatoid arthritis often have significant changes in their hands, but functionally they frequently manage quite well. However, patients are at risk of nerve entrapment syndromes and this woman has bilateral carpal tunnel syndrome, which is worse on the right. The pain is typical, as is the particular muscle weakness (often involves opponens pollicis).

3. Features include:
   - scalp tenderness
   - jaw claudication.

   This is a difficult question, as the overall picture is most consistent with temporal arteritis and you would want to order an urgent ESR and start the patient on steroids (particularly in view of the visual disturbance). However, migraine can occur at any age and the headache is unilateral (as it can be in temporal arteritis). Similarly, patients can have visual disturbance. The features that are much more specific to temporal arteritis are scalp tenderness and jaw claudication.

4. a. **3 is correct.** Of the causes of thirst and polyuria, her diabetes is not poorly enough controlled to account for it, and she is not in particularly severe renal failure. There is nothing to suggest cranial diabetes insipidus. Her blood tests are grossly abnormal, so psychogenic polydipsia would be a silly suggestion. She is very significantly hypercalcaemic, so that is by far the most likely explanation for her symptoms.

   b. **4 is correct.** The most important finding here is the grossly raised ESR. She is obviously very ill and has severe hypercalcaemia. Whilst hyperparathyroidism could cause hypercalcaemia of that degree, a lower serum phosphate might be expected, and hyperparathyroidism does not account for her anaemia and high ESR. Disseminated malignancy often turns out to be the correct diagnosis in this situation.

Data interpretation answers

If this appears difficult, look first at the calcium (high, low, normal?), second at the phosphate (is it changed in the opposite direction from calcium, as might be expected if the primary problem was parathyroid over-or underactivity), then at urea and creatinine to see if there is renal failure (remember this could be the primary disease or a secondary effect of hypercalcaemia) and finally at the alkaline phosphatase (is there bone involvement?).

Patient A The main abnormalities are a raised calcium and lowered phosphate, characteristic of hyperparathyroidism. The raised alkaline phosphatase indicates parathyroid bone disease and the raised urea with normal serum creatinine suggests volume depletion, which could lead to renal failure.

Patient B Here, both phosphate and calcium are high, as are urea and creatinine. There is phosphate retention and renal failure. One interpretation might be tertiary hyperparathyroidism in a patient with longstanding renal failure, but it would be surprising for alkaline phosphatase to be relatively normal. Malignancy such as myeloma is another possibility. An interesting feature of myeloma is that osteoblastic activity is 'paralysed' despite increased osteoclastic activity so alkaline phosphatase may be normal despite widespread bone disease.

Patient C Hypocalcaemia, but serum phosphate is low. This must mean that parathyroid function is intact and tending to correct hypocalcaemia caused by some other disease. A likely cause is vitamin D deficiency. Note that serum alkaline phosphatase is somewhat raised. This is evidence of secondary parathyroid bone disease. Longstanding osteomalacia would be a good explanation for these results.

Patient D Here serum calcium is low and phosphate is high. The diagnosis is hypoparathyroidism.

Patient E In this case, all parameters are normal except alkaline phosphatase. There is increased osteoblastic activity. This would be normal for a growing child or during fracture healing. In an otherwise asymptomatic adult, think of Paget's disease.

Patient F This patient is mildly hypocalcaemic, has moderate hyperphosphataemia, renal failure and a raised alkaline phosphatase. A likely diagnosis is renal bone disease.

Picture answers

1. a. He has a vasculitis with typical localised areas of infarction.

   b. The presence of a vasculitis indicates aggressive disease with a much poorer prognosis.

2. a. He has gout. The site is non-typical, but in a patient who has had multiple attacks, then joints other than the first MTP may be involved.

   b. Allopurinol.

   c. The initial treatment is with NSAIDs. If these cannot be tolerated, then colchicine is an alternative (main side-effects vomiting and diarrhoea). If neither NSAIDs nor colchicine can be used, corticosteroids are effective.

    d. There are a number of causes that might precipitate gout (p. 356). In relation to common factors, ask about change in drug treatment (e.g. prescription of furosemide) or alcohol binges.

    e. Once the attack has subsided then allopurinol should be prescribed (initially under NSAID cover). Main side-effects are rashes (rarely hypersensitivity), dyspepsia, diarrhoea and headache.

3. a. No calcification, therefore probably <40 years.

    b. Abscess (not consistent with lymphadenopathy as variable intensity).

    c. Paraspinal abscess.

    d. No.

    e. Vertebral osteomyelitis.

    f. Most common organisms are *Staphylococcus aureus*, anaerobes and Gram-negative rods such as *Escherichia coli* and *Mycobacterium tuberculosis*.

    g. Aspiration of abscess contents or bone under CT guidance; blood cultures; 'work-up' for cause of infection and tuberculosis, e.g. urine cultures and ultrasound search for dental sepsis, tuberculin skin test, chest X-ray and sputum for acid-fast bacilli, etc.

In fact, this white patient from Salford was 37 years old and had an 18-month history of increasing back pain; he turned out to have a tuberculous paraspinal abscess with osteomyelitis affecting three vertebrae.

4. a. The tibia is bowed and widened, the cortex is thickened and the bone texture is irregular with patchy sclerosis. There is deformity of the knee joint.

    b. Paget's disease of bone.

    c. Raised alkaline phosphatase; raised urinary hydroxyproline : creatinine ratio.

    d. A radionuclide bone scan is the investigation of choice; plain radiography could also be used.

    e. Bisphosphonate therapy reduces bone remodelling and is likely to relieve pain, although the deformity and any secondary osteoarthrosis in the knee will not improve.

Short notes answers

1. You would need information about systemic features, including non-specific symptoms and those pointing to involvement of a particular system (e.g. mononeuritis). You should ask about the family history and any other possible aetiological factors (for example, inflammatory bowel disease). Take great care and time (using the patient's notes and, in many instances, phoning the GP) to document previous drug treatment (p. 346).

2. A patient with suspected temporal arteritis is a medical emergency. The diagnosis is based on the history, examination and very high ESR. If these all fit together, then high-dose steroids should be started *immediately*. The response within 24 hours can be regarded as a diagnostic test. The longer-term management is outlined on page 354.

3. The investigations should include: full and differential blood count, ESR (or plasma viscosity), C-reactive protein, urea, creatinine, rheumatoid factor, antinuclear antibodies, chest radiograph and radiographs of hands and feet. It may be necessary to exclude gout and septic arthritis if a single joint is particularly affected. Details of the abnormalities within these investigations are discussed on page 343.

4. The main concept is overall management of a person with a potentially disabling condition. Adequate opportunity for discussion of the disease and what it means is going to be very important. A team approach is essential and the expertise of the professions allied to medicine must be used. Aids for daily living and mobility may be required. The drug therapy will range from simple analgesia and NSAIDs to suppress inflammation to the introduction of disease-modifying agents. This would involve specialist care and careful monitoring of the disease and response to therapy (p. 347).

5. The history is consistent with a deep vein thrombosis, particularly as the patient may be immobile and inactive with her arthritis. Initial screening is with Doppler ultrasound of the calf. A thrombosis may be ruled out with non-elevation of D-dimers. A venogram is rarely used now. In a patient with osteoarthritis, it is very important to think of a **Baker's cyst** (p. 358). This is best demonstrated using ultrasound or arthrography. The management of a ruptured cyst consists of rest and analgesia.

6. The history is diagnostic of a mononeuritis multiplex. He has involvement of the radial, lateral popliteal and sixth cranial nerve. This, together with the abdominal pain, malaise and weight loss, is consistent with polyarteritis nodosa (p. 358), but it is a rare condition. The diagnosis can be confirmed by arteriography and biopsy.

The more important aspect of this case is recognising the characteristic pattern of a mononeuritis: isolated nerves being 'picked off' which cannot be accounted for by a single lesion. A metabolic (toxic) peripheral neuropathy would cause a symmetrical pattern.

The differential diagnosis should cover the causes of mononeuritis multiplex, of which the most likely is a vasculitis. Diabetes mellitus can cause a mononeuritis and the general features would fit (e.g. malaise, weight loss) so a blood sugar level is needed. However, it would be most unusual for a diabetic patient to develop multiple nerve lesions simultaneously. Many of the connective tissue diseases such as SLE and rheumatoid arthritis may present with a vasculitis. The history, examination and investigations need to be tailored accordingly. A full blood count, ESR, urea and electrolytes (renal impairment), antinuclear antibodies, antineutrophil cytoplasm antibodies (ANCA) and rheumatoid factor should be requested (p. 343).

7. a. See page 360. Think of volume depletion and 'stones, bones and abdominal moans':

   - *Renal*: thirst, polyuria, nocturia, light-headedness (from volume depletion); symptoms of stones in some cases
   - *Intestinal*: nausea, vomiting, constipation, dyspepsia
   - *Neurological*: lassitude, depression and confusion.

   b. See page 363. Approach this by thinking of the factors needed to attain and maintain a normal bone mass — normal sex steroid levels, activity and adequate dietary calcium — and the factors, particularly hormonal, which can reduce bone mass:

   - hypogonadism or early menopause
   - immobility or chronic debilitating disease

   - endocrine excess: corticosteroid therapy, hyperparathyroidism, Cushing's or hyperthyroidism
   - neoplasia, particularly myeloma
   - malnutrition, malabsorption
   - rheumatological disease, particularly rheumatoid arthritis
   - alcohol abuse.

   c. See page 361. This is covered in detail in the text. Priorities are:
   - adequate volume replacement
   - establishment of the diagnosis
   - control of hypercalcaemia with bisphosphonate.

   d. See page 362. You need to know this to the level of detail given in the emergency box, page 362. In summary:

   - Establish venous access and take blood for diagnostic tests.
   - Give 10% calcium gluconate, 10 ml i.v. over 10 minutes.
   - Call for senior help.
   - Repeat i.v. calcium as needed.

Immunodeficiency, HIV infection and allergy

Chapter 9

9.1 Clinical aspects

Learning objectives

You need:
- to understand the major types of immunodeficiency
- to know the major categories of compromised patient
- to recognise serious, persistent, unusual or recurrent infections as a clue to immunodeficiency
- to recognise how specific infections suggest specific immune defects.

Case Study

A 34-year-old Malaysian man presents with pneumonia. He is classified as moderately severe and improves within 48 hours on i.v. antibiotics. He describes three previous hospitalisations with chest infections, one of which was severe. His abdominal examination reveals a midline scar and he reports a severe car accident age 17 years. His immunoglobulins are low at IgG 6.8 g/l, IgM 0.3 g/l and IgA 0.7 g/l.

The immune system is complex but a basic understanding of how the system operates and the related diseases is essential for practising doctors. It is vital for you to have a grasp of the fundamentals so as to recognise immunodeficiency and immune overactivity and then diagnose and treat your future patients effectively. It is possible to grasp and remember the principles with a few key facts and to use this knowledge effectively. In this chapter, the presentation of basic immunology is very clinically orientated to aid memory and understanding.

There are many components of the normal immune system with substantial interactions between them. The immune system can be likened to the nervous system with afferent and efferent arms (Table 80) and specific recognition mechanisms and memory. Some efferent arms are non-specific (phagocytes), others highly specific (e.g. antibody) (Table 81).

Terminology

Immunodeficiency can be classified into primary and secondary forms.

Primary immunodeficiency refers to genetic immune defects such as antibody deficiency, severe combined immunodeficiency (SCID), chronic gramulomatous disorder and other rare syndromes. Most of these patients present in childhood, with the common exception of antibody deficiency.

Secondary immunodeficiency includes acquired immune defects such as acquired immunodeficiency syndrome (AIDS) and medically induced defects such as transplantation, cancer chemotherapy or immunosuppression for immunological diseases such as systemic lupus erythematosus (SLE).

Examples of more subtle forms of secondary immunodeficiency (excluding HIV infection) often combined with defects in barriers to infection are shown in Table 82.

Recognition of immunodeficiency

Clues to the diagnosis of immunodeficiency can be obvious or rather subtle. A way to recall this is with the SPUR acronym referring to infection:

- *s*erious
- *p*ersistent
- *u*nusual (i.e. opportunistic infections)
- *r*ecurrent.

Different types of defect lead to different types of infections. Some immune defects are isolated, others mixed. A clinically useful guide is shown in Box 20.

Defects in humoral immunity

Patients may have complement deficiency (rarely) or immunoglobulin deficiency.

Antibody deficiency

There are four major classes of antibody: IgG, IgA, IgM and IgE. Immunoglobulin deficiencies or dysfunction are relatively common.

Table 80 Afferent and efferent arms of the normal immune system

	Cellular	Humoral
Afferent: antigen presentation	Dendritic cells T cells Macrophages B cells	–
Efferent	T cells Macrophages Monocytes Neutrophils Eosinophils	Complement Antibody Cytokines

Table 81 Key components of the immune system

	Innate defences	Adaptive defences
Cellular	Neutrophils Macrophages Natural killer (NK) cells Eosinophils	T lymphocytes B lymphocytes
Protein humoral	Complement Interferons Cytokines Protective proteins, i.e. mannose-binding	Antibodies
Other	Barriers against infection, e.g. skin	

Table 82 Examples of secondary immunodeficiency problems and risks for specific infection

Underlying conditions	Infections found at higher frequency or in a more severe form
Old age	Pneumonia, urinary tract infection, skin and soft tissue infection, influenza
Pregnancy (2nd–3rd trimester)	Varicella pneumonia, pyelonephritis, serious bacterial infection
Malnutrition	Pneumonia, skin sepsis, *Pneumocystis* pneumonia, measles
Alcoholic cirrhosis	Tuberculosis, pneumococcal and aspiration pneumonia, spontaneous bacterial peritonitis, invasive aspergillosis
Diabetes mellitus	Pyelonephritis, mucosal candidiasis, candidaemia, tuberculosis, cellulitis and osteomyelitis of feet, staphylococcal infection
Influenza	Staphylococcal pneumonia
Chronic renal failure	Tuberculosis, bacteraemia, urinary tract infection, candidaemia
Iron overload/desferrioxamine therapy	*Yersinia* and *Listeria* infections, zygomycosis
Intensive care unit	Ventilator pneumonia, bacteraemia, especially *Staphylococcus*, *Enterococcus* spp., candidaemia, sinusitis
GI surgery	Peritonitis, pelvic or subdiaphragmatic abscess, pneumonia, candidaemia
Pancreatitis	Peritonitis, candidaemia
Burns	Streptococcal, *Pseudomonas* and other bacterial infection, *Candida*, *Aspergillus* and *Zygomyces* spp. infection.

There are a number of immunoglobulin deficiency diseases: some inherited, some acquired and each of variable degree. Some monogenic immunodeficiency conditions have a defined molecular basis. They can be classified as:

- global: X-linked or common variable
- selective: IgA or IgG2.

IgA deficiency

There are two forms of IgA, which can be monomeric or dimeric. Secretory IgA is dimeric IgA (mainly IgA2), to which a secretory piece has been added to retard proteolysis. The first is the predominant form found in serum, making up 15–20% of the total immunoglobulin pool. Secretory IgA is produced by plasma cells in mucosal surfaces and binds microorganisms on the body's surface. Isolated IgA deficiency is found in 1 in 700 Caucasians and only rarely in other groups. Most IgA-deficient individuals lead normal lives but are more prone to develop respiratory, gastrointestinal (GI) and genitourinary tract bacterial infections but not viral infections. A higher incidence of cow's milk allergy, autoantibodies and autoimmune diseases (such as coeliac disease) has been noted. IgA-deficient patients are also much more prone to develop severe transfusion reactions.

IgG subclass and common variable immunodeficiency

IgG comprises the main circulating and extravascular antibody. There are four subtypes: IgG1, IgG2, IgG3 and IgG4. These are present in blood in a ratio of approximately 18:6:2:1, respectively. IgG1 and IgG3 are critically important for activation of complement after antigen binding.

Box 20: Typical infections with different types of immunodeficiency

T cell dysfunction or deficiency

- Intracellular organisms, e.g.
  - *Listeria*
  - *Mycobacteria*
  - *Toxoplasma*
  - Cytomegalovirus
  - Adenovirus
  - Herpes viruses
  - *Histoplasma*

- Fungi
  - Oral candidiasis
  - *Pneumocystis*
  - *Aspergillus*

B cells (antibody deficiency)

- Extracellular bacteria, e.g.
  - *Streptococcus pneumoniae*
  - *Haemophilus influenzae*

- Echoviruses

Complement deficiency

- Bacteria, esp.
  - *Neisseria meningitides*
  - *Streptococcus pneumoniae*
  - *Haemophilus influenzae*

Neutrophil dysfunction or deficiency

- Bacteria, esp.
  - *Streptococcus milleri*
  - Staphylococci
  - Gram-negative rods

- Fungi, esp.
  - *Aspergillus*
  - *Candida*
  - *Mucorales*

Macrophages dysfunction or deficiency

- Mycobacteria
- *Salmonella*
- Fungi

IgG2 is particularly important for defence against bacteria with capsules, such as *Streptococcus pneumoniae*, and deficiency leads to recurrent invasive infections with these organisms. IgG binds efficiently to Gram-positive bacteria but less so to Gram-negative bacteria, which are better bound by IgM.

Common variable immunodeficiency (hypogammaglobulinaemia) presents in adulthood with recurrent or persistent infections. The commonest presentations are:

- chronic sinus and/or pulmonary infections
- bronchiectasis
- acute bacterial infection such as pneumonia, meningitis or septic arthritis.

The organisms involved are usually common bacterial pathogens. However, unusual infections such as *Myco-plasma* or *Giardia* spp. are a clue to the diagnosis. These patients have a low IgA, IgG, IgG2 or pneumococcal-specific antibody. These tests should be done in all patients, with recurrent respiratory infections. Ironically, they may also produce many autoantibodies and have a number of autoimmune diseases such as haemolytic anaemia, pernicious anaemia and alopecia areata. In those with common variable immunodeficiency, there is a 400-fold increase in lymphoma in middle age.

Treatment of patients with antibody deficiency (except selective IgA) requires antibody replacement and often antibiotic prophylaxis, delivered by specialist teams. Immunoglobulin is given either subcutaneously (weekly) or intravenously (3-weekly), usually as home therapy.

Complement deficiency

Complement refers to 19 plasma and about 10 membrane proteins. The plasma complement is mostly produced by the liver. Low complement levels may be found in SLE and are a guide to the activity of disease.

The primary functions of complement are:

- killing of microorganisms, especially bacteria
- clearance of immune complexes.

The complement components form part of cascades leading to immune activation, just like coagulation. The cascades form two separate pathways — the **classical** and the **alternative** — which meet in a **common** third pathway. Deficiencies of the components of the classical pathway lead to both immune complex disease and/or recurrent infection, whereas deficiency of the alternative pathway leads only to recurrent infection (typically with encapsulated bacteria such as *Strep. pneumoniae*). C3 is the anchor for the whole system and, if this is deficient (which is rare), 70–80% of individuals suffer either immune complex disease or recurrent infection, or both. Immune complex disease in complement deficiency includes SLE, glomerulonephritis and vasculitis.

Isolated deficiency of components of the terminal attack complex, C5–C9, also leads to a predisposition to infection. These C5–C9 deficiencies can be screened for simply by measuring total haemolytic complement (CH50), which will be reduced. Infections in C5–C9 deficiency are often caused by *Neisseria meningitidis* and typically manifest as meningitis (on multiple occasions) or a more chronic form known as chronic meningococcaemia (rash, fever and arthritis with positive blood cultures).

Immunodeficiency following splenectomy

The largest lymphoid organ is the spleen, followed by the thymus and then lymph glands and the mucosal lymphoid system. The spleen has three major functions:

- removal of old platelets and red cells from the circulation
- lymphocyte maturation for anti-polysaccharide function (especially antibodies)
- phagocytosis of encapsulated bacteria and fungi.

There are several circumstances in which the spleen is completely or partially non-functional:

Nine

- removal after trauma or for treatment of idiopathic thrombocytopenia
- sickle cell disease (repeated infarction)
- coeliac disease (atrophy)
- SLE.

The haematological features of splenic dysfunction are described on page 264. Patients with no spleen have a 50 times greater risk of developing overwhelming sepsis with encapsulated bacteria such as *Strep. pneumoniae*, *Haemophilus influenzae* and *N. meningitidis* or after a dog bite. Bacteraemia is so rapidly progressive in these patients that 50–80% die, usually within 3–5 days. Protection *must* be given with vaccine and lifelong penicillin, though this is not fully protective.

Cellular immune deficiency

The cellular immune system comprises lymphocytes, monocytes and macrophages, together with neutrophils, with other cells such as eosinophils and natural killer cells playing subordinate roles in most instances. Some of the cells are recognisable morphologically, notably neutrophils; others can best be differentiated by their surface molecules, including the cluster differentiation (CD) ones (Table 83). Probably the most important cell overall is the helper T cell. The cellular immune system is responsible for:

- antigen recognition and processing
- killing most microorganisms
- controlling the immune system.

The major defects in cellular immunity are neutropenia and helper T cell deficiency (AIDS). However, none of these defects is pure as there are so many interdependent immune mechanisms. The next sections cover the major cellular forms of immunodeficiency:

- Helper T cell deficiency (human immunodeficiency virus (HIV) and AIDS)
- phagocyte defects

- rejection and immunosuppression after transplantation.

CD4 T cells: function and deficiency

T cells are thymus-derived lymphocytes. There are two main types. Each type can be distinguished functionally and by CD markers. The main sub-types are:

- Helper T cells (CD4 cells)
- T suppressor and cytotoxic cells (CD8 cells).

Helper T cells have a number of critically important functions in the immune system (Fig. 97). These include:

- recognition of processed antigens from antigen-presenting cells
- overall control of the cellular immune response
- generation of cytokines, which stimulate other cell types
- regulation of IgG production by plasma cells.

Helper T cells are particularly important in recognising and responding to intracellular pathogens such as *Mycobacteria* and herpes virus infection. There are two subtypes of CD4 helper cells known as TH1 and TH2. TH1 cells are critically important in driving the cellular immune response, including the production of proinflammatory cytokines (Fig. 97). TH2 cells are implicated in allergic and hypersensitivity reactions and promote mast cell degranulation and IgE production.

Several disease states cause a fall in helper T cells. The most profound fall is in AIDS, but many severe illnesses will cause them to fall, including, for example, measles. Helper T cell counts are often low in chronically ill patients, especially in patients with lymphoma and sarcoidosis.

Phagocytes: function and deficiency

Phagocytes include neutrophils, monocytes and macrophages. Neutrophils are critically important for handling most bacteria and fungi. Neutropenia and its consequences are discussed on page 275. One genetic defect of phago-

Table 83 Important CD molecules

CD molecule	Expressed on	Role
CD3	All cells	Part of antigen receptor complex and involved in signal transduction
CD4	All helper T cells	Cell adhesion and interacts with class II MHC receptor, HIV receptor
CD8	All cytotoxic cells	Cell adhesion and interacts with class I MHC receptors
Integrins	All leucocytes	Adhesion molecule recognising microorganisms, e.g. *Candida*
CD14	Monocytes	LPS receptor
CD21	B cells	Cell entry molecule for Epstein–Barr virus
CD40 ligand	T cells	Switches B cells from IgM to IgG and IgA production; CD40 ligand deficient in hyper-IgM syndrome
CD95	B cells	Binding triggers apoptosis (programmed cell death); deficient in autoimmune lymphoproliferative syndrome

LPS, lipopolysaccharide; MHC, major histocompatibility complex.

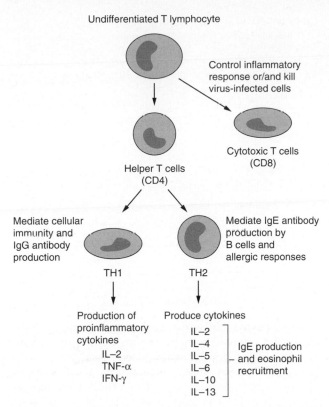

Undifferentiated T lymphocyte

Control inflammatory response or/and kill virus-infected cells

Cytotoxic T cells (CD8)

Helper T cells (CD4)

Mediate cellular immunity and IgG antibody production

Mediate IgE antibody production by B cells and allergic responses

TH1

TH2

Production of proinflammatory cytokines

IL–2
TNF–α
IFN–γ

Produce cytokines

IL–2
IL–4
IL–5
IL–6
IL–10
IL–13

IgE production and eosinophil recruitment

Fig. 97 The role of T cells. IFN-γ, interferon gamma; IL, interleukin; TH1, helper T; TFN-α, tumour necrosis factor alpha.

cytes is chronic granulomatous disease, which leads to recurrent staphylococcal and *Aspergillus* infections.

Monocytes develop into tissue macrophages and, therefore, they can be considered together for clinical purposes. In the brain, microglial cells function partly as macrophages. Macrophages have several functions:

- cytokine production
- phagocytosis of bacteria and fungi
- antigen presentation to T cells.

Phagocytes internalise microorganisms and usually kill them. One particular function that splenic macrophages normally fulfil admirably is the phagocytosis of antibody-coated bacteria. These bacteria are recognised by virtue of a receptor on macrophages (FCγ). An increased number of bacterial infections occurs if this receptor is functionally impaired as in:

- alcoholic cirrhosis
- end-stage renal disease
- SLE.

There are some organisms that are able to evade intracellular killing in macrophages, often because of poor helper T cell function. Examples include *Salmonella*, mycobacteria, *Histoplasma* and *Leishmania* spp. The adaptive mechanisms each organism has developed to achieve this are fascinating. However, the practical consequences of this include:

- carrier states (e.g. typhoid)
- emergence of infection during immunosuppression (e.g. toxoplasmosis)

- long latency between infection and disease (e.g. tuberculosis, histoplasmosis, leprosy)
- need for drugs to penetrate and kill inside the macrophage phagosome.

Neutropenia caused by cytotoxic chemotherapy is also a marker for monocytopenia and, therefore, reduced tissue macrophage numbers. This combined cellular deficiency is partly what makes neutropenic patients so immuno-compromised. In addition, macrophage function is impaired by corticosteroids. Macrophage function is also grossly defective in AIDS, at least partly because of a lack of activation by helper T cells. Macrophage function is substantially improved after activation and, as with neutrophils, interferon gamma is a potent macrophage activator.

Investigating immune deficiency

A careful synthesis of historical information from the patient and the medical notes is the first step in evaluating immune deficiency. You can then arrange appropriate investigations. There is no simple 'immune function screen' that acts like an investigative sieve. A guide to appropriate investigations in patients possibly immuno-deficient is shown in Table 84. These tests should generally be done when the patient has improved from an episode of infection with the exception of an HIV antibody test, which should be done as soon as HIV infection or AIDS is seriously considered. In most cases, these initial screening tests will be normal. You may need to refer the patient to a clinical immunologist or other specialist for further advice.

9.2 HIV infection

Case Study

A nurse from Botswana presents with abdominal pain, fever and nausea. She has no lymphadenopathy palpable, but an abdominal ultrasound reveals extensive retroperitoneal lymphadenopathy. She is moderately pancytopenic at haemoglobin 68 g/l, white cell count 3100×10^6/l and platelets $115\,000 \times 10^9$/l. Her lymphocyte count is 280×10^6/l and her HIV antibody test is positive. An endoscopy shows oesophageal candidiasis.

Table 84 Investigations in suspected immunodeficiency*

Problem	Investigation
Recurrent bacterial infection (e.g. pneumococcal pneumonia, sinusitis)	Igs, IgG subclasses and antipneumococcal antibodies Neutrophil count, mannase binding protein
Progressive (and relatively silent) staphylococcal or other infection (e.g. invasive aspergillosis)	Igs, neutrophil function tests (for chronic gramulomatous disease)
Recurrent meningococcal infection	CH50, Igs
Oral candidiasis, 'pneumonia', other unusual infections with weight loss	T cell subsets, HIV antibody test, Igs
Chronic diarrhoea (? infection) with weight loss	Igs, T cell subsets, HIV antibody test
Unusually invasive or difficult infections	Igs, T cell subsets
Unexplained weight loss (≥10% body weight)	T cell subsets, HIV antibody test

*Remember SPUR, p. 379.
Ig, immunoglobulin; CH50, total haemolytic complement.

HIV infection, leading to AIDS, is now common throughout the world. AIDS was first recognised as a clinical entity in the early 1980s, but is known to have been present since the 1950s. Worldwide, over 35 million people are now infected, 25 million of whom live in Africa. Every day there are 16 000 new infections and AIDS is the fourth most common cause of death worldwide. You must know how HIV and AIDS present clinically and how to handle questions and concerns regarding HIV infection. To do this, you need a basic understanding of how HIV is transmitted and how it causes immune dysfunction.

Epidemiology

The retroviruses

Only four human retroviruses are known: human lymphotrophic viruses (HTLV) 1 and 2 and HIV 1 and 2. It is likely that new human retroviruses will be discovered. They are all single-stranded RNA enveloped viruses. They are called *retro*viruses (i.e. backwards) because they carry an enzyme called reverse transcriptase, which copies the RNA genes of the virus into DNA. This DNA is then integrated into the host cell's chromosomes.

HIV transmission

The primary modes of transmission of HIV are:

* unprotected sex
* blood transmission, e.g. i.v. drug abuse, infected blood products
* mother to child (vertical).

The modes of transmission in individual countries and different social groups within those countries is very variable. In the UK, the majority of HIV cases are in gay men, with a smaller number related to i.v. drug abuse. The most rapidly increasing number of cases is in heterosexuals, some as a result of sexual exposures abroad. In contrast, in France there is a significant heterosexual component to HIV transmission and approximately one-third of French cases are related to heterosexual sex. In Italy, by contrast, the disease is spread primarily in drug addicts and among gay men, with a much smaller heterosexual component. In Africa, heterosexual sex has played the greatest role in transmission, resulting in much vertical transmission (mother to child) and some cases related to blood transmission and/or infected needles. In Thailand and north India, i.v. drug abuse is the primary culprit and in both cases there were explosive outbreaks resulting in several thousand infected individuals in a single year. Many of these individuals are from very poor communities and involved in commercial sex so transmission into the heterosexual population is assured. Vertical transmission can be minimised or prevented with highly effective antiretroviral therapy during pregnancy. Transmission is more likely following vaginal delivery, especially if membranes are ruptured prematurely or if the mother has a high viral load. Breast feeding results in 15% more children being infected.

High-risk behaviour

There are certain aspects of behaviour that increase the risk of transmission. Studies have shown, for example, that the risk of transmission from male to female is greater than female to male. Other factors are:

* higher risk of transmission
  — genital ulceration
  — not circumcised (men)
  — receptive anal intercourse (both sexes)

* lower risk of transmission
  — use of condom
  — vaginal intercourse
  — oral sex, kissing
  — effective antiretroviral therapy.

'Safe sex' denotes stroking and massage, kissing and the use of condoms for any form of penetrative sex. Careful studies have shown that 8% of new HIV infections are acquired by oral sex alone.

Transmission in the health-care setting

For health-care workers who suffer a needle-stick injury, the risk of HIV transmission related to solid needles (such as are used in surgery for sutures) is considerably reduced compared with hollow needles for taking blood or giving i.v. fluids. In addition, the (inadvertent) injection of blood at the same time as a needlestick injury imposes the greatest risk. The overall numerical risk of a health-care worker acquiring HIV following a needle-stick infection is approximately 1 in 250 of such incidents, about 100-fold lower than for hepatitis B. Post-needlestick administration of antiretroviral therapy reduces transmission by at least 80%. A mucosal splash with HIV-infected blood constitutes a negligible risk unless the skin is broken: for example, by eczema.

HIV reproduction

Retroviruses reproduce by utilising the host cell's normal processes of transcription and translation to produce multiple virus particles. Reproduction of the virus proceeds in host cells at a variable pace. HIV may:

- be latent and not reproduce
- reproduce slowly with release of virus from the surface of the cell
- accelerate its own production with death of the host cell.

Understanding what controls the rate of HIV reproduction is central to an understanding of AIDS.

Entry of the virus into host cells requires cell receptors including the CD4 surface molecule on lymphocytes, neural and other cells. About 1 in 10 Caucasians and 1 in 50 black people are relatively resistant to HIV infection, despite exposure, because they lack an essential co-receptor protein called a chemokine receptor. Once the virus has entered the cell and reverse transcriptase has transcribed the viral RNA into the host DNA, that cell is then infected for its life.

Initial infection, so-called primary HIV infection, is characterised by very high levels of circulating virus. As virus reproduction declines, the immune response to the virus accelerates and HIV antibody becomes detectable. At this stage, there is usually only one detectable strain of HIV. As the disease progresses, multiple mutants (strains) of the virus arise, which have different biological properties, including preferences for different cell types (e.g. brain versus lymphocytes). These strains arise because there is no 'proof-reading capability' following RNA transcription during HIV reproduction, so 1–40 DNA base errors are made during each reproduction cycle. Viral mutation has several important consequences:

- Multiple related strains are present in a single person simultaneously
- Different HIV strains are more or less infectious.
- Mutant strains tend to escape the immune response to the virus
- Resistance to antiretroviral therapy may occur quickly.

The amount of circulating HIV can be measured by precisely determining the viral RNA circulating in the

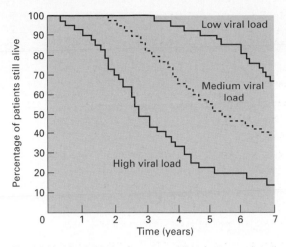

Fig. 98 Viral load shortly after primary HIV infection predicts the development of AIDS and survival. The first deaths in the high viral load group occur within a year of primary infection, whereas in the low viral load groups they start to occur nearly 5 years after primary infection.

blood (viral load). In the first few months after primary infection, determination of the viral load predicts how fast that individual will progress to AIDS (Fig. 98). This has important consequences for when treatment should be started.

Control of HIV infection

For months or years after primary HIV infection, viral replication is partially controlled by mechanisms which are incompletely understood but include cytotoxic T cells. With time, more and more mutants escape protective mechanisms and viral replication increases. The most clinically useful marker of viral reproduction is increasing HIV viral load and later the slow but inexorable decline in the helper T cell count in an initially asymptomatic patient. At the same time, there is gradual destruction of lymph node architecture. Loss of cerebral matter and function is also detectable at lower helper T cell counts (e.g. <100 × 10^6 cells/l).

Clinical stages of HIV infection

There are several stages of HIV infection. Patients may present at any of the stages.

Primary HIV infection

Over 50% of those who acquire HIV infection suffer an illness shortly before seroconversion. This is known as primary HIV infection. The incubation period varies from 7 to 14 days. The clues to the diagnosis include neutropenia, thrombocytopenia, headache and diarrhoea (Box 21). Oral, oesophageal or genital ulceration is also typical and the ulcers are highly infectious.

Diagnosis

At the time of a primary HIV infection, a person's HIV antibody test will be negative, although their HIV viral load will be very high. A retest 2–4 weeks after the primary infection for HIV antibody will usually detect seroconversion, although there are rare instances of delayed seroconversion (retest after 6 months).

Box 21: Clinical and laboratory features of primary HIV infection

Clinical
- Fever*
- Sore throat*
- Myalgia
- Headache*
- Diarrhoea*
- Rash: macular, vesicular*
- Oral, genital or oesophageal ulcers*
- Aseptic meningitis
- Hepatomegaly
- Splenomegaly
- Facial palsy (Bell's)
- Encephalopathy

Laboratory
- Thrombocytopenia*
- Leucopenia*
- Lymphocytic cerebrospinal fluid
- Reduced CD4 cell count
- Negative HIV antibody*
- Positive HIV antigen*
- HIV viral load very high*

*Common.

Management and prognosis

Patients should be treated with combination therapy, certainly until they are improved. Patients who suffer an overt clinical illness of primary HIV infection progress to AIDS more rapidly than those with a silent primary HIV infection. Older patients do much worse.

Asymptomatic and early symptomatic HIV disease

The interval between primary HIV infection (whether overt or not) and development of AIDS is very variable. It varies in untreated patients from 9 months to more than 12 years. One long-term study from San Francisco has shown that 11 years after seroconversion only 60% of the patients had developed AIDS, 20% had AIDS-related complex and 20% were still well.

During the asymptomatic phase of HIV infection, patients are clinically well and have low-grade viraemia and a positive HIV antibody test. They are able to function entirely normally and most do not know they are infected. In the majority of HIV-infected individuals, there is a gradual decline in helper T cell count from around 800×10^6 to $<300 \times 10^6$ cells/l, when symptomatic HIV disease appears. The falling helper T count is a marker, and only a marker, for a general decline in many aspects of immune function. As the helper T cell count falls below 300×10^6 cells/l, opportunistic infections begin to appear.

Symptoms of early HIV infection

Several minor problems herald the later development of AIDS. These include:

- superficial skin problems such as seborrhoeic dermatitis, recurrent staphylococcal skin infections or onychomycosis (fungal nail infection)
- night sweats
- diarrhoea
- unexplained weight loss
- fatigue.

Signs of early HIV infection

Several signs are highly suggestive of HIV infection. These include:

- hairy leukoplakia on the side of the tongue
- lymphadenopathy
- herpes zoster (shingles)
- severe mucosal herpes simplex infection
- oropharyngeal candidiasis (thrush).

Lymphadenopathy is a common feature in HIV infection but is by no means universal and may be found in any of the superficial groups of lymph nodes. Occasionally, lymphadenopathy represents an opportunistic infection, such as tuberculosis, histoplasmosis or lymphoma, but this is unusual. Lymphadenopathy in an at-risk patient should prompt an HIV test.

Laboratory markers of early HIV infection

Clues to the diagnosis of HIV infection include:

- lymphopenia ($<1000 \times 10^6$/l)
- thrombocytopenia
- reduced helper T and elevated cytotoxic T cells.

Thrombocytopenia may be an early manifestation of HIV infection. Patients are frequently asymptomatic, having platelet counts in the 50×10^9 to 120×10^9 cells/l range. Occasionally, symptomatic thrombocytopenia occurs (p. 281).

There are several key helper T cell count landmarks that are used in the management of patients with HIV infection (Fig. 99). The normal count is 800–1200 ($\times 10^6$ cells/l). Management approaches at different levels of helper T cell deficiency vary:

- Arrange 4-monthly checks if ≥500.
- Recommend antiretroviral therapy when <350.
- Start *Pneumocystis* pneumonia prophylaxis when <200.
- Many more opportunistic infections appear when <50.

Patients with higher helper T cell counts (e.g. 400–600) *and* high viral load may also benefit from antiretroviral therapy.

Clinical approach to a newly diagnosed HIV/AIDS patient

When you assess a new HIV/AIDS patient there are certain key aspects to your evaluation. Examination of the mouth and skin is very important.

Your objectives include:

- diagnosis of the current complaint
- assessment of the stage of disease

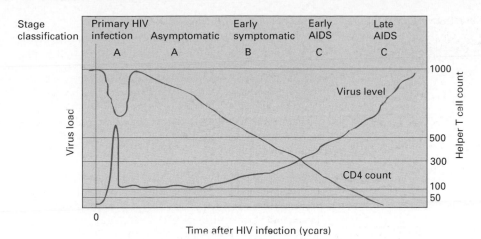

Fig. 99 The relationship between helper T cell counts and the disease stage in HIV infections.

- assessment of the risk of other (future) illnesses (e.g. from prior travel or risk behaviour)
- imparting of confidence to the patient who will need care for many years (e.g. sympathetic, knowledgeable attitude).

You should arrange the following investigations:

- confirmatory HIV test
- helper T cell count
- full blood count
- biochemistry, especially liver function tests
- syphilis serology
- *Toxoplasma* serology
- hepatitis B and C serology
- cytomegalovirus serology
- chest X-ray.

Management of HIV infection (antiretroviral therapy)

The objective of therapy is to reduce circulating viral load to levels undetectable by standard assays (e.g. <50 copies/ml). Once viral load has been completely suppressed, gradual restoration of immune function occurs in almost all patients. If antiretroviral therapy (ART) stops, a rebound of virus is detectable within the blood in days, even after years of successful therapy. For this reason, treatment with current drugs must be lifelong. There are four classes of antiretroviral agent: the nucleoside reverse transcriptase inhibitors (NRTIs) (such as zidovudine, didanosine, zalcitabine and lamivudine), the non-nucleoside reverse transcriptase inhibitors (NNRTIs) (such as nevirapine and efavirenz), the proteinase inhibitors (PIs) (such as saquinavir and ritonavir) and chemokine receptor mimics/fusion antagonists. Resistance appears rapidly with monotherapy and so at least three drugs are now given concurrently. A typical starting combination would be NRTIs with either an NNRTI or a PI. Combination therapy has reduced infection and death rates dramatically (Fig. 100). Problems with compliance, viral resistance and drug toxicity can limit therapy. Recovery of the immune system may be associated with disease, labelled the immune reconstitution inflammatory syndrome' (IRIS).

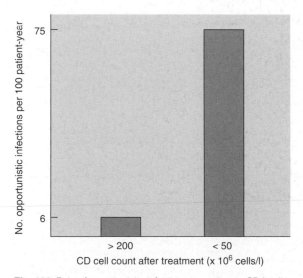

Fig. 100 Rate of opportunistic infections according to CD4 cell count recovery with antiretroviral therapy.

AIDS

AIDS is characterised by being HIV-positive and suffering infections or cancers typical of immunosuppressed patients. The presenting illnesses of AIDS in the UK are shown in Table 85. Each one of these specific diseases represents a marker diagnosis for AIDS and for some is an indicator of helper T cell levels (Fig. 101). The infections in AIDS are generally specific to AIDS, with the exceptions of cryptococcal meningitis, herpes zoster, tuberculosis and several bacterial infections such as salmonellosis. Some infections are more common in Africa (e.g. tuberculosis, pneumococcal pneumonia, salmonellosis) and others may be less common (e.g. pneumonia caused by *Pneumocystis*). A clue to the diagnosis of AIDS is the presence of oral candidiasis or hairy leukoplakia.

Major infections in AIDS

Patients with AIDS suffer from many infections Some of these occur at higher CD4 cell counts, including *Pneumocystis* pneumonia, oesophageal candidiasis and others.

Table 85 Typical presenting illnesses of AIDS in the UK

Illnesses	Percentage presenting
Pneumocystis pneumonia	37
Kaposi's sarcoma	14
Oesophageal candidosis	12
Weight loss (>10% body weight)	6
Lymphoma	4
HIV dementia	3
Cryptococcal meningitis	3
Other infections	21

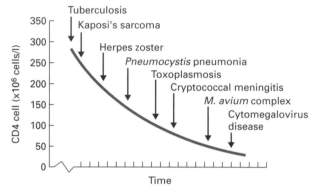

Fig. 101 Occurrence of AIDS-indicating conditions according to CD4 cell count.

Others occur later in the course of AIDS, including cytomegalovirus retinitis and *Mycobacterium avium intracellulare* (MAI) infection. The more common opportunistic infections are covered below; the less common are given in Table 86. Tuberculosis is very common in Africa. Once patients develop an infection, it is almost always recurrent if treatment is stopped unless immune reconstitution has occurred with antiretroviral therapy. Therefore, patients are usually placed on 'maintenance treatment' to prevent recurrence.

Pneumocystis pneumonia

P. jirovecii (an air-borne fungus) is a common cause of pneumonia in AIDS. It presents with:

- dry cough for ≥2 weeks
- intermittent fever and/or night sweats
- recent weight loss
- dyspnoea out of proportion to physical signs
- a normal chest radiograph in 10%.

Pneumocystis pneumonia is best diagnosed by bronchoalveolar lavage or lung biopsy. However, the combination of a low helper T cell count, dyspnoea and cough, a bilaterally hazy infiltrate on the chest radiograph and hypoxaemia is sufficient to suggest the diagnosis. Treatment is with co-trimoxazole in high doses or i.v. pentamidine; corticosteroids are given if the patient is markedly hypoxaemic (Po_2 < 10 kPa (75 mmHg)). The mortality is about 20%.

Oesophageal candidiasis

Oesophageal candidiasis affects about 25% of patients with AIDS. It may be asymptomatic but usually presents with:

- dysphagia
- retrosternal discomfort or pain
- nausea and/or vomiting.

About 30% of patients have no associated oral candidiasis. Diagnosis is best made by endoscopy. Fluconazole is the best treatment.

Cancers in AIDS

There are several cancers almost specific to AIDS or more common (Table 87). Kaposi's sarcoma is caused by a newly discovered herpes virus (KSHV). Cerebral lymphoma is caused by Epstein–Barr virus (p. 419).

Neurological problems in AIDS

About 5% of AIDS patients present with dementia as their AIDS-defining diagnosis. It becomes increasingly common in the later stages of AIDS. It is partially preventable with antiretroviral therapy, even if multiple circulating HIV virus strains are resistant. Other problems include depression and peripheral neuropathy (Table 88).

Prognosis

Prior to the introduction of zidovudine and *Pneumocystis* prophylaxis, most patients would survive 12–15 months following a diagnosis of AIDS. Drug addicts, children under the age of 2 years and those over 50 years tend to have shorter survival times compared with gay men, haemophiliacs and older children. Certain diseases are associated with a good prognosis, e.g. Kaposi's sarcoma and *Pneumocystis* pneumonia, whereas others such as CNS lymphoma have a poor prognosis. Since the introduction of combination antiretroviral therapy and *Pneumocystis* pneumonia prophylaxis, HIV-positive patients will remain well for years if they are compliant with therapy.

HIV antibody testing

The indications for HIV testing in adults are shown in Box 22. Clearly the likelihood of a positive test is higher if your patient belongs to a risk group.

The presence of antibody is a marker of infection and is not protective, unlike in many other infectious diseases where the presence of antibody is both a marker of infection and protective against subsequent infection.

Determining whether a baby is infected if the mother is HIV-positive is more difficult, as maternal HIV antibody is detectable in the baby for about 15 months after birth. Direct viral RNA detection by polymerase chain reaction (PCR) is required.

Counselling

All patients to be tested for HIV antibody must give informed consent. The issues that need discussion before and after HIV testing include life insurance and occupational implications, as well as consideration of who to tell about the result. Some patients prefer to be tested in an anonymous testing clinic. Adequate time should be set aside for both the pre-test counselling and the post-test counselling. This is particularly important if the test comes back positive.

Table 86 Opportunistic infections in AIDS*

Disease	Helper T cell count (×10⁶/l)	Clinical features	Occasional features	Essential investigations	Treatment(s)
Early infections					
Tuberculosis	<300	Cough, fever, weight loss Atypical CXR	Meningitis	Sputum for TB, bacteria, fungi; BAL for TB, fungi; blood culture for TB	Rifampicin, isoniazid, pyrazinamide and ethambutol
Salmonellosis	<250	Fever, diarrhoea, dehydration	Septic shock	Blood culture, stool culture, stools for protozoa, electrolytes and urea	Quinolone or third-generation cephalosporin; rehydration
Mucocutaneous herpes simplex	<250	Painful oral ulceration, pain in perianal area, cold sores	Deep punched-out oesophageal ulcers	None (biopsy/viral culture of blister fluid/lesion)	Aciclovir
Late infections					
Cryptococcal meningitis	<200	Headache, fever, nausea, vomiting	Pneumonia, skin lesions	CT scan of brain, lumbar puncture with opening pressure, fungal blood cultures, cryptococcal antigen	Amphotericin and flucytosine initially, then fluconazole
Toxoplasma encephalitis	<200	Headache, focal neurology, fits	Myocarditis	MR (or CT) scan of brain, *Toxoplasma*, serology	Pyrimethamine and sulfadiazine
Cryptosporidial diarrhoea	<100	Diarrhoea, dehydration	Cholangitis	Stools for protozoa and culture, electrolytes and urea, albumin, liver function tests	Rehydration, experimental antiprotozoal therapy
PML	<100	Focal neurology, fits, abnormal behaviour	–	MR/CT brain scan, lumbar puncture for JC virus PCR	None
Cytomegalovirus retinitis	<100	Visual disturbance	Colitis	Fundoscopy	Ganciclovir, foscarnet or cidofovir
Mycobacterium avium intracellulare	<100	Fever, night sweats, cough, diarrhoea, anaemia	Weight loss	Blood culture for TB	Combination therapy including ethambutol and rifabutin
Invasive aspergillosis	<50	Cough, fever, wheezing, haemoptysis	Tracheobronchitis	CXR, sputum for fungi, BAL for fungi, lung biopsy	Voriconagole

*Not covered in this chapter.

BAL, bronchoalveolar lavage; PML, progressive multifocal leucoencephalopathy; CXR, chest radiograph; TB, tuberculosis; CT, computed tomography; MR, magnetic resonance; JC, Jakob–Creutzfeldt.

Nine

Table 87 Common cancers in AIDS

	Kaposi's sarcoma	CNS lymphoma	Other lymphoma	Squamous cell carcinoma
Organs affected	Skin, gut, lungs	Brain	Lymph nodes, liver, bone marrow, skin	Rectum, uterus, cervix
Typical helper T count ($\times 10^6$ cells/l)	<350	<100	<200	<200
Aetiological agent	KSHV	Epstein–Barr virus	Epstein–Barr virus and probably others	Papilloma virus
Presentation	Purple nodules/plaques on skin/mouth, cough, dyspnoea, peribronchial infiltrate	Focal signs, headache, papilloedema, single enhancing lesion (usually) on CT/MR scan with surrounding oedema	Adenopathy, anaemia, neutropenia, cutaneous abscess	Local pain, bleeding or lump
Management	Chemotherapy and ART	Radiotherapy, dexamethasone	Chemotherapy	Surgery, radiotherapy
Prognosis	Reasonable, one of the less aggressive presentations of AIDS; morbidity high because of unsightly nature of lesions (often on face)	Dismal, most patients die within 3 months	Variable, usually poor; patients tolerate chemotherapy badly because of poor bone marrow reserve	Variable, usually poor as locally invasive at presentation; cervical smears mandatory for HIV-positive women at 6-monthly intervals

CNS, central nervous system; KSHV, Kaposi's sarcoma herpes virus; ART, antiretroviral therapy.

Table 88 Major neuropsychological manifestations of HIV infection/AIDS

Entity	Clinical features
HIV dementia complex	Slowly progressive dementia typically affecting memory and concentration initially, leading to severe dementia over a few months; CT scan shows cerebral atrophy
Depression	Depression is very common in AIDS as in other chronic diseases. Suicide occurs occasionally. Depression may be mistaken for dementia and vice versa
Peripheral neuropathy	Painful or non-painful distal peripheral neuropathy is common. Characteristic are painful soles of the feet with moderate sensory loss. Tends to be progressive and refractory to therapy. May be caused by drugs

CT, computed tomography.

Box 22: Indications for HIV testing in adults

- Patient request
- Organ transplantation
- Blood donation
- Pregnancy (routine antenatal testing)
- Clinical features of AIDS or HIV infection including:
  - Opportunistic infection with no known immunosuppressive disease
  - Unusual lymphoma
  - Squamous cell carcinoma of anus or cervix
  - Early-onset dementia or other unusual neurology
  - Unexplained weight loss
  - Oral candidiasis
  - Night sweats
  - Thrombocytopenia
- Unexplained lymphadenopathy
- Suspicion of primary HIV infection*
- Needlestick injury in health-care worker*
- Rape victim*
- Women with a child with HIV/AIDS

*May not be positive on first test.

Infection control issues

Body fluids from all patients in risk groups and those who are HIV antibody-positive should be handled carefully with gloves on. Gloves should be used for all invasive procedures, including venepuncture, and most surgeons will use two pairs of gloves. Each hospital has detailed procedures for all aspects of handling body fluids. These procedures enable *all* investigations and procedures to be carried out on patients with HIV. The only exception is postmortem, for which few hospitals are adequately equipped. This can pose problems for coroner's cases.

9.3 Transplantation

Learning objectives

You should:
- be able to explain the clinical situations in which transplants are done
- have a working knowledge of graft rejection and tolerance as it relates to transplantation.

Case Study

A 46-year-old with a 1-year-old right single lung transplant is admitted short of breath with a sore throat and bilateral chest infiltrates. His blood and sputum cultures are negative, but his viral polymerase chain reaction test from his throat yields parainfluenza virus type 3. He is very hypoxic.

End-stage organ failure or otherwise untreatable cancer and leukaemia has led to the extensive use of solid organ or stem cell transplantation. Relatively straightforward transplantation *procedures* are corneal, skin and bone transplantation. Liver transplantation is technically challenging but patients need little immunosuppression. In contrast, allogeneic haematopoietic stem cell transplantation is technically straightforward (for the patient) but requires substantial immunosuppression. Some transplantation procedures, such as small bowel, limb, face and skeletal muscle, are essentially experimental at present.

The two major problems with transplantation are organ rejection and infection (often with unusual pathogens). Matching of grafts by human leucocyte antigen (HLA) typing allows more successful transplantation and less immunosuppression to prevent rejection. Identical twin transplants do very well whereas HLA-mismatched (and matched unrelated donor (MUD) transplants) may develop severe rejection early unless the recipient is heavily immunosuppressed (Fig. 102).

Haematopoietic stem cell transplantation (HSCT)

Haematopoietic stem cell transplantation may be either allogeneic (someone else's stem cells) or autologous (own stem cells previously collected). Cells used for transplantation are either circulating stem cells previously collected or bone marrow collected under anaesthetic from multiple iliac crest punctures. Autologous bone marrow transplantation is therefore not formally a transplantation procedure. It is increasingly used to allow increased chemotherapy dose for difficult-to-treat malignancy, such as multiple myeloma. Present indications are shown in Table 89. More recently, reduced intensity and non-myeloablative stem cell transplants have attempted to decrease early mortality in older or sicker recipients, but these approaches may lead to a higher relapse incidence and a higher rate of late infections and are being refined.

Solid organ transplantation

Renal, heart, lung and liver transplantation are now well established for end-stage disease affecting these organs. When these operations are successful, which they increasingly are if performed in large experienced units, patients experience a new lease of life and a longer life. The best outcomes are in renal and heart transplantation, but substantial improvements in both survival and quality of life are now being seen in liver and lung transplant recipients. A young, otherwise healthy recipient of a renal transplant can expect an 80–90% survival over 5 years, which is superior to dialysis. Unlike in other major organ transplants, the kidney can be lost (through rejection) but the patient survives. At 3 years, 80% of kidneys are still functional. Survival for heart transplantation is lower but is still better than 60% at 5 years.

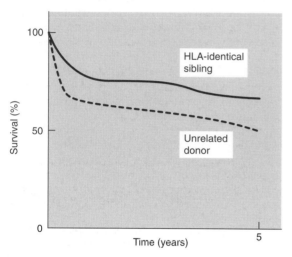

Fig. 102 Survival in HLA-matched and HLA-unmatched transplants.

Rejection

Patients who develop rejection (which most do to variable degrees) receive additional immunosuppressive medication and are much more likely to develop serious infection. Some infections, in particular cytomegalovirus, cause further immunosuppression because of cytokine release and also lead to additional infections.

Pathogenesis of rejection

The pathogenesis of organ (graft) rejection is well understood and reviewed extremely briefly here. Human leucocyte antigens (HLA) are referred to as the major histocompatibility complex (MHC) antigens for the purposes of tissue typing and transplantation. MHC antigens are classified as class I and class II. They form two subsets of three antigens: A, B and C for class I and DR, DQ and DP for class II. There is enormous polymorphism in both class I and class II antigens. Matching MHC class II antigens (DR, DQ and DP) is more important than class I. Some alleles are rare, and finding a matching donor for stem cell transplantation can require screening tens to hundreds of thousands of individuals. International databases have, therefore, been set up to facilitate matching of donors and recipients. Clearly HLA matching in solid organ transplantation from cadavers is necessarily less precise because of the limited time available before the transplanted organ has to be reperfused.

If there is some degree of HLA mismatch, the different HLA type is recognised as different by helper T cells (afferent phase). The efferent phase involves the activation of helper T and cytotoxic T cells, cytokine release and macrophages activation. The graft is damaged by direct cell-mediated cytotoxicity. Apart from attempting to match HLA types, it is important to rule out pre-existing anti-HLA antibodies, which would otherwise destroy the transplanted tissue in minutes. Production of HLA antibodies may follow pregnancy, transfusion or previous transplantation.

Table 89 Indications for stem cell transplantation

Disease	Autologous	Allogeneic
Non-malignant disease		
Aplastic anaemia	Impossible	Possibly*
Thalassaemia major	Impossible	Yes
Inherited immunodeficiencies	Impossible	Yes
Inborn errors of metabolism	Impossible	Yes
Connective tissue diseases	Possibly	Yes
Malignant disease		
Acute and chronic myeloid leukaemia	Possibly	Yes/possibly*
Acute lymphocytic leukaemia	Possibly	Yes
Multiple myeloma	Yes	Possibly
Non-Hodgkin's lymphoma	Probably	Possibly*
Hodgkin's disease after relapse	Yes	Possibly*

*In young adults.

Prophylaxis of rejection

Much attention has been paid by transplant units to the *prophylaxis* of rejection. All units give high immunosuppressive doses during and immediately after transplantation and then gradually reduce the doses according to a set schedule but modified by the patient's course and episodes of rejection. In the early years of transplantation, corticosteroids were the mainstay of immunosuppression. They suppress the immune response: primarily macrophages at modest doses but on T cells as well at high doses. Transplantation was not really successful with steroids alone as they are inadequately immunosuppressives at low doses. Substantial reductions in both infection and rejection rates followed the introduction of ciclosporin, and more recently tacrolimus and sirolimus, and many renal transplant units now reserve steroids for episodes of graft rejection. Ciclosporin works on T cells to prevent the cytokine cascade after stimulation by a new antigen. The major drawback of ciclosporin is toxicity: in particular, nephrotoxicity but also hypertension and neurotoxicity. Serum levels must be monitored. Ciclosporin also has multiple drug interactions. Azathioprine and mycophenolate are also used extensively as immunosuppressants by an anti-proliferative action, especially on T cells.

Monitoring and diagnosing rejection

Monitoring for rejection is relatively simple in renal transplantation; urine output and serum creatinine (or clearance) are good indicators of established rejection. Biopsy is necessary to confirm rejection. In cardiac and lung transplantation, sequential myocardial and lung biopsies are done. Each necessitates an invasive procedure. Monitoring of rejection in liver transplantation requires some liver biopsies and liver function tests. A biopsy is always necessary to confirm rejection and rule out viral infection.

Management of rejection

Drugs used for the treatment of episodes of rejection include methylprednisolone, basiliximab (chimeric anti-CD25 (IL-2 receptor) monoclonal antibody); increased doses of ciclosporin and mycophenolate.

Graft-versus-host disease

Graft-versus-host disease (GVHD) is a form of 'organ rejection' in which transplanted T cells and macrophages react with the tissues of the recipient. The transplantation/transfusion procedures that give rise to GVHD are well recognised:

- allogeneic stem cell transplantation (especially HLA-mismatched grafts)
- transfusion of unirradiated blood products into immunocompromised patients.

The risk of GVHD following bone marrow transplantation depends on the HLA matching of the graft, on whether GVHD prophylaxis is given and on the patient's age. The incidence varies from 10 to 80%.

Acute GVHD is manifest by:

- rash, itchy on palms, soles and ears initially
- intestinal dysfunction, causing diarrhoea
- liver dysfunction.

Acute GVHD leads to profound immunosuppression in and of itself and because the treatment of it with corticosteroids is immunosuppressive. The severity is graded I–IV. Severe GVHD (grades III and IV) carries a high mortality. Chronic GVHD occurs 3 or more months after transplant, with more fibrotic pathology akin to systemic sclerosis/scleroderma. A reduction in the relapse rate of malignancy is associated with GVHD, probably due to a graft-versus-leukaemia effect.

Infection

Patients given immunosuppressive therapy for transplantation (or who receive therapy for other reasons that has a secondary immunosuppressive effect, e.g. radiotherapy) are vulnerable to many of the opportunistic infections seen in HIV-positive patients (see above). Such patients are unable to mount an adequate immune response to certain organisms (particularly T cell and phagocyte responses). The symptoms and signs of infection are more subtle because the usual clinical clues, such as fever, are absent or diminished by immunosuppression. This delays diagnosis and so infections are often severe before they are diagnosed. The poor immune response combined with late diagnosis are the two main reasons why these infections, in general, carry a poor prognosis. Anti-infective prophylaxis is therefore routinely given.

9.4 Allergy

Learning objectives

You should:
- understand the mechanisms, clinical presentation and treatment of anaphylaxis and other allergic phenomena.

Case Study

A 13-year-old collapses in the playground and is brought into accident and emergency ashen-blue with a blood pressure of 60 mmHg palpable. He is successfully resuscitated and after 2 days in the intensive case unit describes how he was taunted with a 'Snickers' bar by older boys in the playground. His Epi-pen was in his school bag and took ages to find.

There are several clinical manifestations of allergy (Fig. 103). These include:

- anaphylaxis
- laryngeal oedema and/or bronchoconstriction
- asthma (p. 89)
- allergic rhinitis/hay fever
- gut allergy: vomiting and/or diarrhoea
- urticaria
- drug allergy manifest as rashes.

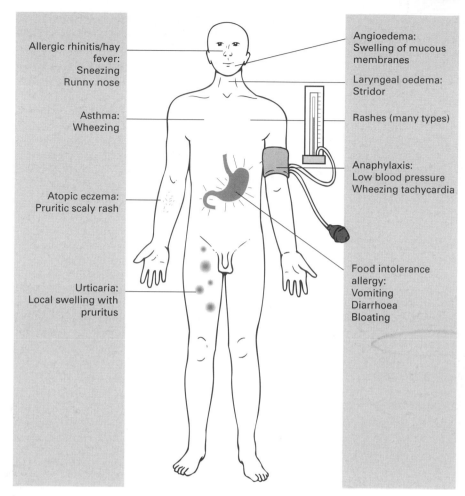

Allergic rhinitis/hay
fever:
Sneezing
Runny nose

Asthma:
Wheezing

Atopic eczema:
Pruritic scaly rash

Urticaria:
Local swelling with
pruritus

Angioedema:
Swelling of mucous
membranes

Laryngeal oedema:
Stridor

Rashes (many types)

Anaphylaxis:
Low blood pressure
Wheezing tachycardia

Food intolerance
allergy:
Vomiting
Diarrhoea
Bloating

Fig. 103 Clinical manifestations of allergy.

Most allergic disease is intermittent and follows exposure to an allergen. Up to 20% of the population suffer from one form of allergy or another. Most individuals have a genetic predisposition, known as atopy. Other risk factors include smoking, high levels of antigen exposure and prenatal factors. Most allergies are manifest in childhood, but some appear in adult life for the first time, particularly drug allergy.

Allergy testing

The rapid-onset and severe allergic syndromes are primarily mediated by IgE, and therefore IgE testing is often helpful in defining the causative allergen(s). A raised total IgE is most consistent with allergy or parasitic infection.

Specific IgE or radioallergosorbent tests (RAST) are available for a large number of allergens, including furry pets, peanut, grasses, *Aspergillus* and other fungi, milk, etc. Skin testing with standardised reagents is also useful. These are intradermal (or prick) tests done on the foream, and the wheal and erythema response 20 minutes after application is compared with the control. Patch testing is a 48-hour test for (usually) contact dermatitis, which reflects a slower type IV hypersensitivity response.

Anaphylaxis

Clinical presentation

Anaphylaxis is life-threatening. It is triggered by exposure to an allergen (e.g. bee sting, penicillin). It is characterised by:

- airway obstruction with stridor/wheezing
- hypotension
- cutaneous reactions, such as pruritus, flushing, urticaria
- GI symptoms, including vomiting and diarrhoea.

Pathogenesis

Immediate hypersensitivity responses are mediated by mast cells and IgE (Fig. 104). Mast cells are derived from haematopoietic precursors and migrate to and mature in connective or mucosal tissue. Mast cells have many granules, which contain histamine, chymase, tryptase (both proteases which directly increase bronchial hyper-responsiveness and bronchial mucus production) and other substances. When released, these substances cause immediate local irritation (wheal and flare reaction) and a late-phase response characterised by infiltration of activated inflammatory cells including T cells. Basophils probably contribute to the immediate hypersensitivity response.

IgE

The most potent stimulus for mast cell degranulation is IgE. IgE comprises less than 0.001% of total immunoglobulin and is produced by B cells. IgE production is stimulated by interleukin-4 and inhibited by interferon gamma and CD8 cells. Preformed IgE binds to mast cells when antigen exposure occurs, leading to mast cell degranulation. Specific IgE — for example, to penicillin — can be detected in blood with a RAST or a skin (prick) test. In prick tests, minute quantities are injected into the dermis and a wheal and flare reaction follows if the person is hypersensitive to that antigen. As exposure to an allergen is necessary to generate a population of B cells and specific IgE, so an allergic response cannot occur on first exposure to an allergen. IgE triggers of mast cell degranulation include complement C3a or C5a and carbohydrates found in some fruits, e.g. strawberries (Table 90).

Management

Treatment of anaphylaxis *must* be immediate (see emergency box below). Patients should be admitted to hospital for several hours after anaphylaxis to observe for relapse. The mortality is about 10% overall but is higher in patients out of hospital. Follow-up to prevent recurrence is essential.

Other allergic diseases

Other diseases mediated by mast cell degranulation include asthma, allergic rhinitis, hay fever and urticaria, and some forms of food allergy other than anaphylaxis. Common allergens include the house dust mite, pets, milk or milk products, eggs and many other foods. In cases of urticaria, for example, identifying the trigger is often difficult and weeks and months of 'detective' work are often unsuccessful. Some cases are caused by pressure on the skin and others result from autoimmunity (IgG antibodies to the mast cell IgE receptor).

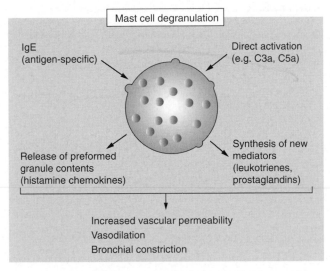

Fig. 104 Hypersensitivity responses mediated by IgE and mast cells.

Clinical Box: Emergency treatment: management of anaphylaxis

Out of hospital

Think of quickest means of acquiring adrenaline (epinephrine): Epi-pen, local doctor, 999 call, direct transport to nearby hospital

If in hospital, act quickly

1. Stop infusions of any blood or drugs
2. Give oxygen by mask in high concentration

Table 90 Causes and mechanisms of allergic symptoms and conditions mimicking allergy

Substance (example)	Mechanism	Symptoms
Venoms (bee sting)	IgE-mediated	Anaphylaxis
Airborne allergens (moulds such as *Aspergillus*, animal dander, pollen)	IgE-mediated	Asthma, rhinitis, hay fever
Foods (peanuts, milk, seafood, egg)	IgE-mediated	Angioedema, anaphylaxis, eczema
Antibiotics (penicillins, sulphonamides)	IgE-mediated	Anaphylaxis, urticaria, angioedema, maculopapular rashes
Drugs and i.v. solutions (opiates, curare, vancomycin, contrast media)	Direct activation of mast cells	
Dialysis membrane and proteins (immunoglobulin, blood products)	Complement activation	
Aspirin, NSAIDs	Build-up of leukotrienes	Rhinitis, asthma, angioedema
ACE inlibitors	Build-up of bradykinin	Angioedema, anaplylaxis

NSAIDs, non-steroidal anti-inflammatory drugs.

Nine

3. Give adrenaline (epinephrine) 0.5–1 ml (1 in 1000) intramuscular; repeat every 10 minutes as necessary

4. Measure blood pressure

5. If hypotensive, give 1–2 litres of colloid (e.g. Haemaccell) quickly.

6. If bronchoconstriction present, use nebulised β_2-antagonists such as salbutamol

7. Give antihistamine i.v. (to prevent relapse)

8. Depending on clinical status and response to treatment, transfer to ward or intensive care unit

9. Give hydrocortisone 100–300 mg i.v. over 1 minute (no immediate effect but will help prevent relapse)

9.5 Immunotherapy

Learning objectives

You should:
- know the indications for immunoglobulin therapy and prevention
- appreciate the wide range of uses to which anti-cytokine monoclonal antibodies and growth factors are put.

Case Study

A 73-year-old retired teacher with severe rheumatoid arthritis has a past family history of tuberculosis. Her consultant wants to start an anti-tumour necrosis factor agent (infliximab). Her tuberculin skin test is negative, but she is on steroids. Her chest X-ray shows apical pleural thickening, and calcification in the right hilar glands.

Various forms of immunotherapy are now a part of routine clinical practice. Passive protection against infection relies on antibody in some situations. Active immunisation is usually a preferable strategy if possible. Other forms of immunotherapy activate or inhibit various arms of the immune system, especially cytokine blockade.

Immunoglobulin

Intramuscular immunoglobulin (gammaglobulin) has several uses. Pooled normal immunoglobulin contains enough antibody for the prevention of hepatitis A, and tetanus and the treatment of tetanus. Hyperimmune globulin is pooled from several donors selected because of high specific antibody titres. It is useful for:

- prevention of hepatitis B in exposed health-care workers (if unimmunised) and newborns
- prevention of varicella in immunocompromised patients
- prevention of rabies after an animal bite in non-immune individuals
- treatment of severe cases of diphtheria
- prevention and treatment of tetanus.

Intravenous immunoglobulin is used to prevent infection in antibody-deficient individuals and for the specific therapy of a few diseases, including Kawasaki disease.

Cytokines, interferons and colony-stimulating factors

Numerous cytokines have been described. Cytokines:

- are inducible proteins
- are largely triggered by infection and other forms of tissue damage
- have immune and non-immune effects
- have paracrine rather than endocrine effects.

Initially all cytokines were described as having immunological functions. This is no longer true; for example, interleukin-1 increases collagen synthesis and wound healing, and neurotrophic factor is a 'survival factor' for many types of neurone. Some cytokines are called growth factors or colony-stimulating factors, but the principles are the same.

Interferons (a type of cytokine) have several effects, which include:

- increased expression of MHC receptors to allow for greater viral antigen recognition
- increased activation of natural killer cells and macrophages
- direct inhibition of viral replication and other viral processes, such as viral penetration of cells
- pro-inflammatory actions and increased TH1 effects (interferon gamma).

Treatment with cytokines

Three interferons and several growth factors that have proven to be therapeutically useful. Interferons have antiviral activity and are given subcutaneously. Colony-stimulating factors are given either intravenously or subcutaneously.

Interferon alpha There are now several indications for the use of interferon alpha:

- treatment of chronic hepatitis caused by hepatitis B or C virus
- eradication of hepatitis B surface antigen (and e antigen) carriage
- hairy cell leukaemia
- Kaposi's sarcoma in AIDS
- renal cell carcinoma
- multiple myeloma.

Interferon beta This reduces the number of radiological exacerbations of multiple sclerosis.

Interferon gamma This cytokine is produced by activated T cells and natural killer cells and acts on lymphocytes, monocytes and some other cells such as microglial and endothelial cells. It increases macrophage and neutrophil activity. It is used for the prophylaxis of infection in chronic granulomatous disease and for interferon gamma deficiency.

Granulocyte colony-stimulating factor A recombinant form is used to shorten the period of neutropenia after cytotoxic chemotherapy, aplastic anaemia or in AIDS. It may also improve neutrophil function and enhance neutrophil longevity.

Granulocyte macrophage colony-stimulating factor This is similar to granulocyte colony-stimulating factor but also acts on the monocyte/macrophage arm to increase the production of cells from the marrow and to improve their function. Its role is less clearly defined.

Cytokine and immunoglobulin blockers

In recent years there have been many cytokine or cytokine receptor blockers developed. They include:

- anti-TNF-α antibodies for the treatment of rhematoid arthritis, Crohn's disease, ankylosing spondylitis and psoriasis.
- IL-1 receptor antagonist for the treatment of rheumatoid arthritis.
- IL-2 alpha receptor antagonist for prevention or treatment of rejection after organ transplantation.
- anti-IgE for the treatment of severe asthma.

Self-assessment: questions

Any or all of each set of five statements may be true or false. Choose your answers and see the reasoning behind the correct answer on pages 403–404.

Multiple choice questions

1. The following are true:
   a. Intravenous immunoglobulin therapy carries a substantial risk of hepatitis B
   b. Splenectomy has no substantial impact on susceptibility to infection
   c. *Neisseria* infections are more common in C6 complement deficiency
   d. Selective IgA deficiency is relatively common in oriental people
   e. Tetanus and diphtheria toxins are directly inactivated by antibody produced after immunisation

2. With respect to phagocytes:
   a. Once a phagocyte has ingested a pathogen (e.g. *Listeria* spp.) progressive infection is arrested
   b. Macrophages directly kill viruses
   c. Interferon gamma has no effect on neutrophil function
   d. Most neutrophils in the body are circulating in blood
   e. The respiratory burst in neutrophils is the primary mechanism for killing bacteria such as *Staphylococcus aureus*.

3. The following are true:
   a. Patients who have had anaphylaxis should wear a Medic Alert bracelet
   b. Hay fever is mediated mostly by switching of neutrophils
   c. High total circulating IgE concentrations can be caused by *Aspergillus*
   d. Radioallergosorbent (RAST) tests are useful for identifying causes of urticaria
   e. The first drug that should be administered to patients with anaphylaxis is an antihistamine

4. With respect to susceptibility to infection the following associations are true:
   a. Diabetes and *Staphylococcus aureus*
   b. Heart transplant recipient and cytomegalovirus
   c. Hodgkin's disease and herpes zoster
   d. Chronic renal failure and bacteraemia
   e. Pancreatitis and candidaemia

5. The following are true:
   a. Specific IgM antibodies are useful for diagnosing recent hepatitis A

   b. Specific IgM antibodies are useful in diagnosis of cytomegalovirus disease in AIDS
   c. IgM binds complement efficiently
   d. IgM antibodies are only found in blood because of their size and not at the site of infection or inflammation
   e. In general, IgM is inefficient at binding Gram-negative organisms

6. The following are true:
   a. HIV-1 infection usually leads to AIDS within 4 years
   b. HIV infects cytotoxic T lymphocytes
   c. Macrophage dysfunction is a common feature of AIDS
   d. HIV may be transmitted by one episode of heterosexual intercourse
   e. Symptomatic HIV disease typically occurs when the helper T cell count falls just below 500×10^6 cells/l

7. Delay in the onset of AIDS-defining illness can be achieved with the following:
   a. Treatment of oral thrush for 7 days
   b. Prophylaxis of *Pneumocystis* pneumonia
   c. Pneumococcal immunisation
   d. Influenza immunisation
   e. Combination antiretroviral therapy

8. Cutaneous manifestations of HIV infection include:
   a. Kaposi's sarcoma
   b. Seborrhoeic dermatitis
   c. Severe mucosal herpes simplex infection
   d. Herpes zoster (shingles)
   e. Onychomycosis

9. Concerning HIV infection and AIDS:
   a. *Pneumocystis* pneumonia is common in Africa
   b. Tuberculosis in AIDS presents like that in non-AIDS patients
   c. Oral candidiasis is a late feature of AIDS
   d. Toxoplasmosis is usually a cerebral disease
   e. Cytomegalovirus retinitis can be treated with aciclovir

10. The following clinical presentations raise suspicion of HIV disease:
    a. Recurrent cold sores on lips
    b. Tuberculosis in an ex-intravenous drug abuser
    c. Non-Hodgkin's lymphoma in a 62-year-old woman
    d. Parents of an adopted child from abroad
    e. Recurrent sinusitis

Extended matched questions

EMQ 1

Theme: Possible diagnoses for patients with infections

Options

1. Acute leukaemia
2. Alcholism
3. Asthma
4. Bronchiectasis
5. Carcinoma of the lung
6. Chronic fatigue syndrome
7. Chronic liver disease
8. Cystic fibrosis
9. Depression
10. Antibody deficiency
11. Influenza
12. HIV infection
13. Meningitis
14. Myeloma
15. Pneumococcal pneumonia
16. *Pneumocystis* pneumonia
17. Splenectomy
18. Systemic lupus erythematosus
19. Tuberculosis
20. Chronic granulomatous disease

For patients A–C, select the most likely diagnosis of the presenting problem *and* the most likely underlying diagnosis.

A. A 42-year-old man has had a chronic productive cough for about 5 years intermittently. Each exacerbation is associated with large amounts of thick green sputum, occasionally tinged pink. His temperature is 36.8°C and respiratory rate 22 breaths/min. He has crackles in his chest on both sides posteriorly. A chest radiograph shows coarse lung markings at both bases, most marked on the left. His complete blood count shows a haemoglobin of 112 g/l, white cell count of 12.8×10^9 cells/l and a platelet count of 440×10^9 cells/l. Liver function tests were normal, albumin was 43 g/l and globulins 28 g/l. His Po_2 is 11.6 kPa (85 mm Hg), Pco_2 4.8 kPa (36 mm Hg), pH 7.41 and base excess +2.

B. A 38-year-old man has had a cough for 4 weeks, productive of small amounts of white sputum. He had a chest infection 9 months ago, associated with chest pain and productive cough that resolved slowly with amoxicillin. He describes weight loss of 3.5 kg over the last 6 months or so, and some tiredness. His temperature is 37.8°C. His chest is normal on examination, except for a respiratory rate of 24 breaths/min. His chest radiograph shows slightly increased lung markings in the left mid-

zone. His blood count shows a haemoglobin of 138 g/l, white cell count of 3.7×10^9 cells/l and a platelet count of 110×10^9 cells/l. His liver function tests are normal, apart from a gamma-glutamyl transferase of 119 IU/l and lactate dehydrogenase (LDH) of 839 IU/l. His albumin is 37 g/l and globulin 51 g/l. His Po_2 is 8.5 kPa (64 mm Hg), Pco_2 4.1 kPa (31 mm Hg), pH 7.47 and base excess +4.

C. A 34-year-old woman is brought in confused and pyrexial. She has been ill for 2 days with 'flu' and become increasingly unwell over the last 8 hours. Prior to this, she was completely well and working, apart from a car accident 3 years ago. Examination shows her to have a pyrexia of 39.3°C and respiratory rate of 32 breaths/min, pulse rate 125 per minute, BP 85/50 mm Hg, Glasgow Coma Scale (GCS) of 11, crackles at the right base and a mid-line abdominal scar, with dusky cold toes and tips of fingers. Her chest radiograph shows consolidation at the right base. Her blood count shows a haemoglobin of 126 g/l, white cell count of 23.7×10^9 cells/l and platelet count of 68×10^9 cells/l. Her liver functions test are normal, apart from an LDH of 720 IU/l; her albumin was 35 g/l and globulin 40 g/l. Her Po_2 was 8.5 kPa (64 mm Hg), Pco_2 4.1 kPa (31 mm Hg), pH 7.28 and base excess of –6.

D. A 74-year-old man with mild emphysema but otherwise well is brought to hospital slightly confused. He was well until 6 days ago, when he, and then his wife, developed fever in association with generalised aches and pains, runny nose and sore thoat. He was quite ill for about 3 days and then improved, but has been worse over the last 24–48 hours. He is more short of breath and is anorexic with some right-sided chest pain. His temperature is 35.3°C, pulse 115 beats/min, respiratory rate 28 breaths/min and blood pressure 140/75 mmHg. Bronchial breathing is apparent at his left base and his left diaphragm is partially obscured on his chest radiograph. His white cell count is 15.3×10^9/l his Po_2 is 8.9 kPa (67 mm Hg), Pco_2 6.1 kPa (46 mm Hg), pH 7.36 and base excess –7. His urea is 10.3 µmol/l.

EMQ 2

Theme: Possible immunological defects

Options

1. None
2. Antibody deficiency
3. T cell defect
4. Phagocyte defect
5. Complement defect
6. Multiple defect

For each clinical scenario below, choose the most likely immunological defect (if there is one). Each option can be selected once, more than once or not at all.

A. A 30-year-old man with cerebral toxoplasmosis
B. A 15-year-old boy with persistent sinusitis

C. A 3-month-old baby with *Pneumocytis* pneumonia

D. A 12-year-old with two episodes of meningococcal infection

E. A 23-year-old woman with pyelonephritis

F. A 7-year-old boy with pneumonia and otitis media

G. A 3-year-old boy with a liver abscess

H. A 16-year-old woman with a subcutaneous abscess containing *Aspergillus*

Objective structured clinical examination (OSCE) stations

OSCE 1

This station deals with the data interpretation of immunoglobulins.

Examiner: You review a 35-year-old patient in outpatients following an admission from the chest unit with pneumonia. This was the third admission over 3 years with a chest infection. A CT scan of the chest was done on an outpatient basis (Fig. 105). What does it show?

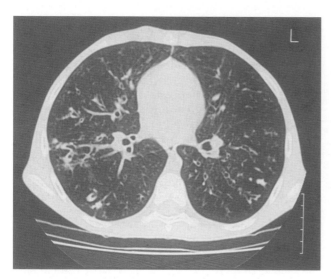

Fig. 105 CT scan of the chest.

Examiner: You are shown only one 'cut' and say the scan is incomplete. You point out some pulmonary consolidation and dilated airways. Are any further tests indicated and, if so, what?

Examiner: Comment on the following results:

IgG	7.1 g/l	(7.68–17.28)
IgA	0.6 g/l	(0.8–4.4)
IgM	2.1 g/l	(0.3–2.7)
IgE	8 IU/l	(<20)
IgG1	5.5 g/l	(4.22–12.92)
IgG2	0.07 g/l	(1.17–7.47)
IgG3	0.92 g/l	(0.41–1.29)
IgG4	0.48 g/l	(0.01–2.91)

OSCE 2

A 10-minute station on chronic viral infection

Examiner: This young man/woman was diagnosed with HIV infection last week and counselled. Additional blood tests were undertaken and he/she has come back today to discuss the results and decide what treatment, if any, is required. The full blood count shows:

Haemoglobin 12.8 g/l
White cell count 3.9×10^6/l
Platelets 185×10^9/l
Neutrophils 2.4×10^9/l
Lymphocytes 0.9×10^9/l
Eosinophils 0.2×10^9/l
Monocytes 0.3×10^9/l
Basophils 0.1×10^9/l
CD4 cell count 130×10^6/l
HIV viral load 280 000 copies/ml ($>10^5$ copies/ml)
Cytomegalovirus IgG antibody +ve
Epstein-Barr virus IgG antibody +ve
Toxoplasma IgG antibody −ve
Hepatitis B core IgG antibody −ve
Hepatitis C antibody +ve
Treponema pallidum haemagglutination assay

Case history questions

Case history 1

A 34-year-old woman is referred to you with tiredness and weight loss of 7 kg over 2 months. She has had a lot of stress at work (advertising) and attributes her symptoms to this and to having no time to cook for herself. There is no significant past medical history apart from pelvic inflammatory disease. She is separated from her husband. Her vital signs are temperature 36.5°C, pulse 92 beats/min, blood pressure 110/70 mmHg, respiratory rate 18/breaths/min. Examination shows her to be thin with several small lymph nodes palpable in the neck and left groin. There are no signs in the mouth or elsewhere.

1. The following tests should be done immediately (true or false?):

    a. Full blood count, differential white cell and platelet count

    b. Biochemistry panel

    c. Chest X-ray

    d. Epstein–Barr virus (EBV) serology

    e. Thyroid function tests

She returns in 2 weeks and is no better. She describes a dull retrosternal chest pain and mild nausea. Her blood results are haemoglobin 117 g/l, white cell count 3.9×10^9 cells/l, neutrophils 2900×10^6 cells/l, lymphocytes 650×10^6 cells/l and platelets 93×10^9 cells/l. She has normal biochemistry and a normal chest radiograph. Her EBV IgM test is negative, IgG positive ('exposure at some time in the past').

2. Now you should do the following (true or false?):

   a. Examine her mouth
   b. Enquire more deeply into HIV risk factors
   c. Arrange an endoscopy urgently
   d. Do an HIV test after obtaining her consent
   e. Treat her with omeprazole empirically

Seven days later, she has had a confirmed positive HIV antibody test and endoscopy shows extensive oesophageal candidiasis. She is at home.

3. Now you should do the following:

   a. Refer her to the local HIV/AIDS unit
   b. Start her on zidovudine therapy
   c. Start her on fluconazole therapy
   d. Arrange admission to hospital
   e. Phone her up to tell her the HIV test result as soon as you receive it.

Case history 2

A 44-year-old man presents to accident and emergency with a 1-week history of breathlessness and cough. Over the last 3–4 weeks he has become increasingly tired, lost 5 kg in weight and had a troublesome boil on his left buttock. On examination, he is breathless when he talks but not at rest, with a dry cough. Vital signs are a temperature of 38.3°C, respiratory rate 30 breaths/min, pulse 110 beats/min, blood pressure 110/85 mmHg. Examination of the chest is otherwise normal and there are no murmurs. Small lymph nodes are palpable in his neck and left groin. There is a small boil on his left buttock but no other skin lesions. There are no signs of i.v. drug abuse. Joints, nervous system and abdomen are normal, as is blood sugar.

1. What additional history should you seek?
2. What important part of the physical examination has been omitted and why might it be important?
3. Give a short differential diagnosis of his pulmonary problem.
4. List two essential investigations which would need urgent results and why.

Case history 3

A 49-year-old female school teacher presents with a long history of eczema all her life, asthma from childhood, hay fever from late childhood, and fish and egg allergy since childhood (angioedema and urticaria minutes after eating). At the age of 42 she develops allergic reactions to avocado, banana and chestnut (facial and pharyngeal angioedema).

1. What is the likely direct link between these foods?
2. What direct question would you ask her?
3. What allergy tests would be most appropriate?
4. What advice would you give?

Picture questions

1. Figure 106 is the appearance of the cerebrospinal fluid (CSF) from an HIV-positive man with a persistent headache and low-grade fever. His last helper T cell count was 123×10^6 cells/l. The CSF showed 10 white cells, all lymphocytes, a protein of 0.6 g/l and a glucose of 3.5 mmol/l. There were <100 red cells.

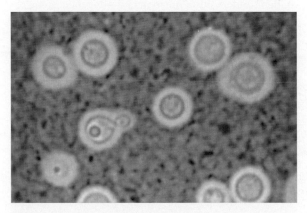

Fig. 106 High power view of cerebrospinal fluid.

   a. What is shown?
   b. What test has been done to show the abnormality?
   c. What other piece of information do you need from the lumbar puncture to manage him properly?
   d. What other tests should be done? (Give four.)
   e. How should he be managed?

2. Figure 107 is the chest radiograph of a heart transplant recipient with fever, shortness of breath and cough. He is 3 months post-transplant and doing reasonably well apart from two episodes of moderate rejection. He is taking anti-*Toxoplasma* prophylaxis as his donor had antibodies for *Toxoplasma* and he did not.

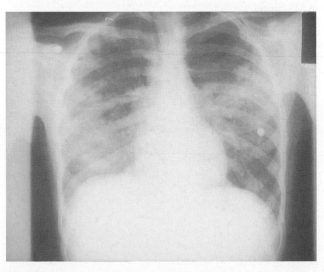

Fig. 107 Chest radiograph in a heart transplant recipient.

a. Describe the abnormality.

b. Give a differential diagnosis.

c. What two investigations should be done urgently?

d. What empirical therapy might you start while waiting for a result?

3. The CT thorax slice (Fig. 108) shows a large nodular area of consolidation in the left lower lobe. The patient underwent a mismatched allogeneic stem cell transplant 9 weeks ago. He then developed a dry cough and a dull ache in the chest, without fever.

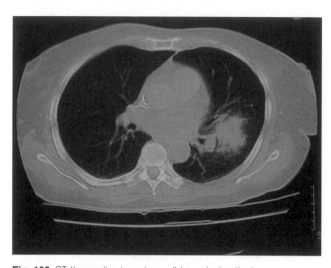

Fig. 108 CT thorax slice in a stem cell transplant patient.

a. Give a differential diagnosis.

b. What tests are likely to be useful?

c. What treatment would you give?

Short notes

1. Write a list of headings you should cover and sketch out the details of the most important points for a discussion group of student nurses that you are leading about the risks of occupational acquisition of HIV.

2. Write short notes on the following:

a. indications for lymphocyte subset determination

b. indications for measuring immunoglobulin levels

c. CD4 cell counts in HIV/AIDS and the rationale for intervention

d. why the development of an HIV vaccine might be difficult

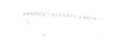

Self-assessment: answers

Multiple choice answers

1. a. **False**. Previous preparations carried a substantial risk of hepatitis C virus but this has been virtually eliminated from immunoglobulin preparations. There is also negligible to zero risk of transmission of HIV via this route.

   b. **False**. Splenectomised patients are at particular risk of overwhelming infection from capsulate organisms including *Streptococcus pneumoniae*. The problem is not only that patients are more likely to develop infections with these organisms but that the infections are likely to be fatal. Splenectomised patients do not respond to pneumococcal vaccine very well. Patients listed for elective splenectomy should be given pneumococcal vaccine at least 10 days prior to splenectomy to protect them against this fatal complication.

   c. **True**. C6 complement deficiency is rare but is associated with either *N. meningitidis* infection or disseminated gonococcal infection.

   d. **False**. Selective IgA deficiency is common in Caucasians, occurring in 1 in 300–700 population. This means that any GP working in a predominantly white neighbourhood will have between three and eight such patients on his list at any one time.

   e. **True**. This is the logic for giving not only tetanus toxoid, to induce the production of antitoxin, but also tetanus immunoglobulin following injury with soil-contaminated material.

2. a. **False**. Some organisms are essentially intracellular organisms (such as *Legionella pneumophila*) and, therefore, thrive intracellularly. Phagocytosis is only one step in the inactivation of an organism; intracellular killing is the next and there are many organisms which have evolved excellent defences for evading this.

   b. **False**. Important viruses may replicate inside macrophages (e.g. HIV) and macrophages may process viral antigens allowing the production of specific antibody and T cell responses to the viruses, but they do not kill viruses directly.

   c. **False**. Interferon gamma upregulates and improves neutrophil function.

   d. **False**. Most neutrophils in the body are contained within the vascular space but exist mainly in what is called the marginating pool. These are 'resting' neutrophils loosely attached to endothelium. A raised white cell count in response to infection reflects the release of neutrophils from the marginating pool. Left shift (or 'bands' in US parlance) reflects the increased circulation of early neutrophils produced from the bone marrow.

   e. **True**. The respiratory burst is a fundamental part of defence against infection and is deficient in chronic granulomatous disease which is why these patients suffer recurrent infection, particularly by *Staph aureus*, *Candida* and *Aspergillus*.

3. a. **True**. Some patients also carry a small preloaded syringe of adrenaline (epinephrine) (Epi-pen) with them, particularly if they are allergic to a common allergen such as peanuts or seafood to which they might be exposed to advertently.

   b. **False**. Neutrophils do not switch and are barely involved in any allergic disease

   c. **True**. Particularly in the context of allergic bronchopulmonary aspergillosis (ABPA), which occurs in asthmatic or cystic fibrosis patients.

   d. **False**. RAST tests are sometimes useful for identifying different causes of anaphylaxis and rarely urticaria.

   e. **False**. Adrenaline (epinephrine) should be the first drug to be administered, followed by steroids and antihistamines.

4. a. **True**.

   b. **True**. Cytomegalovirus causes pneumonitis because of immune suppression; it is frequently fatal if not recognised and treated.

   c. **True**. The increased risk extends to 5 years after the diagnosis of Hodgkin's disease despite the lack of additional chemotherapy or steroids, because of significant depression of cell-mediated (especially T cell) immunity.

   d. **True**. Partly because of frequent use of i.v. catheters but also because of the reduced generalised defence against infection.

   e. **True**. Patients with pancreatitis and those who have had a perforated viscus in the abdomen repaired or removed surgically are at substantial risk for candidaemia.

5. a. **True**. They are also useful for diagnosing recent hepatitis B and other infections: rubella, toxoplasmosis, etc.

   b. **False**. Virtually all AIDS patients are seropositive IgG for cytomegalovirus and the development of disease (such as retinitis or colitis) is not reflected in an increase in the IgM. In addition, in immunocompromised patients, the IgM response may be either blunted or absent. AIDs patients negative for CMV IgG must be given CMV-negative blood, if transfused, or they develop overwhelming CMV infection.

   c. **True**.

   d. **False**. Increased concentrations of immunoglobulin and complement leave the blood space through the vascular endothelium to sites of inflammation and infection.

e. **False**. IgM antibodies are particularly adept at binding Gram-negative organisms, which is why immunoglobulin therapy for patients with recurrent Gram-negative sepsis is less effective than with patients for recurrent Gram-positive sepsis.

6. a. **False**. 60% progress to AIDS over 11 years.

a. **False**. Helper T cells and many other cells are infected but cytotoxic T cells are protective.

c. **True**. AIDS-related infections include toxoplasmosis, salmonellosis, leishmaniasis and histoplasmosis (which are all intracellular pathogens of macrophages). The failure of helper T (CD4) cells to activate macrophages is the primary problem with these infections.

d. **True**. Although the risk is not very high in the absence of genital ulceration.

e. **False**. Typically below 200×10^6 cells/l.

7. a. **False**. There is no evidence for this and prevention of thrush with continuous antifungal therapy may lead to resistance.

b. **True**. Very important; should be introduced when the helper T cell count falls below 200–250 $\times 10^6$ cells/l.

c. **False**. A single episode of pneumococcal pneumonia is not an index disease for AIDS. Immunisation may prevent pneumococcal infection, which is about 100 times more common in AIDS, although it may be less severe.

d. **False**. There is no evidence that influenza is more common or severe in AIDS.

e. **True**. Clearly shown in double-blind controlled trials.

8. a. **True**. Purplish nodules on skin or in mouth.

b. **True**. Common generally but more florid in HIV.

c. **True**. Often rectal/anal and painful.

d. **True**. An indication for an HIV test.

e. **True**. Incidence in general population is 2–3% but in HIV may affect more nails and be recalcitrant to treatment.

9. a. **False**. Less than 10% of patients; pulmonary tuberculosis is much more common and tends to present with higher levels of helper T cells than *Pneumocystis* pneumonia does.

b. **False**. Atypical chest radiograph without cavitation is common, less often smear-positive in sputum.

c. **False**. 90% of AIDS patients develop oral thrush.

d. **True**. Brain and heart. The CT/MR scan usually shows multiple ring-enhancing lesions, which are almost diagnostic of toxoplasmosis in AIDS. Central nervous system lymphomas are usually single. Cardiac toxoplasmosis is usually diagnosed at postmortem.

e. **False**. Only ganciclovir, foscarnet and cidofovir are useful.

10. a. **False**. Recurrent cold sores are common and do not suggest immunodeficiency. Large and painful or prolonged herpes simplex lesions, especially 'below the belt', may constitute an indication for HIV testing.

b. **True**. Tuberculosis is rising throughout the world and any risk factor in association with tuberculosis, or an atypical pattern of tuberculosis, would be an indication for HIV testing.

c. **False**. Non-Hodgkin's lymphoma occurs in AIDS but is more common in non-immunocompromised patients. Only if there is a risk factor would an HIV test be indicated.

d. **False**. Transmission of HIV from child to parents or from child to child is virtually unheard of. Many children from the USA, Romania, Africa and some south-east Asian countries are, however, HIV-positive.

e. **False**. Recurrent sinusitis is a clue to immunoglobulin deficiency, not HIV.

Extended matched answers

EMQ 1

A. **4**, presenting problem; **10**, underlying diagnosis. Most cases of bronchiectasis are not associated with antibody deficiency and measurement of total globulins is a poor means of screening. Immunoglobulins and IgG subsets, should be tested for. If these are normal, functional antibodies to *Pneumococcus* should be tested, and consideration given to DNA testing for adult-onset cystic fibrosis.

B. **16**, presenting problem; **12**, underlying diagnosis. The remarkable hypoxaemia with an almost normal chest X-ray is the clue to the diagnosis. Mild leucopenia and thrombocytopenia with a raised LDH are also typical.

C. **15**, presenting problem; **17**, underlying diagnosis. She also has septic shock and almost certainly pneumococcal bacteraemia Pneumococcal vaccine is partially effective in prevention but difficult to effect after trauma. Life-long oral penicillin is very important for these patients, as is influenza immunisation to reduce the risk of pneumococcal infection.

D. **15**, presenting complaint; **11**, underlying diagnosis. The low temperature, raised urea and metabolic acidosis are signs of a severe infection with a high probability of death. The initial illness is typical of influenza: coryza with fever and generalised myalgia. Community-acquired pneumonia, usually pneumococcal, often follows influenza. Staphylococcal pneumonia is also more common. The raised Pco_2 suggests fatigue and/or type II respiratory failure. He will need admission to the intensive care unit.

EMQ 2

A. **3.** (AIDS)

B. **2.** (hypogammaglobulinaemia)

C. **3.** (AIDS or SCID)

D. **5.**

E. **1.** (consider pregnancy, structural defect of urinary tract)

F. **2.** (hypogammaglobulinaemia) (innate immunity defect also possible such as mannose binding defect).

G. **4.** (chronic granulomatous disease).

H. **4.** (chronic granulomatous disease).

Response to OSCE stations

OSCE 1

The scan shows bilateral bronchiectasis, worse on the right, and 'evolving' consolidation.

Further tests indicated are:

- immunoglobulins for antibody deficiency
- sweat or genetic test for cystic fibrosis
- *Aspergillus* precipitins and IgE for allergic bronchopulmonary aspergillosis (although without asthma, this is unlikely).

The results shows low-normal IgG, low IgA, normal IgM, normal IgE, low IgG2, others normal. The patient has a form of antibody deficiency (specifically IgG2 deficiency) and requires long-term immunoglobulin replacement therapy.

OSCE 2

Results show mild leucopenia, thrombocytopenia, significant lymphopenia and 'CD4-penia', a high HIV viral load, and prior infection with CMV, EBV and HCV but not *Toxoplasma*, HBV or syphilis.

The patient tells you that she learned last week for the first time that her longstanding male partner is bisexual. As he is bisexual, this was a partial surprise but not a complete shock. Now she wants to know how bad her infection is and what is to be done about it.

The points you elicit from the history are as follows:

- Sexual exposure over long period, so time of infection not clear.
- Usually had safe sex but not always.
- All other sexual contacts — UK or European holiday resorts, all Eurasian, no black.
- No i.v. drug use.
- No children.
- Steady partner not yet tested. Not practising safe sex as wants to have a baby (will need preconception counselling).
- Own house and steady job (non-medical, non-caring professional); Some life insurance.
- Strict vegetarian (relevant to *Toxoplasma* risk).
- Blood transfusion after car accident ≃15 years ago (relevant to hepatitis C).

- No pets at home but cats use garden (relevant to *Toxoplasma* risk).

You will gain marks for:

- Expression of sympathy for diagnosis, but positive outlook
- Low CD4 count (±lymphopenia) — at risk of infection
- High viral load — needs anti-HIV treatment
- Had glandular fever (±CMV) previously; no concerns
- Not had toxoplasmosis — needs to avoid undercooked meat, wash all fruit and vegetables thoroughly and not handle cat litter
- Had hepatitis C, possibly from intravenous drug abuse or blood transfusion
- Will need combination (3 drug) antiretroviral therapy
- Combination of two nucleoside reverse transcriptase inhibitors (i.e. AZT + 3TC, zidovudine and lamivudine) and 1 non-nucleoside reverse transcriptase inhibitor (i.e. nevirapine or efavirenz)
- will need primary prophylaxis for *Pneumocystis* pneumonia
- Need to check HCV viral load (if RNA viral replication ongoing)
- Absolute compliance with treatment essential.

Case history answers

Case history 1

1. a. **True.**

   b. **True.**

   c. **True.** She could have a mediastinal lymphoma, sarcoidosis or tuberculosis.

   d. **True.** Glandular fever (infections mononucleosis) is somewhat uncommon at this age, but neck glands and/or fatigue are presentations.

   e. **True.** To rule out thyrotoxicosis (although if her pulse rate was normal and there were no other features of thyroid hyperactivity, not necessary).

2. a. **True.** Key part of assessment: for oral thrush, hairy leukoplakia or Kaposi's sarcoma.

   b. **True.** But sensitively.

   c. **True.**

   d. **True.** After advising her about the benefits to her and her partner(s) of knowing the answer, implications of testing are: mortgages and life insurance and how the test result will be delivered.

   e. **False.** Oesophageal reflux or gastritis are unlikely diagnoses and may make oesophageal candidiasis worse.

3. a. **True.** As she needs their expertise.

   b. **False.** Combination therapy is the appropriate management and the use of zidovudine alone will lose her months or years of life.

   c. **True.**

d. **False.** No need for admission, unless she cannot eat.

e. **False.** The discussion of her result needs to be done face-to-face with someone knowledgeable with the disease area. You need an immediate plan for such a consultation. It should not be done on a Friday or in a rush.

Case history 2

1. His sexual history and possibly his travel history or history of any blood transfusions prior to 1985 in the developed world or more recently elsewhere.

2. The mouth. In particular, there might be oropharyngeal candidiasis, hairy leukoplakia and herpes simplex lesions. Also the genitals. If he is gay, he may have perianal herpes or warts which he has not declared.

3. *Pneumocystis* pneumonia, pneumococcal pneumonia, other community-acquired pneumonia, pulmonary tuberculosis or pulmonary embolism.

4. Chest radiograph and arterial blood gases. The chest radiograph is abnormal in 85–90% of patients with *Pneumocystis* pneumonia and >95% in pneumococcal or other community-acquired pneumonias. Bilateral soft mid- or lower-zone shadows are typical of *Pneumocystis* pneumonia with a ground glass in appearance. Arterial blood gases usually show profound hypoxaemia and hypocapnia which is disproportionately abnormal compared with the patient's appearance. Corticosteroids are absolutely indicated as adjunctive therapy for any patient with *Pneumocystis* pneumonia with a $Po_2 < 10$ kPa (75 mmHg) on air.

Case history 3

1. Latex cross-reaction. The following foods contain latex antigen: avocados, bananas, chestnuts, kiwi, hazelnuts, figs, papaya, peaches, plums, grapes, melons, passion fruit, apples, cherries, nectarines, pears, pineapple, strawberries, carrots, celery, raw potatoes, tomatoes, wheat and rye.

2. Ask her if she reacts to rubber (or latex) gloves. She reports on direct questioning that she gets urticaria and facial swelling from rubber gloves.

3. Skin (prick) tests and RAST tests. Her total IgE is likely to be very high and is not particularly helpful. It is 1000 kiU/l (normal < 200). Her individual allergen results are shown in Table 91.

Table 91 Allergen test results for Case history 3

	Specific IgE (kU$_A$/l) (<0.4)	Skin test result (mm) (<3)
Latex	16	10
Avocado	3	5
Banana	2	2
Chestnut	2	Not done
Hazelnut	4	4
Cod	5	15
House dust mite	44	7
Dog	38	8
Grass	Not done	7

4. Latex allergy management includes:
   - giving written information on latex avoidance
   - writing allergy alert in case notes
   - giving Medic Alert bracelet
   - reducing risk of severe reaction (anaphylaxis)
   - ensuring optimal asthma control with regular inhaled steroids
   - avoiding ACE inhibitors and beta-blockers, if risk assessment justifies it
   - giving rescue self-medication (Epi-pen) (self-treatment of anaphylactic reactions).

Picture answers

1. a. Yeast cells with a capsule characteristic of *Cryptococcus neoformans*.

   b. India ink test.

   c. The CSF opening pressure. Patients with elevated pressure do badly unless the pressure is controlled.

   d. Cryptococcal antigen on CSF and serum, fungal blood culture, CT or MR scan of brain (mass-like lesions caused by *Cryptococcus* are rare, however).

   e. Amphotericin and flucytosine followed by long-term fluconazole.

2. a. Bilateral mid-zone hazy shadowing.

   b. *Pneumocystis* pneumonia cytomegalovirus (CMV) pneumonitis (check his and his donor's CMV status), invasive aspergillosis, pneumonitis caused by *Legionella pneumophila*, *Mycoplasma pneumoniae*, *Strongyloides stercoralis*, etc.

   c. Arterial blood gases and bronchoscopy with bronchoalveolar lavage for diagnosis.

   d. Broad-spectrum antibiotics to include cover for atypical agents, high dose co-trimoxazole (although his anti-toxoplasma prophylaxis makes *Pneumocystis* pneumonia unlikely) and possibly ganciclovir, depending on the serostatus of the donor and patient.

3. a. Pneumonia caused by bacteria (especially *Pseudomonas aeruginosa*), invasive aspergillosis or other filamentous fungus or post-transplant (EBV) lymphoproliferative disorder (PTCD). It is too nodular and large for cytomegalovirus or other virus infections.

 b. Blood culture, *Aspergillus* antigen (blood and bronchoscopy fluid), EBV, PCR, percutaneous biopsy (if not thrombocytopenic), bronchoscopy with transbronchial biopsy, if possible.

 c. Empirical antifungal therapy, probably voriconazole.

Short notes answers

1. Risks include:
 * 1 in 250 for HIV needlestick, much higher for hepatitis B
 * higher risk for HIV if blood injected under skin, slightly higher risk if a hollow needle
 * other viruses, e.g. hepatitis C
 * very low risk for mucosal exposure (≈1 in 5000)
 * no risk in touching patients or clothes/dishes/belongings.
   Protection should involve:
 * Use gloves if you handle any body fluids.
 * Do not resheathe needles.
 * Discard sharps in sharps containers only.
 * Close and discard sharps containers before they are full.
   If exposure occurs:
 * *always* report the incident and see occupational health (no compensation possible otherwise)
 * postexposure prophylaxis is proven (80% protection) but may need combination therapy
 * administer antiretroviral therapy quickly (e.g. within 1 hour of exposure if possible but certainly within 48 hours).

2. a. AIDS/HIV infection, certain intracellular infections, especially if recurrent or severe (SPUR, p. 379), suspected immunodeficiency in childhood and 'opportunistic' infection occurring in patients with no predisposing factors (e.g. cryptococcal meningitis). There are many causes of altered T cell subsets and reduced helper T cell populations. Most of the changes in T cell

subsets are not correlated specifically with clinical disease and are not diagnostically or therapeutically useful.

 b. Suspected immunoglobulin deficiency, e.g. recurrent pneumococcal infection, malabsorption syndrome eluding diagnosis, recurrent sinusitis or pneumonia, some cases of anaphylaxis, in the investigation of myeloma, Waldenström's macroglobulinaemia.

 c. Helper T cell counts ($\times10^6$/l) can be divided into groups:
 800–1200 Normal in adults, higher in babies.
 500 Increase frequency of CD4 cell counts and measure viral load to determine when to start antiretroviral therapy.
 <350 Tuberculosis, Kaposi's sarcoma, herpes zoster and other opportunistic infections start appearing. Patient needs more careful supervision. Start antiretroviral therapy as benefit is likely and toxicity small.
 ≤200–250 Start anti-*Pneumocystis* pneumonia prophylaxis with oral co-trimoxazole.
 ≤50 Most opportunistic infections are much more likely, especially cytomegalovirus retinitis (ask about eyesight regularly), *Mycobacterium avium intracellulare* azole-resistant candidiasis, invasive aspergillosis, adrenal dysfunction, neurological problems.

 d. The main points are:
 * difficult virus to work with as dangerous to staff
 * mutates easily so may escape antigenic determinants selected for vaccine (e.g. influenza vaccine)
 * thousands of subtypes as a result of mutation
 * antibody response to HIV not protective (needs cytotoxic T cells)
 * vaccine should work at mucosal surfaces and in blood
 * live vaccines fraught with uncertainty
 * expensive, difficult animal model (chimpanzee and other primates)
 * difficult to test in the field in humans against placebo, etc.

Infectious diseases

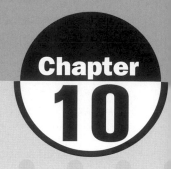

10.1 Clinical aspects

Learning objectives

You should:
- be able to take a history relevant to infectious diseases
- be able to elicit and interpret important physical signs specific for the major infectious diseases
- know how to record body temperature and interpret the value
- appreciate the significance of rigors and know how to act accordingly.

Case Study

A 19-year-old male student is admitted with severe bloody diarrhoea and moderate fever of 9 days' duration. His abdominal radiograph shows some dilatation of the colon. A diagnosis of ulcerative colitis with toxic megacolon is considered, as is colectomy. Detailed history reveals that he has recently moved away from home to student lodgings and is cooking for himself, having never done so previously. He had prepared a chicken by boiling it whole with vegetables in a pot, which he served to some friends. The chicken was undercooked and some had been left over. The pot was too large for the refrigerator and was simply kept in the kitchen. He then finished the chicken off 2 days later on his own. A presumptive diagnosis of severe *Campylobacter* enteritis is made, and he is treated with antibiotics and i.v. fluids and recovers.

Campylobacter is recovered from his stools 3 days after admission. He is given advice on how to prepare food safely.

Infections are common. Viral infections are substantially more common than bacterial infections, which are themselves more common than fungal infections, which, in the Western world, are more common than parasitic infections. In the developing world, parasitic infections are very common and may be chronic. For example, it is estimated that around four billion people worldwide are infected with roundworms.

In this book, the emphasis is on acute rather than chronic infections because it is acute infections that you as a house officer will be expected to manage. For reasons of space, large numbers of infectious illnesses are either completely omitted or dealt with in a cursory fashion and reference books should be used for further information, particularly if knowledge of diseases rarely encountered in the UK is required.

Most infectious diseases are dealt with in this book in their respective organ-based chapters. Here, the focus is on your approach to the patient who may have a life-threatening infection, on generalised infections, classical infectious diseases, genitourinary infections, skin and soft tissue infection and antibiotic therapy. Also described are the legal obligations you are under with respect to infectious diseases.

Taking a history

Infection can arise from many sources. Often a clinical diagnosis can be made with confidence using only a combination of historical data and findings on examination. In addition to the usual details that you should seek regarding the presenting complaint and the review of the systems, other information may be very important in evaluating a patient's illness. These are:

- immunisation history (including travel vaccines)
- travel history
- contact with insects and animals, including reptiles and birds
- whether anybody in the family, at work, or who has attended a recent social gathering is also ill
- the food or water the patient has consumed and how these were prepared

- prior prophylactic therapy or treatment (e.g. malaria prophylaxis)
- sexual history, particularly if the patient is gay
- history of i.v. drug or alcohol abuse
- immunocompromising factors in past medical history (Ch. 9).

Sometimes the key elements of the history are rather subtle and require rather more questioning than might be apparent at first sight. For an example, see the case history above.

Physical examination

A slightly different but complete physical examination is required for patients who may have an infection. This is because large numbers of infections have manifestations outside single organs and because there are many conditions with virtually pathognomonic physical signs. The presence of one of these signs allows a firm diagnosis and suitable treatment. A thorough systematic approach is particularly important.

The key elements of the examination include all parts of the mouth, the ears, the conjunctivae and the skin, a careful search for splenomegaly and, in any patient with neurological symptoms, a detailed neurological examination. Clearly, examination of the respiratory system and a chest radiograph are important to diagnose many forms of pneumonia; auscultation of the heart, electrocardiography (ECG) and echocardiography are important in considering pericarditis and endocarditis; and abdominal examination and ultrasound are important for many reasons. In Table 92 are some examples of findings in the head and neck that may make or suggest a diagnosis which could easily be missed if not actively sought.

Fever, rigors and antipyretics

Body temperature

Body temperature is maintained by a balance between heat production from metabolic processes, particularly in the liver, muscle and brain, and heat loss through the skin. The control of this balance rests in the hypothalamus. There is a normal circadian rhythm of body temperature which varies by about 0.6°C (or 1°F) daily. The lowest body temperature is early in the morning and the high point is in the late afternoon. The implication is that early morning ward rounds may underestimate fever that day, delaying appropriate action. The normal body temperature in any given individual varies between 36.5 and 37.3°C. All patients with a temperature of 37.5°C or above have a fever and some have fever with temperatures of 37°C.

The figures above refer to core body temperature as measured by oral or aural readings. In many wards, axillary temperatures are taken and these are almost always a degree below oral readings. When patients are vasoconstricted, these may be 2 or 3°C below oral readings. You should know how temperature readings are recorded in the ward in order to interpret the charts appropriately.

Two groups of compounds stimulate fever.

Table 92 Contribution of the examination of the head and neck in the diagnosis of infectious disease (examples)

Location	Disease
Ears	
Auroscopy	Bullous myringitis of *Mycoplasma* infection
	Otitis media
	Invasive (or malignant) otitis externa
External ear	Nodules of leprosy on pinna
	Bluish-red skin infiltrate of Lyme borreliosis
Nose and sinuses	Tenderness over the maxillae in sinusitis
	Nasal eschar in invasive fungal infections in neutropenia
Mouth	
Teeth and gingiva	Carious teeth consistent with lack of self-care, endocarditis and tooth abscess
	Gingivitis typical of HIV infection or HSV gingivostomatitis
Tongue	Hairy leukoplakia in HIV infection, bright red tongue of toxic shock syndrome, or Kawasaki disease
Tonsils and pharynx	Exudative tonsillitis of streptococcal pharyngitis, glandular fever or diphtheria
Mucous membranes	Koplick's spots of measles
	Oral candidiasis in HIV infection or Kaposi sarcoma in AIDS
	Ulcers in varicella, primary HIV or HSV infection
	Erythema in toxic shock syndrome
Eyes	Non-purulent conjunctivitis in adenovirus infections, toxic shock syndrome, Kawasaki disease, measles
Neck	Tender lymphadenopathy at the angle of the jaw typical of streptococcal pharyngitis
	Non-tender bilateral lymphadenopathy consistent with glandular fever, toxoplasmosis and HIV infection
	Generally inflamed swollen neck bilaterally consistent with diphtheria
	Localised swelling on one side of the neck consistent with tuberculosis, Hodgkin's disease and streptococcal lymphadenitis

AIDS, acquired immunodeficiency syndromes; HIV, human immunodeficiency virus; HSV, herpes simplex virus.

Exogenous pyrogens For example, Gram-negative endotoxin, enterotoxins of *Staphylococcus aureus*, toxic shock syndrome toxin 1, viruses, yeasts and some drugs (e.g. vancomycin and bleomycin).

Cytokines Especially interleukin-1, tumour necrosis factor, interleukin-6 and interferon gamma.

If these substances are released, particular neurones in the hypothalamus detect them and are stimulated to produce prostaglandin E_2. Other hypothalamic neurones 'reset' the target core temperature for the body. This results in peripheral vasoconstriction, muscle shivering and increased metabolic activity. A 1°C rise in body temperature above 37°C increases total oxygen consumption by 13%.

Hyperpyrexia

Occasionally, hyperpyrexia (>40°C) can be produced because of a lack of heat loss. The causes include heatstroke and malignant hyperthermia, which is precipitated by certain anaesthetics and some neuroleptic drugs in those with an inherited muscle membrane disorder. In addition, the hypothalamic temperature set-point may be elevated following intracranial trauma or tumour or some other hypothalamic dysfunction, e.g. pontine haemorrhage. All of these syndromes are rare apart from heatstroke, in which the history usually makes the diagnosis obvious. It is very important to reduce fever that is above 40°C because permanent brain damage can occur in patients whose temperatures remain sustained above 42°C.

Hypothermia

Occasionally severe infection is accompanied by hypothermia (<36°C) rather than hyperthermia. This is uncommon but carries a poor prognosis if observed. Hypothermia is much more commonly related to excessive heat loss as in exposure, myxoedema or inadequate heating, particularly among the elderly.

Symptoms of fever

A common symptom of fever is chills. An exaggerated form of chills is rigors. The distinction between the two relates to the degree of shaking, which itself is usually related to both the rapidity of rise of pyrexia and its maximum height. Most patients with a significant temperature complain of being cold and wanting to get into bed with their clothes on and extra blankets. They may then lie there shivering, often with their teeth chattering. When this gets to the extent that the whole bed is shaking and their teeth are chattering uncontrollably for 3–10 minutes, that is termed a rigor. Shaking chills and in particular rigors are almost always caused by infection. High fever may occur with other diseases (such as Hodgkin's disease) but shaking chills and rigors rarely do.

Rigors are a distinctive clinic entity and are an absolute indication for admission of a patient to hospital. Common causes of rigors include:

- Gram-negative bacteraemia, especially pyelonephritis and cholangitis
- pneumococcal pneumonia or bacteraemia
- malaria.

Pyrexia makes most patients feel very uncomfortable. Common accompanying features include headache, fatigue, anorexia and irritability. Studies in ferrets and in vitro have shown that many immune responses are augmented by increased body temperature, suggesting that the febrile response is 'good'. However, there are few data suggesting that a *sustained* febrile response is good and so antipyretic therapy is appropriate for the relief of symptoms.

There are two approaches to reducing fever:

- the administration of prostaglandin synthase inhibitors, e.g. paracetamol or aspirin
- direct cooling of the patient by sponging down with cold water.

Naturally patients tend to prefer the former. Corticosteroids should not be used simply for reducing fever. It should be noted, however, that patients taking steroids may have a blunted or absent temperature response to infection, which may mask serious infection and inflammation.

10.2 Serious sepsis and septic shock

Learning objectives

You should:
- know how to distinguish patients with minor infections from those with life-threatening bacterial or fungal sepsis
- be able to diagnose meningococcaemia, serious staphylococcal infection, toxic shock syndrome and septic shock clinically
- know the main complications of serious sepsis and be able to implement the basic management strategies.

Case Study

A day after catheterisation on the elderly care ward, a physically infirm but mentally capable 77-year-old man becomes confused. His blood pressure falls to 90/50 mmHg and he is peripherally warm with a bounding pulse (rate 124/min). His gases show metabolic acidosis and hypoxia, and his creatinine is 190 mmol/l.

Bacterial and invasive fungal infections are frequently life-threatening. Epitomised by bacteraemia and fungaemia they can lead to a cascade of interrelated pathogenetic mechanisms, culminating in hypotension, shock and multiorgan failure. The substances involved besides endotoxin and other products of the microorganisms include tumour necrosis factor, interleukin-1, complement C3 and C5 and several components in the coagulation cascade. In severe cases of sepsis, a cascade of ever worsening host responses is initiated by the above factors, which progresses over hours to days leading to a progressive downhill course. Probably the most dramatic examples are meningococcal septicaemia and toxic shock syndrome and the least dramatic examples are older

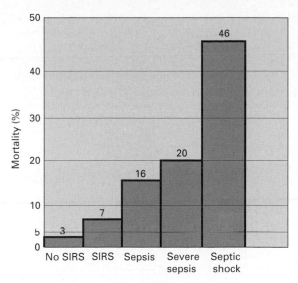

Fig. 109 Mortality in relation to infection with systemic inflammatory response syndrome (SIRS), sepsis and septic shock.

Box 23: Sepsis and septic shock: definitions

Systemic inflammatory response syndrome (SIRS)
At least two of the following:

- Temperature >38°C or <36°C
- Heart rate >90 beats/min
- Respiratory rate >20 breaths/min or PCO_2 < 4 kPa (32 mmHg)
- White blood cell count >12 or <4.0 × 10^9 cells/l or immature neutrophils (left shift or bands) >0.1 × 10^9 cells/l

Sepsis

- SIRS with a confirmed infectious process, e.g. positive blood culture, abnormal chest radiograph, cellulitis, etc.

Severe sepsis

- Sepsis + organ dysfunction, hypoperfusion abnormalities (e.g. lactic acidosis, oliguria, mental status alteration) or hypotension

Septic shock

- Sepsis-induced hypotension (<12 kPa (90 mmHg) systolic) despite i.v. fluids, with hypoperfusion abnormalities, usually accompanied by multiorgan dysfunction or failure

---

patients with bacteraemia from a urinary source or community-acquired pneumonia.

The old terms septicaemia and the sepsis syndrome have been replaced by four more explanatory terms embracing a spectrum of disease directly related to the magnitude of the host response to infection. The mildest form is the **systemic inflammatory response syndrome (SIRS)** and the worst is **septic shock** (Fig. 109). These terms are defined in Box 23. The older dogma is that the severity and mortality of infection are much more likely to be associated with *documented* infection than not, but this is now known to be false. The body's response to infection can occur in the absence of positive cultures, although it is relatively rare to have patients present with these features and have no focus of infection apparent at all. The major exception to this is toxic shock syndrome.

Complications of sepsis

Complications of sepsis include:

- septic shock (see below)
- acute respiratory distress syndrome (ARDS) (see below)
- acute renal failure (p. 179)
- stress ulceration of stomach
- pancreatitis (p. 153)
- disseminated intravascular coagulation (DIC) (p. 285)
- peripheral symmetrical gangrene (see below).

Septic shock

Septic shock occurs as two relatively distinct syndromes.

- **Warm septic shock.** This is manifest by patients with hypotension and a bounding pulse, often with warm but cyanosed peripheries. These patients are alert, anxious and hyperventilating, with a substantial tachycardia.

- **Cold septic shock.** This has a much worse prognosis and is manifest by cold, cyanosed peripheries, an obviously ill and quiet patient who is grey and sweaty, hypotensive, hypoventilating and usually non-communicative.

Patients may progress from the warm phase to the cold phase and this is a bad prognostic feature.

There are two major derangements in the cardiovascular system in septic shock:

- reduced peripheral resistance, leading to a low blood pressure and inappropriate distribution of blood
- myocardial depression leading to a low cardiac output.

In warm septic shock, the first of these is operative and cardiac output is often increased. In cold septic shock, both are operative and the patient is often substantially fluid-depleted and oxygen-deficient in addition.

All patients with septic shock should be monitored extremely closely for respiratory rate, pulse rate, blood pressure, temperature and urine output (e.g. hourly). Arterial blood gases are essential to assess the degree of metabolic acidosis (p. 198) and hypoxia (p. 72). Oxygen should be administered in large quantities as further organ dysfunction can be exacerbated by hypoxia. In addition, ARDS is a common complication and serial monitoring of arterial blood gases will give an early indication of the development of ARDS and, therefore, the need for assisted ventilation. A raised respiratory rate reflects not only hypoxia but also acidosis and you cannot use it as a guide to the need for ventilation in patients with serious sepsis.

Renal dysfunction and, in particular, acute renal failure (p. 179) are common but not universal. Serum creatinine and electrolytes should be measured at least daily in these patients. A fall in the platelet count will give an early indication of DIC, which should prompt the measurement of D-dimers.

Acute respiratory distress syndrome

ARDS is preceded by acute lung injury. There are many causes of acute lung injury, primarily infection, but including hypotension, smoke inhalation and other systemic diseases. The definition of ARDS is:

- ratio of arterial oxygen (Pao_2) to inspired oxygen Fio_2 of ≤200 whether or not positive end-expiratory pressure (PEEP) is used
- bilateral pulmonary infiltrates
- normal or low left atrial pressure (or wedge pressure ≤18 mmHg).

In the early hours after the precipitating event causing ARDS, the chest radiograph may be normal, but diffuse bilateral alveolar infiltrates usually appear within 4–24 hours. The risk of ARDS with some insults is higher than with others. For example, it occurs in 30–40% of patients who aspirate gastric contents but is much less common with cellulitis or *Mycoplasma* pneumonia.

All patients with established ARDS can only be managed in the intensive care unit with assisted ventilation. Patients with mild but acute lung injury may be managed with other forms of oxygen supplementation initially, such as non-invasive ventilation. Intubation and mechanical ventilation are best avoided, if at all possible, in immunocompromised patients. Fluid should be restricted, if possible, to prevent excessive alveolar accumulation of fluid, as there is increased vascular permeability and usually a low serum albumin. The position of the patient should be taken into account, as some patients may not have equal lung injury on both sides and certain positions will allow better ventilation than others.

Most patients with ARDS require 10–20 days of ventilatory support. Corticosteroids may be helpful in infection-free patients who are still dependent on a ventilator after 14 days. A tracheostomy is warranted if patients will require more than 10 days of ventilation, to prevent late strictures of the trachea. Patients who survive ARDS have a good outlook with virtually complete recovery of lung function.

Peripheral symmetrical gangrene

Peripheral symmetrical gangrene is an unusual complication of septic shock, but it is devastating. The patient's fingers, toes and, sometimes, hands and feet, become dusky and cold initially. Then gradually over the next 3–7 days they become obviously gangrenous with a clear demarcation line (dry gangrene). All these patients have DIC. Eventually surgery is required to remove the devitalised digits, if the patient survives.

Management of severe sepsis

The key to the successful management of patients with severe sepsis with or without shock is appropriate antibiotic therapy and excellent supportive care.

Supportive care may mean simply the judicious administration of fluids and oxygen until the septic episode resolves. Alternatively, it may mean full intensive care management requiring ventilation, blood pressure support with pressor agents and haemodialysis or haemofiltration. Clearly, early recognition of sepsis and the prompt administration of appropriate antibiotics can reduce the need for intensive care management.

Recent data show a significant reduction in mortality from sepsis with the use of the recombinant protein, **activated protein C**. The actions of activated protein C, which is downregulated in sepsis, are shown in Figure 110 and

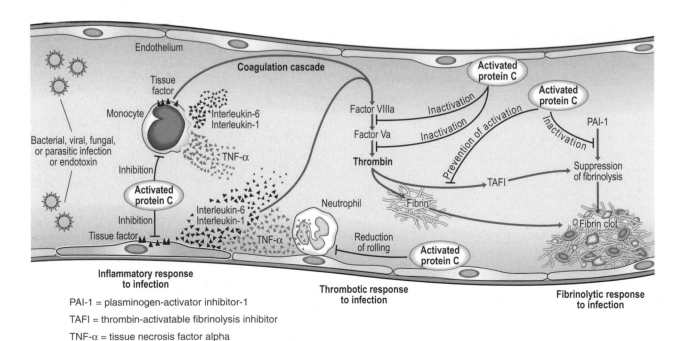

PAI-1 = plasminogen-activator inhibitor-1

TAFI = thrombin-activatable fibrinolysis inhibitor

TNF-α = tissue necrosis factor alpha

Fig. 110 The actions of activated protein C.

Box 24: Actions of activated protein C

Inhibition of coagulation cascade
- Inactivation of factor Va
- Inactivation of factor VIIIa
- Reduction of thrombin production

Enhanced fibrinolysis
- Prevention of activation of thrombin-activatable fibrinolysis inhibitor
- Inactivation of plasminogen-activator inhibitor-1 (from platelets and endothelium)

Anti-inflammatory effect
- Reduced production of TNF-α, IL-1 and IL-6 from monocytes and endothelial cells
- Reduced rolling of neutrophils and monocytes on injured endothelium

---

described in Box 24. It has also recently been shown that modest doses of hydrocortisone improve outcome in severe sepsis and septic shock.

Gram-positive organisms cause 40–60%, Gram-negative organisms 30–45% and fungi approximately 10% of microbiologically documented sepsis in hospital. The mortality is 10–20% for bacteraemia, 40% for fungaemia, 40–60% for severe sepsis and >80% for those with multiorgan failure. Four important examples of sepsis follow.

Meningococcaemia

Neisseria meningitidis is a common Gram-negative bacterium that resides in the nasopharynx in up to 20% of the population. Transmission is greatest between members of the family and can also occur in other closed groups such as school classrooms, military recruits, etc.

The two major manifestations of severe meningococcal disease are:

- meningitis with or without bacteraemia (p. 219)
- meningococcaemia without meningitis.

Clinical presentation

The features of meningococcaemia are variable initially. Early clinical features are:

- fever
- macular rash on the trunk.

As the disease progresses the macular rash, if present, fades (within the first 12–24 hours) and the patient becomes acutely and obviously unwell. Vomiting, pallor, high fever, drowsiness and hypotension are characteristic. There are three clinical features which help to distinguish this infection from other causes of septic shock. These are:

- petechiae and purpuric lesions on the skin and conjunctivae
- rapid onset
- relatively young age of the patient, e.g. child or young adult.

When you are presented with such a very ill patient, it is important to undress them completely to look for pete-

chiae. They are typically 1–2 mm in diameter and found on the trunk, ankles and wrists. They are more likely to be found in clusters where there are areas of pressure applied to the skin by socks or underwear. As the lesions progress, they may coalesce and form large ecchymoses. The lesions may also be found in the conjunctivae. Although difficult to see in black skins, they are usually visible in brown-skinned people.

Investigations

Specific investigations on admission should include a blood culture, an EDTA (ethylenediaminetetraacetic acid) tube of blood for polymerase chain reaction (PCR), a nasal culture, arterial blood gases, urea, electrolytes, full blood count, platelet count and coagulation studies. DIC and thrombocytopenia are common.

Management

The rapid progression of disease is striking and patients may go from first symptoms to death in less than 36 hours. If such a patient presents in general practice, you should give them intramuscular or intravenous penicillin (assuming the patient is not allergic) immediately. All these patients require hospitalisation.

All *N. meningitidis* isolates are susceptible to penicillin and to second- and third-generation cephalosporins (e.g. cefuroxime or cefotaxime). Early administration of antibiotics will reduce the case fatality rate of meningococcaemia from around 100% to around 50%. Patients also need appropriate blood pressure support, possibly artificial ventilation and isolation. If patients are not yet shocked, very frequent and careful observation should be made for the development of shock as this is common and very rapid in onset.

Prevention

All cases of disease produced by *N. meningitidis* are notifiable (p. 429) and this should be done by telephone as soon as the diagnosis is made. If two cases occur that are epidemiologically linked, the episode will be defined as an 'outbreak'. Usually this occurs in the context of a school classroom. In this case, all should receive chemoprophylaxis and possibly immunisation (see below). This will be done by the local Health Protection Unit. In addition, all household members of the patient should be given chemoprophylaxis, as should any other close family contacts who spend a lot of time in the same household. The only health-care staff who require chemoprophylaxis are those who have given mouth-to-mouth resuscitation.

Meningococcal vaccine against the C strain prevents 40% of all cases in the UK. Meningococcal vaccine A&C is indicated in travellers, especially to sub-Saharan Africa and Nepal. Check the most recent recommendations.

Staphylococcal bacteraemia

Staphylococcus aureus and coagulase-negative staphylococcus (including *Staph. epidermidis*) infections are increasing in frequency. Both are major hospital pathogens and *Staph. aureus* is also a major community pathogen. Both are related to intravascular catheter use. Although *Staph. aureus* causes many types of infection, this section will focus on bacteraemia.

Staph. aureus *bacteraemia*

Clinical presentation

Staph. aureus bacteraemia presents in a relatively non-specific way, although some features are distinctive. Virtually all patients look unwell and have fever, usually with chills and/or rigors. Tachycardia, a gallop rhythm murmur and pleural rubs are common. The distinctive clinical features are:

- diarrhoea
- joint pain or pleuritic pain
- cutaneous petechiae or subconjunctival haemorrhage
- confusion (related to 'staphylococcal cerebritis')
- external focus of infection, e.g. infected intravascular catheter site, cellulitis, marks of i.v. drug abuse
- Roth spots in fundi
- *normal* or raised total white cell count (both with marked neutrophilia).

Investigations

The blood culture usually becomes positive within 24 hours, sometimes less. Given that many of the patients have murmurs, it is often difficult to decide whether the patient has endocarditis. Echocardiography is essential for evaluation. If the patient has a prosthetic heart valve, you should assume that the valve is infected (antibiotics and *urgent* surgery) (p. 38).

Management

Flucloxacillin (at least 2 g 6-hourly) is the standard necessary treatment for susceptible *Staph. aureus* bacteraemia. Some isolates (≈10–30%), such as meticillin-resistant *Staph. aureus* (MRSA), are resistant to flucloxacillin, so linezolid, daptomycin or a glycopeptide is required. A shorter course of therapy may be adequate for those with no focal features of disease (e.g. osteomyelitis). Other antibiotics in combination, e.g. rifampicin, gentamicin or fusidic acid, are often used for the more difficult forms of staphylococcal infection. MRSA sepsis with bacteraemia carries a 40% mortality.

Coagulase-negative staphylococcal *bacteraemia*

Clinical presentation

Patients with coagulase-negative staphylococcal bacteraemia are usually not as ill as those with *Staph. aureus* infection and virtually always have one of the following:

- immunocompromised status (e.g. neutropenia)
- indwelling intravascular catheters
- prosthetic intravascular devices, e.g. pacemakers, cardiac valves.

By no means all positive blood cultures for coagulase-negative staphylococci reflect disease. The organism is a normal inhabitant of the skin and improper skin cleaning or a break in aseptic techniques in the laboratory may lead to contamination. Clinical judgement is required.

Management

The principles of management are:

- to remove any infected device or catheter; occasionally cure can be effected with high doses of i.v. antibiotics without removal of a device, but this is rare
- to give appropriate antibiotics.

Like MRSA, coagulase-negative staphylococci are often resistant to flucloxacillin, so vancomycin or teicoplanin is usually used. Linezolid and daptomycin are now an option. The duration of therapy is usually much shorter than with *Staph. aureus* infection, depending on the status of the patient. If longer-term oral therapy is required, this can be quite a problem because of resistance, and it requires detailed microbiological advice.

Toxic shock syndrome

First described in 1978, toxic shock syndrome (TSS) is the archetypal superantigen disease. It is related to toxins produced by *Staph. aureus* or *Streptococcus pyogenes* (group A streptococci). Over 100 cases occur in the UK each year, most related to streptococcal sepsis.

Antigens and antigen-presenting cells

Most antigens are protein molecules that evoke a specific immune response. Sometimes nucleic acids (as in systemic lupus erythematosus (SLE)), glycolipids or small molecules such as metal ions (in combination with protein) act as antigens. Some antigens are more potent than others. Protein antigens can be recognised in either of two ways: as a sequence of 4–6 amino acid residues or as a 3-dimensional small surface site on a globular protein. In the latter case, the components of the antigenic site may be 3–8 amino acid residues separated in terms of sequence but which happen to be together on the surface of the protein as a result of folding.

The majority of protein antigens are not directly recognised by T cells. Instead protein is taken up by an antigen-presenting cell.

Most antigen presentation is done by three cell types:

- macrophages
- B cells
- Langerhans (skin) and dendritic (lymphoid tissue) cells.

Antigen-presenting cells partially digest the antigen and shift the antigenic fragments to the cell surface, adjacent to a major histocompatibility complex (MHC) molecule. The combination of a foreign protein next to an MHC molecule activates T helper cells. A positive feedback loop between the T and B cells is then set up and specific antibody and cellular responses follow. Helper T cells can only recognise antigens presented with MHC class II molecules and CD8 T cells only those presented with MHC class I.

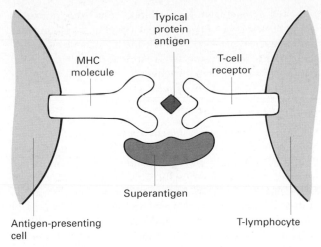

Fig. 111 Toxic shock syndrome. Toxin (superantigen) bridges antigen recognition sites of T cells and antigen-presenting cells to switch on massive T cell proliferation and cytokine release.

Superantigens

A few proteins are able to 'join up' the MHC receptors on antigen-presenting cells with T cells, without being processed (Fig. 111). These are superantigens. The best example is a staphylococcal toxin, TSST-1. Ordinarily, antigen presentation is the rate-limiting step in immune responses. However, superantigens bypass this by activating up to 10% of all T cells, and in this way a vast array of immune responses are rapidly set in motion, which is the main reason these patients get so ill so quickly.

TSST-1 is a protein produced by *Staph. aureus* in the body under favourable conditions (e.g. around a tampon in the vagina during menstruation). Ordinarily antibody is protective but many teenagers have none and so they are at greater risk of disease.

In most cases in women, there is no focus of staphylococcal infection and the organism is a 'commensal' that produces toxin. In a few cases (10% in women and >90% in men) the patients have a focus of infection, such as a wound infection, sinusitis, etc. Streptococcal TSS is related to local streptococcal infection, usually of the skin.

Clinical presentation and investigations

The onset is usually rapid. Feeling as if one is 'getting flu' rapidly progresses to severe illness over 12–24 hours. The key presenting features of staphylococcal TSS are:

- diarrhoea
- fainting, near-fainting or postural hypotension
- high fever with chills and/or rigors
- faint body rash
- drowsiness and/or confusion.

On examination in TSS you will see the following:

- fever >38.5°C
- hypotension or postural hypotension
- macular body rash usually with red cheeks

- erythema of buccal and/or vaginal mucosa
- conjunctivitis.

Investigations show multisystem disease, such as renal dysfunction, raised creatinine phosphokinase (CPK: myositis), thrombocytopenia, etc. The diagnosis is entirely clinical. Sometimes TSST-1-producing *Staph. aureus* can be isolated from the vagina or a wound. In streptococcal TSS, the rash and mucosal erythema may not be present.

Management and outcome

The mortality is approximately 10% for staphylococcal TSS and 30–60% for streptococcal TSS. Treatment is with antibiotics and intensive care. Immunoglobulin infusions may be helpful; non-steroidal anti-inflammatory drugs (NSAIDs) are not.

After 2 weeks of illness, if the patient survives, desquamation of the skin of the hands, soles and body occurs.

Candidaemia

Candidaemia is increasingly common, particularly in patients with cancer or in intensive care units. Unfortunately, only 50–75% of patients with documented invasive candidiasis at postmortem have a positive blood culture before death. Therefore, empiric therapy is frequently justified. There are over 1500 confirmed cases in the UK each year. The major risk factors for candidaemia are:

- perforated gastrointestinal (GI) tract (e.g. faecal peritonitis)
- pancreatitis
- intensive care with central venous catheter
- multiple i.v. antibiotics
- diabetes mellitus
- renal failure or renal replacement therapy.

Clinical presentation

The clinical presentation of candidaemia is very variable. Some patients are acutely ill, others only mildly so. Not all have fever although most do. The following are typical presentations:

- severe sepsis progressing to septic shock (indistinguishable from bacteraemia, but in an at-risk group)
- high fever with skin lesions (typically *Candida tropicalis* infection)
- low-grade fever and leucocytosis in an at-risk patient
- general lack of improvement or deterioration in an intensive care unit patient.

Management and outcome

Some patients have one positive blood culture, others multiple positives; all require therapy. Some species of *Candida* are resistant to fluconazole. The echinocandins (i.e. caspofungin) and amphotericin are the drugs of choice. Venous catheters must be removed or replaced.

The mortality from candidaemia is approximately 40% even if treatment is given early. Half of the deaths are

Ten

attributable to underlying disease rather than directly caused by the candidaemia.

10.3 Skin infections

Learning objectives

You should:
- know the major forms of skin infection, their microbiology and their treatment
- be able to recognise cellulitis and erysipelas and distinguish these from gas gangrene and necrotising fasciitis.

Case Study

A 43-year-old overweight man is admitted with fever, pain in his right calf and circumferential redness over his right lower leg. The edge of the erythema is well demarcated. He also has longstanding athlete's foot (tinea pedis) and glycosuria (?new).

Types of skin infection

There are a number of different skin infections, varying from the trivial, e.g. impetigo and cold sores, to the life-threatening.

Impetigo and localised skin sepsis

Impetigo (pyoderma) is a superficial skin infection usually caused by *Staph. aureus* or streptococci and is common in children. Lesions begin as vesicles and pustules, which then rupture to form characteristic thick, honey-coloured crusts. Topical or oral antibiotics are usually successful. *Staph. aureus* also causes a number of localised infections such as boils, carbuncles and follicultis, which can be appropriately treated with anti-staphylococcal antibiotics and drainage if large.

Erysipelas

Erysipelas is a distinctive type of superficial cellulitis caused by group A streptococci. The most common site is on the lower limbs but the face may be involved. Clinically the skin is somewhat painful, bright red, oedematous and indurated in appearance *with a sharply demarcated border* (Table 93). Virtually all the patients have fever. Only rarely

is the organism grown from a blood culture or from aspiration of skin in the infected area. Therefore, the combination of fever, typical skin lesions and a leucocytosis makes the diagnosis of erysipelas. Treatment is with penicillin, initially i.v. or i.m. and subsequently orally, or with erythromycin or cefuroxime.

Cellulitis

Cellulitis is also an acute infective condition of the skin but extends more deeply to involve subcutaneous tissues. Group A streptococci or *Staph. aureus* are the most frequent causes, but occasionally Gram-negative bacteria or fungi may cause this disease in immunocompromised patients. Unlike in erysipelas, the borders of an area of cellulitis are *not* sharply demarcated. Regional lymphadenopathy and fever are usual (Table 93). Blood cultures are occasionally positive. The diagnosis is a clinical one based on fever, typical appearance of the skin and leucocytosis. Treatment with penicillin i.v. and flucloxacillin or cefuroxime alone is appropriate.

Streptococcal gangrene, gas gangrene and necrotising fasciitis

Life-threatening skin infections include gas gangrene and necrotising fasciitis. Most are caused by *Clostridia* or group A streptococci alone. A few are caused by a mixture of aerobic and anaerobic organisms and the term synergistic necrotising cellulitis is preferred. These include, for example, Fournier's gangrene, occurring in the perineal area in elderly patients, often with diabetes.

Clinical presentation

Characteristic clinical features are:

- local pain which is often severe (Table 93)
- localised oedema of the surrounding area
- brown or black discoloration of the skin
- crepitus of the skin
- foul odour
- severe sepsis ± shock.

Management

There are three major aspects of management:

- antibiotics
- surgical debridement
- management of sepsis (p. 412).

Table 93 Life-threatening skin infections

	Fever	Local pain	Crepitus	Erythema	Dusky/black areas	Systemic toxicity
Erysipelas	++	+	−	+++	−	+
Cellulitis	++	+	−	+++	−	++
Streptococcal gangrene/ necrotising fasciitis	+++	+++	+/−	+/++	++	+++
Gas gangrene	++	++	++	+	+++	++/+++

The antibiotics of choice are i.v. clindamycin or penicillin, metronidazole and a broad-spectrum Gram-negative antibiotic such as ceftazidime. Resection of infected areas is critically important even if mutilating surgery is necessary to save the patient's life. In instances where surgery cannot be completely undertaken without removing vital structures there may be a role for hyperbaric oxygen therapy.

10.4 Classical infectious diseases

Learning objectives

You should:
- know how to diagnose the major classical infectious diseases that occur in adults, including varicella, herpes zoster, rubella, erythrovirus (parvovirus) infection and glandular fever
- know the key clinical manifestations of rarer infectious diseases such as mumps, diphtheria, whooping cough, Lyme disease and leptospirosis
- know how to approach the investigation and management of patients complaining of fatigue
- know which classical infectious diseases are preventable by immunisation.

Case Study

A 19-year-old university student, who grew up in Kenya, complains of sore throat. He is unwell and his tonsils are covered with white exudates. He cannot swallow. He has remarkable lymphadenopathy on both sides of his neck.

In the developed world, most of the major infectious diseases of the last century have now virtually been eradicated. This is, however, not true of the developing world, where these diseases are still common major killers. Measles, in particular, has a major impact on mortality in children in the developing world. This section, therefore, focuses on some of the classical infectious diseases that either are common in the UK or are immunised against. Rabies and tetanus are dealt with on pages 222 and 223 respectively.

Varicella (chickenpox)

Varicella is caused by the herpes group varicella zoster virus (VZV). It is a common infection. Over 60% of the UK population have evidence of prior infection. It is acquired by inhalation of virus particles and is among the most communicable of infectious diseases. If a susceptible individual is exposed to someone infected, they have an 80% chance of contracting varicella. The incubation period is long: 10–21 days.

Clinical presentation

The hallmarks of varicella are fever and a vesicular rash on the trunk.

Fever precedes the rash by 1–3 days and lasts from 5–8 days. There is a wide spectrum of severity, particularly in children, in which the number of skin lesions may range from very few vesicles to complete coverage of the patient. The disease tends to be worse in adults. At least one of the reasons for this is that most adults are secondary cases. Typically the disease is brought home by one of their children who caught it at school or at a friend's house. The child is only mildly ill. However, because the parent is exposed over several days to the infected child, the parent's inoculum is much larger and as a result he/she develops much more severe disease. The same is true for other siblings at home, particularly pre-school children or infants.

Skin lesions

The skin lesions start as small red papules, about 3–5 mm across, and quickly evolve into vesicles containing clear fluid. They are pruritic. Over the next 2–3 days the vesicles rupture and, after 4–6 days, the lesions crust over. Eventually the crust falls off, leaving a slight scar at the site. Lesions are most pronounced on the trunk and head with few lesions on the limbs. In addition, there are usually small ulcers inside the mouth. These ulcers may be profuse and painful, preventing the patient from eating and drinking.

Immunocompromised patients

The illness is much more severe in immunocompromised patients, particularly those with defective T cell immunity, including patients taking steroids. In these patients, fever and back pain are the typical presenting features and the rash may either not be present or be atypical. The mortality of varicella in immunocompromised patients is high.

Management

In hospital, *all* patients with varicella need respiratory isolation and should be managed in an infectious disease unit. Transmission from patients to staff and then to immunocompromised patients, with a fatal outcome, is well documented.

Patients with mild varicella need no treatment other than antipyretics and antipruritics. Immunocompromised patients, secondary cases and those with severe disease should be treated. The drug of choice is aciclovir (i.v. 10 mg/kg every 8 hours) or oral valaciclovir or famciclovir. Aciclovir probably reduces the period of infectivity by 1 or 2 days.

Complications

Complications of varicella are common with severe disease. They include:

- secondary bacterial skin infection
- difficulty swallowing
- pneumonitis (smokers, severe in pregnancy)
- haemorrhagic varicella with or without thrombocytopenia
- congenital varicella syndrome (≈1% risk) if the mother is affected in the first or second trimester of pregnancy
- neurological complications including postinfectious encephalomyelitis, transverse myelitis and cerebral infarction.

Immunisation with VZ immunoglobulin

Passive immunisation of exposed immunocompromised patients (including neonates) can attenuate or prevent infection. Active immunisation with a newly developed vaccine is now possible and may be appropriate for sero-negative health-care staff.

Herpes zoster (shingles)

VZV is a lifelong inhabitant of the body following primary infection. Reactivation occurs from dorsal root ganglia to produce a skin eruption, usually in a single dermatome. Precipitating factors for herpes zoster include immuno-suppression and stressful life events, but in most cases none is found. Herpes zoster may be a presentation of AIDS and may occur during the treatment of lymphoma.

Clinical presentation

The earliest sign of herpes zoster is pain or discomfort in the area infected. This may be present for up to 36 hours before any rash is visible, which makes diagnosis difficult. The rash appears as a vesicular eruption, much like chick-enpox. One of the characteristic features of shingles which distinguishes it from other rashes is the sharp demarcation seen at the midline. Usually there are up to 10 scattered lesions typical of chickenpox in other parts of the body. If there are more than 10 you should consider that the virus has disseminated, which is an indication for hospitalisation and i.v. aciclovir therapy.

As the rash progresses it starts to crust and requires careful dressing if it is extensive. Typically the whole episode is over in about 10–14 days (apart from post-herpetic neuralgia).

Cranial zoster

Occasionally herpes zoster will occur over the cranium in dermatomes C1–C4 or in the distribution of the trigeminal nerve. Some of these patients develop a mild and self-limited form of encephalitis. In patients with infection of the superior branch of the trigeminal nerve (e.g. the fore-head) or the maxillary branch, there is a possibility of corneal involvement as a result of infection of the nasola-bial branch of the trigeminal nerve. As you will recall, the nasolabial branch supplies a small area of sensation at the lateral side of the nose *and* the cornea.

Corneal zoster

Herpes zoster of the cornea is a destructive keratitis that requires aciclovir eye drops for treatment. These patients also develop substantial periorbital oedema which may be bilateral even though there is unilateral skin involvement.

Ramsay–Hunt syndrome

The involvement of the facial nerve can lead to the Ramsay–Hunt syndrome (p. 215) in which skin lesions and pain occur on the pinna and external canal of the ear and there is ipsilateral facial paralysis which rarely recovers.

Management

Non-immunocompromised patients with mild herpes zoster do not require therapy. Immunocompromised patients always require therapy. Therapy may be justified in patients with extensive involvement, although it is sometimes difficult to ascertain the extent of involvement early enough in the illness for therapy to have any impact. At present aciclovir or one of its new prodrugs is the only agent useful for the treatment of shingles. The impact of treatment is to reduce viral excretion and dry up the lesions a couple of days earlier than would be the case without treatment. In the immunocompromised patient, however, varicella zoster can disseminate and cause extensive local disease leading to scar formation. Treatment will prevent this.

Post-herpetic neuralgia

Post-herpetic neuralgia is defined as the persistence of localised pain 4 or more weeks after the rash disappears. The pain can last for months or years and is often severe and resistant to treatment. It is a disease of the elderly patient; there is virtually no risk under the age of 60 but approximately 50% of patients over 60 suffer from it. The cause of post-herpetic neuralgia is not known but it is likely to reflect continuing inflammation in the ganglia. This is supported by finding circulating VZV in mononu-clear cells months after the rash has resolved in those with post-herpetic neuralgia. Famciclovir reduces post-herpetic neuralgia, compared with aciclovir. Steroids are ineffective.

Treatment of the pain of post-herpetic neuralgia differs from the treatment of most other forms of pain. Conventional analgesics are usually ineffective. Tricyclic antide-pressants are of some benefit. Modest doses of gabapentin are usually helpful. Local cutaneous treatments include local anaesthetic patches.

Measles

Measles is caused by an RNA virus for which there is no specific treatment. Immunisation is effective for a popula-tion if uptake is >95% and will reduce the incidence of subacute sclerosing panencephalitis.

Measles can be clinically suspected in adults with five features:

- high fever (100%)
- cough (98%)
- conjunctivitis (96%)
- maculopapular rash on trunk on days 3–5 (100%)
- coryza (84%).

Adults with the disease are often febrile for 10 days or so and are quite ill. Secondary pneumonia and/or otitis media are common. The incubation period is typically 10 days. Patients require respiratory isolation to prevent air-borne transmission. Measles is a notifiable disease.

Mumps

Mumps can be a mild disease with low-grade fever and malaise its only manifestations. Complications include unilateral deafness (1 in 17), aseptic meningitis (p. 219), encephalitis (p. 222), orchitis (1 in 5 adult males), parotitis and pancreatitis (1 in 30). You should consider the diag-nosis in a patient with any of these problems. Immunisa-tion is effective but there is no specific treatment. Mumps is a notifiable disease.

Rubella (German measles)

Without immunisation against rubella, 15–20% of women are at risk of acquiring it in pregnancy. This figure fell to <3% in the 1990s with the success of the measles, mumps, rubella (MMR) triple vaccine. The recent reimmunisation of all schoolchildren against measles and rubella is likely to reduce this figure further. Severe adverse events after the vaccine are rare (1 in 100 000) with no death since 1988.

Rubella is an RNA virus and the incubation period is long, like varicella (10–21 days). There is no specific treatment.

Most patients with rubella have a mild illness, with or without fever but with a rash. The rash is macular, particularly apparent on the trunk and face, and is typically associated with conjunctivitis. Other clues to the diagnosis include lymphadenopathy, especially if suboccipital, and arthritis and/or arthralgia. It is similar to erythrovirus (parvovirus) infection.

The diagnosis is made serologically. This is of critical importance in pregnancy because the risk of fetal infection is 80–90% if rubella is contracted in the first 12 weeks of pregnancy. About 85% of infected infants are damaged. Rubella must be notified.

Erythrovirus (parvovirus) infection (fifth disease)

Erythroviruses (parvoviruses) are small single-stranded DNA viruses that cause erythema infectiosum (fifth disease). In the UK, 50% of adults have evidence of exposure to the virus, mostly in childhood. Unusual features accompany infection in adulthood.

Approximately 20% of infections are asymptomatic. Symptomatic patients typically have:

- low-grade fever
- a facial rash (slapped cheek appearance)
- a reticulated or lace-like rash on the trunk and extremities
- symmetrical, peripheral polyarthropathy or arthralgia.

Symptoms are usually self-limited but may persist for months. Joint symptoms may be the only manifestation of disease.

Complications

In patients with any chronic haemolytic anaemia (e.g. sickle cell disease) and AIDS, erythrovirus can cause severe anaemia. In pregnancy, erythrovirus may cause fetal loss (15–20%), particularly if infection occurs in the first and second trimesters of pregnancy. As the presentation of erythrovirus is similar to that of rubella in pregnancy, blood should be tested for both these viruses in pregnant patients presenting with a fever and/or a rash, particularly if there are any joint symptoms.

Management

The diagnosis of erythrovirus infection can be made either by direct detection of viral DNA in blood or by serology. There is no known treatment, although the chronic anaemia may be successfully treated with immunoglobulin therapy.

Box 25: Glandular fever

Symptoms
- Sore throat
- Malaise
- Mild headache

Signs
- Lymphadenopathy
- Pharyngitis
- Fever
- Splenomegaly

Glandular fever (infectious mononucleosis)

Glandular fever is caused by the Epstein–Barr virus (EBV). It is one particular clinical manifestation of a whole range of diseases caused by the same virus.

Clinical presentation

Glandular fever typically presents over several days with mild chills, sweats, anorexia and, in particular, sore throat (Box 25). Examination reveals non-tender, bilateral and often generalised lymphadenopathy, which is particularly characteristic at the root of the neck. In florid cases, the tonsils or posterior pharynx may be coated with a white membrane, which is often more marked than that seen in streptococcal sore throat and is akin to that seen in diphtheria. However, the presence of splenomegaly and atypical lymphocytosis are features found frequently in glandular fever but virtually never in diphtheria. Most patients do have elevated liver function test results. About 5% of the patients are jaundiced and hepatomegaly is found in about 10%. Virtually all patients have an abnormal lymphocytosis of >10% when ill. More specific tests include the monospot and Paul–Bunnell tests.

Outcome

The majority of cases of glandular fever resolve over 2–3 weeks. Often, however, patients feel tired and unable to concentrate for a much longer period. Occasionally this leads on to typical features of the chronic fatigue syndrome (p. 421). Treatment is usually symptomatic. If amoxicillin or ampicillin is given, this results in a maculopapular eruption in almost all patients. This should not be mistaken as an allergy to these drugs; the mechanism is unclear.

Complications

There are a number of rare complications of glandular fever including:

- splenic rupture (advise no contact sports until the spleen is no longer palpable)
- encephalitis and meningitis
- neurological problems, e.g. peripheral neuropathy
- pericarditis and myocarditis.

Oncogenic potential

EBV infects and immortalises a number of different cell types in the body including B cells and nasopharyngeal epithelial cells. It is clearly associated with a number of different tumours including nasopharyngeal cancer, Burkitt's lymphoma, Hodgkin's disease, non-Hodgkin's lymphoma in patients with AIDS, a rare form of thymic tumour and smooth muscle tumours. It is also responsible for an unusual form of post-transplantation lymphoproliferative disease that is often rapidly fatal. Hairy leukoplakia in AIDS is also associated with EBV. Therefore, EBV is a virus with remarkable oncogenic potential. However, the risk of any of these tumours in a given individual is low.

Diphtheria

Diphtheria is caused by *Corynebacterium diphtheriae*. The manifestations of disease are produced by an exotoxin that is carried on a bacteriophage within the bacterial cell. Therefore, not all strains of *C. diphtheriae* are pathogenic. In the early 1700s, a major epidemic of diphtheria occurred in New England that killed an estimated 2.5% of the population and approximately one-third of all the children. It is for this reason that immunisation programmes are maintained. Immunisation is with a modified toxin (toxoid) and is highly effective.

Clinical presentation

There are several forms of diphtheria. In all cases, *C. diphtheriae* remains superficial (i.e. not invasive) and the organism can be grown from skin, throat or nasal cultures. There are two common forms.

Pharyngeal diphtheria

Symptoms are low-grade fever, sore throat and the development of a 'membrane' on one or both tonsils. It may be mistaken for glandular fever. Cervical adenopathy and local tissue swelling of the neck are common. The membrane can descend to involve the larynx and cause respiratory obstruction.

Cutaneous diphtheria

Indolent skin ulcers sometimes occur with an overlying membrane and are coinfected with other bacteria. Cutaneous ulcers are the major means of disseminating the organism. Chronic skin ulcers in recent immigrants are the most common manifestation of diphtheria in the UK.

Management

Strict isolation in an infectious disease unit is necessary for all patients with possible or confirmed diphtheria. Management of acute disease involves administration of equine diphtheria antitoxin and antibiotics. The best antibiotics appear to be penicillin, erythromycin and clindamycin. Diphtheria is a notifiable disease.

Leptospirosis

Leptospirosis is caused by a number of different varieties (serovars) of *Leptospira*. It is a zoonosis occurring all over the world including in the UK. It is particularly associated with contact with infected water. It is an occupational hazard of sewer workers and canoeists. The most severe form of the disease with jaundice and renal failure is called Weil's disease, but the majority of infections are mild and undiagnosed. It is a cause of aseptic meningitis.

Clinical presentation

The clinical manifestations are not usually specific but, if severe, the initial phase of the illness is like that of dengue fever. It has a sudden onset with headache and myalgia. Usually patients have non-purulent conjunctivitis as well.

Management

The diagnosis can be made by isolation of the organism in the urine but very few laboratories are capable of doing this so a clinical diagnosis is usually appropriate. Serology is available. Patients should be treated with i.v. penicillin for 7–10 days because this causes a more rapid resolution of disease and reduces mortality. Untreated, jaundiced patients have a mortality of 5–30%, usually as a result of renal failure but sometimes through haemorrhagic manifestations.

Rheumatic fever

A scourge of children in the pre-antibiotic era, rheumatic fever would confine children to bed, at home or more likely in sanatoria, for months. It is still common in the developing world. Lack of antibiotics, relative crowding and the prevalence of particular strains of *Streptococcus pyogenes* are responsible for occasional resurgences of disease. Strains such as mucoid M5 seem to be particularly 'rheumatogenic'; others, such as M2, M4 and M12, are not.

Rheumatic fever, like poststreptococcal glomerulonephritis, is a result of cross-reaction of the patient's tissues with certain streptococcal proteins. The sequence of events is as follows. A person has a pharyngitis or tonsillitis caused by one of these unusual streptococci. An antibody response follows, particularly if antibiotic treatment is delayed or inadequate. These antibodies cross-react with the relevant tissues to produce the manifestations of rheumatic fever (or glomerulonephritis).

As rheumatic fever is a clinical diagnosis, with little support from the laboratory (positive antistreptolysin O antibody test only), clinical criteria (the Duckett–Jones criteria) were developed and refined. Major textbooks have a complete list of these. The five major criteria, the presence of any two of which makes the diagnosis, are:

- evidence of heart disease, e.g. new murmur, prolonged PR interval
- polyarthropathy which affects different joints at different times
- subcutaneous nodules (rare)
- chorea (abnormal athetoid movements): St Vitus' dance, a later manifestation, not in adult men
- erythema marginatum: a rapidly expanding circularised rash on the trunk or proximal limbs.

Patients with rheumatic fever need penicillin to eradicate any residual streptococci and anti-inflammatory agents for carditis and arthritis. To prevent relapses, which are common when reinfection with rheumatogenic streptococci occurs, long-term penicillin is advised (>5 years).

Lyme borreliosis

Lyme borreliosis is a multisystem infection caused by the spirochaete, *Borrelia burgdorferi*. It is transmitted by tick bites. It has been reported from most of the North American states, nearly all European countries and throughout Asia. The reservoirs of infection are various small mammals; in addition, birds help to distribute infected ticks during migratory flights. The organism is transmitted by the salivary gland of the tick in the latter part of the 72 hours that the tick is adherent to the skin. Therefore, early removal of the tick is an important part of prevention of the disease. The chance of a person becoming ill after a tick bite in an endemic area is less than 1% in Europe. For this reason, antibiotics are not routinely indicated to prevent Lyme borreliosis after a tick bite.

Clinical presentation and management

There are three clinical stages of disease in Lyme borreliosis and not all of these may appear. Stages 1 and 2 appear within a few weeks or months after infection, stage 3 several months or years later.

Stage 1

Erythema chronicum migrans (ECM) represents stage 1. This is a rash that spreads over some days or weeks and gradually spreads centrifugally. The border of the rash is not usually raised or hot but it does migrate slowly, increasing in size. It will resolve spontaneously in a few weeks or months but more quickly if antibiotic therapy is given. Many antibiotics are effective for ECM including doxycycline, cefuroxime, amoxicillin or azithromycin. Erythromycin is less effective.

Stage 2

Stage 2 disease represents early disseminated infection. The common clinical features include:

- neurological features, e.g. meningoradiculitis, neuritis, meningitis, facial nerve paralysis, etc.
- Lyme carditis, including transient atrioventricular block, rhythm disturbance and myo(peri)carditis
- *Borrelia* lymphocytoma, which is a bluish-red tumour-like skin infiltrate commonly observed in the earlobe or nipples
- arthralgia, myalgia and regional lymphadenopathy.

Effective antibiotics include high-dose i.v. penicillin, ceftriaxone or cefotaxime. Supportive therapy for carditis is appropriate and rarely a permanent pacemaker is required.

Stage 3

Stage 3 disease represents chronic organ involvement, which has a number of clinical manifestations, the commonest of which are:

- arthritis: monoarthritis or oligoarthritis
- acrodermatitis chronica atrophicans, which is a bluish-red discoloration and swelling of the extensor surfaces of the limb (rare)
- Lyme encephalitis and encephalomyelitis, presenting as a spastic paresis and ataxia (rare).

Successful treatment of stage 3 disease is difficult and the resolution of disease is slow. Doxycycline, amoxicillin or cefuroxime is appropriate for cutaneous and joint disease. Neurological involvement requires i.v. penicillin, ceftriaxone or cefotaxime. Failure of therapy or relapse after therapy is frequent and these patients require continued surveillance.

Investigations

The diagnosis of Lyme borreliosis can be made clinically in part, as the cutaneous manifestations are extremely distinctive. Diagnosis of cardiac, joint or neurological involvement requires serology. Unfortunately serology does not distinguish prior infection (without disease) from current active infection. False-positive results occur with positive rheumatoid factor and EBV infection. There are also rare false-negative results.

Chronic fatigue syndrome

Many viral infections lead to malaise and fatigue as part of the manifestations. Usually these features resolve in 2–4 weeks but occasionally it takes as long as 2–3 months for such symptoms to resolve. Since the early 1970s, there has been growing recognition of an entity variously termed myasthenia, Royal Free disease, myalgic encephalomyelitis and, most recently, the chronic fatigue syndrome. The diagnosis is a clinical one and should not be made lightly. You should not make it, for example, simply on the basis of a possible viral infection and a patient who complains of being tired. The reasons for this are twofold. First, the patient may have a treatable medical condition such as hypothyroidism, HIV infection, endogenous depression and many others. In particular, fatigue is highly correlated with emotional stress arising from many different causes. The second reason for not making the diagnosis lightly is that the label chronic fatigue syndrome often sends patients searching medical textbooks and the Internet that may serve to reinforce symptomatology without clear positive benefit to the patient other than being confirmed in their sick role.

Criteria to make the diagnosis are:

- disabling fatigue for at least 6 months
- exclusion of other medical conditions.

The latter requires complete detailed physical examination, exclusion of endocrine disease, neuromuscular disorders such as myasthenia, HIV infection and other chronic infections such as tuberculosis. In particular, patients with associated weight loss need to be very carefully evaluated, even though weight loss is a common manifestation of depression.

Graded exercise therapy and cognitive psychotherapy are the most effective interventions. Depression is common in these patients and they often improve with antidepressant therapy. Other psychological morbidity is a predictor of a low likelihood of improvement. Only 6% of patients are fully recovered at 3 years and the majority are substantially disabled either socially or physically. In addition, many patients have substantial difficulties in concentration and many jobs are frequently beyond them.

10.5 Genitourinary infection

Case Study

A 28-year-old single woman reports a new vaginal discharge. She has been troubled intermittently with this problem and is most concerned that it is smellier than previously. She self-medicated with fluconazole without improvement.

Sexually transmitted diseases are common. Certain patient groups are at high risk; these include gay men, sex workers and young, particularly single, sexually active men and women. Rates of gonorrhoea and syphilis are a useful quantitative guide to unprotected sexual activity and, therefore, are a surrogate marker for HIV transmission rates in populations where HIV exists. Transmission of all sexually transmitted diseases would fall to near zero if condoms were used for all episodes of penetrative sex. However, there are several major factors preventing their use, including lack of availability in many poor, rural parts of the world and inadequate education and protection of teenagers prior to first sexual exposure.

Most sexually transmitted diseases fall into two groups:

- discharges
- ulcers.

The approach taken here, for your ease of learning, is syndromic rather than organism-based. However, control of sexually transmitted diseases is heavily dependent on efficient screening as many are asymptomatic, especially in women.

Discharges

Urethritis (male) and cervicitis (female)

Male urethritis

In men, a discharge from the penis is the most common complaint in genitourinary medical practice. The most common symptoms are:

- discharge from urethra, on underpants or by expressing pus along the urethra
- a stinging or burning sensation on passing urine.

However, you should not take these complaints simply at face value. You should carefully examine the penis and genitals as there is often more than one diagnosis. Rash and joint pain should be carefully sought and you should check the conjunctiva and mouth for features of Reiter's syndrome (p. 352).

Cervicitis in women

In women, the equivalent to urethral discharge is cervicitis. It is commonly asymptomatic or may present with vaginal discharge. The symptoms associated with a vaginal discharge include:

- increased non-menstrual flow
- altered smell or texture of non-menstrual flow.

A significant proportion (about 10%) of women with cervicitis have associated pelvic inflammatory disease. Urethritis in women or the acute urethral syndrome (p. 189) is more commonly caused by the ordinary bacteria that cause bladder infection than by sexually transmitted organisms.

Causes and investigations

The common causes of urethral discharge and cervicitis with their pertinent features are shown in Table 94. For the diagnosis of sexually transmitted disease, high vaginal swabs alone are useless. You should take special *Chlamydia* and *N. gonorrhoeae* cultures directly from the urethra in men, from the cervix and urethra in women, and from the anus if anal intercourse has taken place. Microscopy with Gram stain is desirable for the immediate diagnosis of gonorrhoea.

In about 10–30% of cases of urethral discharge, microscopy culture and specialised tests for *Chlamydia* fail to make a specific diagnosis. Cases without a microbiological diagnosis are termed non-specific urethritis (NSU). Some of these are caused by *Mycoplasma* or *Ureaplasma* spp.

Management

The standard treatment for uncomplicated gonorrhoea in the UK is one dose of cefixime orally with azithromycin (to cover coexisting infection with *Chlamydia*). It is impor-

Table 94 Major sexually transmitted causes of male urethritis and female cervicitis

Cause	Comment
Neisseria gonorrhoeae	Incubation period 2–5 days. 10% have no symptoms. Also found in rectum and throat. Penicillin- and ciprofloxacin-resistant isolates now common
Chlamydia trachomatis	Common cause of urethritis and cervicitis; incubation period 7–14 days
Mycoplasma hominis	Not a cause of urethritis but does cause pelvic inflammatory disease and postpartum fever (15%). Increasing tetracycline resistance
Ureaplasma urealyticum	A relatively common cause of urethritis but may be asymptomatic. Sensitive to erythromycin. A cause of postpartum fever (10%)

tant to screen and treat the partner. Azithromycin and doxycycline are effective for chlamydial infection and most cases of NSU.

Vaginal discharge

If a woman presents with a vaginal discharge, it is important that you ascertain whether she has had a new partner recently or there is any other reason to suspect a sexually transmitted disease. However, increased vaginal discharge alone may be physiological.

Clinical approach to vaginal discharge

There are several causes of vaginal discharge which you can partly distinguish by history.

Vaginal candidiasis Vaginal candidiasis is very common. At least 75% of women suffer it at least once in their lives and about 30% suffer recurrent episodes. Diabetes, pregnancy, antibiotic therapy and cystic fibrosis increase the number of episodes. Some women without the above factors have intractable or frequently recurring vaginal candidiasis for reasons that are not clear. Suspect vaginal candi-diasis if a woman complains of pruritus *and* a non-offensive discharge.

Management In the general practice setting, you can treat with local or oral antifungals without culture or examination on the first occasion. If symptoms do not resolve or they recur quickly, then a full genital examination and microbiological tests are necessary. If a woman complains of discharge without pruritus, consider cervicitis, bacterial vaginosis or *Trichomonas* infection.

Bacterial vaginosis Bacterial vaginosis is the commonest cause of abnormal discharge in woman of child bearing age. Patients complain of a vaginal discharge with a fishy smell.

The characteristics of bacterial vaginosis are a rise in vaginal pH (to ≥4.7), a fall in the numbers of aerobic *Lactobacillus* and a rise in *Gardnarella vaginalis* and 'clue' cells. Clue cells are exfoliated vaginal epithelial cells with a granular appearance because of adherent bacteria. Treat with an anti-anaerobic antibiotic, such as metronidazole.

Trichomonas **infection** *Trichomonas* infection is a sexually transmitted infection of the vagina caused by *Trichomonas vaginalis*, a protozoan. It usually causes a mildly offensive yellow/green, frothy discharge. It is commonly associated with vulval irritation and sometimes dysuria. Organisms can be seen by microscopy in discharge. A single dose of metronidazole (2 g) is curative. Partners need treatment to prevent reinfection.

Genital ulcers

Ulcers of the penis, scrotum, vulva or perineal area are common. Their presence substantially increases the risk of HIV transmission through both heterosexual and homosexual intercourse. Most causes are infectious but there are unusual causes such as Behçet's syndrome, Crohn's disease, Stevens–Johnson syndrome and others.

Ulceration can be divided into multiple painful or solitary non-painful ulcers. In the UK, the most common painful cause is genital herpes and non-painful cause is primary syphilis.

Genital herpes

In a primary attack, patients have multiple, painful ulcers in the vulva, with low-grade fever. They can be so painful in women that walking is impaired or retention of urine follows. The incubation period is 7–14 days. Subsequent episodes are usually less severe than primary attacks and localised to one site, with a characteristic tingling sensation preceding appearance of small, clear vesicles. About one-third of those with genital herpes have recurrent attacks, but asymptomatic shedding of virus is common (30%). If the episode is severe, prolonged or in an unusual site, consider an HIV test.

Genital herpes is a cause of erythema multiforme.

Management

Genital herpes can be treated with aciclovir or valaciclovir orally if started within 48 hours of the lesions appearing. As very frequent recurrences are uncommon, patients are usually treated with intermittent therapy rather than continuously. For patients who have six or more recurrences per year, twice-daily suppressive therapy has been used.

Syphilis

Syphilis is one of the oldest diseases known and has a number of diverse clinical manifestations. It is transmitted by sexual contact, vertically from mother to child or, extremely rarely, by transfusion. Syphilis is caused by *Treponema pallidum*. *T. pallidum* is both a spirochaete and a bacterium. It is not possible to grow it in the clinical microbiology laboratory, although it can be cultured in rabbit testicles.

The disease has four stages although frequently in a given patient only one or two of these will be manifest.

1. primary syphilis (e.g. primary chancre)
2. secondary syphilis (e.g. rash on the palms and soles and oral lesions)
3. latent syphilis (e.g. positive serology)
4. tertiary syphilis (e.g. general paralysis of the insane, syphilitic aortitis, tabes dorsalis or gummas).

Primary syphilis

A primary chancre is a non-painful ulcer up to 1 cm across. The primary chancre in women may be in the vagina or the cervix and as it is painless it is easy to overlook. In men, it is frequently concealed by the foreskin, and in gay men the lesion may be on the anal margin. If the genitals are involved, there is usually painless inguinal lymphadenopathy, which may be the presenting complaint. The incubation period is 9–90 days. Primary syphilis can only be reliably diagnosed by dark ground microscopy or detection of fluorescent treponemal antibody (FTA)-IgM in the serum, as standard serological tests are not positive until 2 weeks after appearance of the chancre.

Secondary syphilis

Secondary syphilis occurs 2–10 weeks after the primary chancre; occasionally both are coexistent. Clinical features are:

- fever and headache
- sore throat
- generalised lymphadenopathy

Ten

- a rash that is non-pruritic and often involves the palms and soles
- snail track ulcers on mucous membranes
- condylomata lata, which are fleshy masses around the anus and vagina similar to soft warts.

Both condylomata lata and mucous membrane lesions are highly infectious. Patients with secondary syphilis may have other organ system involvement, such as hepatitis, meningitis or optic neuritis. The disease of secondary syphilis waxes and wanes over a period of some weeks. The diagnosis is usually made by serology.

Latent syphilis

Latent syphilis has no clinical features and is diagnosed by serology. Many patients in whom primary or secondary syphilis is not diagnosed will in fact have the disease successfully treated inadvertently by a course of antibiotics given for another problem.

Tertiary syphilis

Tertiary syphilis follows primary/secondary syphilis 3–20 years later. The serological tests for syphilis are positive in all forms of tertiary syphilis.

Investigations

The frequency of positivity of serological tests for syphilis is shown in Table 95. The *Treponema palli-dum* haemagglutination assay (TPHA), once positive, stays positive for life. A rise in titre might occur with reinfection. The Venereal Disease Research Laboratory (VDRL) tests for syphilis will rise and fall with infection and treatment, respectively, but slowly. There are occasional false negatives. FTA-IgG is more sensitive than TPHA initially but is then similar to the TPHA. The FTA-IgM is useful as it reflects acute infection and will often rise and fall with each episode of syphilis. It is, however, rather subjective to read in the laboratory and both over-reading and under-reading errors occasionally occur. Occasionally there are false-positive tests in, for example, SLE, but in most cases the disease causing the false positive is apparent.

Management

Syphilis is best treated with penicillin. There is still debate about the best dose, formulation and duration of therapy.

Table 95 The frequency of positive serological results in testing for syphilis

Test[*]	Frequency of positivity (%)			
	Primary	**Secondary**	**Latent**	**Tertiary**
VDRL	75	100	75	75
TPHA	60	100	97	100
FTA-IgG	90	100	97	100
FTA-IgM	90+	100	<10	<10

[*] See text for abbreviations.

The Jarisch–Herxheimer reaction is a reaction to treatment and is manifest as fever and 'flu-like' symptoms 3–12 hours after a dose of penicillin. It occurs following therapy for primary (50% of treatment courses) and secondary syphilis (70–90% of treatment courses). It can usually be managed symptomatically; occasionally steroids are required.

Genital warts

Genital warts are common. They usually present as small (2–5 mm) fleshy protuberances on the skin surfaces of the genitals. They may also appear as flat and slightly pigmented areas of skin. They also occur on the mucosal surfaces but are much harder to visualise and may be 'silent'. Caused by many varieties of papilloma viruses, they constitute a large part of the workload of all genitourinary medicine clinics because they tend to be resistant to treatment.

Papilloma virus infection is a necessary precursor to carcinoma of the cervix and anus, especially in AIDS patients.

Management

Topical podophyllin or podophyllotoxin cream and cryotherapy with liquid nitrogen are the commonest modes of treatment. The former does not work well for established and keratinised warts, and many applications of liquid nitrogen are often necessary for cure of large warts. Other treatments include trichloracetic acid and imiquimod cream Recalcitrant warts may require diathermy or surgery.

Other aspects of genitourinary medicine practice

There are several other major functions besides the diagnosis and treatment of sexually transmitted disease that clinics in the UK undertake. These are:

- HIV counselling, pre- and post-test (p. 388)
- contact tracing
- dealing with psychosexual problems
- medical assessment and counselling after sexual assault
- health promotion and sexual health education
- family planning advice and provision
- screening for cervical precancer and management of abnormal smears in high-risk patients such as HIV-positive women.

All genitourinary clinics hold an independent set of confidential clinic records, as required by law. Names of contacts are recorded if the patient provides details. Staff then contact them discreetly for screening for sexually transmitted infections and appropriate treatment, or the patient encourages their contacts to seek advice.

Psychosexual problems accompanying sexually transmitted disease are common. Examples include:

- concern about repeated transmission of *Candida* (which is not the case), or herpes and warts (which is)
- in the context of a stable relationship, where the infection came from

- feelings of being 'dirty' or 'defiled' leading to a lack of libido and low self-esteem.

Considerable patience, time and skill are required to help affected individuals resume normal sexual relations.

10.6 Imported diseases

Case Study

A couple return from holiday in South-East Asia and the woman develops high fever, myalgia, headache and then a rash similar to sunburn. The man remains well. She requires multiple doses of paracetamol for myalgia. Her doctor checks her bloods but gives her no other therapy.

There are a large number of tropical diseases. Space permits coverage of only a tiny selection. A few others are described in the systems chapters. Consult reference books or knowledgeable clinicians if faced with a diagnostic problem.

Malaria

Malaria is a parasitic disease transmitted by the female *Anopheles* mosquito in most subtropical and tropical countries of the world. There are 100–200 million cases and 1.5–3 million deaths annually from malaria worldwide. There are four major species of parasite infecting humans. *Plasmodium falciparum* is the only one that regularly causes death and the only one that does *not* cause delayed disease months or years after leaving an area endemic for malaria. *P. vivax* and *P. ovale* both have liver and red cell cycles and cause milder infections than *P. falciparum*. *P. malariae* is rare in the UK but may occur decades after leaving an endemic area.

Geography

P. falciparum is found virtually wherever the other three species of *Plasmodium* are found. Areas that are malaria-free include western and eastern Europe, the parts of North Africa that adjoin the Mediterranean, the Middle East, Canada and the USA, Japan, Taiwan, Australia, New Zealand and the southernmost parts of South Africa. The likelihood of becoming infected with malaria in the centre of major cities in Asia and Central America is relatively small even if malaria occurs in these countries. Therefore, malaria prophylaxis is not indicated for a trip to Bangkok or Singapore, for example.

Incubation period

In countries free of malaria, all cases are imported or rarely occur near to airports. *P. falciparum* infection usually presents within a month of returning from an endemic area, but at least 10% of cases occur from 1 to 4 months after leaving an endemic area. Cases involving the other three species of parasite can occur months or years after leaving an endemic area, although most cases of *P. vivax* or *P. ovale* present within 3 years.

Clinical presentation

The clinical diagnosis of malaria can be difficult. Characteristic features include:

- fever and shaking chills and/or rigors
- headache and myalgia
- vomiting and diarrhoea.

The first 1–3 days of a malarial illness are often hard to separate from many other infectious illnesses. After this, the patient typically has paroxysms of fever. These paroxysms comprise three stages, together lasting about 6 hours:

- the cold stage (rigors/chills)
- the hot stage (high fever)
- the sweating stage (defervescence).

After several days of illness in *P. vivax* and *P. ovale* infections, the pattern of paroxysms may develop into the well-described **tertian pattern**, when paroxysms occur every second day. Such characteristic synchrony of fever is uncommon in *P. falciparum* infections, when a more chaotic temperature chart is typical.

Prognostic features

In *falciparum* malaria, the following are poor prognostic features:

- coma
- increased respiratory rate
- oliguria
- high parasitaemia (e.g. ≥10%).

Investigations

All patients who return from the tropics with fever should have a blood culture (for typhoid, etc.) and malaria film taken. You should adopt this rule whether you are working as a GP, in accident and emergency, as a medical house officer or working abroad. Without this, you can miss cases of malaria and typhoid (p. 426). Every year there are about five deaths from malaria in the UK because the diagnosis is considered late or not at all. Do not make this mistake; whenever you see a patient with fever *always* ask if they have been abroad.

Patients with *falciparum* malaria are likely to have a normocytic normochromic anaemia, an elevated reticulocyte count (or polychromasia), a normal white cell count and a reduced platelet count. Careful inspection of the blood film will show parasites in the vast majority of patients on the first blood film. If parasites are not found but symptoms continue, together with anaemia and/or thrombocytopenia, additional films should be sent to the laboratory. In patients taking malaria prophylaxis, it can take 3–5 blood films over the same number of days to make the diagnosis.

The diagnosis of *P. malariae*, *P. vivax* and *P. ovale* infections can be more difficult and repeated films may be necessary.

Management

Falciparum *malaria*

All patients with *falciparum* malaria should be admitted to hospital immediately. You should contact the local infectious disease consultant and it is usual to transfer the patient to the local infectious disease unit for management. The management of *falciparum* malaria is difficult and, improperly managed, the disease carries a high morbidity and some mortality. Ten per cent of adults suffer cerebral damage after cerebral malaria.

Standard therapy for patients with *falciparum* malaria unable to take oral medication is i.v. quinine. The best oral choices are combination tablets; Malarone (proguanil with atovaquone) or Riamet (artemether with lumefantrine). The vast majority of isolates worldwide are resistant to chloroquine, which is why this is no longer used for *falciparum* malaria. *P. falciparum* in Northern Thailand and Myanmar (Burma) is often resistant to both quinine and mefloquine. Mefloquine resistance is spreading.

Patients with parasitaemia above 5% should be actively considered for exchange transfusion depending on how ill they are.

Non-falciparum *malaria*

Patients with *P. vivax*, *P. ovale* and *P. malariae* infections may need admission to hospital for 1–2 days depending on their clinical status but many can be managed as outpatients. They can be treated with oral chloroquine given for 3 days. Patients with *P. vivax* and *P. ovale* infection should then have their glucose-6-phosphate dehydrogenase levels checked. If these are normal, they should then be given 2 weeks of primaquine to eradicate the liver cycle. There are substantial difficulties in the management of pregnant patients with malaria. All forms of malaria are notifiable diseases.

Prevention of infection and prophylaxis

Most *Anopheles* mosquitoes bite at dawn or dusk. If it is possible not to go out at these times, the risk of acquisition of disease is reduced. Long sleeves, socks and long trousers will also reduce the likelihood of being bitten. Insect repellants are useful and should be liberally applied. Travellers should sleep under bed nets, preferably treated with insecticide.

Advice on malaria prophylaxis changes at least annually so check frequently. The choices for prophylaxis are:

- mefloquine *or*
- doxycycline *or*
- atovaquone and proguanil (Malarone), *or*
- chloroquine and proguanil.

All forms of prophylaxis should be taken before leaving the home country for two reasons:

- to make sure that the tablets are tolerated; if they are not, then an alternative regimen can be provided
- to build up tissue levels prior to departure.

In addition, drugs should be continued after return home to prevent late infections.

Typhoid and paratyphoid fever

Typhoid fever is caused by *Salmonella typhi* and paratyphoid fever by *S. paratyphi* A, B or C. These four infections constitute enteric fever. They are usually acquired abroad; most cases of typhoid are from the Indian subcontinent, whereas most paratyphoid fever comes from the Mediterranean basin. Around 17 million cases of typhoid fever occur annually worldwide. All are notifiable diseases.

Clinical presentation

The early features of typhoid or paratyphoid fever are relatively non-specific:

- fever and chills
- headache
- lethargy
- mild cough
- low white cell count.

Examination initially reveals only abdominal tenderness. After 7–10 days, rose spots may become apparent on the skin and are particularly common in paratyphoid fever. Diarrhoea or constipation, and delirium, splenomegaly and hepatomegaly also become detectable. If undiagnosed, the complications of intestinal bleeding, perforation and shock then develop.

Investigations and management

The diagnosis is established by blood culture or stool. False negatives can occur, and so a clinical diagnosis may have to be made. Antibiotic resistance is common. Ciprofloxacin or a third-generation cephalosporin such as cefotaxime is appropriate, for 10 days. Untreated typhoid has a 20% mortality; treated it is <1%.

Chronic carriage

Patients with typhoid require isolation during hospitalisation. All family members should also be screened for stool carriage. After therapy has finished, stool cultures should be checked to ensure that the patient has not become a carrier. This is particularly important in professional food handlers (including those preparing food at home).

Immunisation

A Vi capsular polysaccharide vaccine and an oral live attenuated vaccine are useful in prevention. The first is given parenterally as a single dose. The oral vaccine is given as a three-dose schedule. The efficacy is around 70% for the parenteral vaccines and probably slightly lower for the oral attenuated vaccine. Only those visiting the Indian subcontinent or long-term holidaymakers to the Mediterranean basin, Kenya, Far East and South America require immunisation.

Viral fevers

Dengue fever

Dengue fever (breakbone fever) is caused by one of four viruses transmitted by mosquito bite. It occurs in Central and South America, much of Africa, India and South-East Asia. There are estimated to be 50 million cases worldwide annually. It is a common cause of imported fever in the UK and has an incubation period of 2–14 days. The diagnosis is made by acute and convalescent serology. Treatment is supportive.

Clinical presentation

In older children and adults, dengue produces a characteristic clinical syndrome, the first manifestation of which is the sudden onset of high fever. Dengue causes:

- sudden high fever
- frontal headache
- nausea and vomiting
- backache, and severe muscle and joint pains
- flushing of the face
- non-purulent conjunctivitis
- initial transient macular generalised rash (like sunburn) then a generalised sunburn-like rash.

Viral haemorrhagic fever

There are a number of other viral haemorrhagic fevers (VHFs) which are acquired abroad. The major VHFs are **Lassa fever** and **Ebola fever**, which occur in Africa. They carry a major risk of transmission to health-care workers and especially laboratory staff. Patients with suspected VHF *must* be managed in an infectious disease unit with the appropriate containment facilities. You *must* consult an infectious disease physician if you suspect any VHF.

The maximum incubation period for all viral haemorrhagic fevers is 20 days. Suspect the diag-nosis in anyone with:

- fever following a recent trip abroad
- haemorrhagic manifestations, or coagulopathy without a bacterial cause.

Prognosis

The case fatality rate is lowest for haemorrhagic fever with renal syndrome and dengue fever (1–5%), and highest for Ebola and Crimean-Congo haemorrhagic fevers (55–88%). Lassa fever, and possibly others, can be successfully treated with ribavirin.

Leishmaniasis

Leishmaniasis is an overall term to describe any disease caused by the protozoan *Leishmania*. Visceral leishmaniasis (**kala-azar**) is a common cause of splenomegaly and fever, whereas the cutaneous and mucosal syndromes are chronic. Visceral leishmaniasis is occasionally seen in AIDS. There are ~500 000 cases each year worldwide.

There are a number of different species of *Leishmania* that cause visceral leishmaniasis, particularly *L. donovani*, which can be acquired in the Indian subcontinent, China, Middle East and around the Mediterranean basin, sub-Saharan Africa, Kenya and Ethiopia, Latin America and Brazil.

The incubation period for visceral leishmaniasis is 3–8 months but may be longer. The key manifestations of visceral leishmaniasis are:

- hepatosplenomegaly (sometimes massive)
- fever
- weight loss.

Usually symptoms appear gradually, with a vague abdominal discomfort related to splenomegaly, fever, weakness, weight loss and then the symptoms of anaemia. The fever is low-grade initially but may become high later. Occasionally the symptoms are much more acute, in which case high fever and chills are typical. Hepatosplenomegaly is virtually always found, with the spleen being larger than the liver. In chronic cases, splenomegaly may be massive.

Investigations

A profound normocytic, normochromic anaemia is typical together with leucopenia and sometimes thrombocytopenia. A bone marrow examination, splenic aspirate or liver biopsy will establish the diagnosis.

Management

Treatment is with i.v. liposomal amphotericin, i.v. pentavalent antimony compounds or oral miltefosine.

10.7 Pyrexia of unknown origin

Learning objectives

You should:
- know how to construct a differential diagnosis for pyrexia of unknown origin (PUO)
- be able to develop a rational approach to investigation in patients with PUO.

Case Study

Despite an extensive work-up including cultures, autoantibody tests and a chest X-ray, a 53-year-old man continues to spike temperatures. He is British, but has travelled the world on business and holidays. Apart from a slight hepatomegaly, there are no other findings. An echolucent mass is found in the right lobe of his liver on ultrasound, prompting blood to be sent to the Tropical School and treatment with metronizadole.

PUO also known as fever of unknown origin (FUO) is defined as a fever >38°C (or >1°C above patient's normal temperature) over at least 3 weeks and defying standard diagnostic evaluation (e.g. blood culture, urine culture, chest radiograph, etc). In many cases, the fever has been present for months, perhaps intermittently. The differential diagnosis is wide and the topic is only introduced here.

Clinical presentation

The causes of PUO include those in Table 96. This list is long but not exhaustive.

There are several key points that you need to know about the evaluation of this problem:

Table 96 An incomplete list of the causes of PUO

	Infections	Neoplasms	Other
Common causes	Tuberculosis Occult abscesses (e.g. liver, epidural) Invasive candidiasis AIDS	Hodgkin's disease Non-Hodgkin's lymphoma	Sarcoidosis Drug fever (e.g. vancomycin, bleomycin, rifampicin) Systemic lupus erythematosus (SLE) Vasculitis
Uncommon causes	Subacute bacterial endocarditis Osteomyelitis Brucellosis Psittacosis Relapsing fever Histoplasmosis Cytomegalovirus infection Trypanosomiasis Whipple's disease	Leukaemia Renal cell carcinoma Hepatoma Atrial myxoma	Still's disease Polymyalgia rheumatica Temporal arteritis Granulomatous hepatitis Inflammatory bowel disease Familial Mediterranean fever Fabry's disease Factitious fever

- Confirm the elevated temperature, if necessary by admitting the patient to hospital; some 'cases' are merely exaggerated circadian rhythms, or factitious.
- Repeatedly examine the patient seeking splenomegaly, dental or sinus problems, positional heart murmur (atrial myxoma), thyroid enlargement (thyroiditis) and hyperpigmentation (Whipple's disease).
- Consider a drug cause early in the evaluation, to avoid multiple tests and invasive procedures.
- Do a tuberculin skin test and consider antituberculous treatment early, as up to one-third of PUO cases are caused by tuberculosis.
- Ask for relevant consultant opinions early, particularly if there are abnormalities in one or other body systems.
- Even if patients are not too ill, avoid major invasive procedures (such as laparotomy); rather take a watching brief. 'First do no harm' as a tenet of medical practice applies here, perhaps more than in most other situations.

Important causes of PUO not discussed elsewhere in this book include brucellosis, amoebic liver abscess and factitious fever. These are described briefly below. About 10–15% of genuine cases of PUO are never diagnosed, despite multiple investigations over months or years.

Investigations

Useful tests for PUO include:

- Tuberculin skin test for tuberculosis
- blood cultures with prolonged incubation
- serology for Q fever, brucellosis, cytomegalovirus, HIV, fungi, *Yersinia*, etc.
- computed tomographic (CT) imaging (ultrasound may be falsely negative)
- transoesophageal echocardiography
- white cell scan
- gallium scan
- laparoscopy ± liver biopsy.

White cell scans

White cell scans detect recent large collections of neutrophils. They are particularly useful for intra-abdominal, bone and soft tissue infections. The patient's cells are collected by venepuncture, labelled with [111]indium and reinfused. Patients are scanned 18–24 hours later. Very chronic infections are likely to be falsely negative.

Gallium scans

[67]Gallium is used to label transferrin and lactoferrin at the site of infection. It is more useful for chronic inflammatory, especially granulomatous disease, in identifying either the site of disease or its activity, as the scan abnormality returns to baseline quickly after resolution of disease. Scanning is done daily for 3 days.

Brucellosis

The incubation period of brucellosis, caused by *Brucella abortus* or *B. melitensis*, varies from 1 week to several months. Most patients develop a mild influenza-like illness without complications. The characteristic features of brucellosis include:

- drenching sweats
- chills and fever
- weakness
- myalgia
- back pain.

On examination, lymphadenopathy and splenomegaly are found in up to one-third of patients. Usually the disease resolves spontaneously, although in some instances relapses may occur. Relapse is very unusual if the disease is appropriately treated. The diagnosis can sometimes be made by doing special blood cultures (ask a microbiologist) but is more commonly made by serology.

Complications of brucellosis include sacroiliitis or arthritis, epididymo-orchitis and endocarditis. Brucellosis is also more severe in immunocompromised patients.

Treatment consists of doxycycline plus rifampicin for a minimum of 6 weeks. Relapse occurs in 5%.

Amoebic liver abscess

Liver abscess is a relatively frequent cause of PUO. Bacterial liver abscesses are discussed on page 142. Amoebic liver abscesses occur in returned travellers. Most patients present within 2–5 months of leaving the endemic area, although the presentation can be delayed for years. There are two presentations of amoebic liver abscess:

1. abdominal pain and fever
2. weight loss, low-grade fever and mild or absent abdominal pain.

Diarrhoea is common in both.

Physical examination reveals exquisite point tenderness over the liver. Signs of pleural effusion or infection in the right lung base are common.

Investigations

Virtually all the patients have a peripheral leucocytosis and abnormal liver function tests, in particular a raised alkaline phosphatase. The diagnosis initially should be considered on the basis of travel to any part of the world with poor sanitation, together with tenderness in the right upper quadrant on examination.

Differential diagnosis includes cholecystitis, acute viral hepatitis and a bacterial liver abscess. However, leucocytosis is essentially never found in patients with viral hepatitis and imaging of the liver helps to differentiate cholecystitis from liver abscesses. Travel outside developed countries suggests amoebic liver abscess.

Aspiration of very large abscesses is appropriate, to yield the classical pus (anchovy paste). Cultures of the pus are negative. Amoebic serology is positive in approximately 95% of patients. Stools are usually negative for amoebic cysts.

Treatment with metronidazole is curative and this should be given for at least 10 days. Occasionally, amoebiasis affects other organs of the body, including the brain, skin and genitals.

Factitious fever

Occasionally Munchausen's syndrome manifests as factitious fever. Usually the reading on the thermometer is falsely elevated by rubbing the thermometer or holding it next to a light or hairdryer. To diagnose factitious fever, it is essential to ensure that all temperature readings are directly supervised by the nursing staff. Sometimes patients inject bacteria or yeast into themselves, causing genuine infection.

10.8 Notifiable diseases

Learning objectives

You should:
*   know which diseases are notifiable and how to notify them.

There are several diseases that are notifiable to the local Consultant for Communicable Disease Control (CCDC). You have a legal obligation to notify and specific forms are provided for doing this. There are two diseases that should be notified by telephone and the CCDCs maintain 24-hour cover in order to receive these notifications. These are:

*   meningococcal infection
*   typhoid fever.

The disease should be notified as soon as a clinical diagnosis has been made. If you suspect an outbreak you should phone your local CCDC. There are separate confidential notification systems for AIDS and tuberculosis. Other important diseases to notify include malaria, measles, mumps, meningitis and encephalitis.

10.9 Antimicrobial therapy

Learning objectives

You should:
*   understand the main uses and limitations of each main antibiotic class
*   know key members of each class.

There are many different antibiotics available and this is a subject which is dealt with in both micro-biology and pharmacology texts. The purpose of this short section is to indicate some 'do's and don'ts' and help you to make relatively straightforward treatment choices for most of the common conditions.

Hospital prescribing

In the hospital setting, antibiotic policies are designed to achieve three objectives:

1. the use of appropriate antibiotics and doses for common indications
2. use that reflects the local prevalence of antibiotic resistance
3. to give the pharmacy sufficient buying power to negotiate lower prices for the antibiotics that are used in large volumes.

Endeavour to stick to the antibiotic policy in a hospital as much as possible. However, advice from the microbiologists may suggest a deviation from the policy, especially with very ill patients or unusual problems. 'Allergy' to antibiotics is common, but many cases are not true allergy but merely common side-effects such as nausea. Rash, anaphylaxis, angioedema and bronchoconstriction are legitimate reasons to use an alternative, although a rash many years ago could reflect a coexistent viral infection then or a mild allergy that is no longer present.

Do not prescribe unless there is good evidence for bacterial infection; do not use antibiotics as placebos.

The following section summarises some of the more common antibiotics and their particular uses.

Individual antibiotics

Penicillin

Penicillin is poorly absorbed orally; the only use for penicillin given by mouth is continuation after intravenous or intramuscular therapy for streptococcal sore throat, and for prophylaxis in patients without spleens and after rheumatic fever. Intravenously, it is useful for streptococcal, meningococcal, clostridial and skin infections and for lobar pneumonia. Resistance has not been described in most streptococci or *N. meningitidis* but is found in 5–40% of *Strep. pneumoniae* (the pneumococcus). The normal maximum dose is 4.8 g daily. Penicillin resistance is of little consequence in pneumonia (if i.v. therapy is used) but is critical in meningitis.

Ampicillin/amoxicillin

Previously a very useful antibiotic, **ampicillin** is now of less value. It is a key agent for endocarditis and enterococcal infections, liver and brain abscesses, *Listeria* and gynaecological infections. When combined with clavulanic acid, **co-amoxiclav** (Augmentin) is a useful antibiotic for upper respiratory tract infections including otitis media, sinusitis and bronchitis as well as salpingitis.

Flucloxacillin

Used only for staphylococcal infections, **flucloxacillin** also has efficacy against streptococci. Oral doses are adequate for skin sepsis and continuation after i.v. therapy. Staphylococcal bacteraemia, osteomyelitis, endocarditis and other deep focal manifestations require large i.v. doses (e.g. 8–12 g/day). Activity is enhanced by combination with gentamicin or rifampicin. It is not active against MRSA.

Extended-spectrum penicillins

Examples are **ticarcillin** and **piperacillin**. These drugs offer a greater Gram-negative spectrum, including antipseudomonal activity, but none of them has any antistaphylococcal activity. They do, however, have enterococcal activity, unlike the extended-spectrum cephalosporins. They are used exclusively for patients with hospital-acquired infections, especially those with neutropenia or in intensive care. They are now combined with β-lactamase inhibitors (e.g. Timentin (ticarcillin plus clavulanic acid) and Tazocin (piperacillin plus tazobactam)) to give even more broad-spectrum activity.

Oral cephalosporins

These drugs (e.g. **cefalexin**, **cefaclor** and **cefpodoxime**) have reasonable Gram-positive activity with a limited Gram-negative spectrum (e.g. *E. coli* and most *H. influenzae* isolates). They are, therefore, a useful alternative for mild skin sepsis, respiratory tract infections (especially cefpodoxime) and urinary tract infections. However, resistance rates among urinary pathogens exceed 50%.

Second-generation cephalosporins

These drugs (e.g. **cefuroxime**) have good Gram-positive and moderate Gram-negative activity. Cefuroxime is a useful antibiotic for moderate to severe skin sepsis and urinary tract infections requiring hospital admission. It has no activity against *Pseudomonas*, other resistant Gram-negatives, or *Enterococcus* spp.

Third-generation cephalosporins

These drugs (e.g. **cefotaxime**, **ceftriaxone**, **ceftazidime** and **cefixime** have a broad spectrum of activity for both Gram-positive and Gram-negative pathogens. They have good activity against streptococci, including *Strep. pneumoniae*, and should not be used alone for a serious staphylococcal infection. They have no enterococcal activity and their frequent use has led to the emergence of *Enterococcus* as a major hospital pathogen worldwide. They have little anti-anaerobe activity. Ceftriaxone or cefotaxime is now the agent of choice for meningitis; however, they have no anti-*Listeria* activity.

Cefotaxime and ceftriaxone have no antipseudomonal activity whereas **ceftazidime** is an excellent antibiotic for infections with *Pseudomonas* spp. These are particularly common as urinary pathogens in the intensive care unit, in renal patients and in neutropenia. However, ceftazidime has slightly less Gram-positive activity and that is the reason for preferring ceftriaxone or cefotaxime in the majority of hospital settings.

Quinolones

Norfloxacin is only useful for urinary tract infections. Both **ofloxacin** and **ciprofloxacin** have a broad spectrum. Neither has good activity against *Strep. pneumoniae* and, therefore, they are not good agents alone for the treatment of pneumonia. The newer quinolones, **levofloxacin** and **moxifloxacin**, have sufficient activity to be used for respiratory infection, including that caused by *Legionella*. Ciprofloxacin has slightly greater activity against *Pseudomonas* and some difficult Gram-negative species compared with ofloxacin, but otherwise the spectrum of the two agents is similar. Ciprofloxacin is the agent of choice for typhoid fever and other infectious diarrhoeas. Quinolones have activity against both *M. tuberculosis* and atypical mycobacteria.

Macrolides

Clarithromycin and **azithromycin** are better tolerated and have a broader spectrum than erythromycin. Macrolides have good activity against streptococci and staphylococci and are, therefore, useful agents for the treatment of mild skin sepsis, sore throat, some cases of sinusitis and some staphylococcal infections (but not bacteraemia). **Erythromycin** has no useful activity against the majority of *H. influenzae* isolates but clarithromycin and azithromycin are effective. **Clindamycin** has better anti-anaerobe activity and penetrates well into bone; it is, therefore, a useful antibiotic for the treatment of bone infection caused by staphylococci. Both clarithromycin and azithromycin have antituberculous activity and are now commonly used for atypical *Mycobacterium* infections.

Glycopeptides

Both **vancomycin** and **teicoplanin** have only Gram-positive activity but they cover virtually all Gram-positive organisms, including enterococci. There is slightly more resistance in *Staphylococcus epidermidis* to teicoplanin than to vancomycin, but teicoplanin can be given intramuscularly which vancomycin cannot. Primary uses are the treatment of MRSA, *Staph. epidermidis* and enterococcal infections, and oral vancomycin is used for *Clostridium difficile* infection.

Folate antagonists

Trimethroprim only has a use as a urinary tract antibiotic, with efficacy rates of approximately 75% in uncomplicated cases. **Co-trimoxazole** has a much broader spectrum of activity, including most common Gram-negative pathogens (but not *P. aeruginosa*). It is, therefore, useful for urinary tract infection and also for hospital-acquired Gram-negative pneumonia. It is also the treatment of first choice, in large doses, for *Pneumocystis* pneumonia (p. 398). It has reasonable Gram-positive activity, although a considerable number (>10%) of *Strep. pneumoniae* isolates are now resistant. Toxicity may be a problem, especially in elderly people.

Aminoglycosides

The aminoglycosides (e.g. **gentamicin, netilmicin, tobramycin** and **amikacin**) have an excellent Gram-negative spectrum and good activity against staphylococci. There has been a substantial change in the philosophy of dosing over the last few years, so that they are now generally used in once a day dosing regimens (4–7 mg/kg). This produces higher peak concentrations, which may be more clinically effective, and low trough concentrations, which reduces the risk of toxicity. If once a day dosing is used, levels do not need to be measured unless the patient has impaired renal function, is over 65 years or the course of therapy exceeds 5 days. They also have a particular role as synergistic agents in the treatment of endocarditis caused by streptococci, enterococci and staphylococci, or indeed for other deep-seated, difficult-to-treat infections with these organisms. Resistance is infrequent.

Carbapenems

These antibotics (e.g. **imipenem**, **meropenem** and **ertapenem**) are only given i.v. and are extremely broad-spectrum, including action against anaerobes. Meropenem has less neurotoxicity than imipenem and is indicated for meningitis. Challenging hospital infections are the particular indication for the carbapenems.

Oxazolidinones

Linezolid is the first of a new class of antibiotic primarily active against Gram-positive organisms such as MRSA, especially MRSA pneumonia.

Antifungals

Caspofungin is the first of a new very well-tolerated class of i.v. antifungals, the echinocardins. The antifungal spectrum is limited to *Candida* and *Aspergillus* infections.

Amphotericin is a useful agent for the treatment of most systemic fungal infections, except *Pneumocystis*. It also is effective for leishmaniasis. There are two lipid-associated formulations of amphotericin that are generally less toxic but for these the dose is 3–5 times the standard dose.

Fluconazole is a useful drug for the treatment of mucosal and deep infection caused by *Candida* and *Cryptococcus* spp. It has no activity against *Aspergillus* or many of the other rarer fungal infections such as mucormycosis. Some species of *Candida* are resistant to fluconazole, including *C. krusei*, *C. glabrata* and some isolates of *C. tropicalis*.

Itraconazole is an oral drug for the prevention or treatment of *Aspergillus* infections. It is also effective against *Candida*, skin fungi and other rarer fungi.

Voriconazole is the agent of choice for life-threatening *Aspergillus* infection. It covers many rarer fungi as well. Like itraconazole, it has many drug interactions.

Posaconazole is used for the prevention of fungal infection in leukaemia and after transplantation. It has an extremely broad spectrum of activity.

Flucytosine should only be used in combination with amphotericin or fluconazole for the treatment of cryptococcal meningitis.

Antivirals

Aciclovir is a useful antiviral agent for the treatment of herpes simplex and, to a lesser extent, herpes zoster infections but not cytomegalovirus or Epstein–Barr virus. It is the treatment of choice for herpes simplex encephalitis and other disseminated viral infections caused by these viruses. Resistance is rare except in the context of late-stage AIDS or bone marrow transplantation. Two analogues of aciclovir, **famciclovir** and **valaciclovir**, are superior to aciclovir for treatment of herpes zoster.

Ganciclovir is useful for the prevention and treatment of cytomegalovirus infection in immunocompromised patients.

There are four clinical uses of the teratogenic agent **ribavirin**:

- hepatitis C
- serious respiratory syncytial virus infection
- Lassa fever.

Oseltamivir and **zanamivir** are useful in shortening illness in influenza and reducing transmission of the 'flu virus. However, early use (first few hours) is required for much effect.

Anti-HIV drugs

There are over 19 licensed anti-HIV drugs available, which are always used in combination. The principles of treating HIV infection are described in page 387.

Self-assessment: questions

Multiple choice questions

Any or all of each set of five statements may be true or false. Choose your answers and see the reasoning behind the correct answer on pages 438–439.

1. Penicillin is a good therapeutic choice for the following diseases:
   a. Syphilis
   b. *Escherichia coli* urinary tract infection
   c. Group A streptococcal necrotising fasciitis
   d. *Clostridium* spp. infection, such as tetanus
   e. *Clostridium difficile* causing antibiotic-associated diarrhoea

2. In genitourinary infections:
   a. Vaginal candidiasis is usually transmitted sexually
   b. External anal warts that have just appeared should prompt tests for syphilis
   c. Herpes simplex virus is fast becoming resistant to aciclovir
   d. Chlamydial infections may be asymptomatic
   e. Small multiple painful genital ulcers may be a feature of primary HIV infection

3. Flucloxacillin would be a reasonable choice for treating the following:
   a. *Staphylococcus aureus* endocarditis
   b. Impetigo
   c. Central line infection in an intensive care unit patient with Gram-positive cocci in blood cultures
   d. Osteomyelitis
   e. Gonorrhoea

4. Extended-spectrum penicillins (such as ticarcillin or piperacillin) are generally effective for the following:
   a. *Enterobacter* bacteraemia
   b. Enterococcal endocarditis (e.g. *Enterococcus faecalis*)
   c. Staphylococcal osteomyelitis
   d. *Pseudomonas aeruginosa* urinary tract infections
   e. *Klebsiella* bacteraemia

5. The following would be appropriate indications for vancomycin:
   a. *Staphylococcus epidermidis* central venous line infection
   b. MRSA deep wound infection
   c. Prosthetic hip infection
   d. Endocarditis caused by *Enterococcus faecalis* in a penicillin-allergic patient
   e. Candidaemia

6. There is no specific treatment for the following viral diseases:
   a. Influenza
   b. Lassa fever
   c. Chronic hepatitis B infection of the liver
   d. Respiratory syncytial virus pneumonia
   e. Rubella

7. In treating *Pseudomonas aeruginosa* infections, the following are true:
   a. Ciprofloxacin is more active than ofloxacin
   b. Ceftazidime is more active than cefotaxime
   c. Gentamicin is no longer useful because of resistance
   d. Imipenem and meropenem are 'last resort' antibiotics
   e. Two agents are better than one

8. The following antibiotics have reasonable anaerobic activity (especially against *Bacteroides* spp.):
   a. Ciprofloxacin
   b. Meropenem
   c. Metronidazole
   d. Erythromycin
   e. Cefotaxime

9. The following is true of ciprofloxacin:
   a. It is a good choice for sinusitis
   b. Blood levels following 200 mg i.v. are lower than following 750 mg orally
   c. It is a reasonable alternative therapy for serious staphylococcal infection on its own
   d. It is active against *Mycobacterium* spp.
   e. It is the treatment of choice for typhoid fever

10. The following statements are true:
    a. There is no resistance to quinine in *falciparum* malaria
    b. Mebendazole is effective treatment for all types of GI worm
    c. *Cryptosporidium* infection is as easily treated with metronidazole as is giardiasis
    d. Leishmaniasis is best treated with single doses of ivermectin
    e. Visceral leishmaniasis is best treated with antimonial compounds

11. The following would be appropriate indications for aciclovir:
    a. Viral encephalitis
    b. Shingles
    c. Chickenpox
    d. Prevention of cytomegalovirus infection post-transplant
    e. Chronic fatigue syndrome

12. With respect to treating fungal disease, the following are true:
    a. In oral candidiasis, topical therapy is just as good as systemic therapy
    b. Fluconazole is active against *Cryptococcus* sp.
    c. Fluconazole is active against *Aspergillus* sp.
    d. Voriconazole is the treatment of choice for serious *Aspergillus* infections
    e. Amphotericin and flucytosine together are the optimal initial treatment of cryptococcal meningitis

13. The following statements are true:
    a. It is important to measure trough gentamicin levels to avoid toxicity
    b. In endocarditis, antibiotic levels should be measured to ensure efficacy
    c. Co-trimoxazole is a reasonable choice for a patient aged 60–70 years with an infective exacerbation of chronic obstructive pulmonary disease
    d. Nausea is a common dose-limiting side-effect of co-trimoxazole when used for treating *Pneumocystis* pneumonia
    e. Itraconazole and voriconazole may lead to renal impairment if used with ciclosporin

Extended matched question

Theme: Possible diagnoses in a patient with fever

Options
1. Acute appendicitis
2. Brucellosis
3. Cholecystitis
4. Cryptococcal meningitis
5. Diverticular abscess
6. Endocarditis
7. Enterovirus infection
8. Familial Mediterranean fever
9. Gastroenteritis
10. Lymphoma
11. Malaria
12. Munchausen syndrome
13. Pyelonephritis
14. Salpingitis
15. Toxic shock syndrome
16. Tuberculous meningitis
17. Viral haemorrhagic fever

For patients A–J with fever, select the most likely diagnosis. Each option may be used once, more than once or not at all.

A. A 58-year-old married Pakistani woman with a 1-day history of acute right upper quadrant pain and chills, a fever of 38.6°C, tenderness over the liver and a white cell count of 18.6×10^9 cells/l.

B. A 35-year-old divorced Pakistani woman with a 2-week history of headache and vomiting, a fever of 37.8°C, mild obtundation and neck stiffness, and a white cell count of 10.8×10^9 cells/l.

C. A 35-year-old unmarried black American man with a 2-week history of increasing headache, nausea and sweating, a 2-month history of mild diarrhoea and 4.5 kg weight loss, a fever of 39°C, possible oral thrush and a white cell count of 3.6×10^9 cells/l.

D. A 43-year-old Turkish man with severe night sweats and weight loss for 6 weeks, no cough, a temperature of 38.3°C and a white cell count of 11.2×10^9 cells/l.

E. A 23-year-old white Scottish woman with a 3-day history of bilateral lower abdominal pain 1 week following a holiday in Gibraltar, a fever of 38.3°C, bilateral tenderness and guarding on deep palpation in the left and right iliac fossa (worse on the left) and a white cell count of 16.3×10^9 cells/l.

F. A 33-year-old married black man from the UK with a 7-day history of fever, muscle aches and pains, and sore throat immediately following a trip to Sierra Leone to meet distant cousins. He was fully immunised and took malaria prophylaxis. His fever is 38.8°C, his throat is injected and petechiae are visible on his soft palate. His white cell count is 3.8×10^9 cells/l.

G. A 39-year-old married black man from the UK with a 3-day history of high fever, rigors, nausea and vomiting, following a business trip to the Kolkata area 2 weeks ago. He was fully immunised. His fever is 40°C; he is sweating and shaking and his abdomen is generally tender. His white cell count is 5.6×10^9 cells/l.

H. A 63-year-old white Welshman who has felt generally ill with breathlessness on walking upstairs ever since returning from a holiday in Southern France 3 weeks ago. He has a fever of 37.6°C, pulse rate of 110 beats/min, fine basal crackles at the left base, small inguinal lymph nodes bilaterally, tenderness on deep palpation of the left upper quadrant of the abdomen and a soft systolic murmur in the aortic area radiating to the neck. His white cell count is 13.3×10^9 cells/l.

I. A 23-year-old Pakistani woman with high fever, vomiting and then dizziness for 2 days occurring 2 days after a meal out with friends at a local Chinese restaurant. She has a fever of 39.7°C, blood pressure of 85/50 mmHg, pulse rate of 145 beats/min, dry mucous membranes, reddened pharynx without tonsillar exudate, a faint macular rash over the torso, but no petechiae and generalised muscle tenderness. Her white cell count is 17.1×10^9 cells/l.

J. A 23-year-old white woman from Denmark, who is visiting the UK and has a 3-day illness with increasing headache, fever and nausea. She has vomited once and had one episode of diarrhoea. She has a fever of 38.2°C, blood pressure of 95/70 mmHg, pulse of 92 beats/min, definite neck stiffness and a marked macular rash on the trunk. Her white cell count is 8.3×10^9 cells/l.

Objective structured clinical examination (OSCE) station

This 10-minute station deals with communication using a needlestick injury as a base and a standardised patient.

Examiner: A nurse on your ward pricked herself in the finger with a hollow needle after an i.m. injection on one of your patients. The patient was admitted yesterday with possible staphylococcal endocarditis and has been using intravenous drugs for some years. She is the mother of two children, who have been given up for adoption. You have been phoned by the consultant in microbiology asking you to take blood from the patient for hepatitis viruses and HIV. Please discuss this with the patient.

Case history questions

Case history 1

A 35-year-old man from Malawi presents to accident and emergency with fever of 2 days' duration, rigors and myalgia. He is a businessman based in Kampala and Nairobi who is visiting the UK for the third time in his life. He arrived 6 days ago. Apart from a fever of 38.9°C and a tachycardia, he has no abnormal physical signs. His urine contains blood (++) and protein (++) on dipstick testing.

1. What is the differential diagnosis?
2. List four essential urgent investigations.
3. How should you treat him?
4. What advice (if any) should you give him with respect to his return home?

Case history 2

A 27-year-old Glaswegian with high fever, pain in his toes and left wrist and sweating is admitted to hospital via accident and emergency. He has a fever of 39.3°C, tachycardia of 152 beats/min, blood pressure of 78/53 mmHg and a respiratory rate of 28/min. He has a moderately quiet systolic murmur at the left and right sternal borders, no chest, abdominal or neurological signs and a tender, swollen and red left ankle. Two of his toes show small painful red spots in the pulp.

1. Give a differential diagnosis.
2. List your immediate three most useful investigations.
3. List three investigations for the next morning.
4. Suggest a straightforward management plan.

Case history 3

A 29-year-old artist from Sheffield presents with increasing fever of 5 days' duration. She has lost her appetite and is slightly nauseated. She has a mild cough and her muscles ache slightly. Her travel history reveals a 2-month trip to India, Nepal and Bangkok, from which she returned about 10 weeks ago. She took antimalarial prophylaxis correctly and was immunised against yellow fever, hepatitis A, rabies, meningococcus, typhoid and Japanese B encephalitis. She had one mild bout of diarrhoea when she was away that resolved spontaneously after 3 days.

1. Give a differential diagnosis.
2. Name five key investigations.

Case history 4

The nursing staff in an elderly care ward call you to see an 82-year-old lady admitted with a fall 3 days previously. Before admission, she was well and living independently. The notes indicate that a cardiac cause for the fall is likely, possibly a Stokes–Adams attack. A 24-hour ECG recording has been arranged for the following week. The night sister is concerned because she appears to be drowsy and 'not her usual self'. The pulse rate is 100 beats/min and other observations are unremarkable. When examined she is peripherally shut down, definitely drowsy and orientated only in person.

1. The following would be appropriate immediate actions:
   a. Reassure the nursing staff and leave it to the patient's own medical team to sort out in the morning
   b. Take an oral or aural temperature yourself
   c. Examine her chest carefully
   d. Take a blood culture and full blood count
   e. Do an ECG

An hour later, the following data are available: aural temperature is 37.8°C, blood pressure 85/40 mmHg, white cell count 11.8×10^9 cells/l, 88% neutrophils, ECG showing sinus tachycardia and no additional physical signs.

2. Now the following actions would be appropriate:
   a. Ask the nurse to pass a urinary catheter, send urine for culture and leave the catheter on free drainage
   b. Arrange a CT scan of the head
   c. Do a lumbar puncture
   d. Prescribe oral antibiotics, e.g. amoxicillin
   e. Write out blood request forms for the morning for autoantibodies and complement levels

Case history 5

A 58-year-old hospital patient deteriorates 5 days after a laparotomy and right hemicolectomy. He is breathless, confused and febrile. The patient is a known insulin-dependent diabetic on twice-daily insulin subcutaneously and his blood glucose values (by BM stix) are in the 15–23 mmol/l range despite an increase in insulin yesterday. He is flushed, unwell and restless in bed, with a temperature of 37.8°C, pulse of 110 beats/min, blood pressure of 150/80 mmHg and respiratory rate of 32 breaths/min. His chest has a few crackles in the right midzone (he is a smoker). His abdomen is not diffusely tender and a few bowel sounds are present. His wound is covered with bandages. His chest X-ray is shown in Figure 112.

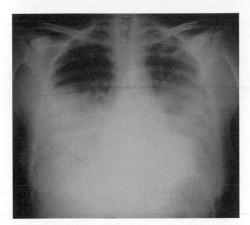

Fig. 112 Chest X-ray retaling to Case history 6.

1. What is the diagnosis?
2. Give five actions that are immediately appropriate.
3. Why are his blood sugars elevated?

Case history 6

A bisexual Londoner, who has visited the genitourinary clinic before, attends accident and emergency after a 9-month interval. He is complaining of penile discharge. He seems rather anxious. On examination there are no abnormalities other than discharge. Gram stain of the discharge shows Gram-negative cocci and white cells.

1. The following are appropriate courses of action:
   a. A prescription for a 10-day course of doxycycline
   b. A blood sample for syphilis serology
   c. Discussion about HIV risk and an HIV test
   d. Refer to genitourinary clinic for contact tracing
   e. Admission to hospital for i.v. antibiotics

You treat him and ask him to come back in 7 days for the results of tests. On return to clinic, the discharge is a little better but not gone. Culture results confirm the diagnosis of gonorrhoea fully sensitive to antibiotics. One of his male sexual contacts is known to the clinic as a highly promiscuous exclusively gay man who was HIV-negative 9 months before.

2. At this stage the following management is appropriate:
   a. Reculture for gonorrhoea
   b. Take samples for *Chlamydia*, *Mycoplasma* and *Ureaplasma* spp.
   c. Treat empirically for syphilis
   d. Refer to urologist for cystoscopy
   e. Encourage him to have an HIV test

He declines an HIV test but takes the course of treatment you prescribed. His most recent female partner is found to have both gonorrhoea and chlamydial cervicitis. They had intercourse again after you treated him but before she was seen. He returns to the clinic 2 weeks later with no discharge. His syphilis tests are VDRL 1 : 8, TPHA positive (both the same as 9 months ago) and fluorescent treponemal antibody-IgM weakly positive.

3. At this point:
   a. There is no need to examine him again
   b. He should be retreated for gonorrhoea
   c. He should be treated for syphilis again
   d. He should have a lumbar puncture done to exclude neurosyphilis
   e. The strength of your recommendation for him to have an HIV test is related to whether he was practising safe sex

Data interpretation questions

Choose the best antibiotic regimen from those given for each of the conditions listed (the route for administration is given if more than one route is possible).

1. Endocarditis, no organism yet isolated, in a patient with a rheumatic mitral valve:
   a. Meropenem and gentamicin
   b. Flucloxacillin (i.v.) and oral rifampicin
   c. Ampicillin and netilmicin (both i.v.)

2. A 60-year-old with severe left leg cellulitis, blood cultures pending:
   a. Oral ciprofloxacin and i.v. gentamicin
   b. Ceftazidime
   c. Cefuroxime (i.v.)

3. A 19-year-old with hypotension, vomiting and purpuric rash:
   a. High-dose i.v. penicillin
   b. Erythromycin (i.v.)
   c. Cefuroxime (i.v.)

4. A 78-year-old man with 3 days of severe diarrhoea and dehydration during convalescence after treatment for pneumonia, stool cultures pending:

   a. Piperacillin/tazobactam and gentamicin (both i.v.)

   b. Oral and i.v. vancomycin

   c. Oral and i.v. metronidazole

5. An intensive care unit patient on renal replacement following a previous episode of septic shock, now with fever and Gram-positive cocci in blood culture:

   a. Cefotaxime

   b. Vancomycin (i.v.)

   c. Flucloxacillin (i.v.)

6. An intensive care unit patient on renal replacement following a prior episode of septic shock, now with fever, raised peripheral white cell count and yeasts in the urine:

   a. Cefotaxime

   b. Caspofungin

   c. Fluconazole (i.v.)

7. A patient with cystic fibrosis, with *Pseudomonas aeruginosa* in sputum and increasing breathlessness and sputum production, sensitivities pending:

   a. Cefotaxime

   b. Oral ciprofloxacin

   c. Ertapenem and ceftazidime

8. Severe sore throat in a 17-year-old who also has tender cervical lymphadenopathy and fever:

   a. Oral erythromycin

   b. Flucloxacillin (i.v.)

   c. Penicillin (i.v.)

9. A 38-year-old gamekeeper from Scotland with chronic monoarthritis of his left knee:

   a. Oral doxycycline

   b. Oral penicillin

   c. Oral erythromycin

10. A 31-year-old with green discharge from one nostril, mild headache and feeling 'off colour':

    a. Oral co-amoxiclav

    b. Cefotaxime

    c. Oral erythromycin

Picture questions

1. Look at the X-ray (Fig. 113).

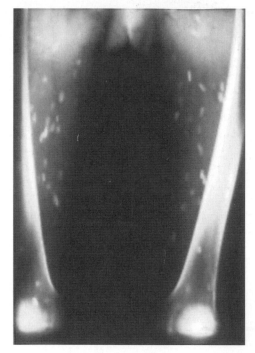

Fig. 113 Plain X-ray of both thighs.

   a. What can you see?

   b. How did this patient probably present?

   c. What is the causative agent?

2. This patient is holding up a specimen of her urine (Fig. 114). She has just recovered from a severe illness:

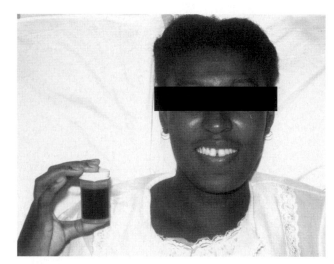

Fig. 114 Patient with urine specimen.

  a. What has she recovered from?

  b. How was the diagnosis made?

  c. Summarise the principles of treatment for this problem.

Short notes

Write short notes on:

1. Management of the febrile shocked patient
2. Fever in a recent traveller from Africa
3. Appropriate investigations for pyrexia of unknown origin.

Self-assessment: answers

Multiple choice answers

1. a. **True.** The treatment of choice, unless allergic.
   b. **False.** *E. coli* are intrinsically resistant.
   c. **True.** Intravenously in large doses, together with surgery.
   d. **True.** Except for *Clostridium difficile*. Metronidazole is also very effective against *Clostridium* infections.
   e. **False.** Oral metronidazole or vancomycin is effective, with a 15% relapse rate (metronidazole is 100 times cheaper).

2. a. **False.** *Candida* resides in the vagina in many women. Occasionally disease appears to follow intercourse, but this reflects a changed vaginal environment rather than transmission.
   b. **True.** Condylomata lata of secondary syphilis can be mistaken for warts.
   c. **False.** A few cases of resistance are reported in patients with AIDS and those who have received stem cell transplants.
   d. **True.** And lead to infertility in women.
   e. **True.** Oral, oesophageal and genital ulceration is one presentation (usually with fever) of primary HIV infection (p. 385).

3. a. **True.** If not MRSA, given with an aminoglycoside or rifampicin.
   b. **True.** Although erythromycin or topical mupirocin would be reasonable alternatives.
   c. **False.** This infection is most likely caused by coagulase-negative staphylococci (e.g. *Staphylococcus epidermidis*) and vancomycin (or teicoplanin) would be the best first choice.
   d. **True.** Although some cases of osteomyelitis are not caused by *Staphylococcus aureus*.
   e. **False.**

4. a. **True.** *Enterobacter* tends to be multiresistant and sensitivity testing is essential to determine the right treatment.
   b. **True.** But only if given with an aminoglycoside. In fact, ampicillin and gentamicin would represent the first choice here.
   c. **False.** All the extended-spectrum penicillins are not active against *Staph. aureus* unless combined with a β-lactamase inhibitor such as sulbactam (tazobactam or clavulanic acid (Timentin)). The combination may be active but it would not be the first choice.
   d. **True.** Slightly more isolates are sensitive to piperacillin than they are to ticarcillin but sensitivity testing will determine this quickly.
   e. **True.**

5. a. **True.** The treatment of choice. Teicoplanin is also effective. Removal of the line is also essential except in exceptional circumstances.
   b. **True.** MRSA stands for both multiply resistant *S. aureus* and meticillin-resistant *S. aureus*. From your point of view these are the same. Resistance to vancomycin has recently been described (glycopeptide intermediate *Staphylococcus aureus* (GISA)). Other good agents are linezolid and deplomycin.
   c. **True.** These infections are most often caused by coagulase-negative staphylococci.
   d. **True.** But only if combined with an aminoglycoside. Given that enterococcal endocarditis has to be treated for 6 weeks, this means treating a patient with two potentially nephrotoxic antibiotics that both need to be assayed for 6 weeks, which is quite a challenge.
   e. **False.**

6. a. **False.** The neuraminidase inhibitors (oseltamivir and zanamivir) are effective if started early enough. Resistance can occur and is conferred by a point mutation. This emphasises the need to collect samples for influenza PCR early. Amantidine may be effective prophylaxis if given before symptoms appear in exposed patients but resistance is now a problem. This is difficult in practice as the incubation time for influenza is only about 3 days and it takes time to prove the diagnosis.
   b. **False.** Ribavirin is partially effective.
   c. **False.** Interferon alpha is often effective (around 30%), as is lamivudine.
   d. **False.** Ribavirin is effective.
   e. **True.**

7. a. **True.** Ofloxacin has very limited activity against *P. aeruginosa*.
   b. **True.** Ceftazidime is one of the most useful drugs in treating *Pseudomonas* infections. Cefotaxime has no activity.
   c. **False.** The prevalence of resistance in *Pseudomonas* spp. depends very much on how frequently drugs are used. In many hospitals in the UK, the aminoglycosides such as gentamicin are used infrequently and so most isolates (e.g. more than 80%) are susceptible.
   d. **False.** Both imipenem and meropenem are highly active against *P. aeruginosa*. There are four major indications for meropenem: (i) resistant organisms susceptible to meropenem; (ii) polymicrobial infection when meropenem alone will be as efficacious as three or four antibiotics together; (iii) in patients who are deteriorating with sepsis with no organism identified and who

are already on broad-spectrum antibiotics (don't forget fungus); (iv) in meningitis.

e. **True.** *Pseudomonas* is notorious for developing resistance on therapy. This is not usually a problem for short courses of therapy for urinary tract infections, etc., but in patients with a difficult infection (e.g. ventilator pneumonia, *Pseudomonas* bacteraemia during neutropenia, etc.) two agents are preferred in the likelihood that the development of resistance will be substantially reduced and activity is slightly enhanced.

8. a. **False.** Ciprofloxacin has no anti-anaerobe activity at all, which is one of its virtues because it disrupts bowel flora less.

b. **True.** Excellent broad-spectrum anti-anaerobe coverage.

c. **True.** Excellent broad-spectrum anti-anaerobe coverage with very little resistance identified. Metronidazole also penetrates very well into abscesses in which anaerobic organisms are often found.

d. **False.**

e. **False.** Some activity against anaerobic streptococci but very little for other organisms.

9. a. **False.** Poor activity against *Strep. pneumoniae* and anaerobes, both common microbial causes of sinusitis.

b. **True.** Oral therapy is preferred for reasons of convenience and cost.

c. **False.** Ciprofloxacin does have reasonable antistaphylococcal activity but it is not a mainstream antibiotic for this organism because it is best used for other indications where its breadth of spectrum is more valuable.

d. **True.** Useful for the treatment of resistant *Mycobacterium* infection including *M. avium intracellulare* in AIDS. Its use can lead to false-negative cultures of *M. tuberculosis.*

e. **True.** *Salmonella typhi* from the Indian subcontinent is now frequently resistant to almost all other drugs apart from the third-generation cephalosporins and ciprofloxacin.

10. a. **False.** Resistance to quinine is rare but does occur around the Cambodian, Thai and Myanmar borders. Resistance may be partial.

b. **False.** Although mebendazole is a good drug for many intestinal parasites.

c. **False.** The response of giardiasis to metronidazole exceeds 90%, whereas there is no useful therapy for *Cryptosporidium* infection.

d. **False.**

e. **False.** This is the old practice and these compounds are somewhat effective. However, i.v. liposomal amphotericin such as AmBisome is highly effective.

11. a. **True.** For all cases, in large i.v. doses.

b. **True.** Of marginal benefit and only indicated if given in the first 48 hours of pain or in an immunocompromised patient.

c. **True.** But only for secondary cases in a household or for immunocompromised patients.

d. **True.** For reasons that are not entirely clear, aciclovir (which has little activity against cytomegalovirus) does seem to prevent or postpone many cytomegalovirus infections after transplantation.

e. **False.**

12. a. **True.** For many groups of patients, e.g. neonates, those who develop candidiasis following antibiotics and patients with AIDS-related complaints. However, in neutropenic patients following radiotherapy to the head and neck, and in late-stage AIDS, systemic therapy is superior.

b. **True.** Fluconazole is the maintenance therapy of choice for cryptococcal meningitis in AIDS.

c. **False.**

d. **True.** Voriconazole levels and liver function tests should be done. Check for drug interactions.

e. **True.** Followed by fluconazole after the acute phase.

13. a. **True.** Trough concentrations of gentamicin above 1 µg/ml and particularly above 2 µg/ml have a much higher incidence of renal toxicity or ototoxicity.

b. **True.** These can be measured directly, as in the case of gentamicin and vancomycin, or indirectly using serum killing levels.

c. **False.** In older people, the incidence of serious and fatal toxicities outweighs the benefits unless there are no alternative agents.

d. **True.** And a reduction in dose to 75% may help and be just as efficacious.

e. **True.** Due to a drug interaction; increased ciclosporin concentrations.

Extended matched answer

A. **3.**

B. **16.**

C. **4.**

D. **2.**

E. **14.**

F. **17.**

G. **11.**

H. **6.**

I. **15.**

J. **7.**

Response to OSCE stations

The risk of transmission by a needlestick injury to a non-immune person is ≈30% if the patient is a carrier for hepatitis B (HBV), ≈3% for a patient positive for hepatitis C (HCV) RNA and ≈0.3% for an HIV-infected patient. A needlestick injury with a hollow needle carries a slightly higher risk than a solid (e.g. suture) needle.

If the nurse is immunised against HBV, as she should be, she will almost certainly be immune. If not, she can be protected with a course of vaccine, given as an accelerated course (three doses at 2-weekly intervals). Some authorities also recommend hyperimmune globulin, which has to be specially ordered. No protection is available for HCV and postexposure prophylaxis is used for HIV.

Check in the patient notes that the tests have not been done on a previous admission. If positive, then repeat tests to determine infectivity status (e.g. HCV RNA) would be appropriate.

Key issues that need to be addressed for all three viruses include:

1. introduction and guarantee of confidentiality
2. discussion of disease including chronicity and infectivity potential if positive
3. what the test result might mean
4. the importance of the result to the nurse
5. discussion of legal, financial and social implications of the test
6. implications for her children
7. request for consent
8. follow-up arrangements.

Introduction and guarantee of confidentiality You and the patient already know each other. Arrange for this conversation to take place in a separate room, not behind curtains on the ward. Ask the patient if she has ever been tested for HBV, HIV or HCV. If she has, then consent has been previously given but must not be assumed for this occasion. If any testing is to be done, informed (verbal) consent is required. Expressly state that you and others will respect her wishes with respect to who to give the result to, if anybody (including the nurse who had the needlestick injury and the Occupational Health Department). Take time to do this — the only urgency is the reassurance of the nurse who had the needlestick injury.

Discussion of the disease See page 143 for HBV, page 144 for HCV and page 383 for HIV.

What the test result might mean A positive result for HBV surface antigen means active infection or carrier status; a negative result means non-infectious. HCV antibodies mean infection and possibly infectious; a positive HCV RNA test means infectious, and negative means non-infectious. A positive HIV antibody test means infected and infectious; a negative test almost excludes infection but a retest in 3–6 months may be appropriate to confirm absolutely that the patient is not 'incubating' infection.

The importance of the test to the nurse A simple explanation that it is important for the nurse to know whether the patient is or is not infected is sufficient. Undue pressure should not be placed on the patient on this point as what has happened has happened and cannot be undone. Furthermore, postexposure prophylaxis should have been administered to the nurse in any case. As the nurse is almost certainly immunised against HBV, this is of less importance.

Legal, financial and social implications of the test See section on page 388. Life insurance issues are generally the most important, but for this patient the immediate social issues are likely to be paramount.

Implications for her children The risk of transmission is very high (≈90%) if the patient is a carrier of HBV, ≈10% for HCV and up to 25% for HIV. Testing should have been done in the antenatal clinic. Positive results would require testing of the children, if not already tested. However, as they have been adopted, it would not be appropriate to attempt to contact them and have them tested. This issue should, therefore, not be raised with the patient at this time, unless she raises it, in which case you should refer to a senior colleague for guidance.

Request for consent See page 388.

Follow-up arrangements HBV surface antigen and HIV antibody test results should be available within 48 hours, when the patient is likely to be in hospital. Giving her these results should also be done in a separate room and, if the HIV test is positive, with the HIV counsellor. The HCV antibody test and HCV RNA test may take a week or more to come back. Arrangements need to be made for communicating the result to the patient and, if positive (which is likely), for assessment of hepatic function and treatment.

Case history answers

Case history 1

1. *Falciparum* malaria, pyelonephritis, community-acquired bacteraemia, e.g. *Pneumococcus*, *Staphylococcus* spp., infection (possibly together) with hypertension or glomerulonephritis.

2. Key investigations: malaria film, blood count, urea/creatinine and blood culture. Other investigations: differential white cell count, electrolytes, urine microscopy (urgent) and culture.

3. With oral malarone for malaria (the diagnosis in this case). If he has a neutrophilia, broad-spectrum antibiotics to include Gram-negative (because of the urine abnormalities) and pneumococcal coverage, e.g. third-generation cephalosporin such as cefotaxime.

4. There is no point giving him prophylaxis against malaria if he intends spending most of his time in Kampala and Nairobi, for two reasons: (i) he will have partial immunity to malaria anyway; (ii) he will be constantly reinfected in Uganda and Kenya and lifelong prophylaxis is not really a tenable option for people living in these countries.

Case history 2

1. Staphylococcal tricuspid valve endocarditis (common in i.v. drug abusers), staphylococcal septicaemia, group A streptococcal sepsis, gonococcal bacteraemia, Henoch–Schönlein purpura. The key factor to elicit on the history is whether he is an i.v. drug abuser or not. If he is, tricuspid

endocarditis is more likely; if he is not, then other diagnostic possibilities are more likely.

2. Blood culture, arthrocentesis of the left ankle and blood gases. Others are full blood count, creatinine, ECG, urethral swab for *N. gonorrhoeae*, chest X-ray, urine microscopy and culture.

3. Echocardiogram, hepatitis B and C antibodies (possibly HIV antibodies) if he is an i.v. drug abuser and antistreptolysin O titre.

4. Assuming he is a drug abuser, the following steps should be taken:

   - Prescribe flucloxacillin in large doses, e.g. 2 g 4-hourly, and a broad-spectrum agent such as cefotaxime to cover other injections. If there is any evidence of a localised abscess (e.g. at an injection site), also prescribe metronidazole.
   - Seek consent from the patient for HIV testing, in a location where your discussion will not be overheard.
   - Ascertain how much heroin he takes and prescribe methadone to prevent withdrawal symptoms.
   - Make provisional plans for central venous line insertion if he has very poor peripheral veins, which is likely.
   - Arrange an echocardiogram urgently.

   If he is not a drug abuser, he would be treated as above but there would be less concern about hepatitis B and C, HIV, etc. Venous access should not be a problem.

Case history 3

1. The most likely diagnosis is amoebic liver abscess. Other possibilities include hepatitis B (unlikely in view of fever), community-acquired infection contracted locally (e.g. *Mycoplasma*), malaria (especially *Plasmodium vivax*), brucellosis and tuberculosis.

2. Blood film for malaria, blood culture, liver function tests, serology for amoebiasis and brucellosis, ultrasound of the liver, chest radiograph.

Case history 4

1. a. **False.** She has clearly had a sudden deterioration and it needs action tonight, not in the morning.

   b. **True.** In many wards axillary temperatures only are measured and when patients are peripherally shut down a pyrexia may fail to be recorded.

   c. **True.** The most common causes of sudden deterioration and fever in elderly people is pneumonia or urinary tract infection. Physical examination is likely to be as sensitive as chest X-ray in the early phases of the disease.

   d. **True.** Although if she has a fever, the full blood count tonight is unlikely to help very much.

   e. **True.** If you did not demonstrate any pyrexia and it appeared that her heart rhythm was

abnormal or very fast and the blood pressure was reduced, then an ECG might be as appropriate as a blood culture because she could be in fast atrial fibrillation or some other tachyarrhythmia. Also consider drugs as a cause of her drowsiness.

2. a. **True.** A disorientated patient on an elderly care ward is highly likely to be incontinent of urine. The catheter allows accurate measurement of urine output, and if this falls, it alerts you to impending renal failure or the need for i.v. fluids. Also she may well be moved less frequently than is desirable and is, therefore, at moderate to high risk of development of pressure sores. The passage of a urinary catheter will reduce the risk of this to some extent, although the nurses should be encouraged to use prophylactic measures to prevent pressure sores as part of a change in the original nursing care plan.

   b. **False.** Unless there are localising neurological signs.

   c. **False.** Unless there is neck stiffness or no other focus of fever is found.

   d. **False.** Given that this rapid deterioration in association with low blood pressure in this patient represents severe sepsis, she requires i.v. antibiotics, not oral antibiotics. In addition, oral amoxicillin will only cover a small number of the appropriate pathogens because resistance is now common in hospital pathogens.

   e. **False.** The acute onset of systemic lupus erythematosus or another connective tissue disease leading to fever and features of sepsis is so unlikely as to be an untenable differential diagnosis. She is so much more likely to have a bacterial infection that these antibody tests do not need to be ordered.

Case history 5

1. Hospital-acquired pneumonia.

2. (i) Administer high-flow oxygen and arrange for his oxygen saturation to be monitored. (ii) Take the bandages off, inspect the wound and take a wound swab (he could have a wound infection too and, if so, consider MRSA pneumonia, especially as he is a diabetic); (iii) arterial blood gases (to check for hypoxia/acidosis); (iv) blood culture (probably infected and may be bacteraemic); (v) blood count and differential white cell count (to check for raised white cell count and anaemia); (vi) urea and electrolytes and blood sugar (for management of raised blood sugar and because he is at risk of acute renal failure); (vii) prescribe and arrange for urgent administration of your hospital formulary antibiotics for hospital-acquired pneumonia including linezolid for MRSA.

3. He has temporary 'insulin resistance' caused by an infection.

Case history 6

1. a. **False.** You have made a diagnosis of gonorrhoea; treat with cefixime 400 mg once, not doxycycline. Cover *Chlamydia*, etc. with azittromycin 1 g or doxycycline.

   b. **True.** For all new presentations, even old patients.

   c. **True.** Clearly an at-risk patient.

   d. **True.**

   e. **False.** Virtually no sexually transmitted diseases require admission to hospital, except HIV and AIDS, and for investigations and treatment of latent or tertiary syphilis.

2. a. **True.** Although it is unlikely to be culture-positive. Between a quarter and a half of patients have continuing discharge despite 'cure', representing another pathogen.

   b. **True.** You did this before, of course, but as the incubation period for these organisms is longer, the results were negative (? falsely negative). Most laboratories only do tests for *Chlamydia*.

   c. **False.** Syphilis does not cause a discharge; await serology.

   d. **False.** Unhelpful in almost all cases of discharge. No bladder symptoms described.

   e. **True.** As before, especially knowing his contact.

3. a. **False.** Syphilis has a longer incubation period and now is the time when you would expect to see a chancre. You also want to reculture his urethral secretions for *N. gonorrhoeae*.

   b. **True.** Clearly history of contact after treatment.

   c. **False.** The VDRL and TPHA titres are stable. The FTA test is read visually and is somewhat subjective. It is only weakly positive. However, he does need follow-up serology in, say, 2 months.

   d. **False.** This is standard practice for new, untreated cases of latent syphilis, but he has been treated before by you.

   e. **False.** Possibly true in general, but you know he was not practising safe sex because he caught gonorrhoea. Patients are not always entirely straight about this.

Data interpretation answers

1. **c is correct.** The combination of ampicillin and an aminoglycoside covers all of the streptococci, enterococci and unusual causes of endocarditis, such as the HACEK (*Haemophilus, Actinobacillus, Cardiobacterium, Eikenella, Kingella*) organisms. In addition, the aminoglycoside has some activity against *Staph. aureus* and about 50% of *Strep. epidermidis* infections. Aminoglycosides are also active against a number of Gram-negative organisms that are occasional causes of endocarditis. It does not matter from the point of view of activity which aminoglycoside is used and gentamicin, netilmicin or tobramycin would all be equivalent. All would require blood levels to be measured.

2. **c is correct.** The most likely pathogen is group A or G streptococci or *Staph. aureus*. Intravenous cefuroxime would treat this well. Ciprofloxacin is not sufficiently active against the streptococci to be useful. Ceftazidime has some streptococcal and staphylococcal activity, but less than that of cefuroxime.

3. **a is correct.** This young man probably has meningococcal septicaemia. Penicillin is the drug of choice, although cefuroxime would be nearly as good. Note that all choices are for i.v. therapy. If you saw this young man at home as his GP, you should give him intramuscular or i.v. penicillin.

4. **c is correct.** The likely diagnosis is *Clostridium difficile* diarrhoea. Piperacillin and gentamicin have no activity against these pathogens. *Cl. difficile* is not an invasive organism and the disease is caused by toxin production. Oral vancomycin is active but only in the lumen of the bowel. Intravenous vancomycin does not penetrate into the bowel and, therefore, is not useful. Vancomycin is expensive for this indication. Metronidazole orally is given for mild cases and in severe cases i.v. metronidazole can also be given, which penetrates extremely well into the wall and lumen of the bowel.

5. **b is correct.** The most likely pathogen is *Staph. epidermidis* or another coagulase-negative staphylococcus. Vancomycin is active against >99% of these organisms, whereas flucloxacillin will only be active against 20–50%. Cephalosporins are not clinically active for *Staph. epidermidis* infection and, therefore, (a) is positively the wrong choice.

6. **b is correct.** As the patient had received multiple antibiotics previously for septic shock, he/she is at risk for candidaemia, particularly as the patient is on haemodialysis and, therefore, has multiple i.v. lines. Fungal blood cultures should be done in this patient but 25–50% are negative even in patients with documented candidaemia at postmortem. A good surrogate marker for candidaemia is candiduria, as in this case. Cefotaxime is clearly the wrong choice. Intravenous fluconazole would be a reasonable alternative but has a 15% lower response rate. Some species of yeast are resistant to fluconazole. All intensive care unit patients with candiduria and any sign of infection or deteriorating clinical status require antifungal therapy.

7. **c is correct.** If these patients can be treated orally this is preferable, although this does depend on the status of the patient. Cefotaxime is not active against *P. aeruginosa*. Ertapenem, ciprofloxacin and ceftazidime would be reasonable choices.

8. **c is correct.** This patient almost certainly has a bad streptococcal sore throat. Intravenous (or

intramuscular) penicillin is preferred because the symptoms resolve much more quickly than they do by giving oral therapy. Around 90% of isolates are susceptible to erythromycin. Intravenous flucloxacillin is not as active as penicillin and, therefore, this is an inferior choice. In mild cases, oral therapy alone suffices. Treatment should be continued for 10 days or recurrence is likely. The switch from i.v. to oral therapy with amoxicillin or co-amoxiclav can be made usually after 1–2 days. There is also some evidence for persistence of streptococci despite therapy. Tonsillar concentrations after *oral* antibiotics are relatively low and further reduced by anaerobic organisms living in the crypts of the tonsils, which produce β-lactamase, inactivating the penicillin or amoxicillin in situ, allowing local persistence and subsequent recurrence. Co-amoxiclav and macrolides may therefore be preferable to amoxicillin. Glandular fever should be excluded to avoid a rash with amoxicillin.

9. **a is correct.** This patient probably has Lyme borreliosis stage 3. Other considerations include tuberculosis or injury-related osteoarthritis. Doxycycline is one of the treatments of choice for Lyme borreliosis. Oral penicillin is inadequately absorbed, although i.v. penicillin might be adequate. Erythromycin is less active (p. 421).

10. **a is correct.** This patient probably has sinusitis. The common causes of sinusitis include *Strep. pneumoniae*, *H. influenzae* and *Staph. aureus*, and, in 30% of cases, anaerobic organisms such as oral *Bacteroides* are also found. Therapy should be directed at these pathogens. Oral co-amoxiclav is a good choice because it will cover all of these commonly occurring organisms. Larger doses are required for sinusitis than for many other indications, because the sinus represents quite a large volume of pus and penetration of the antibiotic into the centre of that pus requires good concentrations. Cefotaxime would be a good choice if the patient was admitted to hospital but it should be given with metronidazole. Although erythromycin may be active against some of the pathogens, it is an inferior choice. Consideration should be given to sinus X-rays and to decongestant therapy.

Picture answers

1. a. Calcified lesions in the muscles of both thighs.
   b. Epilepsy due to cerebral cysticercosis.
   c. *Taenia solium*, larval phase, usually from eating undercooked pork, or food contaminated with animal excrement.

2. a. *Falciparum* malaria (malignant malaria or blackwater fever).
   b. Blood film examination.
   c. See p. 426.

Short notes answers

1. **Initially.** Resuscitate the patient: high oxygen concentrations, i.v. fluids (N/saline and colloid).
   Appropriate key investigations
   - Blood culture
   - Blood count, D-dimers, urea and electrolytes, liver function tests, creatinine phosphokinase, clotting tests
   - Arterial blood gases
   - Urine culture
   - Throat culture and blood (in EDTA tube) for polymerase chain reaction (PCR) if meningococcal infection suspected
   - Respiratory tract culture
   - Chest X-ray.

   Therapy Choose appropriate antibiotic therapy depending on clinical features. These can be obtained by collecting a history from patient, relatives, notes, nursing staff, etc. and by examining the patient carefully, especially skin, chest, abdomen, joints, etc. Choose a broad-spectrum agent with an additional agent if there is an apparent focus, e.g. cefotaxime or piperacillin/tazobactam plus (i) clarithromycin if pneumonia; (ii) flucloxacillin 2 g 6-hourly if features of staphylococcal sepsis (p. 413) or linezolid for MRSA if hospitalised; (iii) metronidazole if an intra-abdominal focus. If in intensive care or a renal patient, use ceftazidime ± vancomycin. Consider treatment with activated protein C. Add i.v. hydrocortisone.

   Management Consider the best care options over the next 12–24 hours:

   - *Anticipate complications*: hypoxia (acute respiratory distress syndrome (ARDS)), disseminated intravascular coagulation (DIC), acute renal failure (p. 179), etc.
   - *Nursing area*. Transfer to intensive care or high-dependency unit or allow to remain on the ward; depends on severity of sepsis, underlying disease, patients' and relatives' wishes, response to initial therapy with oxygenated fluids and decision to resuscitate.
   - *Consult*. Who to advise and seek advice from: your team, microbiologist, intensive care consultant, etc.

2. Must exclude malaria; also consider dengue fever, viral haemorrhagic fever (will need rapid exclusion and strict isolation), tick typhus, HIV, tuberculosis, other viral infections, standard bacterial infections (e.g. pneumonia, urinary tract infection, infectious diarrhoea, etc.).

3. Do investigations depending on clinical findings and differential diagnosis, e.g.

   - tuberculosis: tuberculin skin test, cultures of sputum, cerebrospinal fluid, urine, peritoneal fluid, etc.
   - brucellosis: special blood culture for *Brucella*, *Brucella* serology

- occult abscess: imaging of liver, spleen and kidney, (ultrasound, CT of abdomen), MR of spine for osteomyelitis and epidermal abscess, pelvic ultrasound, white cell and gallium scan
- AIDS: HIV test and helper T cell count
- hypogammaglobulinaemia: immunoglobulins
- autoimmune disease: autoantibodies, erythrocyte sedimentation rate (ESR), plasma viscosity

- endocarditis: blood culture, serology for Q fever, *Candida*, *Bartonella*, *Brucella*, etc.
- tropical diseases: eosinophil count and get advice
- tumours: CT scan, bone marrow, α-fetoprotein
- sarcoidosis: CT of chest; node, liver or skin biopsy
- drug fever: eosinophil count, stop drug, etc.
- seek advice earlier rather than later.

Index

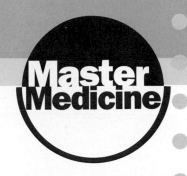

Note: Page numbers in *italics* refer to figures and tables.